Topics in pathophysiology of hypertension

W0050509

DEVELOPMENTS IN
CARDIOVASCULAR MEDICINE

Other volumes in this series:

TOPICS IN PATHOPHYSIOLOGY OF HYPERTENSION

edited by

HERMAN VILLARREAL, MD
Head, Department of Nephrology
Instituto Nacional de Cardiología
Mèxico, DF

&

MOHINDER P. SAMBHI, MD, PhD
Professor and Chief, Division of Hypertension
Sepulveda Veterans Administration Medical Center
UCLA School of Medicine
USA

1984 **MARTINUS NIJHOFF PUBLISHERS**
a member of the KLUWER ACADEMIC PUBLISHERS GROUP
BOSTON / THE HAGUE / DORDRECHT / LANCASTER

Distributors

for the United States and Canada: Kluwer Boston, Inc., 190 Old Derby Street, Hingham, MA 02043, USA
for all other countries: Kluwer Academic Publishers Group, Distribution Center, P.O.Box 322, 3300 AH Dordrecht, The Netherlands

Library of Congress Cataloging in Publication Data

Main entry under title:

Topics in pathophysiology of hypertension.

   (Developments in cardiovascular medicine)
   Includes index.
   1. Hypertension--Addresses, essays, lectures.
2. Physiology, Pathological--Addresses, essays, lec-
tures. I. Villarreal, Herman. II. Sambhi, Mohinder P.
III. Series. [DNLM: 1. Hypertension--Physiopathology
--Congresses. W1 DE997VME v. 31 / WG 340 T6744 1982]
RC685.H8T664 1983   616.1'3207   83-13159

ISBN-13: 978-94-009-6743-4   e-ISBN-13: 978-94-009-6741-0
DOI: 10.1007/978-94-009-6741-0

Copyright

© 1984 by Martinus Nijhoff Publishers, Boston.
Softcover reprint of the hardcover in 1st edition 1984

All rights reserved. No part of this publication may be reproduced, stored in a retrieval system, or transmitted in any form or by any means, mechanical, photocopying, recording, or otherwise, without the prior written permission of the publishers,
Martinus Nijhoff Publishers, 190 Old Derby Street, Hingham, MA 02043, USA.

CONTENTS

III. RECENT ADVANCES IN RESEARCH ON RENIN SYSTEM

IV. RENAL, ADRENAL AND CENTRAL HORMONES IN HYPERTENSION

FOREWORD

It is not often that one one writes the foreword for a book based on a conference which contributed so much to our knowledge in the field of hypertension. During my close association with the International Society of Hypertension from 1978–1982, numerous satellite symposia were held in connection with five international meetings. The specific topics addressed in this volume, the quality of the contributions, and the superb expertise of the contributors make this monograph one of the most outstanding publications that the International Society of Hypertension has sponsored.

Satellite symposia such as the present one serve useful and important functions for our society. They provide a mechanism of getting together the outstanding experts on special subjects for presentation of new data and for a free interchange of ideas. This type of endeavor is one of the most uniquely effective ways of accumulating new knowledge, because the data presented are subjected to critical review and discussion. No textbook or publication in journals can provide the type of critically evaluated information that comes from a small group-meeting of this type. Furthermore, it is a mechanism for scientists to become acquainted or better acquainted with one another. All of this is, of course, very provocative and supportive of high quality research, one of the trademarks of the International Society of Hypertension.

The conference for this book publication was organized by Drs. Herman Villarreal and Mohinder Sambhi, both of whom were also extremely helpful and effective in organizing the Ninth Scientific Meeting of the International Society of Hypertension in Mexico City in February 1982. The contributors to the book are from 13 countries in 4 continents. The topics in this book cover 4 of the major groups of pathogenic mechanisms in hypertension, and several new and important advances are reported in this excellent monograph on hypertension.

JAMES O. DAVIS, MD, PHD
President of International Society of Hypertension (1980–1982)

PREFACE

During the last decade, concepts in pathophysiology of hypertension have made impressive strides. Recent advances in the field have more prominently occurred in the areas of ionic transport across cell membranes, and neural and hormonal mechanisms of blood pressure control, particularly as related to the central nervous system. Although the fundamental fault in this disease with multifaceted presentation remains to be discovered, the view that a generalized or localized defect at the cellular membrane level may be the culprit is receiving attention. Modern sophisticated techniques in molecular biology and genetics are increasingly being applied to these problems. The contents of this volume reflect the recent changes in concepts and directions of research on etiology of essential hypertension.

The opportunity of gathering renowned investigators in the field at a satellite conference held in Acapulco, Mexico was provided by the Ninth Meeting of the International Society of Hypertension.

The selection of the topics and the participants was largely made by the respective session chairmen who also undertook the arduous task of reviewing the manuscripts for publication. We wish to express our gratitude and appreciation to Drs. Daniel Tosteson, Bjorn Folkow, David Bohr and Joseph Hoffman who chaired the session on membrane transport, Drs. Francois Abboud and Willem Birkenhäger who chaired the session on neural control, Drs. Edgar Haber and John Luetscher who chaired the session on renin system, Drs. Jacques Genest and John Laragh who chaired the session on hormones. We are also indebted to Merck, Sharpe and Dohme of Mexico and Merck, Sharpe and Dohme International for their generous and unfailing support. Our sincere thanks also go to the staff of the KPR INFOR/MEDIA Corporation and Martinus Nijhoff Publishers for their patience and cooperation, and for making our editorial task a pleasant one. Finally, we must thank all the contributors for their critical and enthusiastic participation.

HERMAN VILLARREAL
MOHINDER P. SAMBHI

CONTRIBUTORS

Abboud, F.M., MD, Department of Medicine and Physiology, University of Iowa, Iowa City, IA 52242, USA.

Birkenhäger, W. MD, Zuiderziekenhuis, Department of Internal Medicine, Groene Hilledijk 315, 3075 EA Rotterdam, THE NETHERLANDS.

Blaustein, M.P., MD, Department of Medicine, School of Medicine, University of Maryland, 655 West Baltimore Street, Baltimore, MD 21202, USA.

Bohr, D.F., MD, Department of Physiology, Medical School, University of Michigan, Ann Arbor, MI 48109, USA.

Brody, M.J., MD, Department of Pharmacology, University of Iowa, Iowa City, IA 52242, USA.

Bumpus, F.M., PhD, Division of Research, Cleveland Clinic, 9500 Euclid Avenue, Cleveland, OH 44106, USA.

Burke, W., MD, Department of Medicine and Genetics & Center for Inherited Diseases, University of Washington, Seattle, WA 98195, USA.

Corvol, P., MD, Department of Medicine, Institut National de la Santé et de la Recherche Medicale, 17, rue du Fer-à-Moulin, 75005, Paris, FRANCE.

Cusi, D., MD, Universita Degli Studi di Milano, Scuola di Specializzazione in Nefrologia Medica, Via Francesco Sforza 35, 20122 Milano, ITALY.

Denton, D., MD, Howard Florey Institute of Experimental Physiology Medicine, University of Melbourne, Parkville, Victoria, 3052, AUSTRALIA.

Duhm, J., MD, Physiologisches Institut der Universität München, Pettenkoferstrasse 12, D-8000 München 2, FRG.

Dzau, V., MD, Department of Medicine, Brigham and Women's Hospital, 75 Francis Street, Boston, MA 02115, USA.

Eggena, P., PhD, Division of Hypertension, Sepulveda Veterans Administration Medical Center, 16111 Plummer Street, Sepulveda, CA 91343, USA.

Erdmann, E., MD, Ludwig-Maximilians Universität München, Klinikum Grosshadern, D-8000 München 70, FRG.

Folkow, B., MD, Department of Physiology, University of Göteborg, P.O. Box 33031, S-400 33 Göteborg, SWEDEN.

Funder, J., MD, The Panum Institute, Blegdamsvej 3C, DK-22000 Copenhagen, DENMARK.

Ganten, D., MD, Pharmakologisches Institut der Universität, Im Neuenheimer Feld 366, D-6900 Heidelberg, FRG.

Garay, R., MD, INSERM U7, Department of Physiology and Pharmacology, Hôpital Necker, Paris, 75015, FRANCE.

Genest, J., MD, Clinical Research Institute of Montreal, 110 Avenue des Pins Oaest, Montreal, Quebec H2W 1R7, CANADA.

Haber, E., MD, Cardiac Unit, Massachusetts General Hospital, Boston, MA 02114, USA.

Haddy, F., MD, Section of Cardiovascular Sciences, Baylor College of Medicine, Texas Medical Center, Houston, TX 77030, USA.

Haeusler, G., MD, Pharma Research Department, F. Hoffmann-La Roche & Co., Ltd., CH 4022 Basel, SWITZERLAND.

Hoffman, J., MD, Department of Physiology, School of Medicine, Yale University, 333 Cedar Street, P.O. Box 3333, New Haven, Connecticut, USA.

Inagami, T., MD, Department of Biochemistry, Venderbilt University, Nashville, TN 37232, USA

Johnston, C., MD, Monash University, Prince Henry's Hospital, St. Kilda Road, Melbourne, Victoria, 3004, AUSTRALIA.

Jones, A., MD, Department of Physiology, Columbia School of Medicine, University of Missouri, M412 Medical Sciences Building, Columbia, Missouri, USA.

Laragh, J., MD, Cardiovascular Unit, New York Hospital Cornell Medical Center, 525 East 68th Street, New York City, NY 10021, USA.

Langer, S., Dr, Department of Biology, LERS, 58, rue de la Glacière, 75013, Paris, FRANCE.

Luetscher, J., MD, Department of Endocrinology/Hypertension, Stanford University Medical Center, Room M-204, Stanford, CA 94305, USA.

MacGregor, G., MD, Department of Medicine, Charing Cross Hospital, Fulham Palace Road, London W6, UK.

Mark, A., MD, Cardiovascular Division, Department of Medicine, University of Iowa, Iowa City, IA 52242, USA.

Melby, J., MD, Department of Medicine and Physiology, Section of Endocrinology and Metabolism, University Hospital, 75 East Newton Street, Boston, MA 02118, USA.

Meyer, P., MD, Department of Physiology and Pharmacology, INSERM U7, Hôpital Necker, 161 rue de Sèvres, 75015, Paris, FRANCE.

Muirhead, E., MD, Department of Pathology, University of Tennessee, 858 Madison Avenue, Memphis, TN 38103, USA.

Mulvany, M., MD, Institute of Biophysics, University of Aarhus, DK-8000 Aarhus C, DENMARK.

Overbeck, H., MD, Cardiovascular Research and Training Center, School of Medicine, University of Alabama, University Station, Birmingham, AL 35294, USA.

Palkovits, M., MD, Laboratory of Clinical Science, National Institute of Mental Health, National Institute of Health, Building 10, Room 2D47, Bethesda, MD 20205, USA.

Pitcock, J., MD, Department of Pathology, University of Tennessee, 899 Madison Avenue, Memphis, TN 38103, USA.

Postnov, Y., MD, Central Research Laboratories of Ministry of Health, Timoshenko Avenue 21, Moscow, 121359, USSR.

Poulsen, K., MD, The Royal Dental College, Jagtvej 160, 2100 Copenhagen Ø, DENMARK.

Sambhi, M.P., MD, Division of Hypertension, Department of Medicine, UCLA, San Fernando Valley Medical Program, Sepulveda Veterans Administration Medical Center, 16111 Plummer Street, Sepulveda, CA 91343, USA.

Sleight, P., MD, Cardiac Department, John Radcliffe Hospital, University of Oxford, Headington, Oxford, 0X3 9DU, UK.

Starke, K., MD, Alberg Ludwigs Universität, Hermann Herde Strasse, 5, D-7800 Freiburg im Breisgau, FRG.

Tewksbury, D., MD, Marshfield Medical Foundation, 510 North Street Joseph Avenue, Marshfield, WI 54449, USA.

Tobian, L., MD, Department of Medicine, University of Minnesota Hospital, Mayo Box 285, Minneapolis, MN 55455, USA.

Tosteson, D., MD, Department of Physiology and Biophysics, Harvard Medical School,

25 Shattuck Street, Boston, Massachusetts, USA.

Villarreal, H., MD, Department of Nephrology, Instituto Nacional de Cardiología 'Ignacio Chavez', Juan Badiano 1, MEXICO, 14000.

Williams, R., MD, Department of Internal Medicine, University of Utah Medical Center, 50 North Medical Drive, Salt Lake City, UT 84132, USA.

Yamori, Y., MD, Department of Pathology, Shimane Medical University, Japan Stroke Prevention Center, Izumo, JAPAN, 693.

75 Warrick Street, Boston, Massachusetts, USA.

Villacorta, H., MD, Departmental of Cardiology, Instituto Nacional de Cardiología "Juan Chávez", Juan Badiano 1, México, 14080.

Williams, G.A., Department of Internal Medicine, University of Utah Medical Center, 50 North Medical Drive, Salt Lake City, UT 84132, USA.

Yamada, N., MD, Department of Pathology, Shimane Medical University, Izumi-Stroke Prevention Center, Izumo, 69341, USA.

I. TRANSPORT ACROSS MEMBRANES AND HYPERTENSION

INTRODUCTION: MEMBRANE TRANSPORT

D. Tosteson

This part of the Symposium considers possible relations between ion transport across membranes and hypertension. The papers describe investigations of several different ion transport systems, kinds of cells and types of hypertension.

Y. Yamori, Yu. Postnov and D. Bohr provide broad overviews of the subject of membrane abnormalities in essential hypertension in man and several forms of experimental hypertension in animals. These communications convey the considerable range of evidence supporting the view that abnormal membrane function is somehow involved in the pathogenesis of hypertension.

A group of authors (P. Meyer, R. Garay, J. Duhm, M. Canessa, R. Williams, D. Cusi, W. Burke, J. Funder and E. Erdmann) presents papers on various aspects of ouabain-insensitive cation transport in red cells. Both Na-K co-transport (Meyer, Garay) and Na-Na exchange as measured by Na-Li countertransport (Canessa, Williams, Burke and Funder) receive considerable attention. Some investigators (Duhm, Canessa, Cussi) report measurements of both of these modes of cation transport. One paper (Williams) describes the incidence of abnormal maximum rates of Na-Li countertransport in members of different generations of large families in Utah. These data provide the clearest picture so far made of the genetic transmission of this transport system. Burke shows that the maximum rate of Na-Li countertransport declines with age in the normal but not in the hypertensive population. This result emphasizes the importance of care in selecting appropriate control groups when carrying out epidemiological studies of transport systems. Funder's contribution presents evidence suggesting that Na and H compete for the same membrane site in the Na-Li countertransport system. This raises but does not yet answer the interesting question of whether the Na-Li countertransport system also functions as a Na-H exchanger. If this proves to be the situation, many hitherto unsuspected physiological roles of the Na-Na exchange system must be considered.

Several articles in this section (A. Jones, H. Overbeck, and M. Mulvany) explore ion movements in vascular smooth muscle in various models of experimental hypertension. In some cases (Jones, Overbeck), positive correlations between ion movements and concentrations and increased vascular smooth muscle tone are reported. In other cases (Mulvany), no correlation between intracellular sodium and vascular resistance was observed.

Three papers (Haddy, MacGregor, Blaustein) call particular attention to the possibility that a humoral factor that inhibits the Na-K pump is present in increased concentration during volume-expansion hypertension. Haddy describes evidence for such a factor in several different models of experimental hypertension. MacGregor gathers some of the data that he, DeWardener and their colleagues have interpreted to support the presence of such a factor. Blaustein elaborates on the hypothesis that the connection between abnormal Na transport and hypertension is intracellular Ca. He argues that any transport abnormality that leads to increased intracellular Na will pre-dispose to hypertension by leading to reduced extrusion of Ca by the Na-Ca exchange system, thus increasing intracellular calcium concentration and causing increased shortening and tension in vascular smooth muscle fibers.

Taken together, these papers give good reason for continuing to study the relation between ion transport across membranes and hypertension. The story about ouabain-insensitive Na transport in human red cells is by no means clear, although some positive correlations are evident. Most (Canessa, Williams, Burke, Funder, Cussi) but not all (Garay, Duhm) investigators find a greater incidence of *increased* maximum rate of red cell Na-Li countertransport in essential hypertensive, as compared with normotensive human subjects. Most (Meyer, Garay) but not all (Canessa, Kuhm) find reduced outward Na co-transport in patients suffering from essential hypertension. Although some differences in the results are perhaps referable to differences in assay procedures (compare Garay, Canessa, Funder and Duhm), many discrepancies seem to be due to heterogeneity of the patient pool studied. Large variations are observed in the incidence of abnormalities of a particular transport system in different relatively small (20–100) groups of subjects. It follows that interpretations of epidemiological data should be very cautious until a sufficient numbers of subjects has been carefully examined. The studies of large family pedigrees in Utah (Williams) are a good example of what needs to be done.

The growing evidence favoring the existence of an endogenous Na-K pump inhibitor is an important development. Many investigators have searched, in vain, for such a compound. The results reported here suggest that they should not be discouraged but, rather, should press on with vigor. It is entirely possible that such a hormone may play important roles in the regulation of the blood pressure and other physiological processes.

BIOMEMBRANE ABNORMALITIES IN SPONTANEOUS HYPERTENSION

Yukio Yamori, Yasuo Nara, Hiroshi Imafuku, Toshimi Kanbe, Kazuko Mori, Masahiro Kihara, and Ryoichi Horie

INTRODUCTION

Recent studies on spontaneously hypertensive rats (SHR) [1] and strokeprone SHR (SHRSP) [2] have brought us both good news and bad news [3]. The bad news is that hypertension and stroke are definitely determined by genetic factors [4]. On the other hand, the good news is that hypertension and stroke can be prevented by modifying environmental factors or by preventive treatments, even if genetic predisposition is strong [3, 5, 6].

Since hypertensive diseases develop based on genetic predisposition and its interaction with environmental factors, it might be possible to detect the genetic predisposition before the development of these diseases [3]. Such an early detection of predisposition would hopefully contribute to the prevention of hypertension and stroke. Our studies have indicated that biomembrane characteristics may be a hopeful measure to detect the genetic disposition of hypertensive disease [7–11].

IONIC TRANSPORT IN GENETIC HYPERTENSION

We now have eight strains of hypertensive rats in the world. They are: *Dahl salt sensitive strain* [12, 13] or *Sabra hypertensive strain* [14, 15], which develop hypertension when fed on high-salt diet; *genetically hypertensive rats* [16, 17] of New Zealand strain; *Lyon hypertensive rats* [18, 19] or *Münster strain* [20] which develop moderate hypertension but do not develop such marked cardiovascular complications as noted in SHR; *Milan hypertensive rats* [21, 22] which develop mild hypertension; *SHR* and *SHRSP* (Stroke-prone SHRs), which develop moderate to severe hypertension with typical complications of hypertension.

When we review the pathogenic mechanisms of hypertension in all these strains [23], volume expansion is only transiently noted in young Milan hypertensive rats, although deviation of renal function is suggested also in Dahl and Sabra hypertensive rats. Except for young Milan rats, data of hemoconcentration noted in other strains indicates the importance of functional or structural increase in the peripheral vascular resistance. Various types of cellular membrane abnormalities of erythrocytes, such as increased ouabain-resistant Na-transport or permeability in SHR [7, 24] and Sabra rats, a decrease in net Na-flux in SHR and Lyon rats [25], increased Na-K co-transport in Milan rats, and increased Na-concentration of erythrocytes in Münster strain, suggest that these basic alterations may be more or less involved in the pathogenic mechanism of genetic hypertension.

Concerning the deviation of ionic transport in blood vessels, Jones first reported an increased potassium-ion washout from arterial walls in SHR [26, 27], and Hermsmeyer further demonstrated a lower intracellular potassium-ion activity in the vascular muscle cells of caudal arteries in SHR [28]. These findings support the possibility that such an abnormal ionic transport, noted not only in erythrocytes but also in vascular smooth muscle cells, may be of pathogenic importance in hypertension.

PATHOGENIC NATURE OF HYPERTENSIVE VASCULAR LESIONS

Since SHRSP were discovered in 1974, we presumed that there might be some biomembrane abnormalities also in hypertensive vascular lesions, because the cerebral hemorrhage and infarction noted in SHRSP were commonly caused by arterionecrosis. Arterionecrosis is induced by the extensive exudation of plasma into arterial walls, which were damaged by physical or chemical stress. Severe hypertension functionally or hemodynamically reduces regional cerebral blood flow (rCBF) in the predilection sites of stroke lesions that are fed by recurrent arteries. Such chronic mild hypoxia due to the reduction of rCBF increases vascular permeability and finally induces arterionecrosis. Hemorrhage occurs when microaneurysms formed at necrotic arterial walls rupture, and infarction occurs when arteries are occluded with thrombosis at the site of the necrosis or microaneurysms [5, 6].

Increased vascular permeability, one of the basic processes inducing arterionecrosis, is detected by the leakage of horseradish peroxidase or ^{131}I-labelled albumin into the brain through cerebral arteries with a tight blood-brain barrier [23]. Scanning electromicroscopic study on arterial endothelial cells demonstrates small crater formations and abundant villi formations in SHRSP not only in the advanced stage but also in the relatively early stage of hypertension. These morphologically detectable membrane alterations may be based on the more generalized basic membrane abnormality related to genetic pathogenesis of hypertensive diseases.

FRAGILITY, FLUIDITY AND PERMEABILITY OF ERYTHROCYTE MEMBRANE IN SHR AND SHRSP

Since the pathological nature of vascular lesions in hypertension also suggests that the membrane itself is different in SHR and SHRSP, we have further examined erythrocytes, especially the membrane fluidity, osmotic fragility, drug-induced hemolysis, and the permeability of lipophilic ions.

It is already well-documented that the sizes of the erythrocytes from SHR and SHRSP are smaller than that of Wistar-Kyoto (WKY), even at a young age and throughout their life [11].

We applied microviscosimetry (Elscint) to erythrocyte membranes. In SHRSP, but not in stroke-resistant SHR (SHRSR), the membrane viscosity was less [10]; in other words, the membrane fluidity was increased, and erythrocyte membranes might be more permeable in SHRSP. Since membrane fluidity is generally affected by the cholesterol concentration of biomembranes, we examined cholesterol levels of erythrocyte membranes, which were proven to be significantly decreased in SHRSP compared with normotensive WKY. This reduction seems to be related to the lower plasma-cholesterol level in SHRSP. It is interesting that the incidence of stroke, that is, 'arterionecro thrombogenic stroke' but not 'atherothrombogenic stroke,' is high in SHRSP with a lower plasma-cholesterol level as well as in rural inhabitants in Japan with a relatively lower plasma-cholesterol level.

Since sodium permeability and membrane fluidity were different in erythrocytes from SHRSP, we further tested the osmotic fragility of erythrocytes by passing a minute amount of erythrocytes through the osmotic gradient in a thin polyethylene tube of 3 m in length. During coil-planet centrifugation, erythrocytes migrate from high to low osmotic pressure. Both starting and end points of hemolysis were higher in SHRSP, indicating that erythrocyte membranes from SHRSP were more fragile than those from other strains [8, 9].

In order to establish a more simplified technique to detect the altered membrane characteristics, we further observed hemolysis caused by lipophilic reagents [29, 30]. Our scanning electron microscopic observation confirmed that anionically charged anilio nephthalene sulfonic acid (ANS) caused hemolysis by inducing the externalization of the erythrocyte membrane, while cationically charged clemastine hydrogen fumarate causes hemolysis by inducing the internalization of the membrane. Therefore, the acting sites of ANS and clemastine are the outer and inner sides of erythrocyte membranes, respectively.

In 3-month-old rats, ANS-induced hemolysis of erythrocytes from SHRSP was obviously accelerated during the incubation time of 20 to 30 minutes in comparison with those from SHRSR, but the hemolysis in SHRSP was not different from WKY.

The similar acceleration of clemastine-induced hemolysis was observed in the erythrocytes from SHRSP or WKY compared with those from SHRSR during 40- to 60-minute incubation. Therefore, although both SHRSP and SHRSR are hypertensive, hemolysis induced by either ANS or clemastine is accelerated in SHRSP, and this result indicates that the erythrocyte membrane of SHRSP is different in both the outer and inner halves of the lipid bilayer which bind with

ANS and clemastine, respectively. Such lipophilic reagent-induced hemolysis may be applied to detect membrane characteristics related to the stroke-prone-ness.

We have developed a new simple method to detect the permeability of ery-throcytes by using a lipophilic ion, tetraphenyl phosphonium, as an indicator [3, 10]. This method revealed that the membrane potential is significantly greater in SHRSR, while membrane permeability is increased in SHRSP. Since this method detects alterations of erythrocyte membrane in SHRSR and SHRSP as early as 40 days after birth, it may be utilized for the detection of the disposition to hyperten-sion and stroke-proneness.

In summary of the diverse abnornalities noted in the erythrocyte membrane in SHR and SHRSP, there seem to be at least three groups of alterations (Table 1).

Table 1. Biomembrane characteristics of erythrocytes in SHRSP, SHR, and WKY

	Blood Pressure	Na-Ion Permeability	Net Na-Flux	Lipophilic Ion	Osmotic Fragility	Fluidity	Hemolysis with Drug	Membrane Potential
WKY	→ (0)	→	→	→	→	→	→	→
SHR	↑ (5%)	↑	↓	→	→	→	↓*	↓**
SHRSP	↑↑ (90%)	↑↑	↓↓	↑	↑	↑	→	→

(   ): stroke incidence
*: More resistant.
*: Hyperpolarized.

The first group is membrane alterations, such as Na-ion permeability and net Na flux, which are parallel to blood pressure level and thus seem to be more closely related to the pathogenesis of hypertension. The second group of membrane alterations consists of the permeability of lipophilic ions, osmotic fragility, and fluidity determined by microviscosimetry, which are different, especially in SHRSP compared with SHR and WKY, and thus could be related with dispo-sition to stroke. The third group of alterations is noted especially in SHRSR, such as resistance to drug-induced hemolysis which, therefore, may possibly be related to disposition to stroke-resistance. However, erythrocytes themselves are not directly involved in the pathogenesis of hypertension and stroke. Among these membrane abnormalities noted in erythrocytes, the common alterations, if any, noted also in synaptosomes or vascular smooth muscle cells, could be more important in the pathogenesis of hypertension or stroke.

MEMBRANE CHARACTERISTICS OF SYNAPTOSOMES IN SHR

The membrane characteristics of synaptosomes were analyzed further in order to clarify whether or not such a biomembrane abnormality noted in erythrocytes may be a part of more generalized abnormalities in hypertension. We applied microviscosimetry to determine fluidity or fluorochrome method, and labelled norepinephrine uptake or release, to test the synaptosomal membrane characteristics [31].

Fluidity of the synaptosomal membrane was increased in SHRSP but rather decreased in regular SHR. Thus, the alteration of fluidity itself is not closely related to the pathogenesis of spontaneous hypertension itself but may be rather the reflection of diverse membrane alterations. Therefore, in order to detect synaptosomal function, norepinephrine uptake or release was further examined.

The percent release of labelled norepinephrine from synaptosomes was greater in SHRSP than in WKY, especially in response to lower concentrations of potassium ions (Fig. 1). On the other hand, norepinephrine uptake into the synaptosomes, especially in the initial phase, was significantly more in SHRSP than in WKY, and the uptake in SHR was intermediate between them. These findings indicate the possible alteration of synaptosomal functions, which might be related to autonomic nervous function in these hypertensive models.

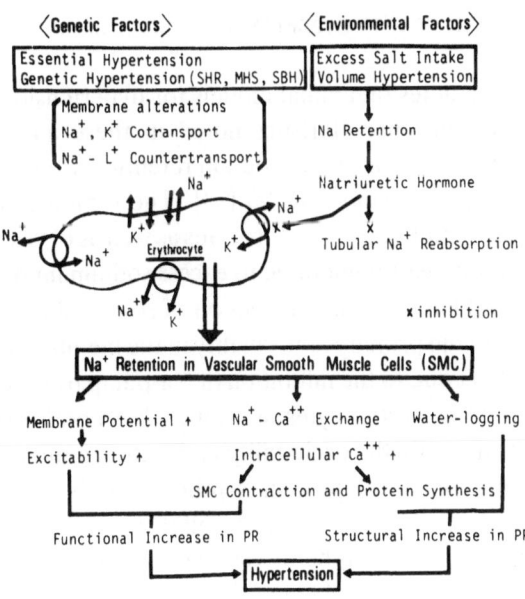

Figure 1. Labelled norepinephrine release from synaptosomes in response to K^+ (25 mM).

MEMBRANE ALTERATIONS OF CULTURED VASCULAR SMOOTH-MUSCLE CELLS FROM SHR

The membrane characteristics of vascular muscle cells were analyzed under tissue culture condition, and the differences in the growth and ionic fluxes, which could be more directly related to the pathogenesis of hypertension, were observed between vascular smooth muscle cells from SHR or SHRSP and those from WKY [32].

Cultured smooth muscle cells from the aorta, which were obtained by an explant method, showed reproducible difference in growth curve among SHRSP, SHRSP, and WKY. Those from hypertensive models grow faster and show greater activity in DNA and protein synthesis.

Labeled Na-influx and labelled K-efflux were both increased in cultured vascular smooth muscle cells under the inhibition of Na-K ATPase by 1 mM ouabain treatment in hypertensive models, especially in SHRSP compared with normotensive WKY (Table 2), indicating that similar membrane abnormalities to those in erythrocytes are noted in vascular smooth muscle cells which seem to contribute to the increased peripheral vascular resistance in hypertension.

Study of labelled Na-uptake also clearly confirmed that ouabain-insensitive Na permeability or transport is increased in SHR and SHRSP. Such abnormality naturally results in intracellular Na-retention, when the compensatory activation in NaK ATPase noted at the early stage of hypertension subsides at the advanced stage.

MEMBRANE ALTERATIONS AND HYPERTENSION MECHANISMS

According to our studies on animal models for hypertension and stroke, among various biomembrane characteristics noted in these animals, the membrane abnormality related to intracellular sodium retention seems to be involved in the pathogenesis of hypertension (Fig. 2) [33]. These models with genetic abnormalities in the cell membrane of erythrocytes as well as of vascular smooth muscle cells are more sensitive or vulnerable to excess sodium intake, which is throught to inhibit Na K ATPase through the action of so-called natriuretic hormone.

Thus, because of the primary abnormality in the membrane and also because of the secondary effect due to the inhibition of Na-pump by excess salt intake, more sodium is retained in erythrocytes as well as in smooth muscle cells. Sodium retention affects not only the excitability and water content of the cells, but also accelerates contraction and protein synthesis, probably through Ca-related mechanisms. Thus, the increment of intracellular Na in vascular wall functionally or structurally raises the peripheral vascular resistance and contributes to the development or maintenance of genetic hypertension.

Table 2. Na$^+$ influx and K$^+$ efflux in cultured smooth muscle cells (SMC) from the aorta of SHRSP, SHRSR, and WKY

		Incubation time after the addition of 1 mM ouabain				turnover/min (n = 6) $p < 0.01$
		0	10 min	30 min	60 min	
Na$^+$ influx	SHRSP	0.193 ± 0.035	0.405 ± 0.046	0.833 ± 0.069	1.018 ± 0.049	
Na$^+$ (µmole/mg protein)	SHRSR	0.208 ± 0.017	0.232 ± 0.076	0.602 ± 0.076	0.968 ± 0.041	
	WKY		0.194 ± 0.028	0.214 ± 0.021	0.508 ± 0.021	0.806 ± 0.028
K$^+$ efflux	SHRSP	0.924 ± 0.01	0.676 ± 0.049	0.347 ± 0.042	0.147 ± 0.020	0.0137
K$^+$ (µmole/mg protein)	SHRSR	0.973 ± 0.058	0.683 ± 0.069	0.476 ± 0.067	0.223 ± 0.024	0.0124
	WKY	0.984 ± 0.056	0.740 ± 0.084	0.458 ± 0.069	0.319 ± 0.046	0.0106

SMC at the 3rd to 7th passages, when they became confluent, was incubated with 1 mM ouabain and at the selected time intervals (10, 30 and 60 min) intracellular Na$^+$ and K$^+$ contents were flame-photometrically assayed, after washing rapidly SMC with cold 0.1 M MgCl$_2$ 6 times and extracted Na$^+$ and K$^+$ with 5% trichlor acetic acid.

Crude synaptosomal fraction was prepared from the forebrain by differential centrifugation. The synaptosomal suspension was incubated with [^{3}H]-norepinephrine (0.4 µCi/mg protein) at 37°C for 15 min under stream of O$_2$:N$_2$ (95:5, v/v), and nonincorporated norepinephrine was removed from the synaptosomal suspension. The norepinephrine-loaded synaptosomal suspension (containing 64 mM NaCl, 40 mM HEPES, 20 mM glocuse, 10 mM KOH, 2.4 mM NaHPO$_4$, 2 mM MgCl$_2$, 2 mM CaCl$_2$, 0.2 mM pargyline, and 2 mM ascorbic acid) was treated with 25 mM or 55 mM KCl solution at 37°C for 5 min. Radioactivity was measured in the synaptosomes after removing released norepinephrine. Norepinephrine release was normalized by adjusting the amount released from the synaptosomes in response to 55 mM KCl solution as 100%.

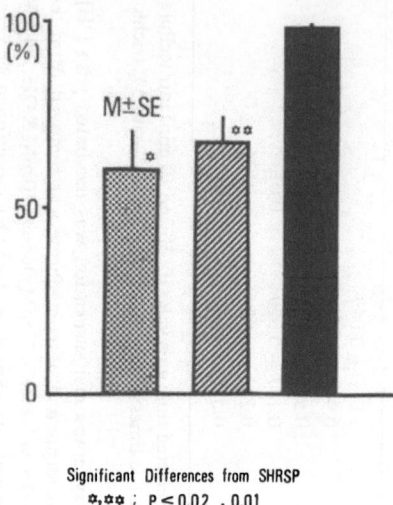

Significant Differences from SHRSP
☆,☆☆ : P < 0.02 , 0.01

Figure 2. Biomembrane alterations and hypertension mechanism.

CONCLUSION

As far as the pathogenesis of spontaneous hypertension is analyzed up to the present, it may be summarized as follows. Spontaneous hypertension is caused by the interaction between genetic and environmental factors. Two main hypertension mechanisms observed up to the present are neural and vascular factors, both of which contribute to the functional and structural increase of the peripheral vascular resistance to establish hypertension in SHR. Generalized biomembrane abnormalities may affect neural factors as well as vascular reactivity or metabolism. It may also affect not only ionic transport to induce intracellular Na retention but also electrolyte balance of the whole body to induce salt retention. Such diverse biomembrane abnormalities noted in vascular smooth muscle cells and synaptosomes may be involved in the basic genetic pathogenesis of hypertension. In the extreme cases, such as in SHRSP, even vascular endothelial cells may also be involved, so that increased vascular permeability causes arterionecrosis, the common basic cerebrovascular lesions both in hemorrhage and infarction in SHRSP.

Biomembrane characteristics noted also in erythrocytes in SHR or SHRSP may be the reflection of diverse membrane abnormalities related to genetic pathogenesis of these hypertensive diseases. Even if these findings are not of pathogenic importance, they may be used as genetic markers of hypertensive diseases and be useful the early detection of the predisposition to these diseases.

REFERENCES

1. Okamoto K, Aoki K: Development of a strain of spontaneously hypertensive rats. Jpn Circ J 27: 283–293, 1963.

2. Yamori Y, Nagaoka A, Okamoto K: Importance of genetic factors in hypertensive cerebrovascular lesions: An evidence obtained by successive selective breeding of stroke-prone and -resistant SHR. Jpn Circ J 38:1095–1100, 1974.

3. Yamori Y, Lovenberg W, Freis ED (editors): Prophylactic Approach to Hypertensive Diseases. New York, Raven Press, 1979.

4. Tanase H, Suzuki Y, Ooshima A, et al.: Genetic analysis of blood pressure in spontaneously hypertensive rats. Jpn Circ J 34:1197–1212, 1970.

5. Yamori Y, Horie R, Akiguchi I, et al.: Pathogenic mechanisms and prevention of stroke in stroke-prone SHR, in De Jong W, Provoost AP, Shapiro APA (editors): Progress in Brain Research. Amsterdam, Elsevier, 1977, pp 219–234.

6. Yamori Y, Horie R, Handa H, et al.: Pathogenic approach to the prophylaxis of stroke and atherogenesis in SHR, in Spontaneous Hypertension. US Dept of Health, Education, and Welfare publication No. (NIH) 77-1179, 1977, pp 269–278.

7. Yamori Y, Nara Y, Horie R, et al.: Ion permeability of erythrocyte membrane in SHR. Jpn Heart J 18:604–605, 1978.

8. Yamori Y, Nara Y, Horie R, et al.: Biomembrane characteristics and chronic effect of tocopherol in models for hypertension and stroke, in De Duve C, Hayaishi O (editors): Tocopherol, Oxygen and Biomembranes. Amsterdam, Elsevier North-Holland Biomedical Press, 1977, pp 247–256.

9. Yamori Y, Nara Y, Horie R, et al.: Biomembrane characteristics in strokeprone spontaneously hypertensive rats (SHRSP). Jpn Heart J 19:597–598, 1978.

10. Yamori Y, Nara Y, Ohtaka M, et al.: Biomembrane characteristics of erythrocytes and platelets in stroke-prone SHR. Trans Soc Pathol Jpn 68:182, 1979.

11. Yamori Y, Nara Y, Horie R, et al.: Abnormal membrane characteristics of erythrocytes in rat models and men with predisposition to stroke. Clin Exp. Hypertens 2:1009–1021, 1980.

12. Dahl LK, Heine M, Tassinari L: Effects of chronic excess salt ingestion. Evidence that genetic factors play an important role in susceptibility to experimental hypertension. J Exp Med 115: 1173–1190, 1962.

13. Rapp JP, Dahl LK: Adrenal steroidogenesis in rats bred for susceptibility and resistance to the hypertensive effect of salt. Endocrinology 88:52–65, 1971.

14. Ben-Ishay D, Saliternick R, Welner A: Separation of two strains of rats with inbred dissimilar sensitivity to DOCA-salt hypertension. Experientia 28:1321–1322, 1972.

15. Ben-Ishay D: Inherited sensitivity and resistance to hypertension in the Hebrew University H and N rats. Jpn Heart J 20 (suppl I):147–149, 1979.

16. Smirk FH, Hall WH: Inherited hypertension in rats. Nature 182:727–728, 1958.

17. Simpson FO: Spontaneous genetic hypertension in rats, in Spontaneous Hypertension. US Dept of Health, Education, and Welfare publication No. (NIH) 77-1179, 1977, pp 254–261.

18. Dupont J, Dupont JC, Fromont A, et al.: Selection of three strains with spontaneously different levels of blood pressure. Biomedicine 19:36–41, 1973.

19. Vincent M, Dupont J, Sassard J: Simultaneous selection of spontaneously hypertensive, normotensive and lowtensive rats. Jpn Heart J 20 (suppl I):135–137, 1979.

20. Wessels F, Samizadeh A, Losse H: Electrolyte metabolism and spontaneous hypertension in rats (SHR, Münster strain). Jpn Heart J 20 (suppl I):141–143, 1979.

21. Bianchi G, Fox U, Imbasciati E: The development of a new strain of spontaneously hypertensive rats. Life Sci 14:339–347, 1974.

22. Bianchi G, Fox U, DiFrancesco GF, et al.: The hypertensive role of the kidney in spontaneously hypertensive rats. Clin Sci Mol Med 45:135a–139s, 1973.

23. Yamori Y, Horie R, Sato M, et al.: Experimental studies on the pathogenesis and prophylaxis of

stroke in stroke-prone spontaneously hypertensive rats (SHR). 1. Quantitative estimation of cerebrovascular permeability. Jpn Circ J 39:611–615, 1975.

24. Postnov YuV, Orlov SN, Gulak PV, et al.: Evidence of altered permeability of the erythrocyte membrane for sodium and potassium ions in spontaneously hypertensive rats. Clin Sci Mol Med 51:196s–172s, 1976.

25. De Mendonca M, Grichois M-L, Garay RP, et al.: Abnormal net Na$^+$ and K$^+$ fluxes in erythrocytes of three varieties of genetically hypertensive rats. Proc Natl Acad Sci USA 77: 4283–4286, 1980.

26. Jones AW: Altered ion transport in vascular smooth muscle from spontaneously hypertensive rats. Circ Res 33:563–572, 1973.

27. Jones AW: Altered ion transport in large and small arteries from spontaneously hypertensive rats and the influence of calcium. Circ Res 34/35 (suppl I):117–122, 1974.

28. Hermsmeyer K: Electrogenesis of increased norepinephrine sensitivity of arterial vascular muscle in hypertension. Circ Res 38:362–367, 1976.

29. Yamori Y, Mori K, Nara Y, et al.: A new technique for detecting erythrocyte membrane characteristics in SHRSP. Jpn Heart J 22:475, 1981.

30. Yamori Y, Horie R, Nara Y, et al.: Genetic markers in spontaneously hypertensive rats. Clin Exp Hypertens 3:713–725, 1981.

31. Nara Y, Yamori Y, Horie R, et al.: Prophylactic trials for stroke in strokeprone SHR (SHRSP). 5 Mechanism of blood pressure reduction by tyrosine administration. Jpn Heart J 21:576, 1980.

32. Yamori Y, Igawa T, Kanbe T, et al.: Mechanisms of structural vascular changes in genetic hypertension: Analyses on cultured vascular smooth muscle cells from spontaneously hypertensive rats. Clin Sci 61 (suppl 7):121s–123s, 1981.

33. Yamori Y: Pathogenic similarities and differences among various strains of spontaneously hypertensive rats, in Proceedings of the 4th International Symposium on Rats with Genetic Hypertension and Related Studies. Stuttgart, Shattauer Verlag, 1982.

DISCUSSION

Discussants: Bohr, Eggena, Yamori, Tosteson, MacGregor.

Bohr: Are there questions either about methodology or about the broad membrane mechanism of hypertension that Dr. Yamori has presented?

Eggena: A quick question regarding the fluidity of membranes: You say the cholesterol incorporation was less. Have you measured circulating lipoproteins in these rats? Are there differences in HDL, LDL, and VLDL?

Yamori: Yes, we checked the lipoprotein fractions, but so far we didn't find any difference in the lipoprotein profiles.

Tosteson: Perhaps you could tell us why you think the chloride and the TPP method differ in the result that they give.

Yamori: TPP is very readily absorbed by cell constituents.

MacGregor: There are many abnormalities in the SHR rat. It may be difficult to know which are related to the rise in blood pressure and which are just inherited abnormalities having nothing to do with the blood pressure. I wonder if you'd like to comment on the kidney cross-transplantation experiments carried out by Kawabe et al. and Bianchi et al. between SHR rats and normotensive rats. This is a critical experiment, indicating that the kidney carries the message.

Yamori: As you said, kidneys transplanted from SHR rats raise the blood pressure in F_1 hybrids of SHR and normotensive rats. Dr. Kawabe performed the experiment when the rats were at 10 or 20 weeks of age. We all know that structural alteration of the blood vessels in the kidney exists already in these young SHR, so the effect of transplanted kidney might result from structural vascular alterations in the kidney. I don't think that Dr. Kawabe's experiment is a definite proof that the kidney is important in the pathogenesis of spontaneous hypertension. As far as the first question is concerned, we detected various kinds of cell membrane abnormalities, but we think that any cell membrane abnormality related to sodium retention in the cell might be related to the pathogenesis of hypertension. The other abnormalities observed in SHR, such as membrane fragility or increased fluidity, might be more closely related to the vascular lesions caused by hypertension.

ERYTHROCYTE NA+ HANDLING IN RAT GENETIC HYPERTENSION

M. DE MENDONCA, M.L. GRICHOIS, K. TOUMI, A. KNORR, P. GUICHENEY, G. Dagher, R.P. GARAY, D. BEN-ISHAY AND P. MEYER

INTRODUCTION

Recent investigations have described various alterations of cation fluxes in the erythrocyte membrane of essential hypertensives (for review, see [1]). Transmembrane pathways in the red cells of genetically hypertensive rats are also altered [2]. This paper summarizes our previous findings on Na+ transport systems in SHR and SbH and reports some new data on the effect of chronic and acute Na+ loads on cellular Na+ handling.

MATERIAL AND METHODS

Rats

The study was conducted on the following substrains of rats (i) Wistar male rats, (ii) Okamoto spontaneously hypertensive rats (SHR) and Wistar-Kyoto normotensive controls (WKY), (iii) Sabra hypertension-prone (SbH) and Sabra hypertension-resistant rats (SbN). All rats were studied at 10-12 weeks of age. Blood pressure values are given in Table 1. The acute Na+ load consisted of an intraperitoneal injection of NaCl 2 mmol/100 g body weight in a volume of 15 ml. Chronic Na+ loading was maintained during 60 days and consisted of 1% NaCl to drink.

Table 1. Blood pressure value measured with tail cuff and pulse transducer (Narco-Biosystems)

Substrains	Wistar	Wistar Chronic Na+ load	WKY	SHR	SbN	SbN
Blood pressure (mm Hg)	111 ± 1.7 (n = 16)	128 ± 4 (n = 9)	137 ± 4 (n = 16)	197 ± 4 (n = 9)	126 ± 2 (n = 9)	146 ± 5 (n = 9)

Blood sampling and erythrocyte Na⁺ and K⁺ transport system measurements

Arterial blood was sampled under pentobarbital anesthesia (25 mg/kg) from a catheter implanted in a cartoid artery. The red cells were washed three times in 155 mM NaCl, and the following parameters were measured according to previously detailed techniques [2]: (i) *intraerythrocyte Na⁺ content*, (ii) *net Na⁺ efflux and K⁺ influx*, in Na⁺-enriched and K⁺-depleted erythrocytes were studied both in Ringer's solution and in plasma at pH 7.40 at 37° C, (iii) ouabain-insensitive Na⁺ outflux was divided into two fractions: one being bumetanide-sensitive, the other bumetanide-insensitive.

RESULTS

Measurements performed under basal conditions

Figure 1 shows that in Ringer's solution, net K⁺ influx is increased and net Na⁺ outflux is decreased in SHR when compared to WKY. The difference in Na⁺ extrusion between SHR and WKY is the same in plasma as in Ringer's solution.

Figure 2 indicates that in SHR the reduction in Na⁺ extrusion stems from a decreased ouabain-resistant and bumetanide-sensitive Na⁺ efflux. It is noteworthy that bumetanide-sensitive Na⁺ outflux is lower in SHR than in Wistar, Wistar Kyoto, SbN, and SbH rats. A difference between SbH and SbN rats was observed concerning the bumetanide-insensitive Na⁺ outflux that we assume represents the passive permeability. These data can be summarized as follows: (i) important differences are observed in genetically hypertensive rats compared to their normotensive controls but the differences are not similar in the various substrains of genetically hypertensive rats, (ii) SHR erythrocytes are characterized by a reduced outward Na⁺ co-transport and possibly an increased Na⁺ pump, (iii) a significantly increased Na⁺ passive permeability is observed in SbH erythrocytes.

Sodium load

(i) *Acute Na⁺ load.* The investigation was performed in SHR and in WKY rats. As illustrated in Figure 3, the erythrocyte Na⁺ content increased four times more in SHR than in WKY rats.

The net Na⁺ and K⁺ fluxes obtained on erythrocytes incubated with Ringer's solution, and with plasma sampled under basal conditions, or with plasma sampled after an acute Na⁺ load are shown in Figure 1.

Plasma sampled after an acute Na⁺ load has a marked inhibitory effect on net Na⁺ extrusion and on K⁺ influx; this phenomenon appears more important in SHR than in WKY rats. Conversely, basal plasma does not alter the values of

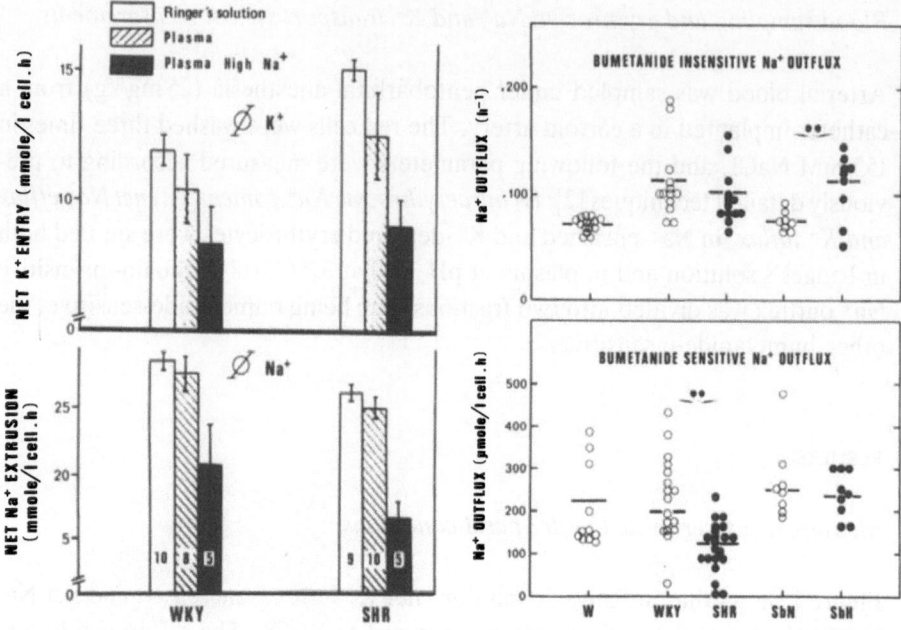

Figure 1. Net Na⁺ extrusion and net K⁺ entry of PCMBS-Na⁺-loaded and K⁺-depleted erythrocytes from WKY and SHR. Measurements were performed in Ringer's solution, 'normal' plasma, and in plasma from rats having received an acute sodium load. Plasma was buffered to pH 7.40 at 37° C. In Ringer's solution, Na⁺ extrusion is lower in SHR than in WKY ($P<0.05$) and K⁺ influx is higher ($P<0.001$). After an acute sodium load, Na⁺ and K⁺ fluxes are lower in plasma than in Ringer's solution ($P<0.01$).

Figure 2. Ouabain-insensitive, bumetanide-sensitive, and bumetanide-insensitive Na⁺ outfluxes of erythrocytes from WKY, SHR, SbN, and SbH. Mean sodium content was 6 to 8 mmole/L cell.
**$P<0.02$.

fluxes measured in Ringer's solution.

(ii) *Chronic Na⁺ load.* Figure 4 shows that, after a chronic Na⁺ load, outward Na⁺ K⁺ co-transport and passive permeability are increased.

DISCUSSION

It is now well established that alterations of Na⁺ transport systems are characteristic of essential hypertension, since they are not obserced in secondary hypertension except at a late stage of renal insufficiency [3]. Studies on renal and spontaneous hypertension in the rat led to similar conclusions [2]. Therefore, an

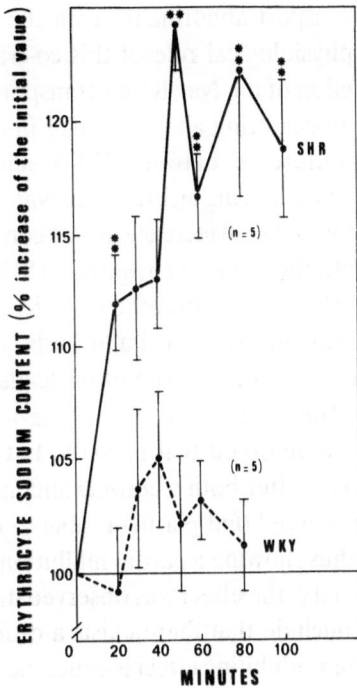

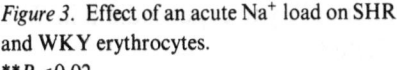

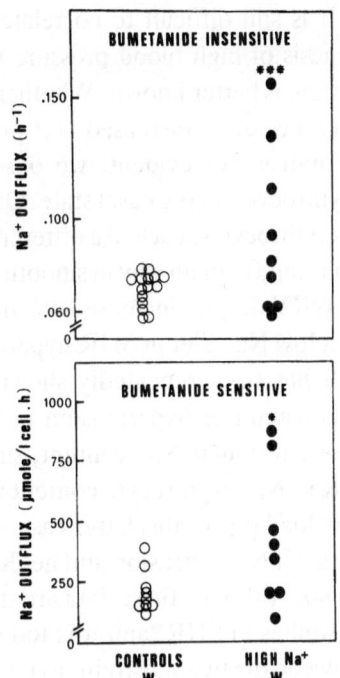

Figure 3. Effect of an acute Na⁺ load on SHR and WKY erythrocytes.
**P <0.02.

Figure 4. Effect of a 60-day high Na⁺ diet (1% saline to drink) on ouabain-insensitive, bumetanide-sensitive, and bumetanide-insensitive outfluxes. Mean sodium content was 6 to 8 mmole/L cell.
*P <0.05
**P <0.01.

abnormal transmembrane Na⁺ transport appears to be related to primary hypertension.

In SHR ouabain-insensitive and bumetanide-sensitive Na⁺ outflux, measured as the rate of Na⁺ enrichment of a Mg^{2+}-sucrose incubation medium, is decreased; in addition, ouabain-insensitive, bumetanide-sensitive K⁺ outflux, measured as the rate of intracellular K⁺, is decreased in Ringer's solution devoid of K⁺ [4]. These observations suggest that Na⁺ K⁺ co-transport is diminished in SHR erythrocytes compared to those of WKY. As K⁺ influx in K⁺-depleted erythrocytes is increased while co-transport is decreased, one may assume that the Na⁺ pump is increased in SHR red cells. The rates of Na⁺ extrusion were similar both in Ringer's solution and normal plasma, thus indicating that plasmatic factors do not have any major action on membrane Na⁺ transport systems in SHR when they are given a standard diet. This result agrees with previous observations of Pamnani [5].

It is still difficult to correlate any co-transport abnormality with the pathogenesis of high blood pressure until the physiological role of this co-transport system is better known. Whether the reduction of the $Na^+ K^+$ co-transport in the presence of an increased Na^+ pump activity can bring about changes in cellular sodium is not evident; we observed no difference between WKY and SHR erythrocytes in the basal state. Other authors measuring an increased Na^+ activity in erythrocytes reached a different conclusion. A small increase in Na^+ concentration could explain why in smooth muscle cells, the Em is less negative in SHR than in WKY despite increased electrogenesis [6]. Furthermore, the beneficial effect of a low Na^+ diet in SHR hypertension could also have a cellular basis [7].

It has been repeatedly shown that excessive Na^+ consumption leads to an aggravation of hypertension in SHR [8]. This could result from long-term increased cellular Na^+ content, since we have observed that in SHR, but not in WKY, Na^+ erythrocyte content was increased after both a chronic and an acute Na^+ load [9]. In this latter case, we have observed that plasma is able to reduce both net Na^+ extrusion and net K^+ influx, thus showing a partial inhibition of the pump. Although these data are still preliminary, the effect was observed in WKY as well as in SHR, and it is too early to conclude that there exists a difference between the two substrains as far as this pump-inhibiting effect is concerned. One may thus speculate that the greater increase in SHR erythrocyte Na^+ content after a sodium load may result from a greater cellular ability to expel sodium in WKY than in SHR when the pump is partially inhibited.

In SbH, co-transport was found to be normal, but the increased passive permeability could explain the increased erythrocyte Na^+ content observed after a chronic Na^+ load. Since in the Milan strain a high co-transport was found [10], it appears that the different genetically hypertensive strains do not exhibit the same membrane abnormalities. It is thus difficult to know how the difference in membrane characteristics observed between hypertensive and normotensive substrains is related to the pathogenesis of hypertension. In Wistar rats, preliminary results obtained after a chronic high Na^+ diet, long enough to renew red cells, suggest that diet can alter the membrane structure, as a marked increase in permeability could be observed in most of the rats. Some data show that dietary sodium may influence membrane protein synthesis [11], and a high sodium intake could therefore affect membrane cell biosynthesis either directly or via a plasmatic factor.

The fact that in rat primary hypertension the Na^+ transport systems are not always modified in the same direction, that dietary sodium may influence membrane characteristics, and that plasma factors may be present, lead one to conclude that the mechanism by which sodium acts at a cellular level to trigger hypertension is complex.

SUMMARY

The erythrocyte Na$^+$ transport systems have been studied in SHR and SbH as well as in Wistar, Wistar-Kyoto, and SbN rats. Measurements were performed in the presence of saline solutions or in the presence of plasma of rats receiving either a standard diet or a Na$^+$ load. Red cell sodium was measured in SHR under an acute Na$^+$ load.

Erythrocyte Na$^+$ content under an acute Na$^+$ load increases slightly in WKY rats and markedly in SHR rats.

A low outward Na$^+$ K$^+$ co-transport and an increased pump activity was observed in SHR red cells, while an increased Na$^+$ permeability was observed in SbH red cells.

The plasma of both WKY and SHR after an acute Na$^+$ load has a Na$^+$ pump-inhibitory effect.

After 2 months of a high Na$^+$ diet, passive Na$^+$ permeability and Na$^+$ K$^+$ co-transport were found to be increased in Wistar erythrocytes.

Thus, the role of Na$^+$ on the onset of high blood pressure may be mediated, at the cellular level, by several complex mechanisms.

REFERENCES

1. Meyer P, Garay RP, De Mendonca M: Ion transport systems in hypertension, in Genest J, Kuchel O, Hamet P, et al. (editors): Hypertension: Physiopathology and Treatment. New York, McGraw-Hill, 1983.
2. De Mendonca M, Knorr A, Grichois ML, et al.: Erythrocyte Na$^+$ transport systems in primary and secondary hypertension of the rat. Kidney Int, in press.
3. Garay RP, Elghozi JL, Dagher G, et al.: Laboratory distinction between essential and secondary hypertension by measurement of erythrocyte cation fluxes. N Engl J Med 302:764–771, 1980.
4. De Mendonca M, Grichois ML, Toumi K, et al.: Furosemide and bumetanide sensitive Na$^+$ fluxes in erythrocytes from genetically hypertensive rats (SHR). Clin Exp Hypertens 3: 885–895, 1981.
5. Pamnani MB, Clough DL, Haddy FJ: Na$^+$, K$^+$ pump activity in tail arteries of spontaneously hypertensive rats. Jpn Heart J XX (suppl 1):228–230, 1979.
6. Losse H, Zidek W, Zumkley H, et al.: Intracellular Na$^+$ as a genetic marker of essential hypertension. Clin Exp Hypertens 3:627–640, 1981.
7. Harsmeyer K: Electrogenesis of increased norepinephrine sensitivity of arterial vascular muscle in hypertension. Circ Res 38:362–367, 1976.
8. Dietz R, Schomig A, Haebara H, et al.: Studies on the pathogenesis of spontaneous hypertension of rats. Circ Res 48:I98–I106, 1978.
9. De Mendonca M, Garay RP, Ben-Ishey D, et al.: Abnormal erythrocyte cation transport in primary hypertension. Clinical and experimental studies. Hypertension 3:I1179–I1185, 1981.
10. Bianchi G: Renal mechanisms in the pathogenesis of essential hypertension, in Frontiers in Cardiology. Punta Ala, Italië, Sept 1981.
11. Devynck MA, Pernollet MG, Matthews PG, et al.: Sodium intake and plasma angiotensin level as modulators of adrenal and uterine angiotensin II receptors in the rat. J Cardiovasc Pharmacol 1:163–179, 1979.

DISCUSSION

Discussants: Bohr, Meyer, Tosteson, Yamori, Denton

Bohr: Were these studies all carried out at 37° C?

Meyer: Yes. The measurements were performed at 37°, and in addition, the plasma experiments were carried out with constant oxygen tension and constant pH.

Bohr: Tell me again, what is being inhibited here–which of the transport mechanisms?

Meyer: I don't know. It's the net active sodium extrusion. Unfortunately, we have no data related to the specific component involved here.

Tosteson: I wonder, what were the conditions used to measure the net sodium extrusion and potassium accumulation?

Meyer: Well, the conditions were the same as those in the other methods using a concentration of 17 micromolar PGMBS. The loading solution had 90 mM of sodium chloride, 50 mM potassium chloride, 1 mM magnesium chloride, 50 mM sucrose, and the osmolality was 320 mosm. The loading solution was removed after 3.5 hr and the loading period was 20 hr. Then the recovery was performed for 1 hr with 150 mM sodium chloride, 5 mM potassium chloride, cysteine, adenine, and inosine in trace amounts, and the osmolality was 292. As I said before, the flux measurements were performed in another solution containing only sodium chloride and potassium chloride – 150 in 5 – and glucose 10. This was performed either in a Ringer solution, or in the presence of plasma sampled in normotensive rats completely replacing this solution. A partial oxygen tension constant at 37° C controlled the PCO_2 and PO_2 levels in the surrounding atmosphere, and the last measurement was performed in the presence of plasma sampled in hypertensive rats or in normotensive rats after acute sodium loading.

Yamori: I am very pleased that you observed the increased sodium content in erythrocytes after chronic sodium loading – 2% sodium in drinking water for 2 months. We observed a similar effect. Membrane abnormalities related to sodium retention appear to be also related to the pathogenesis of hypertension.

Meyer: After 10 days of high sodium diet, we did observe an increase in sodium concentration in hypertensive rats as compared with normotensives. In other words, the sodium content increases specifically in sponstaneously hypertensive rats and in the SBH rats, but not in renin normotensive and respective controls.

Denton: Have you tried that experiment with the high sodium using the plasma from a severely sodium-deficient rat?

Meyer: No, as it is difficult to realize a pure and isolated Na^+ deficit.

CA^{2+} BINDING BY THE ERYTHROCYTE MEMBRANE AND ITS STRUCTURE IN PRIMARY AND SECONDARY HYPERTENSION

YUVENALI V. POSTNOV AND SERGEI N. ORLOV

INTRODUCTION

Recent studies have revealed a number of functional alterations of the erythrocyte membrane in essential hypertension and its experimental analogue – spontaneous hypertension of rats (SHR, Kyoto-Wistar). In particular, it was demonstrated in both forms of primary hypertension that permeability of the erythrocyte membrane for monovalent cations is increased [1–3], and the calcium-binding ability of the inner part of the membrane is decreased [4, 5]. It is natural to suggest that such abnormalities in the erythrocyte membrane function in hypertension are due to certain changes of the membrane structure.

The present investigation deals with the Ca^{2+}-binding ability and certain structural characteristics of the erythrocyte membrane, both in clinical and experimental forms of primary and secondary hypertension.

MATERIALS AND METHODS

Venous blood samples were taken from:

Animals

Spontaneously hypertensive 10-week-old male rats (SHR, Kyoto-Wistar strain) with blood pressure 180–200 mm Hg were used. The normotensive control group (blood pressure 100–120 mm Hg) consisted of Kyoto-Wistar rats (NKWR) of the same sex and age. The animals were kept on standard diet and tap water. The methods of blood sampling and blood pressure measuring were described earlier [1].

Renal hypertension (two-kidney, one-clip Goldblatt-type hypertension) was induced in female Wistar rats 15–16 weeks old) with blood pressure 170–190 mm Hg (duration of hypertension was 4–6 weeks). The control group consisted of intact normotensive female rats of the same weight and age.

DOCA-hypertension was produced in unilateral nephrectomized female Wistar rats (15–16 weeks old) treated by DOCA (crystalline desoxycorticosterone-ace-tate 25 mg, twice with an interval of 10 days, subcutaneously). These rats were kept on a 1% saline solution (blood pressure 175–195 mm Hg, duration of hyper-tension was 4–6 weeks). The control groups for this part of the study were: a) unilateral nephrectomized female Wistar rats kept on a 1% saline solution (blood pressure 125–135 mm Hg); b) unilateral nephrectomized rats (blood pressure 115–125 mm Hg). All rats of control groups were the same age as DOCA-hypertensive rats.

Patients

Subjects consisted of *nine patients with clinically established essential hypertension* (four male and five female, mean age 51, range 38–68 years), hospitalized for chronic ischemic disease (without acute myocardial infarction), frequent crises, or for the examination of causes of high blood pressure. The duration of known hypertension was 4 to 12 years; the blood pressure upon hospitalization was 145–190/90–105 mm Hg. Renal or endocrine pathology, which might have been a cause of secondary hypertension, had been excluded in clinical examination.

A second group of subjects consisted of *11 patients with chronic hypertension of renal origin* (chronic glomerulonephritis or pyelonephritis, three male and eight female, mean age 50, range 35–61 years). The duration of hypertension was 6–15 years; blood pressure was 170–220/100–110 mm Hg.

Controls consisted of *13 normotensive individuals* (six male and seven female, mean age 47, range 32–61 years) without any history of hypertension. Some of them were hospitalized for chronic ischemic desease (without myocardial infarc-tion); the others were healthy volunteers.

Erythrocyte ghosts

The erythrocytes were sedimented by 1,000 × g centrifugation for 10 minutes and washed three times with 150 mM NaCl and 5 mM sodium phosphate solution (pH = 8.0; 0–2° C). The washed erythrocytes were hemolyzed in 20 volumes of 5 mM sodium phosphate buffer (pH = 8.0; 0–2° C) and sedimented (25,000 × g, 30 min.). The sediment was washed three times under the same condition. Lowry's method was used to find the protein concentration [6].

Calcium binding

The method used in this study was described earlier [4]. The incubation medium contained (mM); NaCl-140; EGTA-0.2; $CaCl_2$-0.18; imidazol-HCl-20 (pH = 7.4); $^{45}CaCl_2$-2 μCi/ml; protein concentration 200 μg/ml. The free calcium concentration in the incubation medium, calculated for pK_s Ca...EGTA = 6.3 was $4.5\,\mu M$. After 30 minutes of incubation, the samples were transferred on filters (SM, Millipore) and washed three times with 140 mM NaCl, 20 mM imidazole-HCl solution (pH = 7.4; 0–2° C).

It is known that erythrocyte ghosts contain both right-side-out, inside-out vesicles and unreleased membrane fragments. In order to make both sides of the membrane accessible to calcium, Ca^{2+} ionophore A 23187 $(2\,\mu M)$ was added to the incubation medium.

Fluorescent probes

Two *hydrophobic fluorescent probes* – diphenyl hexatrien (DPHT) and pyrene – were used for the estimation of membrane properties related to its fluidity.

In the case of the DPHT, the intensities of fluorescence at parallel $(F_{\parallel})$ and perpendicular $(F_{\perp})$ orientations of polarization were measured, then both the fluorescence polarization anisotropy $A = (F_{\parallel} - F_{\perp})(F_{\parallel} + 2F_{\perp})$ and the parameter $A/A_o-A)$ were calculated. The parameter $A/(A_o-A)$ is proportional to the microviscosity of the membrane in the probe absorption sites, and A_o^- is the fluorescence polarization anisotropy of immobile and unorientated DPHT molecules $(A_o = 0.362 \,[7])$.

In the case of pyrene, the intensities of monomer $(I^m$ – emission wavelength 373 nm) and aximer $(I^e$ – emission wavelength 450 nm) fluorescence were measured, and the parameter I^m/I^e was calculated. This parameter is also proportional to the microviscosity of pyrene absorption sites in the membrane [8]. The fluorescence of pyrene was excited both directly (325 nm) and indirectly, i.e., by excitation of tryptophane residues in membrane proteins (285 nm). In the first case it is possible to estimate the integral characteristic of pyrene absorption-site microviscosity, while in the second case it is possible to characterize microviscosity of the membrane hydrophobic area near protein molecules only.

The concentration of pyrene was selected so that the quenching of tryptophane fluorescence was 90% of the maximal quenching by pyrene.

The fluorescent probes were dissolved in ethanol. The concentration of ethanol in the measuring cell was no more than 0.2%; the protein concentration was $1 \cdot 10^{-3}\,g/ml$.

The fluorescence measurements were carried out with a Hitachi spectrofluorimeter MPE-4 (Japan). The data are represented as mean $\pm$ SEM. The significance of difference between means was estimated by *t*-test.

RESULTS

The results of the fluorescence polarization anisotropy determination are given in

Table 1. The fluorescence polarization anisotrophy (parameter $A/(A_o\text{-}A)$) of diphenyl hexatrien in erythrocyte membranes of rats

Groups	n	$A/A_o\text{-}A)$
1. Normotensive Kyoto-Wistar rats	10	0.112 ± 0.010
2. Spontaneously hypertensive rats	12	0.180 ± 0.018
3. Rats with renal hypertension	8	0.125 ± 0.011
4. Rats with DOCA hypertension	7	0.119 ± 0.017
$P_{1,2}$		$p < 0.001$
$P_{1,3}$		NS.
$P_{1,4}$		NS.

The incubation medium content (mM); imidazol-HCl-40 (pH 7.4) NaCl-100; $MgCl_2$-5 ($t° = 20°$ C); n is the number of animals; N.S.: not significant

Table 1. These data indicate that microviscosity of the probe absorption sites in the SHR erythrocyte membranes is higher than the control value by 70%. These results are in agreement with data previously obtained in our laboratory [9] and by Montenay-Garestier et al. [10]. There were no differences in the polarization anisotropy of DHTH in erythrocyte membranes of DOCA- and renal-hypertensive rats as compared to corresponding normotensive controls.

No distinction was drawn between the fluorescence spectra of pyrene in SHR and NKWR membrane proparation samples when the excitation wave length was 325 nm, i.e., when the entire pool of bound probe was excited. However, the parameter I^m/I^e was essentially higher in the case of membrane samples from SHR erythrocytes than in the case of control samples when excitation wave length was 285 nm (Table 2). This distinction could be interpreted by the difference of microviscosity of the membrane area localized near protein tryptophane residues (in the limits of Förster radius of migration).

As can be seen from Table 3, Ca-binding ability of the erythrocyte membrane of patients with essential hypertension is reduced by 30% as compared to that of

Table 2. The I^m/I^e ratio of pyrene fluorescence in erythrocyte membranes of rats ($\lambda_{ex} = 285$ nm)

Groups	n	I^m/I^e
1. Normotensive Kyoto-Wistar rats	10	10.05 ± 0.16
2. Spontaneously hypertensive rats	13	12.00 ± 0.09
$P_{1,2}$		< 0.005

The incubation medium contents: 20 mM Na-phosphate buffer (pH 7.2; t = 20° C); n is the number of animals.

Table 3. Calcium-binding ability of the erythrocyte membrane

Groups	n	Ca (nmole/mg of protein)
1. Normotensive patients	13	1.22 ± 0.07
2. Patients with essential hypertension	9	0.87 ± 0.05
3. Patients with chronic renal hypertension	11	1.23 ± 0.10
$P_{1,2}$		<0.005
$P_{1,3}$		N.S.

n is the number of patients; N.S.: not significant.

normotensive controls. The rate of lateral diffusion in the erythrocyte membrane of essentially hypertensive patients is reduced as compared to normotensive patients (an increase of I^m/I^e ratio) (Table 4).

There are no differences in both the Ca-binding ability of the erythrocyte membrane and its structure between patients with chronic renal hypertension and the normotensive group.

As can be seen from Table 4, an increase of Ca^{2+} concentration in the incubation medium results in a change of the lateral diffusion rate of pyrene in the erythrocyte membrane of normotensive individuals and patients with renal hypertension. No influence of Ca^{2+} on the erythrocyte structure of patients with essential hypertension was revealed.

DISCUSSION

The results of the present study confirm the decrease of Ca-binding ability of the erythrocyte membrane previously established in patients with essential hypertension [4] and demonstrate the absence of this alteration in hypertension of renal origin.

It should be noted that the polarization anisotropy of DPHT fluorescence and the ratio of fluorescence intensities of pyrene in the monomer and eximer states evidently reflect two distinct physical properties of the hydrophobic area of the biological membrane: the parameter $A/(A_o - A)$ characterizes the rotational diffusion, while the parameter I^m/I^e characterizes the lateral diffusion [7, 8].

In this connection, we can assume that the rotational diffusion in the whole hydrophobic area, as well as the lateral diffusion in the area of lipid-protein contact in the erythrocyte membrane of spontaneously hypertensive rats, are decreased as compared to the same membrane properties in normotensive control animals.

The study of the fluorescence spectra of pyrene in membrane preparation samples also demonstrates the presence of structural alterations in the ery-

Table 4. The dependence of I^m/I^e ratio of pyrene fluorescence on calcium concentration in the incubation medium

Groups		I^m/I^e			
		$[CaCl_2] = 0$ $[Ca^{2+}] = 0$	$[CaCl_2] = 300\ \mu M$ $[Ca^{2+}] = 0.21\ \mu M$	$[CaCl_2] = 600\ \mu M$ $1Ca^{2+}8 = 0.75\ \mu M$	$[CaCl_2] = 1200\ \mu M$ $1Ca^{2+} = 200\ \mu M$
(a) direct pyrene excitation ($\lambda_{ex} = 325$ nm)					
1. Patients with essential hypertension	9	2.83 ± 0.10	2.82 ± 0.07	2.77 ± 0.05	2.76 ± 0.10
2. Patients with chronic renal hypertension	11	2.14 ± 0.09	2.22 ± 0.07	2.28 ± 0.06	2.46 ± 0.08
3. Normotensive patients	20	2.11 ± 0.06	2.25 ± 0.08	2.33 ± 0.08	2.48 ± 0.09
$P_{1,3}$		<0.005	<0.005	<0.005	<0.05
$P_{2,3}$			N.S.		
(b) Pyrene excitation by tryptophane residues of membrane proteins ($\lambda_{ex} = 285$ nm)					
1. Patients with essential hypertension	9	3.26 ± 0.10	3.25 ± 0.09	3.15 ± 0.12	3.15 ± 0.12
2. Patients with chronic renal hypertension	11	2.30 ± 0.08	2.30 ± 0.10	2.40 ± 0.08	2.46 ± 0.10
3. Normotensive patients	20	2.20 ± 0.06	2.20 ± 0.07	2.40 ± 0.10	2.42 ± 0.08
$P_{1,3}$		<0.005	<0.005	<0.005	<0.005
$P_{2,3}$			N.S.		

The incubation medium content (mM): imidazole-HCl-40 (pH 7.4; t = 37° C) NaCl-140; Mg-140; MgCl$_2$; EGTA-1 CaCl$_2$-1 CaCl$_2$-up to 2, 3; n is the number of patients; [Ca^{2+}] is free calcium concentration in the incubation medium; N.S.: not significant.

throcyte membranes obtained from essentially hypertensive patients, but not in those with renal hypertension.

It has become evident that the membrane defect in erythrocytes, which we viewed as a part of widespread membrane alteration [11, 12], is inherent only to primary hypertension. This assumption is supported by experimental studies in which decrease of calcium-binding ability [4] and alteration of monovalent cation permeability [13] were revealed in spontaneouly hypertensive rats, but were not present in rats with renal and DOCA-salt hypertension. This suggests a profound pathogenetic similarity between human essential hypertension and spontaneous hypertension of rats (Kyoto-Wistar hypertensive rats).

Comparing the data on direct and indirect excitation of fluorescent pyrene (Table 4), one can notice a certain irregularity in the structural alteration of the membrane. It is known that in the case of the sarcoplasmic reticulum of skeletal muscles, the rate of pyrene lateral diffusion at physiological temperature (37° C) in the lipid bilayer and in the annular lipids region are equal [14]. This feature was also observed in our study of erythrocytes, both in normotensive and renal hypertensive patients. On the contrary, in the case of essential hypertension, the rate of lateral diffusion of pyrene in the annular lipid regions was decreased considerably as compared to the lipid bilayer. This indicates that the protein molecules in the erythrocyte membrane of these patients are functioning in structurally different lipid environments.

As can be seen from Table 4, the increase of Ca^{2+} concentration in the incubation medium (accompanied by increasing membrane-bound Ca) results in a decrease of the rate of pyrene lateral diffusion, both in the erythrocyte membrane of normotensive and renal hypertensive patients. This phenomenon might be caused by the clostration of acid lipids induced by calcium [15]. In the case of essential hypertension, where lateral diffusion in the membrane is initially decreased, this phenomenon cannot be clearly seen. This may demonstrate the existence of altered interaction of membrane lipids with calcium ions.

Further studies should reveal the specific mechanism responsible for the formation of the structural defect in the erythrocyte membrane and, probably, in the plasma membrane of other types of cells, as well as prove its connection with membrane function alterations in essential hypertension.

SUMMARY

1. Ca^{2+}-binding ability and some biophysical characteristics of membrane structure of red blood cells in patients with essential and renal hypertension and in rats with spontaneous, renal, and DOCA hypertension were studied by means of $^{45}Ca/^{40}Ca$ exchange and by the method of membrane fluorescent probes, respectively.

2. Ca^{2+}-binding ability of the erythrocyte membrane of patients with essential

28

hypertension was found to be reduced by 30% as compared to that of normotensive controls, while there was no difference in Ca^{2+}-binding in the erythrocyte membrane of patients with chronic renal hypertension.

3. Microviscosity of hydrophobic areas of erythrocyte membrane of spontaneously hypertensive rats was found to be increased as compared to that of normotensive controls. The rate of lateral diffusion of pyrene in the region of annular lipids in the erythrocyte membrane of spontaneously hypertensive rats is lowered.

4. The rate of lateral diffusion of pyrene in the erythrocyte membrane of patients with essential hypertension is lowered, both in the lipid bilayer and in the region of annular lipids, as compared to that of normotensive patients.

5. There are no differences in erythrocyte membrane structure both in the clinical and in the experimental forms of secondary hypertension under investigation.

ACKNOWLEDGMENT

The authors are grateful to Dr. A.M. Adler and Dr. Ilya Yu. Postnov for the clinical examination of the patients. We thank Dr. N.I. Pokudin and Z.V. Karagodina for their help.

REFERENCES

1. Postnov YuV, Orlov SN, Gulak PV, et al.: Evidence of altered permeability of the erythrocyte membrane for sodium and potassium ions in spontaneously hypertensive rats. Clin Sci Mol Med 51:160s–172s, 1976.
2. Postnov YuV, Orlov SN, Shevchenko AS, et al.: Altered sodium permeability, calcium binding and Na-K-ATPase activity in the red-cell membrane in essential hypertension. Pflugers Arch 371:263–270, 1977.
3. Cannessa M, Adragna N, Solomon HS, et al.: Increased sodium-lithium countertransport in red cells of patients with essential hypertension. N Engl J Med 302:772–776, 1980.
4. Postnov YuV, Orlov SN, Pokudin NI: Decrease of calcium-binding by the red cell membrane in spontaneously hypertensive rats and in essential hypertension. Pflugers Arch 379:191–195, 1979.
5. Devynck MA, Pernollet MG, Nunez AM, et al.: Calcium-binding alteration in plasma membrane from various tissues of spontaneously hypertensive rats. Clin Exp Hypertens 3:797–808, 1981.
6. Lowry OH, Rosebrough NJ, Farr AL, et al.: Protein measurement with Folin phenol reagent. J Biol Chem 193:265–275, 1953.
7. Vladimirov YuA, Dobretsow GE: Fluorescent probes in study of biological membranes (in Russian). Moscow, Nauka, 1980, pp 32–36, 122–136.
8. Galla HJ, Luisetti J: Lateral and transversal diffusion and phase transition in erythrocyte membranes. An eximer fluorescent study. Biochim Biophys Acta 556:108–117, 1980.
9. Orlov SN, Gulak PV, Karagodina ZV, et al.: The properties of erythrocyte membrane structure in spontaneous genetic hypertension (in Russian). Cardiology (Moscow) 21 (11):108–112, 1981.
10. Montenay-Garestier T, Aragon I, Devynck MA, et al.: Evidence for structural changes in

erythrocyte membranes of spontaneously hypertensive rats. A fluorescence polarization study. Biochem Biophys Res Commun 100:660–665, 1981.

11. Postnov YuV: Essential hypertension as a membrane pathology (in Russian). Cardiology (Moscow) 15 (8):18–23, 1975.

12. Postnow YuV, Orlov SN: Alteration of membranes control over intracellular calcium in essential hypertension and in spontaneously hypertensive rats, in Zumkley H, Losse H (editors): Intracellular Electrolytes and Arterial Hypertension. Stuttgart, George Thieme Verlag, 1980, pp 144–151.

13. Orlov SN, Postnov IYu: The permeability of the red blood cell membranes for sodium in different types of chronic experimental hypertension (in Russian). Cardiology (Moscow) 21 (7):33–36, 1981.

14. Litvinov IS, Obraztsov VV: Lateral diffusion of pyrene in membranes of sarcoplasmic reticulum (in Russian). Biophysika (Moscow) 27:65–70, 1982.

15. Ohnishi S, Ito T: Calcium-induced phase separations in phosphatidylserine-phosphatidylcholine membranes. Biochemistry 13:881–887, 1974.

DISCUSSION

Discussants: Meyer, Postnov, Tosteson, Witowsky

Meyer: I would like to congratulate you on your data and say that we can confirm all the data you presented. In addition, there is another membrane which is very sensitive in the rat: the platelet membranes, which give results similar to those of erythrocytes. My question is related to essential hypertension. We had some difficulties and I would like to know what your experience is, in reproducing the rat data in essential hypertensives in terms of calcium-binding and fluorescence studies. Our studies are still not complete, but they seem to be more difficult in human beings than in the rat. Do you have the same impression?

Postnov: Yes. There are some differences in humans compared with rats because of the rate of fluidity of the erythrocyte membrane and its calcium-binding ability. The membrane in man is more rigid than in rats, and its calcium-binding ability is higher in these animals.

Witowsky: Do you, or anyone else, have data enabling you to be sure that the defects you show are primary in the red cell, and not secondarily induced by cross-transfusion experiments? What are the data on the primary nature of these membrane defects?

Postnov: We have no experience with cross-transfusion, but we have some experience showing that in the prehypertensive stage in rats with spontaneous hypertension there are membrane alterations. I know that Dr. Meyer has results on very young prehypertensive animals – is that right?

Meyer: Yes, and in addition I'd like to stress the point that in Wistar rats, in renal hypertensive rats, we don't have these alterations.

Postnov: In DOCA hypertensive rats there are no differences – I mean there are no such membrane alterations. Salt loading by a 1% NaCl solution during 3 months doesn't cause hypertension, of course, but there is also no difference in membrane fluidity in these rats.

Tosteson: Do you know whether the increased calcium accumulation in mitochondria is calmodulin-dependent?

30

Postnov: There are no data on calmodulin-dependent calcium transport in mitochondria. I hope that the main events concerning calmodulin occur in plasma membranes.

CALMODULIN-DEPENDENT CALCIUM TRANSPORT IN ERYTHROCYTES IN PRIMARY HYPERTENSION

S.N. ORLOV, N.I. POKUDIN AND YU.V. POSTNOV*

INTRODUCTION

The alteration of membrane handling of intracellular calcium recently found in different types of cells in primary (essential) hypertension and its experimental model (spontaneous hypertension in rats) gives grounds to regard primary hypertension in humans and rats as a certain form of membrane pathology.

The first data obtained on hypertensive rats by Aoki et al. showed a decreased rate of ^{45}Ca accumulation and an increased Ca-Mg-ATPase activity in the crude microsomal fraction of aortal smooth muscle and cardiomyocytes [1]. However, because of the functional overloading of cardiovascular contracting cells and their hypertrophy in chronic hypertension, it was difficult to regard these abnormalities of membrane transport as primary to hypertension.

The fact that these membrane alterations are widespread and not of secondary nature in these forms of hypertension, follows from data on cells other than the contracting cells of the cardiovascular system. In particular, the decrease of Ca-binding ability in erythrocyte membranes [2, 3], the rise of intracellular exchangeable Ca content in adipose tissue [4, 5] in both forms of hypertension, as well as the reduction of Ca-binding by plasma membranes of adipocytes [6], hepatocytes, and synaptosomes [7] were revealed in the last few years. However, it is not clear at present if these membrane abnormalities actually cause the alteration of intracellular Ca^{2+} concentration. Erythrocytes are the most suitable object for the purpose, because the electrochemical gradient in these cells is created by one system only, namely Ca-Mg-ATPase [8]. It is known that the activity of this system is determined by the Ca^{2+}-dependent protein regulator, calmodulin [9]. The plasma membrane vesicles, turned inside-out, constitute an excellent model for the study of the Ca-pump activity as well as its interaction with calmodulin [10, 11].

In the present investigation, we use this model for the study of Ca transport in erythrocytes of patients with essential hypertension and of spontaneously hypertensive rats.

MATERIALS AND METHODS

Animals

Male, spontaneously hypertensive Kyoto-Wistar rats (SHR) (aged 14 weeks, weight 270–290 g, blood pressure 180–200 mm Hg) and normotensive Kyoto-Wistar rats (NKWR) (the same age, blood pressure 110–130 mm Hg) used in this study were obtained from inbred colonies maintained in our laboratory. The aminals were kept on standard diet and, 24 hours before the experiment, were starved with free access to water.

Patients

Subjects consisted of 10 patients with clinically established essential hypertension (four male and six female, mean age 50, range 38–64 years) hospitalized for chronic ischemic disease (without acute myocardial infarction), frequent crises, or hospitalized for examination of causes of high blood pressure. The duration of known hypertension was 4 to 12 years; the blood pressure upon hospitalization was 145–190/90–105 mm Hg. Renal or endocrine pathology, which might have been a cause of secondary hypertension, had been excluded in clinical examination. The patients had received antihypertensive drug treatment nonsystematically; none of them received any diuretics 3 to 4 days before the study.

Controls consisted of 11 normotensive individuals (five male and six female, mean age 48, range 32–58 years) without any history of hypertension. Some of them were hospitalized for chronic ischemic disease (without myocardial infarction); the others were healthy volunteers. Blood samples (8–9 ml) were taken on an empty stomach in the morning, using a test tube wetted with heparin solution (25 U/ml). Erythrocytes were sedimented by centrifugation at 1,500 × g for 5 minutes (0–2° C), plasma and white cells were removed, and samples were washed three times with iso-osmatic solution: 150 mM NaCl, 5 mM Na-phosphate buffer (pH 8.0).

Erythrocyte ghosts were obtained by hemolysis of 1 volume of packed erythrocytes in 20 volumes of 5 mM sodium phosphate buffer (pH 8.0) and sedimented (30,000 × g, 25 min). The sediment was washed three times under the same conditions.

Enrichment of membrane fractions by inside-out vesicles (IOV) was made by additional washing of erythrocyte ghosts in 20 volumes of 0.5 mM sodium-phosphate buffer (pH 8.0; 90 min) with a subsequent sedimentation (30,000 × g, 60 min), homogenization, and washing in 10 mM imidazol (pH 7.4). In some cases the 0.5 mM sodium-phosphate buffer contained 0.2 mM EGTA.

The amount of IOV in membrane fractions was measured according to [12]. Lowry's method [13] was used to find the protein concentration.

The rate of calcium accumulation by IOV was determined by means of ^{45}Ca and membrane filtration [6]. The samples on the filters (HA-Millipore) were washed three times with 5 ml of 140 mM NaCl, 1 mM EGTA, and 10 mM Tris-HCl solution (pH 7.4; 0–2° C). The incubation medium contents are given in the figure and table captions. In all cases the calcium uptake was linear up to 10 minutes. For the determination of the rate of calcium accumulation, the incubation time was limited to 5 minutes. The data were computerized, and Lineweaver-Burk plots were used to estimate the maximum rate of calcium transport and its affinity to Ca^{2+}.

Bovine brain calmodulin was obtained from V.A. Tkachuk's laboratory (Biological department of Moscow University).

RESULTS

Spontaneous hypertension in rats

There was no difference in the Ca-pump activity of erythrocytes between hypertensive and normotensive rats when the free calcium concentration was less than 4.5 μM (Fig. 1a). These data agree with earlier reports on Ca-Mg-ATPase activity in the erythrocyte membrane in primary hypertension [14, 3]. However, when a

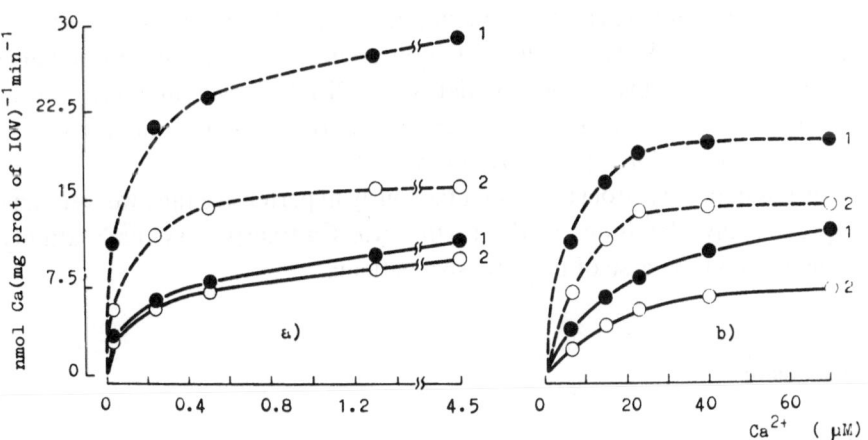

Figure 1. The dependence of the rate of calcium uptake by inside-out vesicles of the erythrocyte membranes on free calcium concentrations. 1 – normotensive control rats; 2 – spontaneously hypertensive rats. (——) without calmodulin; (---) with calmodulin (2 μg/ml). The incubation medium content (mM); imidazole-HCl-40; NaCl-120; MgCl$_2$-5; ATP · Na$_2$-4; ^{45}CaCl$_2$-up to 0.18 (a) or up to 0.25 (b); EGTA-0.2 (a) or without EGTA (b) (pH 7.4 t° = 37° C); protein of the erythrocyte membrane – 50 μg/ml.

saturated concentration of calmodulin is added to the incubation medium, the rate of calcium accumulation by the insideout vesicles of SHR is twice as low as that in normotensive rats. As can be seen from Table 1, both the affinity of calmoculin-activated calcium transport to Ca^{2+} and the maximal rate of calcium uptake in the erythrocytes of SHR are diminished as compared to normotensive control rats.

There was no difference between both groups of animals in the affinity to calmodulin ($K_{0.5}$ about 90 ng per ml).

When EGTA was absent in the incubation medium, the calcium concentration varied from 7 to 70 μM. Under these conditions, the Ca-pump activity in erythrocytes of SHR was diminished both in the absence of calmodulin and when calmodulin was introduced in the medium in saturated concentration (Fig. 1b).

The only possible cause of the differences revealed in the study is the decrease of the maximal rate of calcium transport (V_{max}) (see Table 1).

Essential hypertension

Unlike spontaneously hypertensive rats, essentially hypertensive patients have a lowered Ca-pump activity in erythrocytes in the absence of exogenous calmodulin when EGTA is present in the incubation medium (Fig. 2a). This feature is due to the 2-fold decrease of the Ca-transport system's affinity to Ca^{2+} (Table 2). It should be noted that the decrease in the activity of the Ca-pump in erythrocytes of hypertensive individuals, occuring when exogenous calmodulin is introduced, is due to the decrease of the maximal rate of Ca-transport.

The treatment of erythrocyte membranes by EGTA, in the process of turning their vesicles inside out, abolishes the differences in Ca-transport rate between normotensive and hypertensive patients (Fig. 2b). However, in this case also, the calmodulin-stimulated increase of Ca^{2+}-transport rate in the inside-out vesicles is considerably less for hypertensive individuals.

Just as in the erythrocytes of spontaneously hypertensive rats, we were unable to detect any alterations in the erythrocyte Ca-transport system's affinity to calmodulin in the case of hypertensive patients.

DISCUSSION

The results of our investigation confirm the presence of two Ca-binding centers in Ca-Mg-ATPase in the erythrocyte membrane. For the erythrocytes of rats, the affinity of these centers to Ca^{2+} undergoes a decrease in the presence of exogenous calmodulin (K_m 30 μM and 12 μM for one center, 0.16 and 0.08 μM for the other, in the absence and presence of exogenous calmodulin respectively see Table 1). For unknown reasons, the Ca-transport system's affinity to Ca^{2+} in the

Table 1. The affinity of calcium uptake to Ca^{2+} (K_m) and its maximal rate (V_{max}) in the erythrocyte membranes of spontaneously hypertensive rats

Groups	n	EGTA in the incubation medium (mM)	Calmodulin in the incubation medium (μg/ml)	K_m (μM)	max nmol Ca/mg prot. of IOV/min
1. Normotensive Kyoto-Wistar rats	6	0	0	33.52 ± 1.90	13.56 ± 0.70
2. Normotensive Kyoto-Wistar rats	6	0	2	11.78 ± 0.93	26.90 ± 0.99
3. Normotensive Kyoto-Wistar rats	6	0.2	0	0.163 ± 0.005	13.78 ± 1.01
4. Normotensive Kyoto-Wistar rats	6	0.2	2	0.078 ± 0.003	29.25 ± 1.25
5. Spontaneously hypertensive rats	6	0	0	32.40 ± 1.78	9.51 ± 0.66
6. Spontaneously hypertensive rats	6	0	2	11.59 ± 0.88	15.00 ± 0.69
7. Spontaneously hypertensive rats	6	0.2	0	0.159 ± 0.006	12.03 ± 0.79
8. Spontaneously hypertensive rats	6	0.2	2	0.099 ± 0.003	16.98 ± 1.53
$P_{1,5}$				N.S.	<0.01
$P_{2,6}$				N.S.	<0.005
$P_{3,7}$				N.S.	N.S.
$P_{4,8}$				<0.01	<0.005

The incubation medium content is given in the caption to Fig. 1; n is the number of animals; N.S.: not significant.

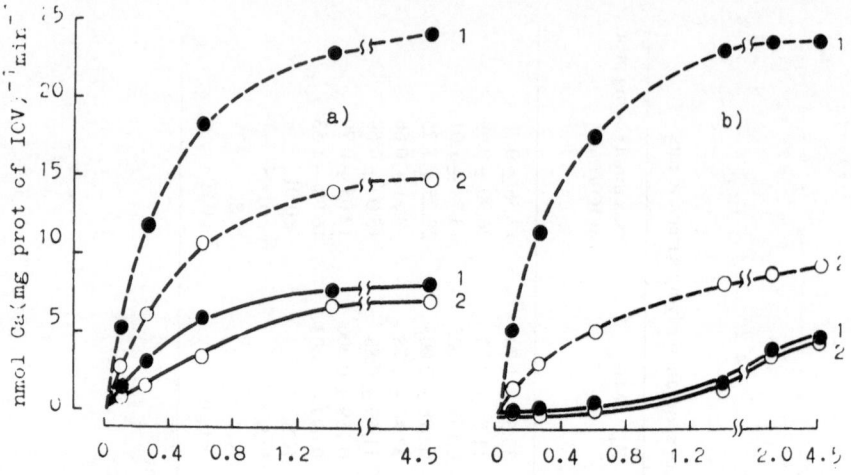

Figure 2. The dependence of the rate of calcium uptake by inside-out vesicles of the erythrocyte membranes on free calcium concentration 1 – normotensive patients; 2 – patients with essential hypertension (——) without calmodulin; (---) with calmodulin (2 μg/ml). The incubation medium content (mM): imidazole-HCl-40; NaCl-120; $MgCl_2$-5; ATP $\cdot Na_2$-4; EGTA-0.2; $^{45}CaCl_2$-up to 0.18 (pH 7.4; $T° = 37°$ C); protein of the erythrocyte membrane 0 50 μg/ml; inside-out vesicles were prepared without (a) or with (b) EGTA treatment.

erythrocytes of humans in the presence of calmodulin is four times less than of rats (Tables 1 and 2). The data in Table 1 show that Ca-Mg-ATPase activity with low affinity to Ca^{2+} in the erythrocytes of hypertensive rats is considerably decreased. Differences in the Ca-pump's activity between hypertensive and normotensive rats occur only in the presence of exogenous calmodulin. This fact is particularly interesting if we note that it is precisely ATPase with high affinity to calcium that functions *in vivo* ($Ca^{2+}_{i\ n} = 10^{-6}-10^{-7}$ M).

It can be assumed that the Ca-pump's activity under low calcium concentrations is due to the presence of calmodulin in the erythrocyte membrane. Indeed, the affinity of purified Ca-Mg-ATPase to Ca^{2+} is 10–14 μM, but becomes less than 1 μM when exogenous calmodulin is added [15]. One of the methods for removing endogenous calmodulin is to treat the membrane by EGTA [16]. In our case, such treatment brought about a five to six-fold decrease of the Ca-pump's affinity to Ca^{2+} (Table 2).

After EGTA treatment, there are no differences between normotensive and hypertensive individuals in Ca-pump activity (Fig. 2b). It may therefore be assumed that the decreased Ca-pump activity in erythrocyte membranes not treated by EGTA of hypertensive patients is related either to a lower content of calmodulin in this membrane, or to changes in the interaction of calmodulin with Mg-Ca-ATPase. We feel that the second alternative is more probable. Indeed, the decrease of the Ca-pump's activity in both forms of primary hypertension is observed in the presence of saturated calmodulin concentrations.

Table 2. The affinity of calcium uptake to Ca^{2+} (K_m) and its maximal rate (V_{max}) in the erythrocyte membranes of patients with essential hypertension.

Groups	n	EGTA treatment of membranes	Calmodulin in the incubation medium (μg/ml)	K_m (μM)	V_{max} nmol Ca/mg prot. of IOV/min
1. Normotensive patients	11	–	0	0.33 ± 0.02	8.51 ± 0.80
2. Normotensive patients	11	–	2	0.35 ± 0.03	24.03 ± 1.44
3. Normotensive patients	11	+	0	1.72 ± 0.09	5.32 ± 0.61
4. Normotensive patients	11	+	2	0.33 ± 0.04	25.11 ± 1.77
5. Essentially hypertensive patients	10	–	0	0.61 ± 0.05	7.99 ± 0.58
6. Essentially hypertensive patients	10	–	2	0.33 ± 0.02	15.01 ± 0.90
7. Essentially hypertensive patients	10	+	0	1.68 ± 0.10	4.98 ± 0.50
8. Essentially hypertensive patients	10	+	2	0.52 ± 0.04	10.32 ± 0.71
$P_{1,5}$				<0.001	N.S.
$P_{2,6}$				N.S.	<0.001
$P_{3,7}$				N.S.	N.S.
$P_{4,8}$				<0.001	<0.001

The incubation medium content is given in caption to Fig. 2.; n is the number of patients; N.S.: not significant.

The causes of the alterations in calmodulin and Ca-Mg-ATPase interaction are unknown. There are data, however, showing the important role played by hydrophobic forces in this interaction [17]. In this connection, data on the increase of the microviscosity of hydrophobic regions in erythrocyte membranes [18, 19] and the decrease of the lateral diffusion rate obtained by the fluorescent probe method [18] are especially interesting.

It is known that calmodulin concentration in the erythrocyte cytoplasm considerably exceeds the value needed to saturate the Ca-pump [20]. Hence it may be assumed that the decrease in the calmodulin-dependent Ca-transport determines the increase of intracellular calcium recently detected in the erythrocytes of spontaneously hypertensive rats [21]. If this membrane alteration is not limited to erythrocytes (apparently, this is indeed the case), it may be viewed as the main cause of calcium overload in other tissues (e.g., the increase of exchangable calcium content in adipocytes of spontaneously hypertensive rats [4] and patients with essential hypertension [5]).

SUMMARY

1. Calcium transport in inside-out vesicles (IOV) of the erythrocyte membranes of spontaneously hypertensive rats (SHR) and patients with essential hypertension was studied.
2. The activity of calcium pump with low affinity to Ca^{2+} in IOV of SHR is decreased as compared to normotensive controls. There are no differences in the activity of calcium pump with high affinity to Ca^{2+}.
3. The activity of calcium pump with high affinity to Ca^{2+} in IOV of patients with essential hypertension is decreased as compared to normotensive controls. This difference is absent after EGTA treatment of the erythrocyte membranes.
4. The effect of the saturated concentration of calmodulin on calcium transport in IOV of SHR and patients with essential hypertension is two to four times lower as compared to normotensive controls.
5. It is suggested that the alteration of interaction between Ca-Mg-ATPase and calmodulin may be a cause for the increase of intracellular calcium content in both forms of primary hypertension.

REFERENCES

1. Aoki K, Ikedo N, Yamashita K, et al.: Cardiovascular contraction in spontaneously hypertensive rats: Ca^{2+} interaction of myofibrils and subcellular membrane of heart and arterial smooth muscle. Jpn Circ J 38:1115–1119, 1974.
2. Postnov YuV, Orlov SN, Pokudin NI: Decrease of calcium binding by the red blood cell membrane in spontaneously hypertensive rats and in essential hypertension. Pflugers Arch 379:191–195, 1979.

3. Devynck MA, Pernollet MG, Nunez AM, et al.: Analysis of calcium handling in erythrocyte membranes of genetically hypertensive rats. Hypertension 3:397–403, 1981.

4. Postnov YuV, Orlov SN: Features of intracellular calcium distribution in the adipose tissue of spontaneously hypertensive rats (SHR). Experientia 35:1480–1481, 1979.

5. Postnov YuV, Orlov SN, Pokudin NI: Alteration of intracellular calcium distribution in the adipose tissue of human patients with essential hypertension. Pflugers Arch 388:89–91, 1980.

6. Postnov YuV, Orlov SN: Evidence of altered calcium accumulation and calcium binding by the membranes of adipocytes in spontaneously hypertensive rats. Pflugers Arch 385:85–89, 1980.

7. Devynck MA, Pernollet MG, Nunez AM, et al.: Calcium binding alteration in plasma membrane from various tissues of spontaneously hypertensive rats. Clin Exp Hypertens 3:797–808, 1981.

8. Schatzmann HJ: Active calcium transport across the plasma membrane of erythrocytes, in Carafoli, et al. (editors): Calcium Transport in Contraction and Secretion. Amsterdam, Oxford, 1975, pp 45–49.

9. Sarkadi B, Szacz I, Gardos G: Calcium and calmodulin in the regulation of blood-cell function. Haematologia 14:121–136, 1981.

10. Macintyre JD, Green JW: Stimulation of calcium transport in inside-out vesicles of human erythrocyte membranes by a soluble cytoplasmic activator. Biochim Biophys Acta 510:000–000, 1978.

11. Orlov SN, Pokudin NI, Gulak PV, et al.: The mechanism of ATP-dependent calcium uptake by plasma membranes (in Russian). Proc USSR Acad Sci 262:482–485, 1982.

12. Steck TL: Preparation of impermeable inside-out and right-side out vesicles from erythrocyte membranes, in Korn ED (editors): Methods in Membrane Biology. New York, Plenum Press, 1974, vol 2, pp 245–281.

13. Lowry OM, Rosebrough NJ, Farr AL, et al.: Protein measurement with Folin phenol reagent. J Biol Chem 193:265–275, 1981.

14. Postnov YuV, Orlov SN, Shevchenko AS: Ca^{2+}-binding alteration and features of Na-K-ATPase activity in the erythrocytes of patients with essential hypertension (in Russian). Bull Exp Biol Med (Moscow) 84:41–44, 1977.

15. Niggli V, Adungah ES, Penniston JT, et al.: Purified $(Ca^{2+}-Mg^{2+})$-ATPase of the erythrocyte membranes. Reconstitution and effect of calmodulin and phospholipids. J Biol Chem 256:395–401, 1981.

16. Roufogalis BD, Maud D: Regulation by calmodulin of the calcium transport ATPase in human erythrocyte. Can J Biochem 58:922–927, 1980.

17. Tanaka T, Hidaka H: Hydrophobic regions function in calmodulin enzyme(s) interactions. J Biol Chem 255:11078–11080, 1980.

18. Orlov SN, Gulak PV, Karagodina ZV, et al.: The properties of erythrocyte membrane structure in spontaneous genetic hypertension (in Russian). Cardiology (Moscow) 21 (11):108–112, 1981.

19. Montenay-Garestier T, Aragon I, Devynck MA, et al.: Evidence for structural changes in erythrocyte membranes of spontaneously hypertensive rats. A fluorescence polarization study. Biochem Biophys Res Commun 100:660–665, 1981.

20. Schreiber WE, Gentry R, Fisher EH: Calmodulin and cyclic nucleotide phosphodiesterase activities in erythrocytes from normal and schizophrenic subjects. Biochem Biophys Res Commun 100:1415–1421, 1981.

21. Losse H, Zidek W, Zumkley H, et al.: Intracellular Na^+ as a genetic marker of essential hypertension. Clin Exp Hypertens 3: 627–640, 1981.

THE Na+/K+ CO-TRANSPORT SYSTEM IN ERYTHROCYTES FROM ESSENTIAL HYPERTENSIVE PATIENTS

RICARDO PABLO GARAY

INTRODUCTION

The ionic leak across human red cell membranes is very small and close to the ground permeability of an artificial lipid bilayer [1]. Transmembrane ionic movements are allowed by genetically coded transport systems. Regarding Na+ and K+ transport, most of the carrier-mediated fluxes are catalyzed by the Na+/K+ pump [2]. This system catalyzes the exchange of intracellular Na+ by extracellular K+ coupled to the hydrolysis of ATP, thus generating electrochemical gradients of Na+ and K+ across the cell membrane (Fig. 1). The stationary gradients (and thus the intracellular Na+ concentration) result from the balance between the pump

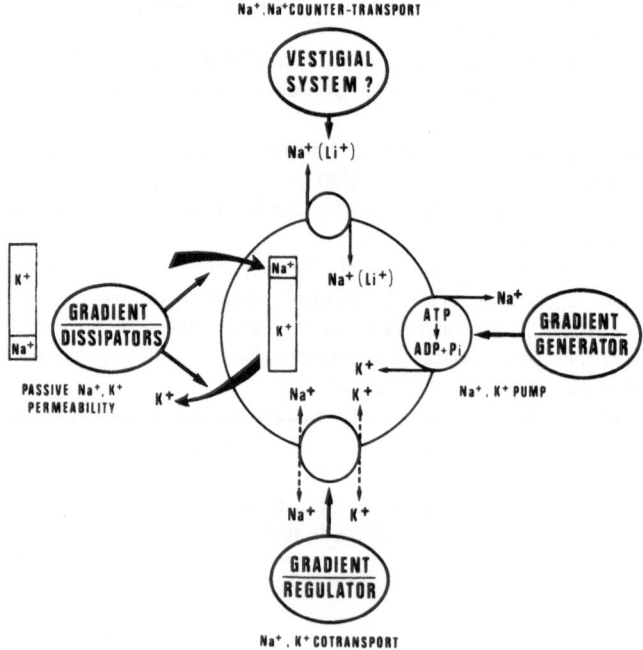

Figure 1. A model of Na+ and K+ transport in human red cells.

fluxes and the Na$^+$ and K$^+$ leaks that continuously dissipate a small part of this electrochemical energy (Fig. 1). This same electrochemical energy in other cells may serve several vital functions, particularly the action potential in excitable cells or the coupled transport of metabolites. Recently, the development of methods for measuring small fluxes revealed the existence of other transport systems independent of the Na$^+$/K$^+$-pump (Fig. 1): 1) a furosemide-sensitive Na$^+$/K$^+$ co-transport system, which catalyzes a simultaneous influx [3] or efflux [4] of both Na$^+$ and K$^+$; and 2) a ouabain-resistant, one-to-one Na$^+$:Na$^+$ exchange, which can be detected using Li$^+$ as a tracer [5]. The physiological role of the Na$^+$/K$^+$ co-transport system seems to be the 'buffering' of any change in physiological intracellular Na$^+$ concentration [6] (Fig. 1). The physiological role of the Na$^+$:Na$^+$ exchange is unknown.

The above transport systems have been studied in erythrocytes from essential hypertensive patients. A study of essential hypertensive patients from Paris showed *low outward Na$^+$/K$^+$ co-transport fluxes* in a high fraction of subjects [7, 8]. On the other hand, Canessa et al. reported an *increase* in Na$^+$/Li$^+$ countertransport fluxes in a high fraction of essential hypertensives from Boston [9]. A comparison of data obtained in different laboratories (Table 1) suggests that, with the exception of Caucasian hypertensives from Boston, more than 50% of essential hypertensive patients show *low* outward co-transport fluxes. On the basis of a comparative study of co-transport and countertransport fluxes on the same patient, in Paris and in Boston, Canessa proposed that the population of essential hypertensive patients is heterogeneous, having hypertensives with low co-transport (Co ⊖ hypertensives) and others with high countertransport (Counter ⊕ hypertensives) [10]. This paper is mainly concerned with methodological aspects and kinetic characterization of hypertensives with low co-transport fluxes (Co ⊖ hypertensives).

PATIENTS

Outward Na$^+$/K$^+$ co-transport fluxes have been studied in erythrocytes from 149 essential hypertensive patients (70 males, 79 females; aged 1–76, mean 40) and compared to 125 normotensive controls devoid of familial hypertension (67 males, 58 females; aged 19–65, mean 36). Details for the selection of patients can be found in [8].

METHODS

The stimulation curves of outward Na$^+$/K$^+$ co-transport by intracellular Na$^+$ have been measured using a similar procedure to that described in [4].

A previous screening of hypertensives with low co-transport fluxes has been

Table 1. Outward Na$^+$/K$^+$ co-transport in essential hypertension

Investigators	Normotensive controls	Essential hypertensives	Percent of subject with abnormal Co-transport*	
			Normotensive controls	Essential hypertensives
Garay et al. (Boston, 1980)	520 ± 150 (5)	210 ± 147 (149)	9.2	71.2
Garay et al. (Paris, 1980)	463 ± 126 (98)	322 ± 193 (49)	25.0	56.0
Cusi et al. (Milan, 1981)	438 ± 147 (31)	295 ± 170 (28)	31.2	64.3
Davidson et al. (Capetown, 1981)	403 ± 182 (48)	251 ± 75 (30)	0	81.5
Brunois et al. (Reims, 1981)	607 ± 162 (33)	212 ± 114 (7)	0	85
Herubel et al. (Rouen, 1981)	577 ± 174 (18)	193 ± 88 (9)	33.3	88.9
Ghione et al. (Pisa, 1981)	394 ± 201 (9)	351 ± 224 (24)	25	50
Meckler & Ben-Ishay (Jerusalem, 1981)	416 ± 170 (12)	500 ± 300 (11)	35.7	0.0
Adragna et al. (Boston, 1981)	310 ± 112 (14)	230 ± 80 (20)	33.3	55.0
Canessa et al. (Philadelphia, 1981)**	450 ± 275 (21)	159 ± 60 (13)	56.3	100.0
Gless et al. (Heidelberg, 1981)	287 ± 65 (16)			

Values are mean ± SD of the bumetanide- or furosemide-sensitive Na$^+$ efflux into a Mg^{2+} sucrose medium and are expressed in μmol/L cells/h.

* Co-transport lower than 300 μmol/L cells/h.

** The subjects included in this study were all blacks.

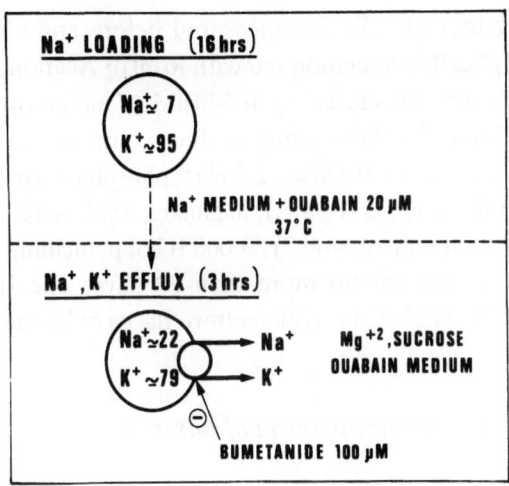

Figure 2. A new Na$^+$/K$^+$ co-transport assay for essential hypertension.

done using a previous co-transport assay [8] simplified here in order to obtain greater accurancy and to permit the analysis of more subjects per day (Fig. 2).

Preparation of red cells

Venous blood, 3–5 ml collected in heparinized tubes, was centrifuged at 1750 × g for 10 minutes, and the plasma and buffy coat were aspirated. The delay between the collection of blood and the aspiration of buffy coat never exceeded 90 minutes. During this time interval, the blood was kept in the cold. Once the buffy coat was removed, the red cell pellet was used immediately or stored at 4° C for no more than 4 days in a preserving solution containing (mM) 140 KCl, 10 NaCl, 1 MgCl$_2$, 2.5 Na$^+$ phosphate (pH 7.2 at 4° C).

Loading of red cells with Na$^+$

The kinetic study reported here shows that the major co-transport abnormality in essential hypertensive patients is a half-maximal co-transport stimulation of about 20 mmol intracellular Na$^+$ cells as compared to 9–16 mmol/L cells in normotensive controls. Thus, outward Na$^+$/K$^+$ co-transport fluxes were measured in erythrocytes loaded to an intracellular Na$^+$ concentration of 20–25 mmol/L cells. This is the intracellular Na$^+$ concentration giving maximal variation between normotensives and hypertensives.

Before loading, red cells were washed twice with isosmotic NaCl. The hemoglobin content per liter of cells was measured before and after loading. (An aliquot of 15–30 μl of cells was hemolyzed with 10 ml of Acationox 0.02% and the hemoglobin absorbance was measured at 540 nM.) One ml of washed red cells was suspended in 50 ml of a Na$^+$-loading medium containing 1) 45 ml of a 'basal' solution (mM):120 NaCl, 75 sucrose, 2.5 Na$^+$ phosphate (pH) 7.5 at 37°C), 1 MgCl$_2$, 10 Na$^+$-MOPS (pH 7.5 at 37°C), 10 glucose, 0.02 ouabain; 2) 5 ml of fetal calf serum without complement; and 3) 50,000 IU of penicillin. The Na$^+$-loading medium was kept frozen for no more than 20 days. The suspensions were incubated 18–20 hours at 37°C in tissue-culture flasks of 75 cm^2 surface area.

Preparation of red cells for measurement of fluxes

Na$^+$-loaded erythrocytes were washed five times with 110 mM MgCl$_2$. After the last wash, the red cell pellet was resuspended to a hematocrit of 20–25% with 2 ml of efflux media. The efflux media contained (mM) 75 MgCl$_2$, 85 sucrose, 0.1 ouabin, 10 Tris-MOPS (pH 7.4 at 37°C), 10 glucose. A portion of this suspension was set aside to measure hematocrit. In addition, 100 μl of the suspension was hemolyzed with 7 ml of Acationox 0.02% in order to measure hemoglobin per liter of cells by spectrophotometry and intracellular Na$^+$ and K$^+$ by flame photometry. The intracellular Na$^+$ concentration after loading was 23 ± 2 mmol/L cells. The change in hemoglobin per liter of cells is inversely correlated to the change in cell volume. Cell volume after loading was in all the cases 0 to 5% less than before loading. This prevents the inhibition of co-transport fluxes by cell swelling (Fig. 3).

Measurement of fluxes

Of the cell suspensions, 0.5 ml was added to two tubes, each containing 2 ml of efflux media, and to two other tubes, each containing 2 ml of efflux media with 0.1 mM bumetanide neutralized with Tris. (A stock solution of bumetanide was freshly prepared by diluting 8 mg of bumetanide ClH in 100 μl DMSO and 20 μl Tris and then adding distilled water to a final volume of 2 ml.) The tubes were incubated for 3 h at 37°C with continuous agitation and 'vortexed' every 20–30 minutes. (Control experiments showed that the fluxes were linear up to 4–6 hours. Fig. 4.) After incubation, the tubes were transferred to 4°C and spun down for 4 minutes at 1750 × g at 4°C. The supernatant was carefully removed (avoiding pellet contamination), and the Na$^+$ and K$^+$ concentrations were measured by flame photometry. All assays were performed in duplicate.

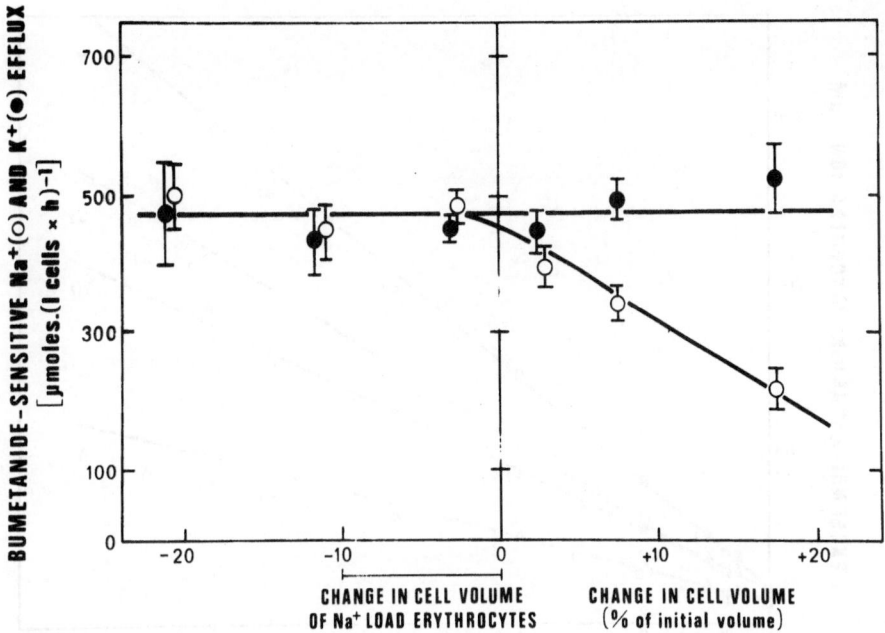

Figure 3. The effect of a change in cell volume on outward Na⁺/K⁺ co-transport fluxes. Human erythrocytes from a normotensive control were loaded to 23.5 mmol intracellular Na⁺/L cells using the technique described in Methods. The cells were then incubated in Mg⁺ sucrose medium, in which the osmolarity and cell volume were varied by changing the sucrose concentration. Under cell swelling, there is an inhibition of bumetanide-sensitive Na⁺ efflux, as previously described by Adragna et al. (Fed. Proc. 39: 1237,1980). Na⁺ loading in the presence of ouabain results in minimal cell shrinkage that does not affect co-transport fluxes.

Calculation of bumetanide-sensitive Na⁺ and K⁺ effluxes

The outward fluxes catalyzed by the Na⁺/K⁺ co-transport system correspond to the bumetanide-sensitive Na⁺ and K⁺ effluxes. These fluxes were obtained by subtracting the amounts of external Na⁺ and K⁺ determined in the presence of bumetanide from those measured in its absence (DNa), in accordance with the following formula:

$$\text{Flux} = \frac{(\text{DNa}) \times (1\text{-final hematocrit})}{3 \times \text{final hematocrit}}$$

Fluxes were expressed in μmol/L cells/h.

Kinetic features of the Na⁺/K⁺ co-transport assay

A recently proposed Na⁺/K⁺ co-transport assay [8] has now been modified. At

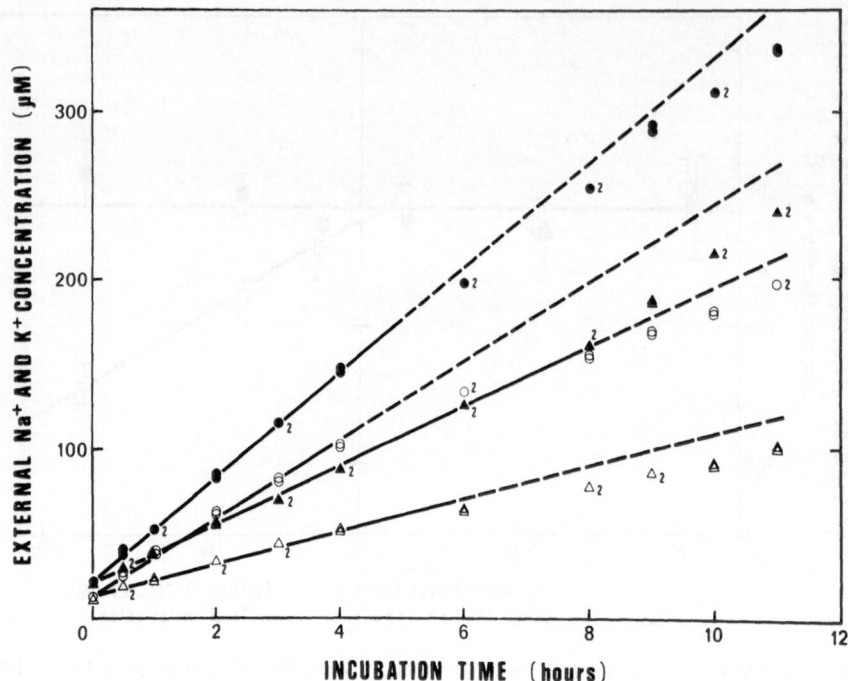

Figure 4. Time dependence of the Na$^+$ and K$^+$ efflux from Na$^+$-loaded human erythrocytes in a Mg^{+2} sucrose and ouabain medium. Cells were loaded using the ouabain method up to 21.9 mmol/L cells of intracellular Na$^+$. Na$^+$ efflux in the presence ($\triangle$) and absence ($\bigcirc$) of 0.1 mM bumetanide, and K$^+$ efflux in the presence ($\blacktriangle$) and absence ($\bullet$) of bumetanide.

least in normotensive controls, the co-transport fluxes measured with both methods seem quite similar (Fig. 5). In addition, the new co-transport assay is less arduous and more precise: 1) the Na$^+$ loading with ouabain at 37° C avoids the use of PCMBS and thus the recovering step of PCMBS treatment [for unknown reasons, Na$^+$ loading with ouabain at 37° C requires the presence of 10% fetal calf serum in order to preserve a functional co-transport. (Fig. 5)]; 2) the replacement of 1 mM furosemide by 0.1 mM bumetanide avoids the transient increase on the passive K$^+$ permeability by furosemide observed in some susceptible individuals; 3) the measurement of outward co-transport fluxes over a long period of time diminishes experimental error and decreases the number of incubation tubes. The experimental range of variation of the co-transport fluxes in now less than 5% (Fig. 4 and 5).

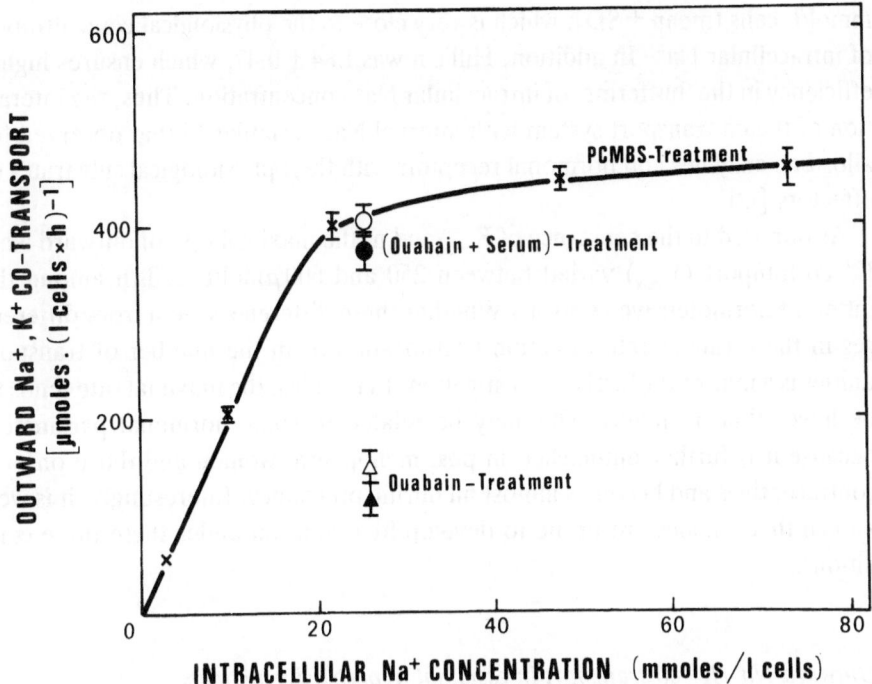

Figure 5. A comparison between outward Na$^+$/K$^+$ co-transport fluxes in Na$^+$-loaded erythrocytes by PCMBS technique (◯) and by the ouabain method with (◯, ●) and without (△,▲) 10% fetal calf serum. In PCMBS-treated erythrocytes, the measured fluxes correspond to the stimulation by intracellular Na$^+$ of bumetanide-sensitive Na$^+$ efflux (ref. 4). In ouabain-treated cells, but bumetanide-sensitive Na$^+$ (◯,△) and K$^+$ (●,▲) efflux were measured.

RESULTS

Kinetic characteristics of outward Na$^+$/K$^+$ co-transport fluxes

It has been previously reported [4] that in normal subjects the interaction between the rate of outward co-transport (V) and the intracellular Na$^+$ concentration (Na$_i$) can be described by the equation:

$$V = \frac{V_{max}}{1 + (K_{50\%}/Na_i^+)^n} \qquad (1)$$

where $K_{50\%}$ represent the intracellular Na$^+$ concentration required for half-maximal stimulation of the outward co-transport, n is Hill's n, a parameter which depends on the co-operative interactions between binding sites [11], and V_{max} is the maximal rate of outward co-transport.

In 42 normotensive controls studied here, we obtained $K_{50\%} = 12.8 \pm 2.3$

mmol/L cells (mean ± SD), which is very close to the physiolgical concentration of intracellular Na^+. In addition, Hill's n was 1.84 ± 0.47, which ensures higher efficiency in the 'buffering' of intracellular Na^+ concentration. Thus, the interaction of the co-transport system with internal Na^+ is similar to that observed for allosteric enzymes and hormonal receptors with their physiological substrates or effectors [12].

As opposed to the constancy of $K_{50\%}$ and n, the maximal rate of outward Na^+/K^+ co-tranport (V_{max}) varied between 250 and $600\,\mu mol/L$ cells/h among the different normotensive controls. Whether these differences stem from differences in the turnover rate of cation translocation or in the number of transport unities is a matter for further investigation. In females, the maximal rate tends to be lower than in males. This may be related to some hormonal parameter, because it is further diminished in post-menopausal women and those on oral contraceptives and becomes almost nil during pregnancy. Interestingly, it is well known that females are prone to develop hypertension under these three conditions.

Outward Na^+/K^+ co-transport in essential hypertensive patients

In essential hypertensive patients, equation (1) may also fit the curves of stimulation for the outward Na^+/K^+ co-transport by intracellular Na^+. However, each one of the three kinetic constants of equation (1) and particularly the half-maximal stimulation ($K_{50\%}$) were abnormal in a large percentage of hypertensives. In 45 out of 54 essential hypertensive patients (83.3%), $K_{50\%}$ was higher than 16 mmol/L cells. Such abnormal values were only rarely seen in normotensive controls (4 out of 42). A significant loss of cooperativity (Hill's n lower than 1.4) and a decrease in V_{max} further characterize some of these hypertensive patients (35.2 and 50% respectively). However, three male hypertensives showed V_{max} higher than $800\,\mu mol/L$ cells/h as previously observed by Adragna et al. [13].

None of the abnormalities seen in hypertensives showed any correlation with severity of high blood pressure, age, or sex.

The main kinetic abnormality in most of the hypertensive patients studied thus appeared as a $K_{50\%}$ of 18–21 mmol/L cells vs. 10–13 mmol/L cells in normotensive controls. This seems to characterize Co ⊖ hypertensives from a kinetic point of view. On the other hand, this result indicates that maximal differences between normotensives and hypertensives may be found in erythrocytes loaded to 20–25 mmol/L cells of intracellular Na^+.

A Na^+/K^+ co-transport assay for the detection of Co ⊖ hypertensives

Outward Na^+/K^+ co-transport fluxes were measured in erythrocytes loaded up to

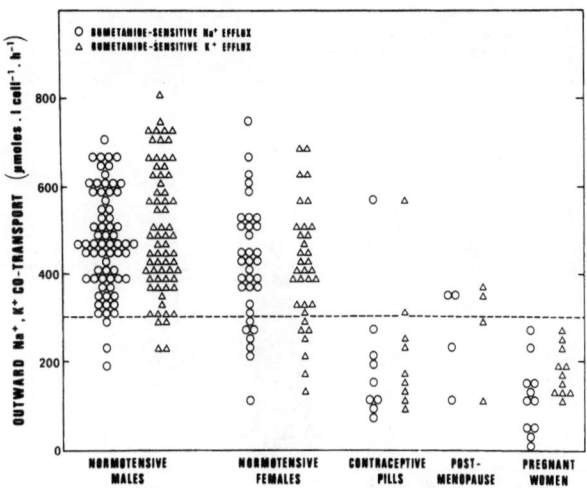

Figure 6. Individual values for outward Na$^+$/K$^+$ co-transport fluxes in normotensive subjects of familial hypertension.

22 ± 2 mmol intracellular Na/l cells. Figure 6 shows that most of the normotensive controls showed outward co-transport fluxes higher than $300\,\mu$mol/L cells/h. In fact, only 3 out of 67 normotensive males (4.5%) and 7 out of 34 females (20.6%) showed co-transport fluxes lower than $300\,\mu$mol/L cells/h. On the other hand, normotensive females who are pregnant, postmenopausal, or take contraceptive pills showed low co-transport fluxes (Fig. 6). As shown before, this is the consequence of a decrease in the maximal rate of outward co-transport fluxes. Thus, excluding the normotensive woman under these three circumstances, only 10 of 101 normotensive controls (9.9%) showed co-transport fluxes lower than $300\,\mu$mol/L cells/h.

Figure 7 shows that 106 out of 149 essential hypertensive patients (71.2%) are characterized by outward co-transport fluxes lower than $300\,\mu$mol/L cells/h. Some of these patients were studied by the previous kinetic method showing, in almost all cases, high $K_{50\%}$ of co-transport stimulation by intracellular Na$^+$. Thus, they correspond to our previous definition of Co $\ominus$ hypertensives.

DISCUSSION

It is reported in this paper that a high fraction of Caucasian hypertensives from Paris (Co $\ominus$ hypertensives) are characterized by a low apparent affinity of the Na$^+$/K$^+$ co-transport system for intracellular Na$^+$. This is accompanied by a tendency for a loss of co-operativity and low maximal co-transport rate. The final result is a relative loss of the regulatory properties of the Na$^+$/K$^+$ co-transport system on cell Na$^+$ content [6]. Results obtained in other laboratories show that

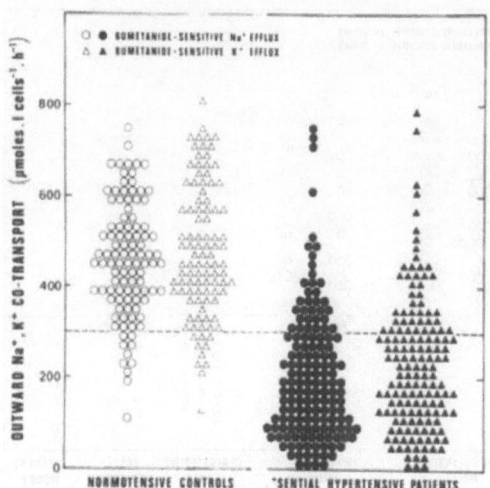

Figure 7. Individual values for outward Na⁺/K⁺ co-transport fluxes in Caucasian essential hypertensive patients from Paris compared to normotensive controls. Females under oral contraceptives, postmenopausal, or pregnant were excluded from this figure.

Co ⊖ hypertension is very frequent (Table 1). These Co ⊖ hypertensives seem different from those studied in Boston by Canessa and Adragna et al., which seem characterized by high Na⁺/Li⁺ countertransport and high Na⁺/K⁺ co-transport fluxes (counter ⊕ hypertensives) [9, 10, 13]. Thus, in a given population sample, a variable proportion of hypertensives with low co-transport (Co ⊕ hypertensives) or high countertransport (Counter ⊕ hypertensives) may be found (Fig.8).

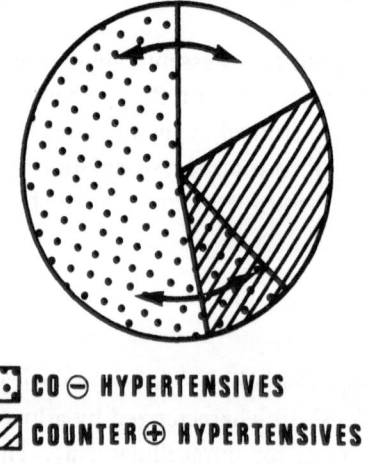

CO ⊖ HYPERTENSIVES

COUNTER ⊕ HYPERTENSIVES

Figure 8. A model of Na⁺ transport in erythrocytes from essential hypertensive patients. Essential hypertensives fall into at least two categories (Co ⊖ and Counter ⊕ hypertensives). The fraction of each category of hypertensive differs according to the sample population.

Regarding Co ⊖ hypertensives, the results in erythrocytes cannot be easily extrapolated to other cells, particularly excitable cells or Henle's loop cells. In these cells, instead of the K$^+$ gradient, the Cl$^-$ gradient may be the driving force for net Na$^+$ movements through a Na$^+$/K$^+$/Cl$^-$ co-transport [14], and the co-transport system may regulate Na$^+$ and Cl$^-$ gradients. Another difference arises from the fact that most of the intracellular Na$^+$ regulation in erythrocytes is mediated by the pump that catalyzes fluxes one order of magnitude higher than the co-transport system. In other cells, such as vascular smooth muscle cells, the co-transport and pump fluxes seem to be of the same order of magnitude [15], indicating that the co-transport system may be the physiologic regulator of the intracellular Na$^+$ concentration in target cells for hypertension.

In Co ⊖ hypertensives, an abnormal co-transport function may be a crucial derangement resulting in dysregulation of disturbances in cell Na$^+$ concentration secondary to excess Na$^+$ intake, particularly in vascular smooth muscle cells and catecholaminergic neurons, which are excitable cells of high surface/volume ratio. Indeed, a temporary Na$^+$ retention following an acute Na$^+$ load was observed in erythrocytes from genetically hypertensive rats [16]. This Na$^+$ retention may increase vascular resistance through noradrenaline release from adrenergic neurons [17] or by activation of Na$^+$/Ca^{2+} exchange in vascular smooth muscle cells [18]. Before the development of clinical hypertension, a slight increase in pump activity may compensate for the co-transport abnormality [7].

SUMMARY

A Na$^+$/K$^+$ co-transport assay applied to erythrocytes from 44 Caucasian essential hypertensive patients has previously shown that 86.4% are characterized by abnormally low outward co-transport fluxes [8]. Several laboratories have since confirmed that more than 50% of essential hypertensives are characterized by low outward co-transport fluxes (Co ⊖ hypertensives). However, Caucasian hypertensives from Boston seem to be characterized by increased fluxes of a different transport system: Na$^+$/Li$^+$ countertransport (Counter ⊕ hypertensives). As suggested by Canessa, the two classes of hypertensives seem to be different [10].

The detection of Co ⊖ hypertensives is in part limited for methodological reasons. Thus, the previous co-transport assay has been modified in order to obtain greater accuracy and to permit the analysis of more subjects per day. In 149 hypertensive patients analyzed here, the frequency of Co ⊖ hypertension was 71%.

A detailed kinetic study of Na$^+$/K$^+$ co-transport in essential hypertensives showed that the most characteristic abnormality of Co ⊖ hypertension is an abnormally low apparent affinity for intracellular Na$^+$. In fact, the intracellular Na$^+$ concentration giving half-maximal co-transport stimulation was higher than

16 mmol/L cells in 83% of 54 hypertensive patients. The apparent affinity for Na^+ was normal in 38 out of 42 normotensive controls (90.5%). In some hypertensives, the outward co-transport shows an abnormally low maximal rate and loss of co-operativity (50 and 35.2% of the patients, respectively). The final result is low outward co-transport fluxes (Co $\ominus$ hypertensives) when the physiological intracellular Na^+ concentration is near normal. This indicates a relative loss of the regulatory properties of the co-transport system on cell Na^+ content. This abnormality may be a crucial factor accounting for the disturbance of homeostasis in cell Na^+ content as a result of excess Na^+ intake in excitable cells of high surface/volume ratio such as vascular smooth muscle cells and adrenergic neurons.

ACKNOWLEDGMENTS

I wish to express my gratitude to C. Nazaret for technical help; to P. Meyer, J.P. Grunfeld, M. Bellet, and J.L. Elghozi for their careful clinical selection and management of hypertensive patients; to G. Dagher and P. Hannaert for their interest; and to M. Price (Baylor College of Medicine, Houston) for help with the English language.

REFERENCES

1. Lew W, Beauge L: Passive cation fluxes in red cell membranes, in Giebisch, Tosteson, Ussing (editors): Membrane Transport in Biology, ed 2. New York, Springer-Verlag, 1979, pp 81–115.
2. Garay RP, Garrahan P: The interaction of sodium and potassium with the sodium pump in red cells. J Physiol (Lond) 231:297–325, 1973.
3. Wiley JS, Cooper RA: A furosemide-sensitive co-transport of sodium plus potassium in the human red cells. J Clin Invest 53:745–755, 1974.
4. Garay RP, Adragna N, Canessa M, et al.: Outward sodium and potassium co-transport in human red cells. J Membr Biol 62:6–12, 1981.
5. Sarkadi B, Alfinoff JF, Gunn RB, et al.: Kinetics and stoichiometry of Na-dependent Li transport in human red blood cells. J Gen Physiol 72:249, 1978.
6. Garay RP, Hannaert P: Third International Congress on Na^+, K^+-ATPase. New Haven, CT, Yale University Press, 1981.
7. Garay RP, Dagher G: Erythrocyte Na and K transport systems in essential hypertension, in Losse H, Zumkley H (editors): First International Symposium on Intracellular Electrolytes and Arterial Hypertension. Stuttgart, Georg Thieme Verlag, 1980, pp 69–76.
8. Dagher G, Garay RP: A Na^+, K^+-cotransport assay for essential hypertension. Can J Biochem 58:1069–1074, 1980.
9. Canessa M, Adragna N, Solomon H, et al.: Increased sodium-lithium countertransport in red cells of patients with essential hypertension. N Engl J Med 302:772, 1980.
10. Canessa M, Bize I, Solomon H, et al.: Na countertransport and co-transport in human red cells: Function, dysfunction and gene in essential hypertension. Clin Exp Hypertens 3:783–795, 1981.
11. Garay RP: Thermodynamic restrictions on the allosteric models through an analysis of the free energy of interaction between sites. J Theor Biol 63:421–441, 1976.
12. Monod J, Wyman J, Changeux JP: On the nature of allosteric transitions: A plausible model. J

Mol Biol 12:88–118, 1965.

13. Adragna N, Tosteson DC, Canessa M: Simultaneous measurements of Li-Na countertransport and Na-K co-transport in red cells of patients with essential hypertension. Eighth Scientific Meeting of the International Society of Hypertension, Milan, June 1981.

14. Haas M, McManus T: Effect of anion substitution and membrane potential on Na/K co-transport in duck red cells. Fed Proc 40 (30):484, 1981.

15. Tuck M, Garay RP, Russo-Marie F, et al.: Na^+, K^+ co-transport system in vascular smooth muscle cells. Ninth Scientific Meeting of the International Society of Hypertension, Mexico 1982.

16. De Mendonca M, Garay RP, Ben-Ishay D, et al.: Abnormal erythrocyte cation transport in primary hypertension. Clinical and experimental studies. Hypertension 3:I179–I183, 1981.

17. Nakazato Y, Ohga A, Onoda Y: The effect of ouabain or noradrenaline output from peripheral adrenergic neurons of isolated guinea pig vas deferens. J Physiol 278:45–54, 1978.

18. Blaustein MP: Sodium ions, calcium ions, blood pressure regulation and hypertension: A reassessment and a hypothesis. Am J Physiol 232(3):C165, 1977.

DISCUSSION

Discussants: Jones, Garay, Sleight, Meyer, Denton, Dulm, Sambhi

Jones: We've been using furosemide and we can identify furosemideinhibitable sodium, potassium, and chloride fluxes in rabbit carotid. When you inhibit this co-transport system, do you find a change in the cell sodium concentration? In other words, do you think this is a mechanism for regulating cell sodium concentration, or is that mainly dependent on the pump-leak mechanisms?

Garay: I have no evidence to suggest a regulator role for intracellular sodium concentration of the sodium-potassium co-transport in vascular smooth muscle cells.

Jones: Are the cell sodium levels in patients that have low co-transport any different from those with normal co-transport?

Garay: No.

Jones: So there's no evidence there either.

Garay: The cell sodium concentration in hypertensives seems to be very close to normotensive controls. In our hands, perhaps there is a difference in the mean – 5 or 10 percent difference – but the interindividual variation in intracellular sodium concentration is higher than the difference in mean value between hypertensives and normotensives. This is not surprising because in human red cells co-transport fluxes are very low compared to pump fluxes.

Jones: The eletrochemical energy gradient under normal conditions for chloride is about one-fifth that for sodium. Now, if you square five, the numbers will work out. But actually you'd need five chlorides to move out of the cell to be able to carry with it one sodium against this electrochemical gradient under normal conditions. Under the conditions you showed us, were those cells sodium-loaded, or did they contain the normal 10–15 millimolar cell sodium from vascular tissues?

Garay: Normal.

Jones: That's all right, because we had difficulty finding a furosemide-inhibitable sodium efflux under those conditions. We had to raise the cell sodium into the 50–60 millimolar range, and then we could see a rather nice furosemide-inhibitable sodium efflux. If we had no potassium in the cell, we couldn't see it either

Garay: Did you have sodium in your medium?

Jones: Yes, we had some sodium.

Garay: We have no sodium in our medium, just magnesium and sucrose. Thus, sodium moves downhill.

Jones: Our tissues tend to shrink in that medium.

Garay: We work in magnesium-sucrose at room temperature. In addition, a mild shrinkage does not change co-transport fluxes in human erythrocytes.

Sleight: I wonder how you characterized your hypertensives; you said that there were 20 percent in whom you could find neither high nor low co-transport. The reason I ask is that when we studied a group of about 60 patients we thought hypertensive, and then monitored them intra-arterially away from hospital for 24 hr, we found about 30 percent of this group of mild-to-moderate hypertensives to be completely normal away from doctors. You may therefore have some noise in your data, a sort of pseudo-hypertension. I might say that one of the things that really seemed to separate the two groups was that people with target-organ damage were much more likely to correspond to their cuff pressures, whereas in people without target-organ damage, about half didn't have hypertension.[1]

Meyer: I just want to say that these patients had moderate high blood pressure, which is arbitrarily defined as being more than 160 mm Hg over 95 for at least two consecutive visits. They were on a sodium-free (Author: Not sodium free?) diet but were not treated, and all of them had a routine investigation ruling out the possibility of secondary hypertension. I'd like to stress the point that since we perhaps observed an interference of sodium balance on the activity of the outward co-transport in the rat, it might be important to correlate the measurement of fluxes observed in various areas with urinary sodium output.

Denton: Can you tell us something of the interrelations of these systems under normal physiological conditions? Can you assign a quantitative role to each one in the final dynamic equilibrium that exists?

Garay: Yes. I have the impression that the actual data indicate that the sodium-lithium countertransport and the sodium-potassium co-transport are two different systems. For instance, if you look at sensitivity to drugs, sodium-potassium co-transport could be achieved by loop diuretics, but sodium-lithium countertransport would not be inhibited – or there is a difference in the dose-response curve. If you look at the effects of different diuretics on sodium-potassium co-transport, there is a very close correlation between the capacity to achieve a co-transport and the diuretic activity, but that's not the same for the sodium-lithium countertransport. On the other hand, if you look at kinetic affinities, for instance, the affinity for lithium of the sodium-lithium countertransport is very high and the affinity for lithium in the co-transport is low. If you look at a more profound analysis of kinetics, the kinetics of sodium-lithium countertransport are very simple – it's Michaelian kinetics. For instance, the stimulation of sodium-lithium countertransport by intracellular sodium is Michaelian, but the stimulation of sodium-potassium co-transport by intracellular sodium is sigmoidal.

There are many other arguments, and another investigator is going to speak about that. The sodium-lithium countertransport performs a 1:1 sodium-sodium exchange; so it seems very hard to

[1] Flores et al: Lancet, 1981.

imagine a physiological role for a system that performs a 1:1 sodium-sodium exchange. Dr. Tosteson suggested that it is just a vestigial system. For instance, it could be a vestige of sodium-calcium exchange in some excitable tissues. My impression is that the intracellular sodium concentration in human erythrocytes depends on the equilibrium between the sodium-potassium pump and the potassium-sodium permeability, but the sodium-potassium co-transport and the sodium-sodium countertransport are vestigial systems that do not change intracellular sodium concentration. The co-transport system may play a regular role in other cells.

Duhm: Dr. Garay, may I ask you for your opinion concerning the diagnostic value of the determination of red cell co-transport and countertransport acitivity? Can you distinguish people who are prone to develop hypertension later in life or not? Can you distinguish essential hypertensives from secondary hypertensives by means of determination of the two transport activities?

Garay: We must wait to answer this question. We have performed sodium-potassium co-transport and countertransport assays in families, but we don't know now if they will become hypertensives or not. In genetically hypertensive rats, the abnormalities seem to precede the development of hypertension. At least from this point of view, it may be a useful test. These tests in secondary hypertension will only be useful for those secondary hypertensives without familial hypertension. But, at this time I cannot give a definite answer on the applicability of these tests in clinics.

Sambhi: I think the question that Dr. Sleight asked is a very important one for those of us who are not involved in the field directly. It gets very confusing for us. Are these abnormalities more prominent in people with higher grades of hypertension with target-organ damage? Dr. Meyer said that his patients had moderate hypertension, but he defined it as a diastolic level of 95 and a systolic of 160. Now that would be mild hypertension by all standards. And data on that type of population certainly are subject to a good deal of noise. So can we have one definite answer – are these abnormalities more prominent in people with established hypertension with target-organ damage?

Meyer: Yes, the answer is that the electrolyte change occurs in 40 percent of normotensive, non-selected populations on the basis of heredity and in about 70 to 75 percent of people having high blood pressure. It is not influenced at all under our conditions by the severity of the high blood pressure.

SODIUM, LITHIUM, AND POTASSIUM CO- AND COUNTER-TRANSPORT IN ERYTHROCYTES AND ITS RELATION TO ESSENTIAL HYPERTENSION

Jochen Duhm

INTRODUCTION

Results presented in 1980 seem to indicate that the Na^+/Li^+ exchange activity in erythrocytes of essential hypertensive patients is two to three times greater than in red cells of nonessential hypertensive individuals. Relatively no overlap was observed between the two groups [1]. Furthermore, the idea has been put forward that measurement of red cell Na^+/Li^+ exchange may be a useful tool in differentiating between essential and secondary hypertension and in identifying those normotensive individuals who are predisposed to developing essential hypertension later in life [1–3].

The data and ideas are as provocative as was the earlier hypothesis of a red cell Li^+ transport defect being related to the occurrence of affective disorders [4]. The latter hypothesis prompted intensive research, which resulted in the characterization of the Na^+/Li^+ exchange system in human erythrocytes [5–9], but failed to demonstrate a diagnostically valuable difference in red cell Li^+ transport between control subjects and patients suffering from affective diseases [10–13].

As a second red cell cation transport abnormality, characteristic for essential hypertensive patients, a reduction of the chloride-dependent Na^+/K^+ cotransport system to one fourth [14] or one half [15] of the normal value has been reported. The potential diagnostic value of this finding was highlighted [15–17], and the hypothesis was developed that a Na^+/K^+ co-transport defect might be casually responsible for the development of essential hypertension [14, 18, 19]. This hypothesis if based on the theory that the main function of the Na^+/K^+ co-transport system in nonepithelial tissues is to extrude Na^+ from the cells – the driving force being provided by the outwardly directed K^+ gradient. A defect of such a mechanism would then result in accumulation of cellular Na^+ in the smooth muscle cells of resistance vessels. According to the Na^+/Ca^{2+} exchange concept, even a small increase in Na^+ should cause a rise in the basal cellular concentration of free Ca^{2+} [20] and thus result in an increase in contractile tone of the smooth muscle cells and a rise in peripheral resistance, respectively.

The basis for the hypothesis outlined above is deduced from studies of furosemide-sensitive outward cation movements in human erythrocytes (14, 18, 21]. However, the system operates bidirectionally [22–25], and its role in the maintenance of the steady-state cellular Na^+ and K^+ contents is by no means understood.

In the present paper, some kinetic properties of inward co-transport are described, and inward and outward co-transport are compared in human erythrocytes with different activities of this transport system. Furthermore, an attempt is made to evaluate the physiological role of the co-transport system in human red blood cells. Simple tests to assess the Na^+/K^+ co-transport and Na^+/Li^+ exchange system are described and applied to essential hypertensive patients. Finally, red cell Na^+/K^+ co-transport is studied in some models of experimental hypertension in rats.

RESULTS

Furososemide-sensitive inward transport of Rb^+

The Na^+/K^+ co-transport system is operationally defined here to mediate ouabain-resistant cation translocation which is sensitive to inhibition by furosemide. To assess inward K^+ co-transport, Rb^+ was used as a tracer, since Rb^+ is known to effectively replace K^+ at the external aspect of the transport system [26, 27]. The dependence of ouabain-resistant Rb^+ uptake of external Rb^+ at a fixed concentration of 145 mM Na^+ in the medium for human and rat erythrocytes is shown in Figure 1. In each species, two red cell specimens are studied, one with a high and another with a low co-transport activity. In the presence of furosemide, Rb^+ uptake rose lineally with rising Rb^+ in both species. This fraction of Rb^+ uptake (resistant to ouabain and furosemide) is attributed to a leak which is four times greater in rat than in human erythrocytes (0.08 as compared to 0.02 μmoles Rb^+ uptake per ml cells per hour per 1 mM increase in external Rb^+). In the absence of furosemide, Rb^+ uptake showed a tendency to saturate in both species. Double reciprocal plots of furosemide-sensitive Rb^+ uptake were analyzed by linear regression analysis, yielding apparent K_m values for external Rb^+ of 4.5 to 5 mM in human and 3 to 4 mM in rat erythrocytes. Thus, the apparent affinities for external Rb^+, which are in the same range as those for K^+ [26, 27], were similar among the red cell specimens studied in Figure 1. However, the apparent maximum velocities of furosemide-sensitive Rb^+ uptake, being greater in rat than in human erythrocytes, was four times higher in the faster rat than in the slower human specimen.

The dependence of inward Rb^+ co-transport on external Na^+ at a fixed Rb^+ concentration of 5 mM is examined in Figure 2, with the erythrocytes of the two human donors studied in Figure 1. External Na^+ was replaced by choline. A small furosemide-sensitive Rb^+ uptake is seen in the absence of external Na^+ and cannot be attributed to co-transport. This fraction was reduced (but not abolished) when choline was replaced by Mg^{2+} [28], which particularly inhibits inward co-transport [29].

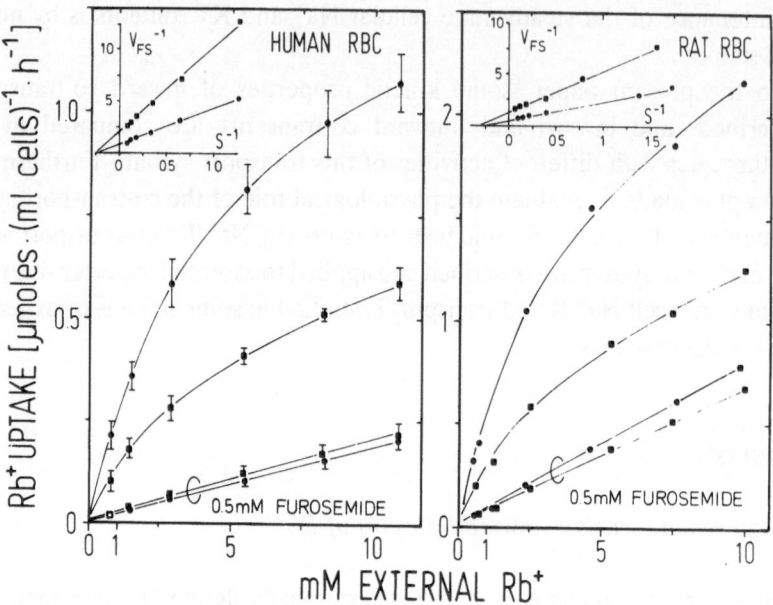

Figure 1. Dependence of ouabain-resistant Rb$^+$ uptake in 145 mM Na$^+$ medium on external Rb$^+$ concentration in human (n = 3, ±S.D.) and rat erythrocytes. In both species, two red cell specimens with high (●) and Low (■) co-transport activity are studied with and without 0.5 mM furosemide. The inserts show double reciprocal plots of furosemide-sensitive Rb$^+$ uptake (^{V}FS) versus external Rb$^+$ concentration (S).

Blood was drawn into heparin and the red cells were washed three times with 145 mM NaCl. After 15 minutes of preincubation (37° C, pH 7.4, hematocrit 1–2%, 0.2 mM and 5 mM ouabain with human and rat erythrocytes, respectively), RbCl was added to yield the Rb$^+$ concentrations denoted at the abscissa. One hour later, the red cells were washed three times with 150 mM choline chloride in the cold and hemolyzed with bidistilled water containing 6% 1-butanol (vol/vol). Cation concentrations of the hemolysates were measured by atomic absorption spectrometry. All values given in Figures 1–9 refer to 1 ml of original cells as calculated on the basis of hemoglobin determinations. In addition to the components listed, all media contained 5 mM glucose, 1 mM inorganic phosphate, and 10 mM MOPS-Tris (pH 7.4 at 37° C).

With rising external Na$^+$, furosemide-sensitive Rb$^+$ uptake increased, the shape of the dependencies being entirely different in the two donors (Fig. 2). In the faster transporting erythrocytes, the increase is hyperbolic. The slowly transporting cells show a sigmoidal rise of furosemide-sensitive Rb$^+$ uptake with external Na$^+$, this curve can be fitted by the Hill equation, yielding a Hill coefficient 'n' of about 1.6. A similar sigmoidal activation by Na$^+$ has been seen with furosemide-sensitive Na$^+$ release in human erythrocytes [21].

Relation between inward and outward co-transport

The relationship of inward to outward co-transport is shown in Figure 3, with

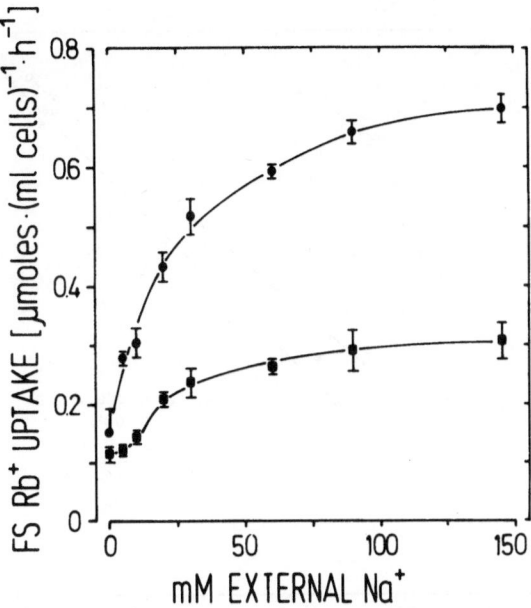

Figure 2. Dependence of furosemide-sensitive (FS) Rb$^+$ uptake at 5 mM Rb$^+$ on external Na$^+$ with the two human red cell specimens studied in Figure 1. External Na$^+$ was iso-osmotically replaced by choline. For further experimental details, see legend of Figure 1. Mean values ±S.D. from three experiments.

erythrocytes from 13 donors selected on the basis of their known differences in inward co-transport. Furosemide-sensitive Rb$^+$ uptake was determined in 145 mM Na$^+$ and 5 mM Rb$^+$ media. Outward co-transport was assessed by measuring furosemide-sensitive Na$^+$ and K$^+$ release into a Mg^{2+} medium with cells loaded by the PCMBS-technique. The cells contained approximately 50 μmol/ml of Na$^+$ and 50 μmol/ml of K$^+$. Inward Rb$^+$ transport showed a highly significant correlation to outward co-transport of both Na$^+$ and K$^+$. This finding demonstrates that *interindividual variations in outward co-transport are paralleled by corresponding variations of inward co-transport.*

Co-transport in essential hypertension

The close correlation found between inward and outward co-transport shown in Figure 3 provided the basis for applying a simple inward co-transport assay in a comparative study done on erythrocytes of normotensive and essential hypertensive individuals. In summary, the tests consisted in measuring furosemide-sensitive Rb$^+$ uptake in fresh erythrocytes incubated for one hour in media containing 145 mM Na$^+$ and 5 mM Rb$^+$ (Table 1, flasks A and B). Thus, the overnight contact with PCMBS and the subsequent rejuvenation procedure necessary for the cation

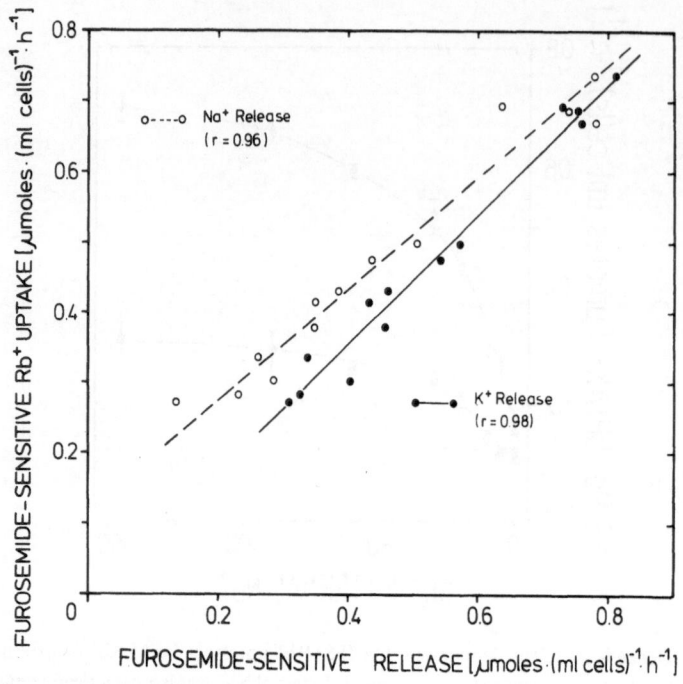

Figure 3. Relation between furosemide-sensitive Rb⁺ inward co-transport and furosemide-sensitive outward co-transport of K⁺ (●) and Na⁺ (○) (human erythrocytes). Inward co-transport was assessed in 145 mM Na⁺–5 mM Rb⁺ media as described in Table 1, and outward co-transport was determined with Na⁺–5 mM Rb⁺ media as described in Table 1, and outward co-transport was determined with Na⁺-loaded cells in Mg²⁺ media according to Dagher and Garay (15). The Na⁺ and K⁺ contents were 40 ± 5 and 61 ± 6 μmol/ml cells after the PCMBS-loading procedure performed in a 100 mM Na⁺-40 mM K⁺ medium.

release technique proposed by Dagher and Garay [15] are avoided.

The inward co-transport rates obtained from red cells of 38 normotensive subjects – 18 with well-established essential hypertension and five with renal hypertension – are summarized in Figure 4 (left-hand panel). The data for women and men are given separately (except in the case of renal hypertension). No significant difference is seen between the three groups. The mean values or Rb⁺ inward co-transport are slightly higher in the essential hypertensive patients than in the other two groups, this trend being opposite to that expected from the data of Garay et al. [14, 19]. Among the 18 essential hypertensive patients, six were classified as being of the low-renin type. Four of them had a very low co-transport activity, while two showed high co-transport rates.

It is thus concluded that the *Na⁺/K⁺ co-transport system is not altered in erythrocytes of essential hypertensive patients* living in the Munich region. Furthermore, no consistent relationship of co-transport and plasma renin activity seems to exist.

Table 1. Uptake tests to assess the Na^+/K^+ co-transport and Na^+/Li^+ exchange system of human erythrocytes

10 ml fresh blood (Na^+-heparin)	HK	Hb	MCHC
Wash red cells 3 × with chlorine	Na^+	K^+	Rb^+

4 Tubes, 25 ml medium each
(37° C, 0.2 mM ouabain, 5 mM glucose, 10 mM MOPS/TRIS pH 7.4)

NaCl(145)-RbCl(5)   MgCl$_2$(71)-Sucrose(85)
                                     RbCl(5)-LiCl(2)

A	B	C	D
	0.5 mM		0.1 mM
	Furosemide		Phloretin

Start by adding appr. 0.6 ml cells
1 h incubation (37° C)
Wash cells 3 × with chlorine (0° C)
Hemolyze ca. 0.25 ml cells with 1.6 ml 6% butanol (duplicates)
Measure Rb^+ and Li^+ (AAS) and Hb

Furosemide-sensitive   Phloretin-sensitive
Rb^+ Uptake Li^+ Uptake

Activity of the Na^+/K^+ Activity of the Na^+/Li^+
Co-transport System   Exchange System

Na^+/Li^+ exchange in essential hypertension

Parallel to the determination of inward co-transport, the activity of the Na^+/Li^+ exchange system was assessed in all probands by a simple assay. The test measures phloretin-sensitive inward Li^+ transport in Mg^{2+} media as described in Table 1 (flasks C and D). It was demonstrated earlier that the rats of inward Li^+ transport show a highly significant correlation to Li^+ outward transport by the exchange system [6, 9, 28].

No significant differences in mean values of inward Li^+ exchange are observed between the control probands and the essential and renal hypertensive patients (Fig. 4, right-hand panel). The variability was similar among the three groups. A slight but not significant trend towards lower exchange rates is observed in the essential hypertensive subjects. This trend is the reverse of that to be expected from the data of Canessa et al [1–3]. Four of the six patients with low renin hypertension had the slowest exchange rates found among the essential hypertensive probands (three of the four also had a low co-transport rate).

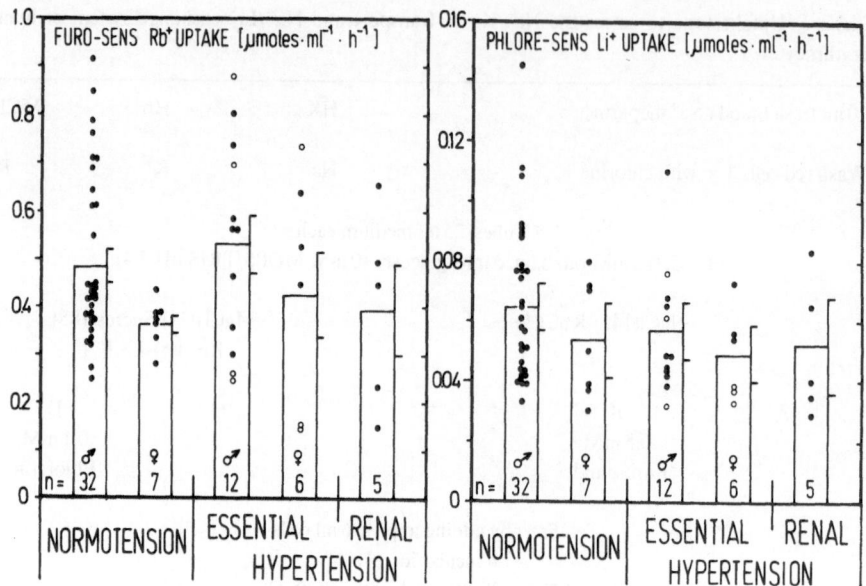

Figure 4. Na⁺/K⁺ co-transport (left) and Na⁺/Li⁺ exchange (right) in normotensive, essential hypertensive, and renal hypertensive individuals. The transport rates were determined by the uptake assays described in Table 1.

The *control group* (BP 123 ± 12 (systolic) to 80 ± 9 (diastolic) mm HG ± S.D., 37 ± 9 years) comprises two individuals with familial history of hypertension.

The *essential hypertensive* patient (BP 164 ± 24 to 104 ± 11 mm Hg after 2 hours of recumbency, 43 ± 12 years) had no antihypertensive medication for at least 2 weeks prior to the experiments. Cases of secondary hypertension are excluded. The six probands indicated by open symbols (O) showed a low-renin hypertension (basal PRA below 1 ng AI/ml plasma/h, increase in PRA upon i.v. administration of 40 mg furosemide plus active orthostasis less than twofold).

The *renal hypertensive* patients (BP 173 ± 26 to 103 ± 6 mm Hg, 47 ± 15 years, plasma creatinine values above 1.5 mg/dl) had intrarenal vascular stenosis, unilateral kidney atrophy, and unilateral pole resection, respectively.

The red cell Na⁺ contents were slightly higher in the essential hypertensive than in the normotensive probands, the difference not being statistically significant (7.8 ± 1.75 as compared to 7.36 ± 1.02 μmol/ml cells). Since inward Li⁺ transport by the exchange system is known to show a transacceleration by internal Na⁺ [5, 9], the higher Na⁺ content in the essential hypertensives should have accelerated Li⁺ uptake. Therefore, the slightly lower Li⁺ uptake in essential hypertension cannot be attributed to differences in red cell Na⁺. (For further discussion of the effect of internal Na⁺ on the Li⁺ uptake assay, see [30]).

Both the exchange and the co-transport system tended to exhibit lower transport rates in red cells of females than in red cells of male donors – in the normotensive as well as in the essential hypertensive group (Fig. 4).

Comparison of co-transport and exchange

If Na⁺/K⁺ co-transport and Na⁺/Li⁺ exchange were two different functions of one and the same system, one would expect that the two transport activities show a strict positive correlation to each other. On the other hand, the reports of a low co-transport [14] and a fast exchange [1] in essential hypertension, and the reverse relationship in normotensive individuals suggest a negative correlation between the two transport systems. However, all possible combinations are found, i.e., red cell specimens with high, medium, or low activities of both transport systems or with high activity of the one and low activity of the other system(Fig. 5). This is also seen in patients with low-renin hypertension. The data in Figure 5 are more suggestive of a random distribution than of a strict relationship between the two transport systems and indicate that the two transport activities are loosely coupled to each other. A linear-regression analysis of the widely scattered data in Figure 5 yields a weak positive correlation between the two transport systems, both in normotensive and essentially hypertensive individuals. No significant differences between the two groups were observed. Similar results have been obtained by Cusi et al. [31, 32].

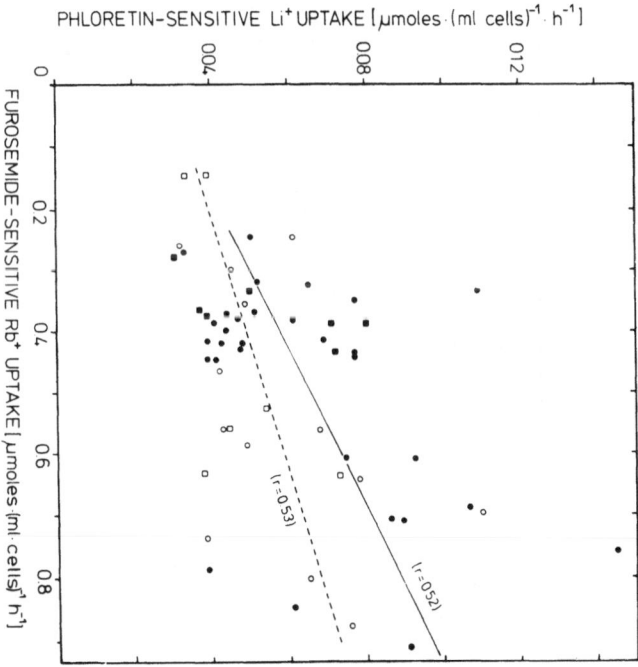

Figure 5. Relation between Na⁺/Li⁺ exchange (ordinate) and Na⁺/K⁺ co-transport (abscissa) in erythrocytes from normotensive individuals (●——■) and essential hypertensive patients (○----□). Women are denoted by ■, □, and men by ●, ○. The data are the same as in Figure 4.

Co-transport in rat hypertension

The possible alterations in red cell cation transport properties were also studied in some models of rat hypertension. As shown in Figures 1 and 6, rat erythrocytes show an interindividual variability in Na^+/K^+ co-transport similar to that found in human erythrocytes. However, rat erythrocytes do not exhibit a typical Na^+/Li^+ exchange system comparable to that found in human red blood cells [33]. Therefore, only the co-transport system was examined.

Four types of hypertension were included in the study: DOCA, DOCA-salt, one-clip, two-kidney hypertension in Sprague-Dawley rats, and spontaneous hypertension in Wistar-Kyoto rats. The values for furosemide-sensitive Rb^+ uptake are summarized in Figure 6 – data on red cells Na^+, plasma K^+, and mean blood pressure are included. Drinking water containing 1% NaCl over 6 weeks did not alter inward co-transport, red cell Na^+ or blood pressure, respectively. In

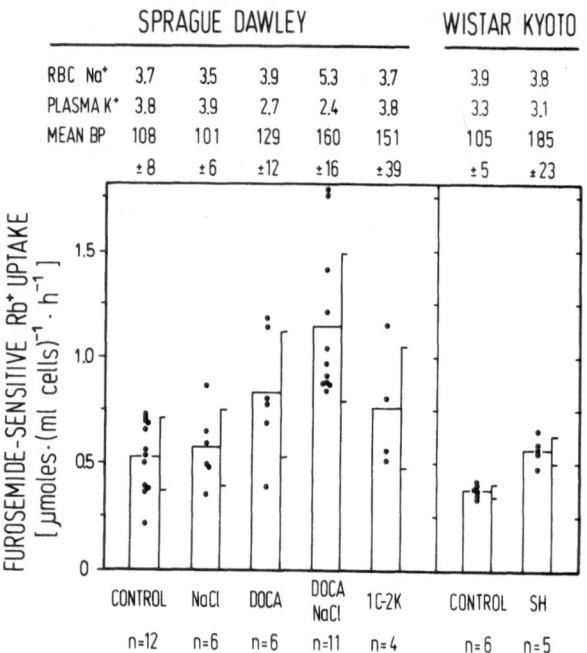

	SPRAGUE DAWLEY					WISTAR KYOTO	
RBC Na⁺	3.7	3.5	3.9	5.3	3.7	3.9	3.8
PLASMA K⁺	3.8	3.9	2.7	2.4	3.8	3.3	3.1
MEAN BP	108	101	129	160	151	105	185
	±8	±6	±12	±16	±39	±5	±23

CONTROL   NaCl   DOCA   DOCA NaCl   1C-2K   CONTROL   SH
n=12   n=6   n=6   n=11   n=4   n=6   n=5

Figure 6. Inward co-transport activity in rat hypertension. DOCA was administered for 4 to 6 weeks (25 mg s.c., six times per week), with and without 1% NaCl in drinking water, and renal hypertension was induced by clipping the left renal artery for 10 to 16 days. Blood pressure was measured in the left femoral artery during slight ether anesthesia, blood being drawn from the abdominal aorta. The red cells were washed three times in a medium containing 145 mM NaCl, and resuspended in the same medium (hematocrit 2–4%) with and without 5 mM ouabain plus 0.5 mM furosemide, respectively. After 15 minutes of preincubation, Rb^+ was added at a final concentration of 2 mM, and samples were taken after additional 30 and 60 minutes of incubation. For further experimental details, see legend for Figure 1.

DOCA-salt hypertension, however, a twofold increase in inward co-transport is observed with no overlap between the control and the DOCA-salt group ($P<0.001$). The acceleration in co-transport was associated with a significant increase in red cell Na^+ ($P<0.001$) and the expected fall in plasma K^+. DOCA alone caused a moderate increase in co-transport and blood pressure. In one-clip, two-kidney hypertension, the co-transport was not significantly altered.

In Wistar-Kyoto control rats, the rates of Rb^+ uptake were slightly lower than in Sprague-Dawley rats. In the spontaneous hypertensive animals, the co-transport rate was significantly elevated by about 50% ($P<0.001$) and the red cell Na^+ content was not altered (Fig. 7).

Ouabain-sensitive Rb^+ uptake, a measure of the Na^+/K^+ pump activity, was $4.6 \pm 0.4\,\mu$moles/ml cells/h for the control Sprague-Dawley rats in the 145 mM Na^+–2 mM Rb^+ medium. The pump rate was significantly increased by 40% in the DOCA-salt rats ($P<0.005$) but not essentially altered in the animals treated with either salt or DOCA alone or in the one-clip, two-kidney hypertensive animals. The increase in the pump rate in the DOCA-salt rats is paralleled by an elevated red cell Na^+ content (see Fig. 6). In the spontaneous hypertensive rats, ouabain-sensitive Rb^+ uptake was 15% higher than in the Wistar-Kyoto control rats, the difference from the control value not being statistically significant.

The leak pathway for Na^+ and K^+, as assessed by Na^+ and Rb^+ uptake in the presence of ouabain plus furosemide, was elevated by 19 and 26% in the DOCA-salt rats. In the spontaneous hypertensive rats, the Na^+ leak was not enhanced

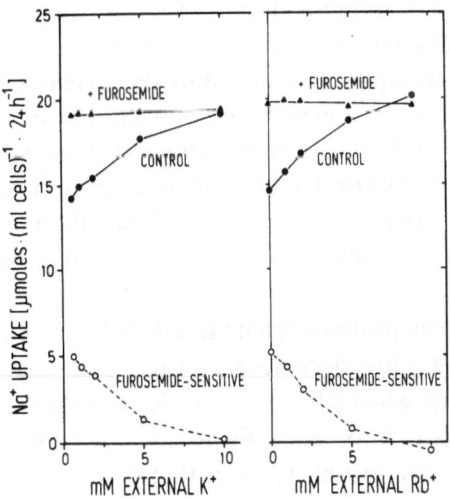

Figure 7. Effect of external K^+ and Rb^+ on ouabain-resistant Na^+ gain over 24 hours in human erythrocytes with and without 0.5 mM furosemide. Single experiment with red cells of the donor studied in Table 2 and Figures 1 and 2 (●), representative of eight experiments with red cells of other donors.

when Rb[+] leakage was increased by about 50% above the value found for the normotensive Wistar-Kyoto strain ($P<0.001$).

Role of the Na[+]/K[+] co-transport system for red cell Na[+] and K[+]

To study the role of the furosemide-sensitive transport system for red cell Na[+] and K[+], cation net movements were examined during prolonged incubation of human erythrocytes with ouabain in 145 mM Na[+] medium containing either 5 mM K[+] or 5 mM Rb[+] (Table 2). Ouabain-resistant Na[+] net uptake in the presence of 5 mM K[+] was about 20 μmol/ml cells in 24 hours, the uptake not being significantly altered by furosemide (Table 2, see references 22, 23). A similar result was obtained for Na[+] gain when the 5 mM K[+] was replaced by Rb[+].

Net loss of K[+] following incubation in the medium containing K[+] was slightly reduced in the presence of furosemide (13%, p<0.01). The furosemide-induced K[+] retention was more pronounced in the presence of 5 mM Rb[+] (33%, p<0.001). In the 145 mM Na[+]–5 mM Rb[+] medium, furosemide-sensitive K[+] retention and furosemide-sensitive uptake of Rb[+] were nearly identical numerically (Table 2).

To gain further insight into the physiological role of the furosemide-sensitive transport system, ouabain-resistant Na[+] and K[+] movements were studied in Na[+] media of varying K[+] and Rb[+] content. Figure 7 shows results obtained for ouabain-resistant Na[+] net uptake in 24 hours. The Na[+] gain rose with rising concentrations of both K[+] and Rb[+]. In the presence of furosemide, the Na[+] uptake was independent of external K[+] and Rb[+] and remained at the value seen in the absence of furosemide, with 5 to 10 mM of K[+] or Rb[+] in the medium.

No effect of furosemide on Na[+] gain at 5 to 10 mM of external K[+] or Rb[+] does not mean that no Na[+] transport is mediated by the system, but rather indicates that the rates of unidirectional inward and outward movements are identical. Accordingly, the data in Figure 7 demonstrate that outward Na[+] transport exceeds inward Na[+] transport by the furosemide-sensitive system at low, but not at normal, external K[+] (Rb[+]) concentrations. Thus, the red cell co-transport system serves as a Na[+] extruding mechanism at lowered, but not at normal, external K[+].

A similar conclusion can be drawn from the data in Figure 8 concerning the net effect on cell K[+]. Net K[+] loss decreased with rising external K[+]. However, it remained at a high value when Rb[+] instead of K[+] was the second cation in the medium. In the presence of furosemide, the K[+] loss was reduced, independent of external K[+] and Rb[+]. The overall result is that of a furosemide-sensitive K[+] retention, which decreases with rising external K[+] but is not altered by Rb[+]. Furosemide-sensitive Rb[+] uptake is also depicted in Figure 8 (right-hand penal). It rises with increasing external Rb[+] and is similar in magnitude to the furosemide-sensitive K[+] retention at 5 and 10 mM external Rb[+].

Table 2. Ouabain-resistant cation net-movements during 24 h of incubation (pH 7.4, 37° C, 0.2 ml ouabain, hematocrit 1%) in 145 mM Na⁺ media containing either 5 mM K⁺ or 5 mM Rb⁺. The K⁺ concentration in the Rb⁺ media rose from 0.03 to 0.3 mM during the 24 h of incubation. The data are given in μmol/ml cells/24 h and are means ± SEM from the number of experiments indicated on red cells of one donor with a furosemide-sensitive one-hour Rb⁺ uptake in 145 mM Na⁺-5 mM Rb⁺ medium of 0.71 ± 0.04 μmol/ml cells/h.

	Na⁺ Gain Control	Furosemide	Furosemide	K⁺ Loss Control	Furosemide	Furosemide	Rb⁺ Gain Control	Furosemide	Furosemide
5 mM K⁺ (n = 5)	20.1 ± 1.4	19.4 ± 1.4	− 0.7 ± 1.4	19.4 ± 1.3	16.9 ± 1.4	− 2.5 ± 1.5			
5 mM Rb⁺ (n = 7)	20.3 ± 1.0	20.6 ± 1.0	+ 0.3 ± 0.3	23.8 ± 1.3	15.6 ± 1.4	− 8.2 ± 0.3	10.4 ± 0.2	1.6 + 0.2	8.8 + 0.2

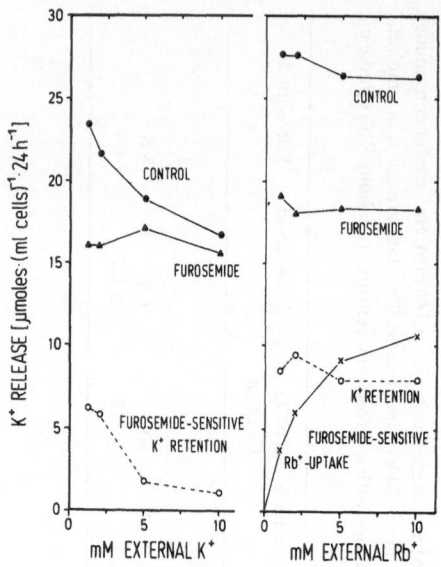

Figure 8. Effect of external K^+ and Rb^+ on ouabain-resistant K^+ loss over 24 hours. The experiment was done on the cells of the same donor as in Figure 7.

As already shown in Figure 1, at low external K^+ (Rb^+) there is low inward K^+ (Rb^+) co-transport. The reduction of K^+ loss due to furosemide at low external K^+, seen in Figure 8, is to be attributed, therefore, to inhibition of outward K^+ transport. At higher external K^+ (Rb^+), the rates of furosemide-sensitive K^+ (Rb^+) inward and K^+ outward movements become about equal.

From these results it is concluded that *the furosemide-sensitive transport system serves to promote a net extrusion of Na^+ at low but not at normal or elevated external K^+ concentrations. A second function, more important quantitatively, is a K^+ extrusion which increases upon lowering of external K^+ but is also seen at normal external K^+ concentrations.* These conclusions are in accordance with earlier studies on Na^+ and K^+ net movements in human erythrocytes during prolonged incubation with ouabain [22–25].

The so-called Na^+/K^+ 'co-transport' system is dependent on the simultaneous presence of Na^+, K^+, and Cl and is inhibited by furosemide [22–26]. Evidence has been presented [21] for furosemide-sensitive cation movements with a $Na^+:K^+$ stoichiometry of 1:1 (see also Fig. 3). However, the $Na^+:K^+$ ratio of furosemide-sensitive transport falls down to 0.2:1 for inward movements in a 145 mM Na^+ and 5 mM K^+ medium [26] and to 0:1 for inward K^+ (Rb^+) transport in choline or Mg^+

media (Fig. 2, [28]). Thus, it remains unclear whether the coupling ratio of the co-transport system is variable, or whether there are two furosemide-sensitive transport systems, one mediating a 1:1 Na^+/K^+ co-transport in the usual sense, and the other a K^+ transport with the potential capacity for both unidirectional K^+ movements and for bidirectional 1:1 K^+/K^+ exchange (see [27]).

Physiological role of the furosemide-sensitive cation transport system of human erythrocytes

The present study revealed that the bidirectionally operating furosemide-sensitive transport system of human erythrocytes is functionally almost silent, with respect to net-translocation of Na^+, at normal external Na^+ and K^+ concentrations (Fig. 7, Table 2). The only significant effect of furosemide seen in media of normal cation composition containing ouabain is a small retardation of K^+ loss (Fig. 8, Table 2).

In contrast, in Na^+ media with lower than normal K^+ concentrations, the overall effect of bidirectional transport by the system is a net extrusion of both K^+ and Na^+, the loss of K^+ exceeding that of Na^+ (Figs. 7 and 8). The question thus arises whether the biological function of the furosemide-sensitive transport system of human erythrocytes is not only related to cellular K^+ and Na^+, but also to the homeostasis of plasma K^+.

Obviously, at lowered external K^+ there is a significant K^+ loss from the cells. Thus, the system can contribute to maintaining the external K^+ concentration constant by placing the great internal K^+ pool at the disposal of the external space when external K^+ tends to fall. In this respect, the increase seen in red cell co-transport activity in DOCA-treated rats (Fig. 6) needs to be considered.

Administration of DOCA or DOCA plus salt substantially reduced plasma K^+. The acceleration of K^+ loss through the co-transport system expected under these conditions was associated with a small but not significant lowering of red cell K^+ from 107 ± 2 to 103 ± 9 μmoles/ml cells in the DOCA-salt rats. Possibly, the fall in red cell K^+ was counteracted *in vivo* by an increased K^+ uptake through the Na^+/K^+ pump. In fact, an enhanced ouabain-sensitive Rb^+ uptake was seen *in vitro* in these cells. This can be attributed to an activation of the pump by the elevated red cell Na^+ content.

Another finding indicating a role of the co-transport system in K^+ homeostasis is the highly significant negative correlation ($r = -0.55$) of K^+ content to the activity of the co-transport system seen in erythrocytes of 66 human donors (Fig. 9). Thus, the co-transport system seems to contribute to establishing the steady-state K^+ level in human erythrocytes. Of interest in this context is the observation that a mutant mouse fibroblastic cell line deficient in the co-transport system can maintain cell K^+ at normal values even at such low external K^+ concentrations, where normal fibroblasts lose substantial amounts of K^+ and eventually die [34].

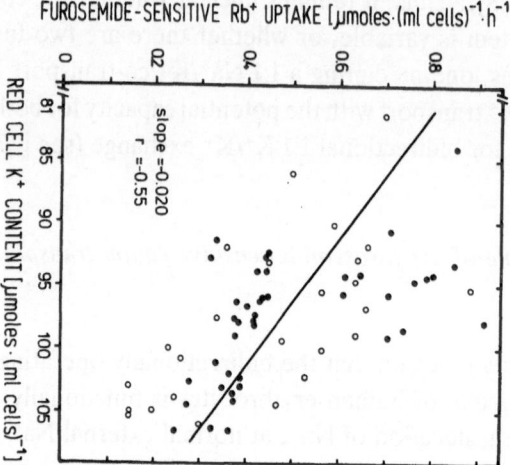

Figure 9. Relation between K⁺ content and furosemide-sensitive Rb⁺ uptake determined as described in Table 1 in human erythrocytes (n = 66). The correlations for red cells from essential hypertensive (○) and normotensive individuals (●) were not significantly different from the correlation for all probands shown in the figure.

The second aspect is the red cell Na⁺ content. In this study, no relationship exists between red cell Na⁺ content on co-transport activity. However, from experiments on cation release, it was concluded by Garay et al. that the function of the co-transport system is to extrude Na⁺ when cellular Na⁺ is elevated [14, 19], at least at external K⁺ concentrations below 20 mM [18]. This conclusion provided the basis for the idea that a reduction in co-transport activity may be related to the genesis of essential hypertension [14, 18, 19]. The present studies (Table 2, Fig. 7) and earlier results [22, 23] demonstrate that the co-transport system of human erythrocytes does not promote a Na⁺ net extrusion in Na⁺ media of physiological K⁺ concentration, even in red cells with twice the normal Na⁺ content. The co-transport system mediates uphill Na⁺ net extrusion only at lower than normal external K⁺ (Fig. 7).

Whether a similar Na⁺ extruding mechanism sensitive to inhibiton by furosemide exists in cells other than erythrocytes is not well established. Therefore, further research is needed to understand the role of the co-transport system in cellular Na⁺ and K⁺ homeostasis and its dependence on external K⁺.

Na⁺/K⁺ co-transport and Na⁺/Li⁺ exchange in hypertension

In the earlier reports of Garay et al [14, 17] and Canessa et al [1], drastic differences in Na⁺/K⁺ co-transport and Na⁺/Li⁺ exchange were observed in erythrocytes of normotensive and essential hypertensive individuals. No or very minimal, overlap between the two groups was seen [1, 14, 17]. In later reports from the same authors, the differences were found to be much smaller and a substantial overlap was observed [2, 3, 18, 19]. A trend similar to that initially reported was found in other laboratories. The transport rates, however, overlapped to a great extent between the two groups [31, 32, 35, 36].

The procedure proposed by Canessa et al. to measure the Na^+/Li^+ exchange rate [1, 31] can be adopted relatively easily. The only major modification that was proposed concerns the loading process (see Dr. Funder's contribution in this volume). The PCMBS cation loading technique, however, has been modified several times by the Garay group [14-17, 38]. This is not easy to replicate in other laboratories due to several variabilities affecting the loading process, such as the ratio of PCMBS to hemoglobin, the source of choline chloride, and the Ca^{2+} contamination of the materials used to prepare the incubation media.

To avoid the laborious and sometimes failing loading procedures, simple uptake tests were developed to assess the activities of the two transport systems [28]. These consist in measurement of furosemide-sensitive Rb^+ uptake and phloretin-sensitive Li^+ uptake over one hour with fresh erythrocytes (see Table 1). The most important question for evaluation of the assays was whether interindividual differences in the transport activities are reflected in both inward and outward cation movements. As evidenced by the data in Figure 3, a highly significant positive correlation is found between outward and inward cation transport rates by the co-transport system. A similar positive correlation was observed for Li^+ transport by the Na^+/Li^+ exchange system in the two directions [28].

Accordingly, results obtained with our uptake test can well be compared with data on cation release as assessed by the release techniques. No significant differences were found, for either Na^+/Li^+ exchange or Na^+/K^+ co-transport, between red cells of 18 essential hypertensive probands, 38 normotensive individuals, and 5 patients suffering from renal hypertension (Fig. 4). These observations demonstrate that alterations in the two transport systems cannot serve as a general criterion for detecting essential hypertensive individuals. The possible reasons for the disrepancy between our results and those of Canessa et al. and Garay et al., such as differences between the populations studied [18, 39, 40] or the renin status, have been discussed in detail earlier [30].

A further argument to be considered in interpretation of the results comes from studies on co-transport in rat erythrocytes. As shown in Figure 6, the co-transport activity can increase up to twofold upon treatment with DOCA or DOCA plus salt. Whether this acceleration of co-transport is a direct result of mineralocorticoid action or an event secondary to lowering of plasma K^+ or alteration of some other plasma factor(s) is not yet known.

To date, data on co-transport and exchange mechanisms have been interpreted with the tacit assumption that the activities of the transport systems remain constant within single individuals. In fact, a remarkable stability of the two

72

transport systems has been observed in single individuals [6, 15, 28, 38], indicating that the transport activities in each individual are either genetically determined or governed by a plasma factor that remains stable over long periods of time.

However, the red cell co-transport activity can change (Fig. 6). Thus, the question arises as to whether the transport activities in the human populations studied by the different authors happened to be altered *in vivo* prior to the assay. Factors to be considered in this context are drugs, dietary regimen, and any medication causing a lowering of plasma K^+ such as treatment with diuretics or laxatives (see contribution of Dr. Erdmann in this volume).

In our study, only patients whose antihypertensive medication was omitted for diagnostic reasons for at least 14 days prior to the experiments were included. Data for plasma K^+ are available for 10 of the 18 essential hypertensives. A negative correlation between furosemide-sensitive inward co-transport and plasma K^+ is found ($r = -0.20$) and is not statistically significant. Thus, in future research on red cell cation transport in hypertension, not only a familial history and the renin status need to be considered, but also other parameters such as plasma K^+ concentration and premedication.

SUMMARY

Reliable and simple uptake tests are applied to assess the activities of the Na^+/Li^+ countertransport and the Na^+/K^+ co-transport system of human erythrocytes. The uptake rates determined over 1 hour with fresh cells truly reflect the release rates determined with the more difficult and laborious cation release techniques proposed by Canessa et al. [1] and Garay et al. [14, 15].

No significant differences in mean value of transport rates for the two systems are observed between 38 normotensive individuals, 18 hypertensive, and 5 renal hypertensive patients. Four out of a total of six low-renin essential hypertensive patients exhibited some of the lowest transport rates for both systems among all individuals examined. It is concluded that determination of red cell Na^+/Li^+ exchange and Na^+/K^+ co-transport is not a useful tool for the diagnosis of essential hypertension.

The co-transport activity was negatively correlated to the red cell K^+ content of 66 donors ($r = -0.55$), indicating a possible role of the co-transport system in cellular K^+ homeostasis. No relationship between co-transport and red cell Na^+ content was observed.

The co-transport system mediates Na^+ net extrusion in Na^+ media only at lower than normal external K^+ concentrations. A small K^+ net extrusion by the system is seen in media of normal Na^+ and K^+ content, the K^+ extrusion substantially increasing at lowered external K^+.

The stoichiometry of furosemide-sensitive Na^+ and K^+ movements varies between 1:1 and 0:1, possibly due to the existence of a furosemide-sensitive K^+/K^+ exchange system.

DOCA-salt hypertension induces a twofold increase in Na^+/K^+ co-transport activity of Sprague-Dawley rat erythrocytes.

A possible role of plasma K^+ in influencing the red cell Na^+/K^+ co-transport system *in vivo* is discussed.

ACKNOWLEDGMENTS

The excellent technical assistance of Mrs. Jutta Kronauer and Mrs. Brigitte Göser is most gratefully acknowledged. The author thanks B.O. Göbel for cooperation in the experiments, Drs. P.C. Weber and R. Lorenz for selecting the essential hypertensive patients, Dr. F.-X. Beck for the cooperation in the study with hypertensive rats, and Dr. D. Ganten for the gift of spontaneous hypertensive and normotensive Wistar-Kyoto rats. The work was supported in part by the Wilhelm-Sander-Stiftung.

REFERENCES

1. Canessa M, Adragna N, Solomon HS, et al.: Increased sodium-lithium countertransport in red cells from patients with essential hypertension. N Engl J Med 302:772–776, 1980.
2. Canessa M, Adragna N, Bize I, et al.: Ouabain-insensitive cation transport in the red cells of normotensive and hypertensive subjects, in Zumkley H, Loss H (editors): Intracellular Electrolytes and Arterial Hypertension. Stuttgart, Thieme, 1980, pp 239–250.
3. Canessa M, Bize I, Solomon H, et al.: Na countertransport and co-transport in human red cells: Function, dysfunction and genes in essential hypertension. Clin Exp Hypertens 3:783–795, 1981.
4. Mendels J, Frazer A: Intracellular lithium concentration and clinical response. Towards a membrane theory of depression. J Psychiatr Res 10:9–18, 1973.
5. Duhm J, Eisenried F, Becker BF: Studies on the lithium transport across the red cell membrane. I. Li^+ uphill transport by the Na^+-dependent Li^+ countertransport system of human erythrocytes. Pflugers Arch 364:147–155, 1976.
6. Duhm J, Becker BF: Studies on the lithium transport across the red cell membrane. IV. Interindividual variations in the Na^+-dependent Li^+ countertransport system of human erythrocytes. Pflugers Arch 370:211–219, 1977.
7. Haas M, Schooler J, Tosteson DC: Coupling of lithium to sodium transport in human red cells. Nature 258:425–427, 1975.
8. Pandey GN, Sarkadi B, Haas M, et al.: Lithium transport pathways in human red blood cells. J Gen Physiol 72:233–247, 1978.
9. Sarkadi B, Alifimoff JK, Gunn RB, et al.: Kinetics and stoichiometry of Na-dependent Li transport in human red blood cells. J Clen Physiol 72:249–265, 1978.
10. Greil W, Besker BF, Duhm J: On the relevance of the red blood cell/plasma lithium ratio, in Cooper TB, Gershon S, Kline NS, et al (eds): Lithium, Controversies and Unresolved Issues. Amsterdam, Excerpta Medica, 1979, pp 209–217.
11. Pandey GN, Dorus E, Davis JM, et al.: Lithium transport in human red blood cells. Genetic and clinical aspects. Arch Gen Psychiatry 36:902–908, 1979.
12. Ramsey TA, Frazer A, Mendels J, et al.: The erythrocyte lithium-plasma lithium ratio in patients with primary affective disorder. Arch Gen Psychiatry 36:457–461, 1979.

13. Rybakowski J: Pharmacokinetic aspects of red blood cell lithium index in manic-depressive psychosis. Biol Psychiatry 12:425–432, 1977.

14. Garay R, Dagher G, Pernollet M-G, et al.: Inherited defect in a Na$^+$-K$^+$ co-transport system in erythrocytes from essential hypertensive patients. Nature 284:281–283, 1980.

15. Dagher G, Garay RP: A Na$^+$, K$^+$ co-transport assay for essential hypertension. Can J Biochem 58:1069–1074, 1980.

16. Garay R, Meyer P: A new test showing abnormal net Na$^+$ and K$^+$ fluxes in erythrocytes of essential hypertensive patients. Lancet 1:349–353, 1979.

17. Garay RP, Elghozi J-L, Dagher G, et al.: Laboratory distinction between essential and secondary hypertension by measurement of erythrocyte cation fluxes. N Engl J Med 302:769–771, 1980.

18. Garay RP, Dagher G: Erythrocyte Na$^+$ and K$^+$ transport systems in essential hypertension, in Zumkley H, Losse H (editors): Intracellular Electrolytes and Arterial Hypertension. Stuttgart, Thieme, 1980, pp 69–76.

19. Garay RP, Mannaert P, Dagher G, et al.: Abnormal erythrocyte Na$^+$ K$^+$ co-transport system, a proposed genetic marker of essential hypertension. Clin Exp Hypertens 3:851–859, 1981.

20. Blaustein MP: Sodium ions, calcium ions, blood pressure regulation and hypertension: A reassessment and a hypothesis. Am J Physiol 232:C165–C173, 1977.

21. Garay R, Adragna N, Canessa M, et al.: Outward sodium and potassium co-transport in human red cells. J Membr Biol 62:169–174, 1981.

22. Dunn MJ: The effects of transport inhibitors on sodium outflux and influx in red blood cells: Evidence for exchange diffusion. J Clin Invest 49:1804–1814, 1970.

23. Dunn MJ: Ouabain-uninhibited sodium transport in human erythrocytes. Evidence against a second pump. J Clin Invest 52:658–670, 1973.

24. Sachs JR: Ouabain-insensitive sodium movements in the human red blood cell. J Gen Physiol 57:259–282, 1971.

25. Wiley JS, Cooper RA: A furosemide-sensitive co-transport of sodium plus potassium in the human red cell. J Clin Invest 53:745–755, 1974.

26. Dunham PB, Stewart GW, Ellory JC: Chloride-activated potassium transport in human erythrocytes. Proc Natl Acad Sci USA 77:1711–1715, 1980.

27. McManus TJ, Schmidt WF III: Ion and co-ion transport in avian red cells, in Hoffman JF (editors): Membrane Transport Processes. New York, Raven Press, 1978, vol 1, pp 79–106.

28. Duhm J, Gobel BO: Sodium-lithium exchange and sodium-potassium co-transport in human erythrocytes. I. Evaluation of a simple uptake test to assess the activity of the two transport systems. Hypertension, in press.

29. Ellory JC, Flatman PW, Stewart GW: Inhibition of human red cell sodium and potassium influxes by external divalent cations. J Physiol 307:37P–38P, 1980.

30. Duhm J, Gobel BO, Lorenz R, et al.: Sodium-lithium exchange and sodiumpotassium co-transport in human erythrocytes. II. A simple uptake test applied in normotensive and essential hypertensive individuals. Hypertension, in press.

31. Cusi D, Barlassina C, Ferrandi M, et al.: Familial aggregation of cation transport abnormalities and essential hypertension. Clin Exp Hypertens 3:871–884, 1981.

32. Cusi D, Barlassina M, Ferrandi M, et al.: Relationship between altered Na$^+$-K$^+$ co-transport and Na$^+$-Li$^+$ countertransport in the erythrocytes of essential hypertensive patients. Clin Sci 61: 33s–36s, 1981.

33. Duhm J: Lithium transport pathways in erythrocytes, in Lux HD, Emrich HM (editors): Basic Mechanisms in the Action of Lithium. Amsterdam, Excerpta Medica, in press.

34. Jayme DW, Adelberg EA, Slayman CW: Reduction of K$^+$ efflux in cultured mouse fibroblasts, by mutation or by diuretics, permits growth in K$^+$-deficient medium. Proc Natl Acad Sci USA 78:1057–1061, 1981.

35. Canali M, Borghi L, Sani E, et al.: Increased erythrocyte lithium-sodium countertransport in essential hypertension: Its relationship to family history of hypertension. Clin Sci 61:135–155, 1981.

36. Swarts HGP, Bonting SL, DePont JJHHM, et al.: Cation fluxes and Na^+-K^+ activated ATPase activity in erythrocytes of patients with essential hypertension. Clin Exp Hypertens 3:831–849, 1981; Hypertension 3:641–649, 1981.
37. Canessa ML, Tosteson DC: Determination of the sodium-lithium countertransport system of human erythrocytes, in Cooper TB, Gershon S, Kline NS, et al. (editors): Lithium, Controversies and Unresolved Issues. Amsterdam, Excerpta Medica, 1979, pp 978–982.
38. Garay RP, Elghozi J-L, Dagher G, et al.: Abnormality of net Na^+ and K^+ erythrocyte fluxes in human hypertension: Latest developments, in Zumkley H, Losse H (editors): Intracellular Electrolytes and Arterial Hypertension. Stuttgart, Thieme, 1980, pp 212-221.
39. Garay RP, Nazaret C, Dagher G, et al.: A genetic approach to the geography of hypertension: Examination of Na^+-K^+ co-transport in Ivory Coast Africans. Clin Exp Hypertens 3:861–870, 1981.
40. Woods KL, Beevers DG, West MJ: Racial differences in red cell cation transport and their relationship to essential hypertension. Clin Exp Hypertens 3:655–622, 1981.

DISCUSSION

Discussants: Garay, Duhm, Brody, Tosteson.

Garay: The sodium-potassium co-transport system, and particularly the Na^+ fluxes catalyzed by this system, are very labile. If you incubate human erythrocytes at 37° C in a physiological Ringer medium containing potassium 4.2 millimolar, sodium 140 millimolar, with ouabain, glucose, and penicillin for 24 hours, the co-transport is inhibited.

Duhm: We took cells incubated in potassium medium for 24 hours and measured co-transport activity and found it had not changed after 24 hours of incubation with glucose.

Garay: When we added 10 percent of fetal calf serum, we prevented inhibition of the co-transport. Furthermore, a 24 hour incubation with furosemide increases passive potassium permeability. You need to use another diuretic which is less toxic for the passive permeability.

We ran this experiment with bumetanide in the presence of 10 percent serum, and in at least 60 experiments we observed a statistically significant difference between control and bumetanide. The net Na^+ effusion by the Na^+, K^+ co-transport system was about 0.1 to 0.2 mmoles per hour. Maybe you can run this same experiment with 0.1 bumetanide in the presence of 10 percent calf fetal serum and obtain a statistically significant difference under these conditions.

Duhm: You have 4.2 millimolar potassium in the Na^+ medium, and I agree that there is a small sodium extrusion by the co-transport system under these conditions, which is hard to measure. Twenty-four hours of incubation are needed to get significant differences. The point I wanted to make is that the furosemide- or bumetanide-sensitive potassium net movements exceed the sodium net movements, especially at lowered external K^+ concentrations.

Garay: Regarding your results in hypertension, I would like to know if you have other results performed in our experimental conditions. It is very difficult for me to compare results obtained with different techniques because the kinetics of the sodium-potassium co-transport and sodium-lithium countertransport are very complicated. Thus, the reported differences between hypertensive and normotensive depend on the kinetic conditions.

Duhm: May I propose that you apply our test in Paris. We have demonstrated that the results obtained by your and our tests show a highly significant correlation to each other, with a correlation coefficient of over 0.9.

Brody: I wish not to enter into this controversy, but to ask a totally different question. Your experiments with DOCA-salt animals, I think, give an opportunity to test for cause-and-effect relationships. There are at least three interventions or experimental situations that we know will prevent the development of DOCA-salt hypertension. These are central administration of 6-hydroxydopamine, use of the vasopressin-deficient Brattleboro rat, and our lesion in the anterior hypothalamus. It would be very interesting to test whether or not each of these interventions, which block the development of hypertension also alter the effects on co-transport. Any one, or, especially, all of those tests might give some indication whether this alteration is fundamental to the hypertensive process or only secondary to it.

Duhm: We have preliminary results strongly suggesting that the increase in red cell co-transport activity in the DOCA-salt hypertensive rats is not related to the hypertensive process as such, but rather secondary to the lowered plasma K^+ levels. In DOCA-salt hypokalemia, the cells tend to lose K^+ and shrink a little bit, as indicated by the increase in mean cellular hemoglobin content (MCHC) we have seen in these animals. Rat erythrocytes differ fundamentally from human red cells since their co-transport activity depends strongly on cell volume, a phenomenon not seen in human erythrocytes. A shrinkage of the rat red blood cell by 15% induces a ten-fold increase in co-transport activity, and the 3–5% of shrinkage we observed in the DOCA-salt hypertensive rats may well explain the doubling of co-transport rate in these animals. May I add that, in my opinion, any data on co-transport activity of rat erythrocytes can only be interpreted when the cell volume (MCHC) is known. An increase in co-transport activity of rat erythrocytes is only a real increase when a cell shrinkage (and also a cell swelling) is excluded. Thus, I do not assume any cause-and-effect relationship between hypertension and red cell co-transport activity in the rat. Rather, there is a causal relationship between red cell volume (or red cell K^+) and co-transport. The co-transport rise seen in erythrocytes from DOCA-salt rats can be reversed by reswelling the cells, it can be prevented by supplementing the diet with extra K^+, and it can be mimicked by feeding the rats with a K^+-deficient diet.

Tosteson: With regard to the furosemide-sensitive rubidium uptake as an assay of co-transport, I would like to have your thoughts about the possibility that a substantial part of that could be rubidium-potassium exchange that is furosemide-sensitive. I'm sure you know that there is a very prominent component of K^+-K^+ exchange in which rubidium can participate in bird red cells, for example, where the co-transport system is much more active than it is in human red cells. How can we be sure that a significant fraction of what you're observing isn't this K^+-K^+ exchange system?

Duhm: What we have is a furosemide-sensitivity of Rb^+ uptake in NaCl media which is not seen in nitrate media. Commonly, furosemide-sensitive Rb^+ (or K^+) movements in human red blood cells are attributed to the so-called Na^+-K^+ co-transport system which is chloride dependent. However, there is certainly a K^+-K^+ exchange and other phenomena which are inhibited by the drug. At present, the question whether there is one system with more than one function (e.g., 1:1 Na^+-K^+ co-transport and 1:1 K^+-K^+ or Na^+-Na^+ exchange) or whether there are several systems with different functions which are all inhibited by furosemide is only subject to speculation. I prefer to assume that there is one furosemide-sensitive system which has the following potential capacities:
(1) 1:1 Na^+-K^+ co-transport in both directions
(2) 1:1 K^+-K^+ exchange (dependent on Na^+)
(3) 1:1 Na^+-Na^+ exchange (dependent on K^+)
(4) unidirectional k^+ transport (in both directions, in the absence as well as in the presence of Na^+)
(5) unidirectional Na^+ transport (in both directions, independent of K^+).
There seems to be no obligatory 1:1 coupling unidirectional Na^+ and K^+ movements or of the exchange

phenomena. The actual mode of operation seems rather to depend on the availability of cations on the two sides of the membrane. The data in Figure 8 certainly suggest that the predominant action of the so-called 'co-transport' system is a K^+-K^+ exchange in media of physiological cation composition.

Tosteson: That leaves open the possibility that there are two different systems of unknown relationship that we're looking at, and that would require sorting out in making any of these correlations.

FAMILIAL AGGREGATION OF SODIUM COUNTERTRANSPORT AND CO-TRANSPORT AND ESSENTIAL HYPERTENSION

MITZY CANESSA, HAROLD SOLOMON, BONITA FALKER, NORMA ADRAGNA AND R. CURTIS ELLISON

INTRODUCTION

Inherited biochemical differences among individuals and among populations have been related to differences in susceptibility to disease as well as to differential human survival.

As an attempt to define susceptibility to hypertension in the human population, we have proposed to investigate the genetic polymorphism of red cell Na-transport systems. This can be instrumental in explaining why, in the same habitat, two or more discontinuous forms of Na-transport traits may have different susceptibility to elevated blood pressure. Evidence has been collected to support that three systems which transport Na in red cells largely vary in man: the Na-pump, the Na/Na exchange, and the Na/K co-transport [1, 2, 3].

The polymorphism of red cell Na-transport systems might help to (1) investigate inherited differences in distinct populations to provide answers to the epidemiologists' questions about the prevalence of hypertension in certain human populations; (2) uravel the causes of family resemblances in blood pressure; (3) provide an estimate of hypertensive risk early in life; (4) design adequate preventive nonpharmacological management at the individual level.

Several observations have indicated that heredity is involved in the pathogenesis of hypertension in man. Population and family studies in relatives, young siblings, newborns, twins, adoptees and spouses [4, 5, 6] have underligned human hypertension as a distinct genetic trait. However, the controversy initiated by the work of Platt [7] and Pickering [5] about the mode of inheritance and the number of genes involved in the disease remains unsolved.

Several epidemiological studies have contributed a great deal of information to assess the contribution of genetic factors to the incidence and prevalance of the disease in several populations [6]. More importantly, epidemiological studies have established risk factors such as age, weight, sex, and race [8]. The investigation of the relationship between the polymorphism of red cell Na-transport systems in essential hypertension can fill the existing gap in the middle-ground between human genetics and the epidemiology of hypertension.

Two membrane transport proteins translocating Na across the red cell membrane, the Na/Na exchange and the Na/K co-transport, are altered in individuals and families with essential hypertension. Both transport proteins can be distinguished operationally by their different properties. In agreement with this finding, the Na/Na exchange system appears altered in certain populations and the Na/K co-transport in others. Notably, both disturbances seem to have different geographic and ethnic distributions as well as strong familial aggregation, as previously found for other genetic traits. In order to deal with populations of genes rather than individual genes, population genetics will define this phenomenon as panmictic units or demes of Na transport.

Family resemblance is in the middle-ground of genetics and epidemiology and can be used to identify environmental causes of human diseases.

Familial aggregation of blood pressure has been adequately documented by several studies [11–14]. The present study presents evidence of familial aggregation of Na countertransport and Na/K co-transport in two different populations. In this research project, we have investigated 23 Caucasian families and 10 black families, each with a minimum of two adolescent offspring.

The present results indicate that: (1) Na countertransport and co-transport display statistically significant familial aggregation; (2) the aggregation of elevated blood pressure correlates with elevated countertransport in the Caucasian and black families studied; (3) there are population differences in the type of Na transport alteration in families with essential hypertension. While Caucasian families have marked elevations of countertransport and Na/K co-transport, a reduced K co-transport was the main defect in black families.

The ethnic differences found in the familial aggregation of the Na transport system as well known characteristics of genetic traits. The polymorphism of red cell Na transport can be an adequate tool to assess individual and population differences in the prevalence of hypertension.

FAMILIAL RESEMBLANCE IN LI/NA COUNTERTRANSPORT AND NA/K CO-TRANSPORT

We studied 23 Caucasian families composed of two parents and a minimum of two offspring. The age of the offspring varied between 10 and 20 years. The families were classified into three groups: *Group 1:* The parents were documented normotensives. The family history of the grandparents was negative for hypertension as established by records of their age, age of death, cause of death, treatment for hypertension, stroke and heart trouble. *Group 2:* The parents were normotensive but the grandparents had family history of hypertension. *Group 3:* One or both parents were hypertensive. In the case of the black families, groups 1 and 3 above were composed of only one parent (usually the mother).

Random or Assortative Marriage

In the study of intrafamilial correlation coefficients for a given genetic trait, the absence of correlation between spouses gives evidence for random marriage in the population. In our sample of Caucasian families, we found significant correlation between diastolic blood pressure, Li/Na countertransport and Na/K co-transport between husband and wife (Table 1). In the black families, this parameter could not be computed since only the mother could be included in the study. Several interpretations can be derived from this finding. Inasmuch as the couples with teenage offspring had lived together for at least 20 years, this may indicate the presence of a large environmental factor in both transport systems. Notably, in studies on the genetics of hypertension, correlation between blood pressure of husbands and wives has been highly significant in some but not all studies [11–13]. In the twin study of Rose et al. [13], the correlation of blood pressure between the twin's spouse and the co-twin's spouse was nearly as high as that found between husband and wife. As an explanation for this finding, Rose [13] proposed that the spouse aggregation cannot be solely attributed to a shared household. It may reflect, as well, social homogamy of morphological factors which mediate blood pressure such as homogamy for body size, similarities in age, race, social class, or cultural traits such as drinking and dietary preferences. Rose [13] also established that important additive genetic effects might be present after the elimination by covariance of the correlation with body size. It was proposed that social homogamy arising from assortative marriage may contribute to the familial aggregation of blood pressure [13].

In order to investigate the causes of the significant correlation found between husband and wife for countertransport and co-transport, correlation coefficients for blood pressure, body weight and age were also determined. Covariance analysis showed that blood pressure and age correction eliminated the correlation between spouses. In an additional sample of 34 spouses included in the analysis, the intraspouse correlation coefficient was not significant (Table 1).

Table 1. Correlation coefficients between husband and wife in 24 Caucasian families

	n	r	p
Weight	24	0.61	<.005
Age	24	0.88	<.0005
Diastolic blood pressure	24	0.62	<.005
Li_i/Na_o countertransport	24	0.71	<.005
	37	0.34	<.025

n = number of subjects.

INTRAFAMILIAL CORRELATION COEFFICIENTS FOR Li_i/Na_o COUNTERTRANSPORT IN CAUCASIAN FAMILIES

Table 2 shows that several intrafamilial coefficients for Li_i/Na_o countertransport are statistically significant in the 23 Caucasian families studied. All of them are significantly different from zero which is the maximal value expected for one-half the genes in common. The intrafamilial correlation coefficients for Na/K co-transport were also statistically significant.

The systolic and diastolic blood pressure significantly correlated with Li_i/Na_o countertransport ($p<0.001$) in the Caucasian families. Weight and blood pressure were also family-aggregated in our sample. Familial aggregation of blood pressure seems to be mediated at least partly by aggregation of body size. Blood pressure was highly correlated with body size indices in the twin study of Rose [13] as well as in our study.

POPULATION DIFFERENCES IN RED CELL Na TRANSPORT AND ESSENTIAL HYPERTENSION

The frequency distribution of Li_i/Na_o countertransport in Caucasians and American blacks from Philadelphia appear to be different. Sixty per cent of the blacks have countertransport values below 0.2 mmol/liter cells × hour. The American black population studied in collaboration with Dr. B. Falkner shows a reduction in Na/K Co-transport in the hypertensive patients but with a large crossover with the normotensive controls. Notably, the furosemide-sensitive component of K efflux in significantly higher than Na efflux in the normotensive subjects. The coupling ratio between furosemide-sensitive Na and K fluxes is significantly lower than one in Caucasian normotensives.

These findings deserve further studies in larger samples as well as further characterization of K-transport pathways using other cell-loading techniques.

Table 2. Intrafamilial correlation coefficients for Li_i/Na_o countertransport in Caucasian families

	Number of subjects	r	p
Parent-offspring	74	0.67	<.0005
Father-offspring	37	0.66	<.0005
-sons	19	0.82	<.0005
-daughthers	17	0.65	<.005
Mother-offspring	51	0.43	<.0005
-sons	18	0.73	<.0005
-daughters	18	0.62	<.005

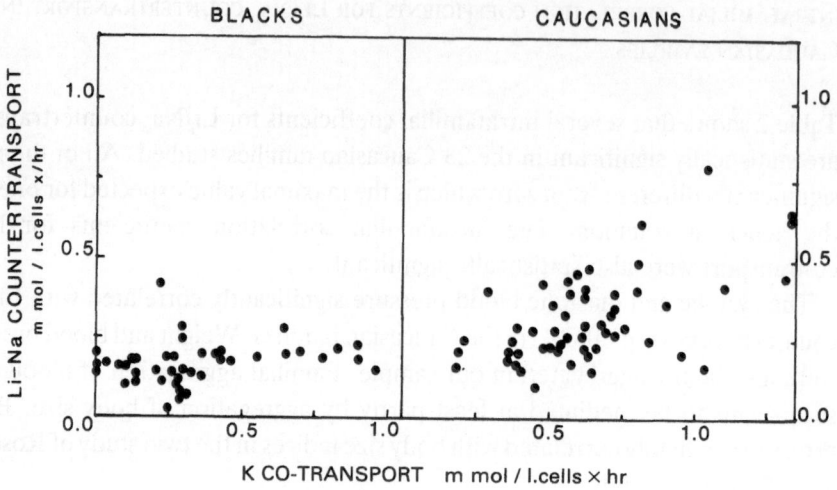

Figure 1. The relationship between the maximal rate of K co-transport and Li-Na$_o$ countertransport in the members of black and Caucasian families.

Caucasians: $Y = 0.14 + 0.28X$; $n = 57$; $r = 0.57$; $p < .001$.

Blacks: $Y = 0.15 + 0.06X$; $n = 44$; $r = 0.26$; $p < .1$.

THE RELATIONSHIP BETWEEN Na COUNTERTRANSPORT AND CO-TRANSPORT

Figure 1 shows a plot of the relationship between K co-transport and Na countertransport found in members of Caucasian and black families. In both groups, there is significant correlation between both transport systems. However, the slope of the regression line found in the Caucasian families was significantly higher than in the black families. We have not compared our data with those obtained in Paris and Milan since not all of the co-transport measurements had determined the maximal rate. Cusi [12] reported a slope of Na countertransport and Na co-transport which was significantly higher in hypertensive than normotensive subjects as Dagher has found in Paris [10]. The data collected by the Milan [16], Boston [18], and Paris [10] groups agree, therefore, in the marked correlation between countertransport and co-transport in the overall population and in the hypertensive population.

Several hypotheses can be raised to explain the present results. The highly significant regression of countertransport and co-transport may indicate that they are simultaneously regulated in essential hypertension. Such a regulation seems to be markedly reduced in the black population [21] that we have studied, while appearing significantly active in Caucasian families, and at intermediate values in Caucasians living in Paris and Milan. We have not found in the literature reliable data on racial differences of the Na pump, despite the claims that blacks have higher cellular Na. Unfortunately, the data collected by Woods on the racial differences in the ouabain-insensitive Rb influx [15] were done at external Rb concentrations of 4 μM. This concentration is 1000 times lower than the $K_{0.5}$ for ouabain-sensitive Rb and K influx and three orders of magnitude lower than the physiological plasma levels of K.

Cusi [16] and Garay [17] have measured the maximal rate of the ouabain-sensitive Na efflux in PcMBS loaded cells. Both groups found large interindividual variation without significant differences between normotensive and hypertensive patients. We still have few data on the maximal rate of the Na-pump in red cells loaded by the nystatin procedure that can complete our picture of the Na-pump.

THE RELATIONSHIP BETWEEN BODY WEIGHT, LI/NA COUNTERTRANSPORT, AND NA/K CO-TRANSPORT

A number of epidemiological studies have documented the relationship between overweight and hypertension [19]. Recent studies by De Luise et al. have raised the possibility that a genetically-determined lower number of ouabain-sensitive Na-pumps might be the characteristic of a subgroup of morbidly obese patients [3].

The present study conveys evidence for a relationship between weight gain, increased blood pressure and alterations in Na countertransport and Na/K co-transport in two different populations.

Table 3 shows that elevated countertransport strongly correlates with body weight index in a Caucasian population; while in blacks the reduction in the furosemide-sensitive K efflux correlated strongly with overweight. Most of the hypertensive black patients with low co-transport were over 25 kg/m². Notably, the black adolescents born to hypertensive parents that had low K co-transport were not overweight, while their blood pressure was in the borderline for hypertension. The data suggest that it is worthwhile to investigate whether subjects with K co-transport lower than 0.2 mmol/liter cells x hour may remain normoten-

Table 3. The relationship between weight gain, Na countertransport, and co-transport

	Number of subjects	Li/Na countertransport		Number of subjects	Na/K co-transport	
		r	p		r	p
Cancasians	61	0.38	<.005	52	0.23	N.S.
Blacks	48	0.13	N.S.	43	−0.3	<.005

Cation fluxes expressed in mmol/liter cells × hour.
Weight expressed in Kg/m².

sive if they maintain normal weight. Similarly, it will be important to investigate whether hypertensive subjects who are overweight will reduce their elevated countertransport and blood pressure while undergoing weight-reduction therapy. We are currently investigating this matter in the hopes that it may allow the design of nonpharmacological preventive maneuvers for individuals according to their pattern of red cell Na transport polymorphism.

POSSIBLE MEANING FOR THE GENETIC POLYMORPHISM OF NA TRANSPORT FOR ESSENTIAL HYPERTENSION

In studying red cell Na transport in hypertension, we have uncovered a high degree of heterogeneity in the human populations affected by essential hypertension [22] and in the members of their families [23]. Very often a peculiar syndrome (diabetes, mania, anemia) which was at first thought to be a descrete entity has turned out to represent a variety of distinct disorders. The degree of genetic heterogeneity (Table 4) expressed in essential hypertension by studying red cell Na transport is in agreement with the epidemiological and clinical finding that hypertension is not homogeneous in different populations.

From the operational point of view, Na countertransport and Na/K co-transport seem to behave as two different transport proteins. The significant correlation between both systems found in different populations affected by essential hypertension suggests the possibility that both proteins might be similarly regulated. If this is so, it is the regulation of these proteins that is altered in most of the patients with essential hypertension. Two types of alterations in certain loci may produce elevated co-transport and countertransport such as we see in certain Caucasian populations, as well as the reduced co-transport and low countertransport observed in other populations, such as American blacks and Mediterranean Europeans.

Table 4. Na transport in essential hypertension

	Li_i/Na_o Countertransport	Na/K Co-transport	Li Leak	Na-pump
Caucasians				
Boston	Elevated	Elevated	Normal	Normal
Paris	Normal	Reduced Na = K	Normal	Elevated turnover
Blacks				
Philadelphia	Reduced	Reduced Na > K	High	Reduced ?

It is tempting to promote discussion on the significance of the differences in Na-transport polymorphism and the prevalence of hypertension. An interpretation, probably too audacious at this stage of our research, would be that the elevated countertransport and Na/K co-transport found in some subjects and populations are protective traits. The very low doses of Na countertransport and Na/K co-transport which we found in the American blacks with essential hypertension may suggest that in this ethnic group the regulation of the Na and K gradients is hampered. Even though Caucasians have a reduced Na/K co-transport, blacks seem to have more of a reduction in K co-transport than Na co-transport.

Alternatively, the elevation in countertransport can be considered to be linked to different clinical forms of hypertension such as mild, labile, severe, or established, which may be differentially distributed in several populations. To complete our picture of the relationship between the polymorphism of red cell Na transport as a susceptibility factor in human hypertension, it is very important to determine the distribution of these transport systems in unselected populations.

At this stage of the research on membrane epidemiology, it is probably wiser to develop more thoughtful experiments than more theories of hypertension.

SUMMARY

We have studied in 33 families (normotensives, NT, plus hypertensives, HT) the correlation between the maximal rate of Li/Na countertransport (CT), outward Na/K co-transport (CO), diastolic blood pressure, and body weight.

Several intrafamilial correlations are statistically significant for Na countertransport and Na/K co-transport in the Caucasian families. The data provide quantitative evidence for familial resemblances in Na transport and in blood pressure.

Ethnic differences were found in the type of alteration of red cell cation transport. While hypertensive Caucasian families have a marked elevation of countertransport and Na/K co-transport, reduction of K co-transport and normal countertransport were found in black families.

Elevated countertransport correlated with weight index (Kg/m^2) in Caucasian families, while in the black families, reduced K co-transport correlated with weight gain. Na countertransport and Na/K co-transport were found significantly correlated in the members of black and Caucasian families. The slope of the regression line between both Na transport systems is significantly lower in the black families than in the Caucasians. These findings are tentatively interpreted as an expression of a defective regulation of these transport systems in the black population.

ACKNOWLEDGMENTS

This work was supported by NIH grants GM-25686 and HL-25064.

REFERENCES

1. Canessa M, Adragna N, Solomon H, et al.: Increased Li/Na countertransport in patients with essential hypertension. New Engl J Med 302:772 (1980).
2. Garay RP and Meyer P: A new test showing abnormal net Na and K fluxes in erythrocytes of essential hypertensive patients. Lancet 1:349 (1979).
3. De Luise M, Blackburn GL, and Flier JS: Reduced activity of the red cell Na-K pump in human obesity. New Engl J Med 303:1017 (1980).
4. Yamori Y: Heredity of hypertension. In: Arterial Hypertension; (editors): F Gross and JS Robertson. Boston: G.K. Hall Medical Publishers (1980).
5. Pickering G: High Blood Pressure. London: JA Churchill, Ltd. (1968).
6. Report of the Hypertension Task Force, Pediatric and Genetic Subgroup. Vol. 6, NIH Publication No. 79–1628 (1979).
7. Platt R: Heredity in hypertension. Lancet 1:899 (1963).
8. Paul O: Epidemiology of hypertension. In: Arterial Hypertension; editors: F Gross and JS Robertson. Boston:GK Hall Medical Publishers (1980).
9. MacMahon B: Epidemiological approaches to family resemblance. In: Genetic Edpidemiology; editors: NE Morton and ChS Chung. New York: Academic Press (1978).
10. Canessa M, Bize I, Solomon H, et al.: Na countertransport and co-transport in human red cells: Function, dysfunction and genes in essential hypertension. Clin. Exp. Hyperten. 3:783 (1981).
11. Miall WE, Heneage P, Khosla T, et al.: Factors influencing the degree of resemblance in arterial pressure of close relatives. Clin. Sci. 33:271 (1967).
12. Annest JL, Sing ChF, Biron P et al.: Familial aggregation of blood pressure and weight in adoptive families. Am. J. Epidemiol. 110:479 (1979).
13. Rose RJ, Miller JZ, Gunn CE et al.: Aggregation of blood pressure in the families of identical twins. Am. J. Epidemiol. 109:503 (1979).
14. Stini WA: Association of early growth patterns with the process of aging. Fed. Proc. 40:2588 (1981).
15. Woods KL, Beeve DG and West M: Familial abnormalities of erythrocyte cation transport in essential hypertension. Brit. J. Med. 282:1186 (1981).
16. Cusi D, Barlassina C, Ferrandi M, et al.: Familial aggregation of cation transport abnormalities and essential hypertension. Clin. Exp. Hyperten. 3:871 (1981).
17. Garay RP, Hannaert P, Dagher G, et al.: Abnormal erythrocyte Na/K co-transport system: A proposed genetic marker of essential hypertension. Clin. Exp. Hyperten. 3:851 (1981).
18. Adragna N, Tosteson DC and Canessa M: Simultaneous measurements of red cell Li/Na countertransport and Na/K co-transport in patients with essential hypertension. VIII Scientific Meeting, International Society of Hypertension, Milan (1981).
19. Kotchin JM: Effect of relative weight on familial blood pressure aggregation. Am. J. Epidemiol. 105:214 (1977).
20. Garay RP, Nazaret C, Dagner G, et al.: A genetic approach to the geography of hypertension, examination of Na/K co-transport in Ivory Coast Africans. Clin Exp. Hyperten. 3:861 (1981).
21. Canessa M, Adragna N and Falkner B: Measurements of Na transport in red cells of Black patients with essential hyperytension. Fed. Proc., 41:1661 (1982).
22. Canessa, M., Adragna, N., Solomon, et al.: Red cell Na transport polymorphism and essential hypertension. Clin. Res., 30:334a, 1982.

23. Adragna, N., Ellison, C., Solomon, et al.: Intrafamilial correlation coefficients for Na countertransport and co-transport in essential hypertension. Clin. Res., 30:333a, 1982.

RED CELL SODIUM-LITHIUM COUNTERTRANSPORT IN HYPERTENSION

W. Burke, S. Hornung, B.R. Copeland, C.E. Furlong and A.G. Motulsky

INTRODUCTION

We are exploring the role of major genes in the pathogenesis of common diseases [1]. The role of heredity in control of blood pressure is evidenced by familial aggregations of blood pressure levels [2]. Correlations of systolic (S) and diastolic (D) blood pressure in identical twins (S: .55, D: .58) are significantly higher than among unidentical twins (S: .25, D: .27) [3]. Adoption studies suggest more resemblance between biologic sibs and their parents than between adopted sibs and their adoptive parents, suggesting that genetic factors rather than a common environment alone account for the familial aggregation of blood pressure levels [4].

Blood pressure is a graded trait. In population studies, no bimodality of blood pressure levels distinguishing normals from hypertensives can be discerned. To account for underlying genetic factors, it has been suggested that hypertension is a multifactorial trait caused by the interaction of an unknown number of undefined genes with various environmental factors [5]. Since it can be shown that a relatively small number of genes can produce bell-shaped distribution curves such as observed for blood pressure [6], it is worthwhile to search for identifiable genes that may be related to hypertension.

The demonstration of red cell membrane abnormalities affecting ion transport, which are correlated with essential hypertension, is an exciting lead for the genetic exploration of hypertension [7, 8]. Red cells can be obtained easily, and the red cell membrane may be a model for inherited membrane defects of vascular smooth muscle cells affecting electrolyte transport. Such defects may mediate vasoconstriction that causes hypertension [9]. We have used a sodium-lithium countertransport assay [8] to estimate the frequency of abnormal red cell countertransport in an unselected population and to assess whether this frequency changes with age.

MATERIALS AND METHODS

Countertransport assay

Assay of sodium-lithium countertransport in red cells was done by a method slightly modified from that of Canessa et al. [8] with incubations done at 37.8° C instead of 37° C. Blood (7 ml) was drawn into heparinized vacutainer tubes. Red cells were separated by centrifugation at 4° C (3000 g for 5 min), and all plasma and buffy coat were rigorously removed. The remaining packed red cells were incubated in a shaking-water-bath (40 oscillations/min) for 3 hours at 37.8° C in medium containing lithium chloride (150 mM), glucose (10 mM), TRIS [Tris (hydroxymethyl)aminomethane] (10 mM), and MOPS [3-(N-morpholino) propane sulfonic acid] (10 mM), pH 7.4 at 37.8° C.

Cells were then centrifuged at 4° C (7500 g for 2 min) and washed 3 times in a solution containing $MgCl_2$ (75 mM), sucrose (85 mM), TRIS (10 mM), MOPS (10 mM), ouabain (0.1 mM), pH 7.4 at 4° C (washing buffer).

A 1:1 dilution of washed red cells was made in washing buffer and maintained at 4° C. Part of this cell suspension (1.2 ml) was mixed with 4.8 ml of sodium-free medium containing $MgCl_2$ (75 mM), TRIS (10 mM), MOPS (10 mM), glucose (10 mM), sucrose (85 mM), and ouabain (0.1 mM). A second part (1.2 ml) of this cell suspension was mixed with 4.8 ml of sodium-containing medium containing NaCl (150 mM), TRIS (10 mM), MOPS (10 mM), glucose (10 mM), and ouabain (0.1 mM). Both media had a pH of 7.4 at 37.8° C.

These cell preparations were distributed into individual microcentrifuge tubes in 1- to 1.5-ml aliquots and incubated at 37.8° C without shaking. At 15-, 30-, and 45-minute intervals, tubes were removed, and cells were separated for 3 minutes in an Eppendorf microcentrifuge. The supernatant was removed carefully and transferred. Lithium was measured in supernatants by atomic absorption spectrophotometry (Hitachi Model 180-70). Standards contained lithium chloride (15–150 mM) in either $MgCl_2$ (75 mM) or NaCl (150 mM). The increase of lithium in the supernatant with time (expressed as mmol lithium/L RBC hour) was linear. Sodium-lithium countertransport was expressed as the difference between the slopes for the two incubation media used (sodium-free and sodium-containing).

Subjects

Subjects for the unselected population study were sought by notices announcing the opportunity to donate blood for unspecified research in the following locations: selected clinics and laboratories of the University of Washington Affilated Hospitals; two local residences for senior citizens; and in a downtown Seattle office building.

Each subject had his or her blood pressure measured, a brief family and personal medical history was taken, and blood was drawn for sodium-lithium countertransport measurements. Only data from Caucasian subjects were used.

Subjects were defined as normotensive if they had a diastolic blood pressure of 90 mm Hg or less, a mean arterial pressure of less than 110 mm Hg, and absence of hypertension in their personal history.

Subjects were considered hypertensive if they met any of the following criteria: (1) a personal history of hypertension and current treatment with antihypertensive drugs; (2) a personal history of hypertension, not currently on antihypertensive medication, with a diastolic blood pressure of more than 90 mm Hg and a mean arterial pressure of more than 110 mm Hg; (3) no personal history of hypertension but a diastolic pressure of more than 100 mm Hg and a mean arterial pressure of more than 110 mm Hg. A small number of subjects could not be definitively categorized as either normotensive or hypertensive and were termed 'borderline.'

In addition, we measured sodium-lithium countertransport in red cells of eight subjects enrolled in an experimental biofeedback program for control of hypertension. Based on blood pressure readings prior to the onset of the program, six of these subjects could be defined as 'hypertensive' by our criteria, and two were categorized as 'borderline.'

The data reported here include 120 normotensive subjects and 29 hypertensive subjects.

Normotensive subjects were further categorized according to their family history of hypertension: 25/120 or 21% were unable to give a family history; 46/93 or 49% had a positive family history, defined as having a first-degree relative with hypertension (parent, sib, or child); 16/93 or 17% had a negative family history, defined by the absence of hypertension or stroke in grandparents, parents, sibs, or children. An additional 17/93 or 18% had a negative family history, but did not know the health status of their grandparents; 16/93 or 17% had negative family histories except for the presence of hypertension or stroke in one or more grandparents.

RESULTS

Age and sex distributions for our subjects are shown in Table 1. Among normal subjects, we studied more females (73) than males (47). There was no significant difference (t test and regression analysis) in red cell Na-Li countertransport between males and females in all studied subpopulations (Table 2).

Table 3 shows the frequency of hypertension observed in unselected subjects (excluding subjects on biofeedback treatment). The prevalence of high blood pressure increased with age, and the frequencies observed were similar to those described in previous surveys [10, 11].

The results of red cell Na-Li countertransport of all subjects studied are shown

Table 1. Demography of study population

Group	No.	Male	Female	Age range	Mean age
Normals					
Age 20–39 years	66	27	39	20–39	29
Age 40–59 years	26	10	16	40–59	47
Age 60 and above	28	10	18	<60	74
Family history negative	16	8	8	21–50	34
Family history positive	46	13	33	22–81	38
Family history not fully available	58	26	32	20–86	44
Total	120	47	73	20–86	52
Hypertensives					
On medication	18	6	12	32–87	62
Off medication (unselected)	5	2	3	30–62	47
Off medication (biofeedback)	6	6	0	31–50	43
Total	29	14	15	30–87	55

Table 2. Red cell sodium-lithium countertransport (mmol lithium/L RBC/h). Lack of correlation with sex

		Means ± SD		
	No.	Males	Females	*t*-test
Normals				
Total	120	0.33 ± 0.11 (47)	0.32 ± 0.11 (73)	NS
Age 20–39	66	0.35 ± 0.11 (27)	0.34 ± 0.13 (39)	NS
40–59	26	0.34 ± 0.11 (10)	0.32 ± 0.09 (16)	NS
60-above	28	0.27 ± 0.09 (10)	0.30 ± 0.10 (18)	NS
Hypertensives				
Total	29	0.48 ± 0.15 (14)	0.56 ± 0.20 (15)	NS
Age 20–39	5	0.50 ± 0.20 (4)	0.58 (1)	–
40–59	13	0.48 ± 0.15 (8)	0.48 ± 0.16 (5)	NS
60-above	11	0.45 ± 0.02 (2)	0.61 ± 0.22 (9)	NS

Numbers in parentheses ( ) refer to total number in each subgroup.
NS: Not significant.

Table 3. Frequency of hypertension in unselected Caucasian subjects by age

Unselected subjects	No.	% Hypertensive
Age: 20–39	71	5.6%
40–59	39	20.5%
60-above	40	27.5%
Total	150	15.2%

in Figure 1 and Table 4. A highly significant difference ($P = 0.001$) between normotensive (0.33 ± 0.11) and hypertensive (0.52 ± 0.18) subjects was apparent, although significant overlap in countertransport status was noticed (Fig. 1). Borderline subjects (0.37 ± 0.06) were statistically indistinguishable from the normotensive group.

Table 5 shows results of countertransport determination for several hypertensive subgroups. There were no statistically significant differences between those on antihypertensive medication, those on no treatment, and those on biofeedback treatment. The mean values for countertransport, however, were somewhat lower for the biofeedback group.

Figure 2 shows subjects with negative and positive family histories (as defined in the section on Materials and Methods) in comparison to hypertensive subjects. The mean result for countertransport among normals with a negative family history was 0.30 ± 0.09 (SD). The mean value for countertransport among those

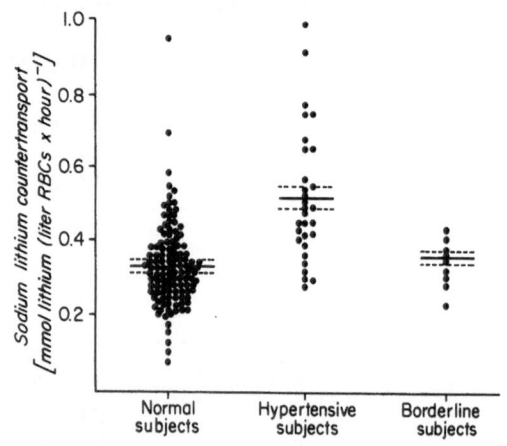

Figure 1. Comparison of sodium-lithium countertransport values for 120 normal subjects of all ages, 29 hypertensive subjects, and 9 borderline subjects. Mean values ± standard error of the mean (SEM) are indicated. For normal subjects, the mean ± SEM is .33 ± 0.01; for hypertensives, 0.52 ± 0.03; and for borderline subjects, 0.37 ± 0.02. (Standard deviations are given in Table 4.)

Table 4. Red cell sodium-lithium countertransport (mmol lithium/L RBC/h)

Blood pressure status	No.	Mean counter-transport ± SD
Normals	120	0.33 ± 0.11*
Hypertensives	29	0.52 ± 0.18*
Borderline individuals†	9	0.37 ± 0.06⁺

* P = 0.001 for normal vs hypertensive subjects.

† See Methods for definition of borderline hypertension.

⁺ P = 0.02 for borderline vs hypertensive subjects.

Table 5. Red cell sodium-lithium countertransport (mmol lithium/L RBC/h). Hypertensive subgroups

	No.	Mean counter-transport ± SD
On medication*	18	0.54 ± 0.16
Off medication (unselected)	5	0.53 ± 0.26
Off medication (biofeedback)	6	0.46 ± 0.17†

* 13/18 on thiazides; 5/18 on beta-blockers; 4/18 on triamterene; and 4/18 on other drugs (prazosin, reserpine, hydralazine).

† Difference not statistically significant (P = 0.34 for the biofeedback group compared with other hypertensives).

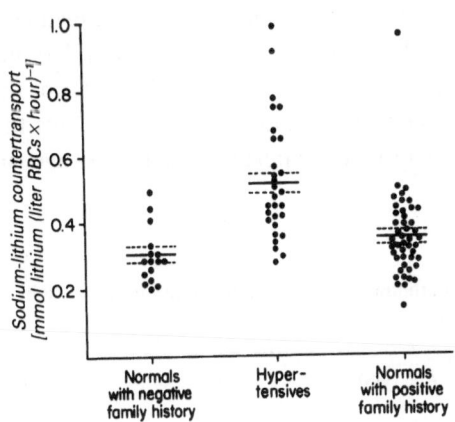

Figure 2. Comparison of sodium-lithium countertransport values for 16 normal subjects with negative family history, 29 hypertensive subjects, and 46 normal subjects with positive family history. Mean values ± standard error of the mean (SEM) are indicated. For normal subjects with a negative family history, the mean ± SEM is 0.30 ± 0.02; for hypertensives, 0.52 ± 0.03; and for normal subjects with a positive family history, 0.35 ± 0.02.

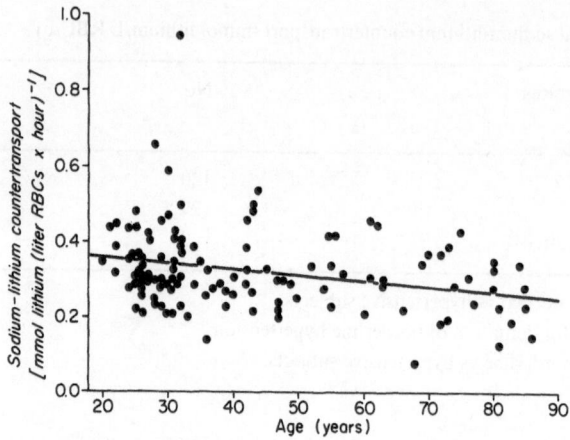

Figure 3. Plot of sodium-lithium countertransport versus age for 120 normal subjects. The slope derived from a regression analysis is shown; the value of the regression coefficient is 0.0015.

with a positive family history was 0.35 ± 0.13, suggesting weak statistical significance at a level of $P = 0.06$. Not unexpectedly, these data suggest that overlap in countertransport values between normotensive and hypertensive subjects may be decreased when only normotensive subjects with a negative family history are considered.

We also examined red cell countertransport as a function of age (Fig. 3). A regression analysis showed a significant decrease of countertransport with age ($P = 0.005$). This age trend could also be demonstrated by examining mean countertransport values at different age groups (Table 6). Normotensive subjects who were 60 years or older had a significantly lower mean countertransport than younger individuals without hypertension ($P = 0.02$). No such age-related differences could be seen among hypertensives: 0.49 ± 0.17 for those 20–39 years old, 0.48 ± 0.15 for those 40–59 years old, and 0.58 ± 0.21 for those 60 years old and above. Regression analysis for hypertensives against age (not shown) indicated

Table 6. Red cell sodium-lithium countertransport (mmol lithium/L RBC/h). Age group analysis of normal subjects

Group	Age (yrs)	No.	Mean Counter-transport $\pm$ SD
A	20–39	66	$0.35 \pm 0.12*$
B	40–59	26	0.33 ± 0.09
C	60-above	28	$0.38 \pm 0.10*$

* $P = 0.02$ for group A vs group C.

no relationship between age and countertransport among hypertensives.

We interpret these data to mean that some younger individuals who are not yet hypertensive have countertransport abnormalities. With advancing age, such individuals will no longer be included among normotensives, since they will have become hypertensive. Thus, an older normotensive group will be a more appropriate control group, since it is less likely to include prehypertensives with abnormal countertransport. Since mean countertransport falls with age in normal subjects, comparisons of older hypertensives with younger normal subjects (as we have done in our total populations) minimizes the real differences.

DISCUSSION

We have reproduced the observation of Canessa et al. [8] that mean red cell countertransport in hypertensive individuals is significantly increased. We have also shown that mean countertransport tends to be lower in normotensive individuals with no family history for hypertension when compared with normotensives who have a family history of hypertension. These results are expected if abnormal countertransport values would be found more frequently among normotensives with a family history for hypertension.

In keeping with the hypothesis that a high countertransport value may identify individuals who are likely to develop hypertension, we predicted that countertransport would fall with age in normotensive but not in hypertensive subjects. This relationship between age and countertransport could be clearly demonstrated (Fig. 3; Table 4). We suggest that the decrease in countertransport with age seen in the normotensive population represents the progressive loss of normotensive individuals who have become hypertensive. If this interpretation is correct, a 'high' countertransport value in a young normotensive individual suggests that such an individual may be at risk to become hypertensive in later life. The use of this laboratory assay for clinical prediction of hypertension is limited, however, by the overlap in countertransport values between normotensive and hypertensive populations. This overlap remains considerable even if observations are limited to normotensive subpopulations that are considered more appropriate controls than the normotensive group as a whole, i.e., normotensives with no family histories for hypertension or normotensives in older age groups (Fig. 4).

Several explanations can be postulated for this overlap. It is possible that some low countertransport values among certain hypertensive subjects represent undiagnosed secondary hypertension. Furthermore, high countertransport values in some normotensives with a negative family history may represent young individuals who will ultimately become hypertensive. High countertransport values in the older normotensive group could represent susceptible individuals who remain normotensive, perhaps because the necessary environmental factors

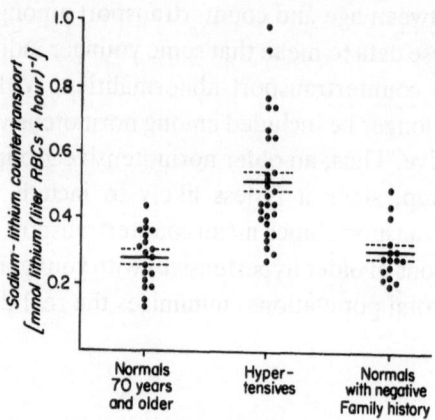

Figure 4. Comparison of sodium-lithium countertransport values for 19 aged, normal subjects (70 years and above), 29 hypertensive subjects, and 16 normal subjects with a negative family history for hypertension. Mean values ± standard error of the mean (SEM) are shown. For normal subjects aged 70 and above, the mean ± SEM was 0.28 ± 0.02; for hypertensives, 0.52 ± 0.03; and for normal subjects with negative family history, 0.30 ± 0.02.

for expression of hypertension are lacking. In addition, it is quite likely that essential hypertension is the end result of several pathophysiologic mechanisms. While a determinant affecting membrane transport may be an important underlying mechanism in many patients with hypertension, other mechanisms not affecting membrane transport may apply in a significant number of hypertensives. With this formulation, an unequivocal distinction between normals and all hypertensives could never be achieved.

These considerations make it difficult to set a definite cutoff value for countertransport values between normals and hypertensives. It can be estimated from our data, however, that the frequency of normotensive individuals with elevated countertransport values, in whom there is an increased risk for hypertension, is high – perhaps as high as 30–40% in an unselected population.

SUMMARY

Red cell sodium-lithium countertransport was determined among 120 normotensives and 29 hypertensives of European origin. Red cell countertransport was identical in males and females. Hypertensives had statistically significant increased countertransport when compared with normotensives. Normotensives with a family history of hypertension had higher countertransport values than those without such a family history.

Red cell countertransport among normotensives, but not among hypertensives, decreased with age.

These results are interpreted to mean that red cell Na-Li countertransport is abnormally elevated not only among hypertensives but also among some pre-hypertensive normotensive subjects. With advancing age, a significant number of prehypertensives become hypertensive and are no longer included when sampling aged normotensive individuals. This presumably accounts for the decline of countertransport with age.

ACKNOWLEDGEMENT

Aided by grant GM 15253 and fellowship AI 06058 to B.R.C.

REFERENCES

1. Motulsky AG: The genetics of common diseases, in Morton NE, Chung DS (editors): Genetic Epidemiology. New York, Academic Press, 1978, pp 541–548.
2. Murphy EA: Genetics in hypertension. Circ Res 32 + 33 (suppl 1):129, 1973.
3. Feinleib M, Garrison RJ, Fabsitz R, et al.: The NHLBI twin study of cardiovascular disease risk factors. Am J Epidemiol 106:284, 1977.
4. Mongreau J-G, Biron P, Bertrand D: Familial aggregation of blood pressure and body weight, in Levine MI, Levine LS (eds): Juvenile Hypertension. New York, Raven Press, 1977, p 39.
5. Pickering G: The inheritance of arterial pressure, in Stamler J, Stamler R, Pullman TN (editors): The Epidemiology of Hypertension. New York, Grune & Stratton, 1967, p 18.
6. Motulsky AG: Multifactorial inheritance and heritability in pharmacogenetics. Hum Genet (suppl) 1:711, 1978.
7. Garay RP, Elghazi J-L, Dagher G, et al.: Laboratory distinction between essential and secondary hypertension by measurement of erythrocyte cation fluxes. N Engl J Med 302:769–771, 1980.
8. Canessa M, Adragna N, Solomon HS, et al.: Sodium-lithium countertransport in red cells of patients with essential hypertension. N Engl J Med 302:772–776, 1980.
9. Garay RP, Dagher G: Erythrocyte Na$^+$ and Li$^+$ transport systems in essential hypertension, in Zumkley II, Losse H (editors): Intracellular Electrolytes and Arterial Hypertension. New York, Thieme-Stratton, 1980, pp 69–76.
10. Page LB: Hypertension and atherosclerosis in primitive and acculturing societies, in Hunt JC (editor): Hypertension Update. Bloomfield, NJ, Health Learning Systems, Inc, 1979, pp 1–10.
11. Harris L, et al.: The Public and High Blood Pressure, US Dept of Health, Education, and Welfare publication No. (NIH) 74–356, 1973, pp 80–86.

DISCUSSION

Discussants: Williams, Burke, Motulski, Devine, Haber, Abboud

Williams: Obviously our interests overlap considerably. You showed some differences between countertransport in individuals with a positive family history. Can I assume that those were all adults with a positive family history? Or have you looked at children with positive family histories too?

Burke: We have looked at no one under the age of 20.

Williams: O.K. Have you tried making your age correlation sex-specific?

Burke: I should have mentioned that. We've actually looked very carefully at whether there are any differences between sexes and we've done that in two ways. We've looked at all normals and all hypertensives – one sex compared to another – and we've also done that within each age group – 20 to 39, 40 to 59, and 60 and above. We find no significant difference, so that's actually a way in which our data diverge from yours. At no point do we see a significant difference between males and females.

Williams: Never?

Burke: Never.

Williams: You say that you feel that there's still evidence of a major gene effect. What evidence do you have that there's a major gene effect?

Burke: I didn't mean to imply that we see evidence. I only meant to imply – and I'm sorry if I over-represented – that we still feel that one can entertain that hypothesis – only, though, if one accepts that there are significant modifying factors and, clearly, those modifying factors could be genetic.

Williams: Suppose it's polygenic. What would that mean for your 2D electrophoresis?

Burke: It would be much harder to see something.

Motulski: I would like to stress the problems one faces in genetically oriented research on hypertension. We are looking at a 'quantitative' trait and are making arbitrary cut-offs in blood pressure levels beyond which we call some people hypertensives. This somewhat artificial dichotomization of the data is one of the major difficulties in this work. One can postulate that at this upper level of high blood pressure, there may be some major gene product involving ion transport that strongly affects blood pressure by a specific mechanism as discussed at this conference. Such a major gene hypothesis is in contrast to the concept that postulates the interaction of many undefined genes of small effect.

Concerning Dr. Williams' interpretation of the polygenicity of countertransport: Polygenicity can be mimicked if there is overlap between the effects of single genes such as multiple alleles, each with a characteristic quantitative effect. It is more difficult to work with a 'genetic marker' that is far removed from gene action. Unless a test can be found that is better than the test systems we are discussing today, genetic analysis will be difficult even if there is major gene action. However, should a major gene defect somehow be identified, one can go much further, such as isolating the gene. If it turns out that ion transport abnormalities in hypertension are the end effect of multiple genes influenced by the environment, the research and practical significance of ion transport abnormalities become less exciting. The challenge to me is that in common diseases there may be major genes involved. Hypertension is a good example, and the ion-transport systems we are discussing are good candidates for major gene action.

Devine: If identical twins have a correlation coefficient of .5 for blood pressure, doesn't that signifty that the genic involvement must be pretty major? Would you comment on that?

Burke: The caveat one would always have to throw in is that even though identical twins share a genotype, and almost certainly share environment, the classic study with identical twins separated by adoption, to control completely for environmental effects, versus nonadoptive twins, to my knowledge has not been done with hypertensives. However, I think that, in general, a correlation of .55 is suggestive that both environmental and genetic factors are important.

Williams: In Dr. Feinlib's *NHLBI* Twin study of about 500 twin pairs, analyses have been done with and without a correction for common environmental effects. In both cases, the estimated heritability was about 60 percent for systolic and about 40 percent for diastolic blood pressure. But, as was already pointed out in the previous presentation, that's looking at the genetics of blood pressure per se, not necessarily the genetics of hypertension. I'm very concerned, as are the Seattle group, that we may be dealing with two different things.

Haber: In searching for a specific gene product rather than screening all the proteins that are present in the membrane, would it not be more direct to go after the protein that might be involved in the actual process? Can you identify a drug involved in the particular co-transport system or sodium-lithium transport system you're looking at that might be the best candidate for binding to at least part of that channel, which then might be used in an approach to find the protein involved in the channel itself?

Burke: I agree with you that this is an approach that would be very effective. Dr. Furlong is actually investigating that and feels there may be a possibility of getting some, perhaps iodinated, compounds that would specifically bind to that sodium-lithium countertransport. That's at this point, as far as I understand it, in a pretty speculative stage, but I agree that would be a very effective method.

Haber: Well, which are the drugs?

Burke: I'm sorry I can't tell you the specific products.

Abboud: Do you think you might be able to separate the populations a little better by stressing the individuals with a sodium load? Does excessive sodium intake increase the countertransport, for example, and if it does would you be able to get better separation?

Burke: I think that's a very interesting question, and I'm sure a lot of people working in this area are interested in that kind of approach, to control in some way for salt intake. Most people on a normal American diet have a pretty impressive salt intake, of course. It may be that we're dealing with salt-loaded people in general. It's a more elaborate experiment to deliberately give people high-salt diets that you control and then measure urine sodium excretion, but it could be done. Another approach that we've considered is to try to isolate populations. Sometimes these are available in communal situations where certain kinds of strict health food laws are observed. Such populations are different from the typical American population in having very low salt intake, and we're interested in pursuing that possibility to see if mean countertransports are different.

HYPERTENSION: MULTIPLE MEMBRANE MALFUNCTIONS

D.F. Bohr, A.L. Harris, C.C. Guthe and R.C. Webb

INTRODUCTION

In the past decade, two major developments have focused research interest on the cell membrane for the role it may play in the pathogenesis of hypertension. One development is based on the finding that the sensitivity of vascular smooth muscle increases in experimental hypertension. This increase is due to an altered membrane function of this tissue [1]. It may be responsible for the increase in total peripheral resistance that causes the arterial pressure elevation. The second development is the evidence that the membrane abnormality in hypertension is present in many tissues [2, 3]. The membrane of the red blood cell has been mostly studied as a readily available marker for the disease and as a tool for study of the characteristics of the membrane malfunction.

This manuscript will present evidence supplementing both of these developments. It will conclude with arguments supporting the hypothesis that the membrane malfunction that really initiates hypertension is in a pressure-regulating center in the hypothalamus. Evidence will be drawn from each of the three common forms of experimental hypertension: genetic, renal, and mineralocorticoid. Cell membrane abnormalities, although they may differ with the form of hypertension, have been described for each. However, one defect that may be common to all is an abnormal relationship between the membrane and the calcium ion.

METHODS

Blood pressures

Blood pressures were measured indirectly by the tail cuff method. To do this, a Narco Pneumatic pulse transducer was recorded on a Grass polygraph. Triplicate readings were taken and averaged for each rat.

Red blood cells

Rats were anesthetized with 50 mg/kg of sodium pentobarbital i.p. The abdominal aorta was cannulated, and 10 cc of blood were drawn into a syringe containing 100 units of sodium heparin. It was centrifuged for 10 minutes at $1000 \times g$, and the plasma and buffy coats were removed. Red blood cells were washed three times at room temperature in physiological salt solution (PSS) containing (mM):NaCl, 140; KCl, 5; $MgSO_4 \cdot H_2O$, 1.22; $NaH_2PO_4 \cdot 7H_2O$, 1.19; $CaCl_2 \cdot H_2O$, 1.6; dextrose, 11.1; morpholino propane sulphonic acid, 20; fraction V bovine albumin (0.25%). The pH was adjusted at room temperature to 7.4. After each wash, the cells were centrifuged and the PSS discarded. Packed red blood cells, 1 or 1.5 ml, were resuspended in an equal volume of PSS in a 25-ml siliconized glass Erlenmeyer flask and incubated with gentle shaking to prevent sedimentation. Before and after incubation, hematocrit values were measured for each sample. After incubation, the samples were centrifuged and the incubation PSS separated for final Na^+ and K^+ concentration determinations. Final hemoglobin concentrations were also measured in the PSS. Ionic flux was measured as a change in the ion concentration (expressed as mEq/L packed cells/unit time) in the PSS and adjusted for red blood cell volume shifts as measured by hematrocrit changes. The following formula was used:

$$\text{IONIC FLUX} = \frac{[\text{ion}]a\,(1 - H_a) - [\text{ion}]b\,(1 - H_b)}{H_b}$$

where $[\text{ion}]a$ = ion concentration in the PSS after incubation
        $[\text{ion}]b$ = ion concentration in the PSS before incubation
and H_a = value of hematocrit after incubation
        H_b = value of hematocrit before incubation.

Hematocrits were determined using microhematocrit tubes centrifuged at $4500 \times g$ for 2 minutes.

Albumin and dextrose were added to the PSS to minimize hemolysis during the washing and incubation. The percentage of lysis was calculated by dividing the concentration of hemoglobin in the PSS after incubation by the hemoglobin concentration of the erythrocyte suspension in PSS before incubation. Hemoglobin concentrations were measured by the cyanohemoglobin method. Hemolysis rarely exceeded 1.3% and never exceeded 2.0%.

Vascular smooth muscle

Two-kidney one-clip (2K-1C) renal hypertensive rats were prepared with a silver block (0.2-mm slit) on one renal artery. Rats were used 3 to 4 months after this procedure at a time when their tail blood pressures exceeded 175 mm Hg. Control Sprague-Dawley rats had pressures below 130 mm Hg. All animals were killed by a blow to the head and aortae; mesenteric and tail arteries were excised. The arteries were stored in PSS and cut into helical strips, which were mounted vertically on a glass holder in a tissue bath containing PSS. The upper ends of the strips were connected to a force transducer, and the resting tension was adjusted to give a maximum active-force generation for each strip. The bathing medium was maintained at 37° C and aerated with a mixture of 95% O_2 and 5% CO_2. The pH of the solution was 7.4, and it had the following composition (mM): NaCl, 130; KCl, 4.7; NaH_2PO_4, 1.18; $MgSO_4 \cdot 7H_2O$, 1.17; $CaCl_2 \cdot 2H_2O$, 1.6; $NaHCO_3$, 14.9; dextrose, 5.5; and $CaNa_2$ EDTA, 0.03. Solutions of varying calcium concentrations were made by adding the appropriate amount of $CaCl_2$ to PSS, which had been made up without calcium.

The technique devised by Karaki et al. [4] was used to characterize the calcium storage sites responsible for the phasic response induced by norepinephrine in vascular smooth muscle in normotensive and in 2K-1C hypertensive rats. The technique is illustrated in Figure 1. Following stimulation of the muscle with a concentration of norepinephrine that gave a maximum response, this agonist was rinsed from the bath with calcium-free PSS containing 1 mM EGTA. After several rinses and 10 minutes exposure to this calcium-free solution, the vascular smooth muscle no longer contracted in response to this concentration of norepinephrine. After 10 minutes in this calcium-free solution, it was replaced with PSS containing calcium, ranging in concentration from 0.025 to 2 mM. These calcium-containing solutions were left in the bath for 5 minutes to 'load the calcium stores.' It was then again replaced with the calcium-free, EGTA-containing solution. After 1 minute, the vascular smooth muscle was again stimulated with a maximum concentration of norepinephrine. The magnitude of response was used as a measure of the amount of calcium that has been stored in the pool, which is available for norepinephrine stimulation.

The statistical significance was assessed by Student's t test. $P < 0.05$ was considered significant. Data are expressed as mean ±S.E.M.

RESULTS

Red blood cells

Preliminary studies demonstrated that the flux of sodium and potassium were significantly greater in red blood cells from spontaneously hypertensive rats (SHR) than they were from three stains of normotensive rats: Long-Evans (LE), Sprague-Dawley (SD), and Wistar-Kyoto normotensive (WKY) (Fig. 2). These studies were carried out at 4° C, and hence the fluxes were passive with Na^+ and K^+ moving down their concentration gradient.

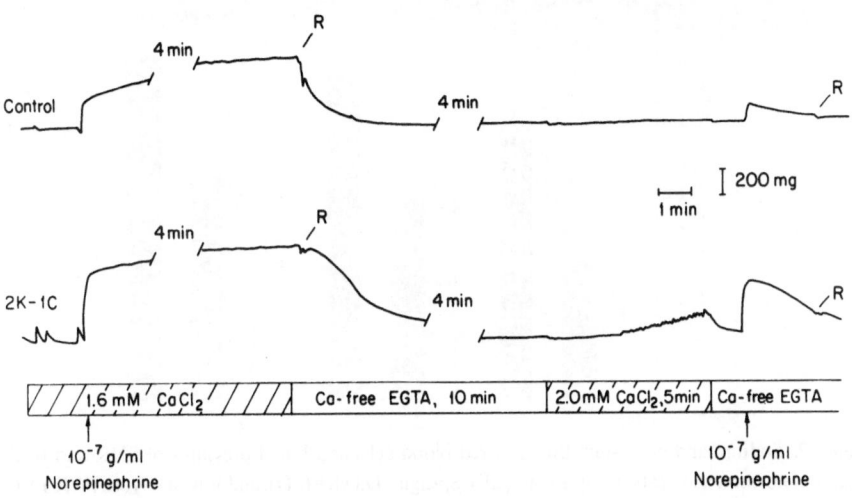

Calcium Store for Norepinephrine Response – Rat Aorta

Figure 1. Calcium store for norepinephrine response (aortic strips). Helical strips of aortae from normotensive control and 2K-1C hypertensive rats were made to contract in response to 10^{-7} g/ml norepinephrine in normal PSS containing 1.6 mM $CaCl_2$. After the contractile response had reached a plateau, the strips were placed in calcium-free PSS containing 1 mM EGTA for 10 min (depletion of calcium store). Following the calcium-free EGTA treatment, the strips were placed in normal PSS containing 2.0 mM $CaCl_2$ for 5 min (calcium loading). At the end of the calcium-load period, the strips were again placed in calcium-free PSS containing 1 mM EGTA (1 min), and 10^{-7} g/ml norepinephrine was added to the muscle bath. The magnitude of this second response to norepinephrine was larger (on a percentage basis) in aortic strips from 2K–1C hypertensive animals than in those from normotensive animals. Presumably, a store of calcium that can be mobilized by norepinephrine is filled during the loading procedure (5 min, 2.0 mM $CaCl_2$); this store is more rapidly filled in the aortic strips from hypertensive animals. Note that aortic strips from hypertensive rats contracted during the calcium-loading procedure, whereas those from normotensive rats did not (see Fig. 4). R = rise.

In Table 1 are presented the results of similar studies carried out at 37° C, in the absence and presence of ouabain. In control and ouabain-insensitive and sensitive fluxes, there was no difference in the red blood cells from SHR compared with those from the WKY. Since this was at variance with the observations made at 4° C, studies were next carried out at temperatures ranging between 4° C and 37° C, all in the presence of ouabain. This study demonstrated that as the temperature was cooled from 37° C to 15° C, the flux decreased. However, as the temperature was decreased from 15°C to 4°C, there was a reversal in this decrease so that the flux at 4° C was greater than that at 15° C. In Figure 3, it is demonstrated that whereas there is no difference between the red blood cell fluxes of SHR and WKY at 15° C, the difference is significant at 4° C.

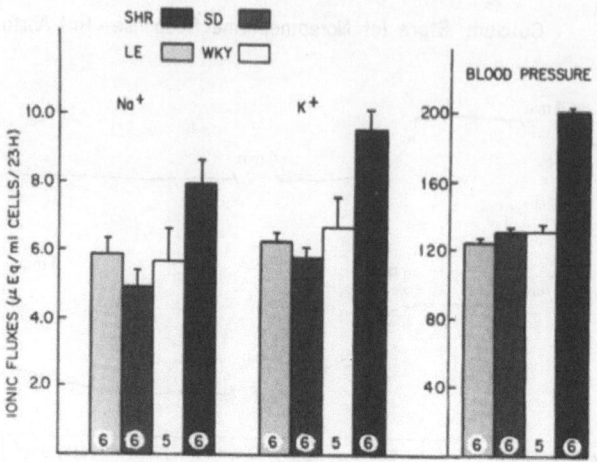

Figure 2. Sodium and potassium fluxes of red blood cells and blood pressures of SHR and of three strains of normotensive rats: Long-Evans (LE), Sprague-Dawley (SD), and Wistar-Kyoto (WKY). Cells were incubated for 23 hours in physiological salt solution (PSS). Fluxes represent the decrease in sodium and increase in potassium content of the PSS that occurred during this period. In all three parameters, the SHR is significantly greater. Data represent the mean and standard error of the number of animals indicated at the bases of the columns.

Vascular smooth muscle

Figure 1 illustrates the technique used to characterize calcium storage in vascular smooth muscle. In this experiment, aortic strips from a normotensive and from a 2K-lC hypertensive rat were mounted in the same bath. Following a 10-minute

Table 1. Sodium and potassium fluxes in red blood cells at 37° C. Negative numbers represent fluxes against concentration gradients. None of the flux differences between SHR and WKY are significant. Numbers range from 2 to 8 rats for each determination.

		Control Flux	Ouabain-Insensitive Flux	Ouabain-Sensitive Flux	Na:K of Ouabain-Sensitive Flux
CONTROL WKY	Na	− 2.26 ± 1.76	8.09 ± 1.00	− 10.35	1.56
	K	2.31 ± 0.21	9.86 ± 0.39	− 6.65	
SHR	Na	− 2.40 ± 1.15	7.67 ± 0.88	− 10.07	1.42
	K	3.46 ± 0.76	10.55 ± 0.53	−7.09	

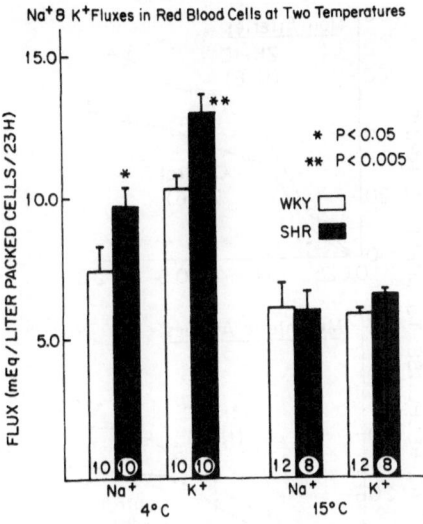

Figure 3. Passive fluxes of sodium and potassium in red blood cells from SHR and WKY at 4° C and 15° C in the presence of 3 mM ouabain. Fluxes of all cells are greater at 4° C than at 15° C. There is no difference between fluxes in cells from SHR and WKY at 15° C, but fluxes of both cations are significantly greater in red blood cells from SHR than from WKY when they are studied at 4° C. Columns represent mean fluxes with standard errors of the mean of the numbers of rats indicated at the base of the columns.

period of calcium depletion, they were exposed for 5 minutes to PSS containing 2 mM calcium. This solution was replaced with the calcium-free solution, and 1 minute later the strips were tested for the amount of available calcium by stimulation with a maximum concentration of norepinephrine. The response of the muscle from the hypertensive rat was clearly greater than that from the normotensive control. Results of these studies are summarized in Figure 4 for various loading concentrations of calcium in vascular smooth muscle from the three arteries. In every comparison, the magnitude of the response in this test of calcium loading was greater in the muscle from the hypertensive rats. The order of the magnitude of storage in the three vessels for both normotensive and hypertensive rats was: tail artery, mesenteric artery, aorta.

The possibility that the differences in these responses were due to differences in the rates of unloading calcium stores was tested by comparing contractile responses to norepinephrine of these muscles in calcium-free solution following the initial response to a maximal concentration of norepinephrine. Data quantifying these contractile responses indicate that there was no difference in rates of calcium depletion between the smooth muscle from control and 2K-1C rats.

Using this Karaki technique, there was a second interesting and striking difference between the vascular smooth muscle from the normotensive and hypertensive rats. After the initial 10-minute period in the calcium-free solution,

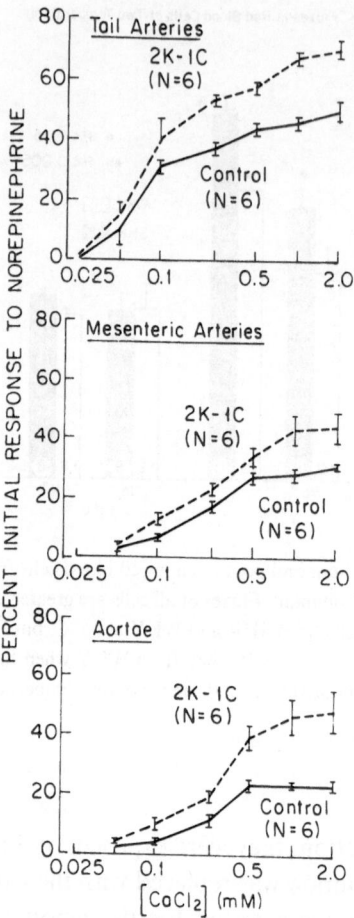

Figure 4. Calcium store for norepinephrine response: dose-response relationship. Helical strips of aortae and tail and mesenteric arteries from normotensive control and 2K-1C hypertensive rats were subjected to the procedure of calcium depletion and calcium loading as described in Figure 1. The concentration of calcium added back to the PSS during the loading procedure was varied from 0.025 mM to 2.0 mM. The magnitude of the norepinephrine response (expressed as a percentage of the initial response to nore-pinephrine in normal PSS, 1.6 mM $CaCl_2$) following the loading period was greater in arteries from hypertensive rats relative to that in arteries from control rats at all concentrations of calcium tested. Values are the mean ± S.E.M. for six normotensive rats and six hypertensive rats.

the vascular smooth muscle from the hypertensive rat contracted slowly on exposure to calcium; that from the normotensive control did not (Figure 1). A summary of this comparison is presented in Figure 5. The period in the calcium-free solution appears to have altered the membrane of the vascular smooth muscle from the hypertensive rat in such a way that it leaks calcium. The order of the magnitude of this leak in the three vessels is: aorta, mesenteric artery, tail artery. The leak does not occur in normal vascular smooth muscle.

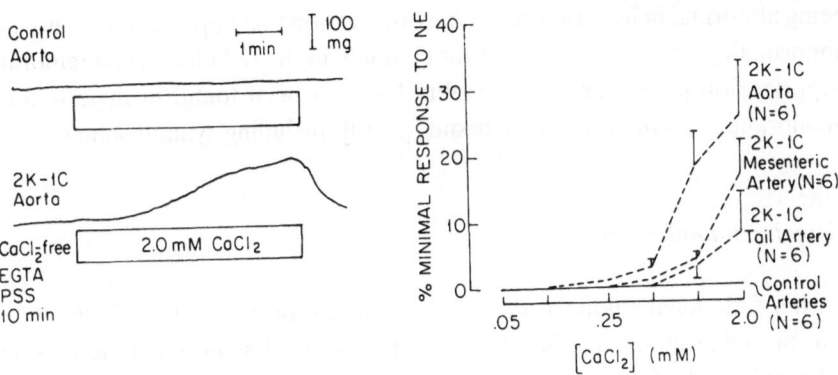

Figure 5. Contraction following exposure to calcium-free PSS, 1.0 mM EGTA. Arterial segments from 2K-1C hypertensive rats contracted in response to calcium following treatment with calcium-free PSS, 1.0 mM EGTA, whereas those from normotensive rats did not contract (left panel). The magnitude of the contractile response was greatest in aortic strips from hypertensive rats and least in tail arteries from these animals; mesenteric arteries were intermediate in contractile magnitude (right panel). Values are the mean $\pm$ S.E.M. for 6 hypertensive rats and 6 normotensive rats.

DISCUSSION

These observations form a basis for the consideration of three specific questions: 1) What is the nature of the generalized membrane change? 2) What characterizes the membrane change in vascular smooth muscle? 3) How might a membrane change initiate the hypertension?

Red blood cells

Results of the studies reported here confirm earlier work by Freidman et al [5]. They emphasize that there is a difference between the red cell membrane of SHR and WKY that can be unmasked by reducing the temperature to a level below 15° C. At these low temperatures, the membrane characteristics of both types of cells change so that fluxes to sodium and potassium increase. This change is significantly greater in the membrane from SHR. Livne (personal communication) has recently observed temperature-dependent differences between red blood cell membranes from patients with essential hypertension and those from normal subjects. Although the increase in permeability of the red blood cell membrane at low temperatures has been known for over 10 years [6], the molecular basis for the increase remains obscure. It does appear to be a substantial lead in the problem of understanding the membrane abnormality that is found in the red blood cell in hypertension.

Other studies have identified specific channels, such as the sodium-potassium co-transport system [7] or the sodium-lithium countertransport system [8], as being abnormal in hypertension. One observation that appears to be basic in this abnormality is a deficiency in calcium binding in the red blood cell membrane in hypertension [2, 9]. This abnormality has also been found in hypertension in membranes of numerous other tissues [3, 10], including synaptosomes.

Vascular smooth muscle

Earlier functional studies with vascular smooth muscle gave evidence that was interpreted as indicating that this tissue had fewer than normal binding sites for calcium in each of.the three types of experimental hypertension [11]. Calcium was less effective in stabilizing the membrane of this muscle from the hypertensive models than it was in stabilizing that from normal control animals.

In the studies reported here, two additional types of evidence are presented which indicate that the vascular smooth-muscle membrane from the renal hypertensive rat differs from that of its normotensive control. When the membranes of these muscle preparations have been sensitized by incubation in a calcium-free solution, those from the hypertensive animals leak calcium upon subsequent exposure to this cation; those from the normotensive control do not. It was also demonstrated that the muscles from hypertensive animals store calcium more readily in pools that are available for activation by norepinephrine. These differences are illustrated schematically in Figure 6. Both differences would be expected to cause vascular smooth muscle from the hypertensive animal to be more responsive and hence to cause a greater increase in vascular resistance than would the normal muscle. It is unlikely that these two abnormalities reflect a single defect, since calcium storage is greatest in the tail artery and least in the aorta (Fig. 4), whereas the calcium leak is greatest in the aorta and least in the tail artery (Fig. 5).

Possible membrane changes in hypothalamic centers

Studies of the red blood cell membrane in SHR have identified a possible marker for hypertension and an abnormal membrane that is readily accessible for study. The observed increase in leakiness to calcium of the vascular smooth-muscle cell membrane in renal hypertension has exemplified a possible mechanism for the increased sensitivity of this tissue in hypertension and hence for the increase in total periperal resistance. Finally, this discussion will review evidence relating to the action of mineralocorticoids on cell membranes. It will conclude by supporting a hypothesis that mineralocorticoids cause hypertension by their action on cell membranes in a hypothalamic center.

Calcium Handling by Membrane of Normal and Hypertensive Vascular Smooth Muscle

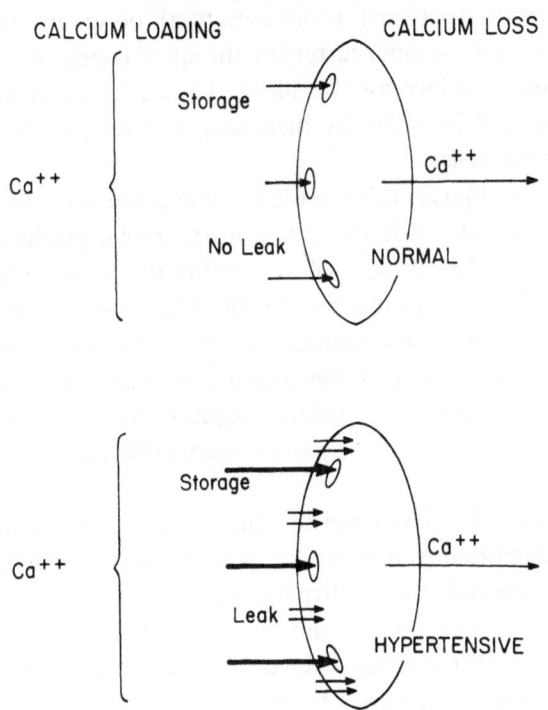

Figure 6. Schematic model showing differences between calcium handling by vascular smooth muscle of normotensive and of renal hypertensive rats. Storage of calcium in pools available to norepinephrine activation is greater in the hypertensive animal. The vascular smooth-muscle membrane of the hypertensive animal leaks calcium following a period of calcium depletion; that of the normotensive control does not. Rate of calcium loss of the cells from control and hypertensive is not diffferent.

A deficiency of calcium-binding sites is clearly implicated in the membrane abnormality of the red blood cell and of the vascular smooth muscle. The observation that there is a reduced number of calcium-binding sites on synaptosomal membranes from SHR [3] suggests that this calcium abnormality may also be implicated in the central nervous system in hypertension.

In 1958, Friedman and Friedman [12] studied the effects of aldosterone on human red blood cells loaded with sodium by 24 hour storage at 4°C. They observed net efflux of sodium after the cells had been rewarmed to 37°C. In untreated blood, there was a rapid increase in sodium concentration in the plasma, demonstrating the activity of the Na^+-K^+ ATPase sodium extrusion pump. In blood treated with aldosterone, there was an initial further *decrease* in plasma sodium before the onset of a gradual rise. Although these results could have been caused by an inhibition of the Na^+-K^+ ATPase by aldosterone, it seems more likely that the membrane permeability was increased by aldosterone, permitting further passive influx of sodium down its concentration gradient.

Recently, Dawson (personal communication) observed that aldosterone caused an increase in the sodium current on the apical membrane of the epithelial cell of turtle colon. This increase was blocked by amiloride, demonstrating that aldosterone produced its effect by increasing sodium channels in the apical membranes of these cells.

Petty, Kokko, and Marver [13] reported a similar action of aldosterone on the corticle-collecting tubule. Adrenalectomy in the rabbit produced an 86% decrease in Na^+-K^+ ATPase activity (Pi release) in this tissue. The decrease was reversed within 3 hours after treatment with aldosterone, yet this reversal was prevented when sodium entry through the luminal surface was blocked with amiloride. They concluded that the increase in Na-K ATPase activity with aldosterone 'appears to be a secondary adaption that is dependent on an aldosterone-enhanced increase in the passive entry of Na across the luminal membrane.'

Strong support can be developed for the possibility that mineralocorticoids have a similar membrane action on a hypothalamic center that is capable of causing hypertension [14]. DOCA hypertension does not occur in an animal in which this region has been treated with the neurotoxin, 6-OH dopamine [15] or when a localized AV3V region has been destroyed [16]. In DOCA hypertension in the pig, arterial pressure seems to be the regulated variable, since it is elevated in a very reproducible fashion, whereas its two determinants, cardiac output and total peripherial resistance, are highly variable in the contribution that each makes to the pressure elevation [17]. It is as if the mineralocorticoid has produced a resetting of a pressure-regulating center. In this animal there is a parallel resetting of the thirst center, which is evidenced by a marked increase in water turnover. Water intake increased from 4 L per day to over 20 L per day, while the mean arterial pressure rose from 100 mm Hg to 140 mm Hg.

The role of sodium in this resetting was evidenced by the parallel reversal of both the hypertension and the polydypsia when the pig was placed on a low-salt diet [18]. It is as if deoxycorticosterone had produced an increase in the sodium channels of the cell membrane in these centers, but when the animal was made sodium deficient, the resetting induced by the mineralocorticoid could not be sustained.

These arguments support the hypothesis that mineralocorticoids cause an increase in sodium channels of the membranes of the cells or hypothalamic pressure-regulation center as they are known to do in membranes elsewhere in the body. With this membrane change and sufficient body sodium, the set point of the center is raised to a higher level. Hypertension then develops because of altered activity of neural or humoral efferent systems regulated by this center.

ACKNOWLEDGEMENTS

This study was supported by a grant from NIH (HL-18575) and the Michigan Heart Association. R.C. Webb is a recipient of an RCDA (HL-00813).

REFERENCES

1. Webb RC, Bohr DF: Recent advances in the pathogenesis of hypertension: Consideration of structural, functional, and metabolic vascular abnormalities resulting in elevated arterial resistance. Am Heart J 102:251–264, 1981.
2. Devynck MA, Pernollet MG, Nunez AM, et al.: Analysis of calcium handling in erythrocyte membranes of genetically hypertensive rats. Hypertension 3:397–403, 1981.
3. Devynck MA, Pernollet MG, Nunez AM, et al.: Calcium-binding alteration in plasma membrane from various tissues of spontaneously hypertensive rat. Clin Exp Hypertens 3:797–808, 1981.
4. Karaki H, Kobuto H, Urakawa N: Mobilization of stored calcium for phasic contraction induced by norepinephrine in rabbit aorta. Eur J Pharmacol 56:237–245, 1979.
5. Friedman SM, Nakashima M, Rosemary AM: Glass electrode measurement of net Na^+ and K^+ fluxes in erythrocytes of the spontaneously hypertensive rat. Can J Physiol Pharmacol 55:1302–1310, 1977.
6. Wieth JO: Paradoxical temperature dependence of sodium and potassium fluxes in human red cells. J Physiol 207:563–580, 1970.
7. Garay RP, Dagher G, Pernollet MG, et al.: Inherited defect in Na^+, K^+-co-transport system in erythrocytes from essential hypertensive patients. Nature 284:281, 1980.
8. Canessa M, Adragna N, Solomon HS, et al.: Increased sodium-lithium countertransport in red cells of patients with essential hypertension. N Engl J Med 302:772, 1980.
9. Postnov YV, Orlov SN, Pokudin NI: Decrease of calcium binding by the red blood cell membrane in spontaneously hypertensive rats and in essential hypertension. Pflugers Arch 379:191–195, 1979.
10. Postnov YV, Orlov SN: Evidence of altered calcium accumulation and calcium binding by the membranes of adipocytes in spontaneously hypertensive rats. Pflugers Arch 385:85–89, 1980.
11. Holloway ET, Bohr DF: Reactivity of vascular smooth muscle in hypertensive rats. Circ Res 33:678–685, 1973.
12. Friedman SM, Friedman CL: Effect of aldosterone and hydrocortisone on sodium in red cells. Experientia 12:452–454, 1958.
13. Petty KJ, Kokko JP, Marver D: Secondary effect of aldosterone on Na-K ATPase activity in the rabbit cortical collecting tubule. J Clin Invest 68:1514, 1981.
14. Bohr DF: What makes the pressure go up? Hypertension 3 (suppl II):160–165, 1981.
15. Hauesler G, Finch L, Thoenen H: Central adrenergic neurons and the initiation and development of experimental hypertension. Experientia 28:1200, 1972.
16. Brody MJ, Fink GD, Buggy J, et al.: The role of the anteroventral third ventricle (AV3V) region in experimental hypertension. Circ Res 43 (suppl I):I-2.
17. Miller AW, Bohr DF, Schork AM, et al.: Hemodynamic responses to DOCA in young pigs. Hypertension 1:591–597, 1979.
18. Cohen DM, Grekin RJ, Mitchell J, et al.: Hemodynamic, endocrine, and electrolyte changes during sodium restriction in DOCA hypertensive pigs. Hypertension 2:490–496, 1980.

PRELIMINARY ANALYSIS OF SODIUM-LITHIUM COUNTER-TRANSPORT AND BLOOD PRESSURE IN UTAH PEDIGREES

ROGER R. WILLIAMS, STEVEN C. HUNT, MARY M. DADONE, SANDRA HASSTEDT, JEAN B. SMITH, K. OWEN ASH AND HIROSHI KUIDA

INTRODUCTION

Essential hypertension is a major health problem worldwide. It is one of the strongest and most prevalent risk factors leading to early heart attacks, strokes, kidney failure, and blindness. Prospective heart studies have indicated a gradient of increasing risk for coronary and cerebral vascular diseases, with some apparent increase at diastolic blood pressure (DBP) of about 85 to 95 mm Hg and dramatically increased risk for persons whose DBP exceeds 110 mm Hg [1]. Two large clinical trials have now documented a significant reduction in these problems when DBP is lowered to 90 mm Hg [2, 3].

Important questions need to be answered to further refine the definition of essential hypertension. Could further benefit result from lowering blood pressures to a DBP of 85 mm Hg? Do some individuals have 'normal blood pressure' in the sitting position but above normal levels when they are standing, walking, working, or exercising? What additional criteria for identifying persons with unhealthy blood pressure could be obtained from measurements taken during exercise, in the standing position, or during ambulatory blood pressure monitoring? These and other important questions are summarized in Table 1.

What causes essential hypertension? Family, twin, and adoption studies indicate that genetic factors play an important role in the control of blood pressure in the normal population. Heritability estimates of about 50% have been obtained for systolic and diastolic blood pressure [4]. Hypertension has been less well defined genetically. It has been shown to aggregate strongly among relatives of hypertensive individuals. Whether hypertension is a major gene or polygenic trait has been argued for many years. Good pedigree-analysis data are not yet available to answer that question.

Sodium intake has also been documented as a major factor [5]. It would appear that many individuals who get essential hypertension have a genetic predisposition that requires a high sodium intake for its expression. The exact pathophysiological mechanisms and biochemical factors involved are currently being investigated but are not fully defined. It seems likely that among the large number of individuals with essential hypertension, several major subgroups should emerge with distinguishing characteristics and distinct pathophysiologic and genetic mechanisms.

Table 1. Essential hypertension

1. What is it?	Organ damage
	Sitting DBP > 90 mm Hg
	Others BPs?
2. Causes?	Genes and environment?
	Pathophysiology?
	Subgroups?
3. Detect better?	Earlier?
	More accurately?
	Markers?
4. Treat better?	Tighter control?
	Better criteria?
	Tailored?
5. Prevent or delay?	Find predisposed?
	Modify risk?

Could new methods be devised for earlier and more accurate detection of hypertension? Data in this report indicate that some individuals with dramatic early expressions of the harmful effects of hypertension were treated for the hypertension only 4 or 5 years before the occurrence of early heart attacks and strokes. Other members of their families with suggestive indications of early hypertension are being followed by physicians but not treated, because sitting blood pressures are not always elevated (DBP>90 mm Hg on three visits).

It is possible that special blood pressure tests such as standing, ambulatory, or exercise measurements would help define individuals who need treatment at an earlier stage? Could cation flux tests or other biochemical measures help identify individuals with genetic predisposition to hypertension?

Might it also be possible to prevent problems by controlling blood pressure more carefully? Data from a clinical trial [2] indicate that carefully maintaining DBP below 90 mm Hg will prevent a substantial number of cardiovascular problems. Might criteria be established for even tighter control? Once pathophysiologic mechanisms are known, it is possible that treatment could be more specific and tailored to the exact type of hypertension detected. Special tests to evaluate patients already taking antihypertensive medication may help identify those who could now maintain healthy blood pressure without medication.

Ultimately, might it be possible to prevent or substantially delay the onset of hypertension? To do so will require reliable methods for finding those predisposed. Cation flux tests have provided one of the most promising avenues for detection of hypertension-prone individuals at an early stage so that the risk of hypertension could be potentially modified.

Answers to the above questions are being sought in a prospective study of members of pedigrees prone to hypertension in Utah. The data presented in this report represent a preliminary analysis of subjects screened during the first year of operation. Over the next 4 years, the sample size will be increased fourfold and subjects will have been screened twice, increasing the reliability of results obtained. Consequently, the information presented here is to be considered preliminary. These data are presented mainly to pose important questions for other researchers to consider and to document our approach. We describe the type of variables collected and type of analyses carried out to seek answers to the questions posed above.

METHODS

Study subjects were members of pedig. es prone to hypertension and its complications, including early strokes and heart attacks. Several large population-based files for Utah residents have been entered into a computer at the University of Utah, making it possible to identify new pedigrees to study or to extend those already identified. These files, as described in Table 2, include approximately 30% of current Utah adults and their ancestors extending back four to six generations. Linked to these massive computerized genealogies are death certificates for the entire state of Utah for a 20-year-period, of which 12,000 coronary deaths and 3,500 stroke deaths have been linked to pedigrees. Clusters of early atherosclerotic problems within the same pedigree identify interesting population-based kindred for detailed clinical studies.

A current study of hypertension-prone pedigrees will include a screening examination and evaluation for 2,500 individuals each screened twice by the end of 1985.

Results for 384 individuals studied so far are given in this report. For 181 individuals, the careful construction of pedigree information and analysis of sodium-lithium countertransport (SLC) within pedigrees are also presented. As

Table 2. Utah pedigrees in computer

---

1. 1.2 million persons in four- to six-generation pedigrees (1970–1960)
   over 90% of Utah residents from 1880 census
   About 30% of current Utah adults
2. 140,000 death certificates (1956–1975)
   12,000 coronary deaths in pedigrees
   3,500 stroke deaths in pedigrees
3. Screening hypertension-prone pedigrees
   2,500 twice each by 1985
   600 screened in 1981
   181 in pedigree analysis (half youth)
   302 adults in other analyses

Table 3. Subjects studied in Utah

Type of Subjects	Four Study Pedigrees	Other Adults	Total
Normotensive			
Youth (3–17)	82		82
Adults (18–82)	79	154	233
Hypertensive			
On Rx	10	20	30
Borderline	10	29	39
Total Studied 184 M, 200 F	181	203	384

shown in Table 3, most of the study subjects were healthy adults and youth, but as shown in subsequent pedigree examinations, a strong loading of atherosclerotic problems and hypertension in their pedigrees indicate that their future chance of these problems is markedly elevated.

Once living members of high-risk families were identified, they were contacted by phone and mail to inform them of the study objectives and to request their participation. Current participation rate is well over 90% of those invited. Participants were scheduled for clinic visits approximately 1 to 2 months in advance. To further prepare them for their visit, questionnaires were mailed to them and brief home visits were made to deliver and retrieve containers for the collection of three 12-hour overnight urine specimens.

During a clinic visit of approximately four to six hours, the individual questionnaires were collected and reviewed, and many additional data items were collected, as summarized in Table 4. Information from personal questionnaires,

Table 4. Variables collected in screening clinic (4–6 hours)

A. Personal questionnaire (114 items)

Identifiers	Genetic traits & illnesses
Demographics	Personality type
Socioeconomic status	Life stress
Religious activity	Menstruation, pregnancy, hormone use
Height & weight history	Diet, exercise, tobacco, alcohol
HBP Dx and/or Rx	Medications & hospitalizations

B. Genealogical charts (five generations, about 100 persons)
Names, dates, and places for eight nuclear families: own, parents, grandparents, great-grandparents

C. Medical family history (45-min. interview)
(for all 1st- and 2nd-degree relatives, 20–40 persons)

Vital status, sex	Cause & place of death
Age now or at death	Age at first detection of:

Table 4. Continued.

	Marriage & offspring	CHD HBP Breast CA
	Weight & smoking status	CVA DM Other CA
		Any major illness
D.	Fasting blood & plasma tests (24)	
	Chloresterol	19 standard chemistries
	Triglycerides	Hematocrit
	HDL	Plasma renin
E.	Erythrocyte tests	
	Li-Na Countertransport	
	Intracellular Na, K, & Li (pre-load & post-load)	
	'Sodium slope'	
	'Magnesium slope'	
F.	Three 12-hour overnight urine tests (9)	
	Volume, specific gravity	
	Na, K, creatinine,	
	Hb, protein, glucose,	
	Kallikrein, calcium	
G.	Blood pressure & heart rates (21)	
	(systolic, 4th & 5th phase diastolic)	
	Lying (2)	Tilted 50° (5)
	Sitting (6)	Grip 2 min. (2)
	Standing (2)	Blood draw (3)
	Pulse obliteration (1)	
H.	Clinic measurements	
	Height	Standard ECG
	Weight	32 lead surfacemap ECG
	Abdominal girth	Grip strength
	Skinfolds (3)	
	Wrist	
I.	Physician's history and physical exam	
	Cardiovascular disease	Heart & lungs
	Other major illnesses	Funduscopic
	Medications	Pulses
	Family history review	
J.	Tests to be added this year	
	Na-K Co-transport	
	Ouabain binding	
	Blood pressure & pulse during:	
	Bicycle ergometer exercise	
	24-hour Holter monitor (8 per hour)	

genealogical charts, medical family history, blood analyses, urine tests, and clinic measurements were carefully recorded on standardized forms for entry into a Data General computer system dedicated to medical genetic studies at the University of Utah. Statistical analyses were carried out using extracts of standard statistical software packages (BMD), and genetic analyses were executed using programs and methodologies specifically developed at the University of Utah [6, 7].

A laboratory for the determination of SLG has been established by Dr. Smith and Dr. Ash at the University of Utah with extensive help from Dr. Canessa at Harvard. Details of the procedure as it is currently employed are summarized in Table 5. Water-bath temperature appears to be the most critical variable influencing the outcome of the tests. Length of lithium-loading time can also have some influence on the results. As indicated, samples drawn from the same subjects show good reproducibility, and results from Utah correlate well with the results from Boston using duplicate samples. There was a slight but consistent bias (Utah results consistently lower than Boston results).

To maintain laboratory standardization, a control subject whose blood had been previously analyzed, was reanalyzed with each set of determinations. It had been initially hoped that a frozen unit of blood could be used to serve as a laboratory standard control. As indicated in Table 5, freezing red blood cells markedly increased the lithium leak and resulted in an unreliable SLC value after less than one month of frozen storage.

Most blood pressure measurements were recorded using an automated infrasound blood pressure recording device. Korotkoff sounds were recorded visually on a disk and all read by the same technician after the subjects had left the clinic. The deflation rate of the blood pressure cuff was maintained at a 2-mm drop per heart beat to allow the measurement of blood pressures within an accuracy of ±2 mm Hg. To allow direct comparisons of the automated device (Physiometrics SR 2) with ordinary blood pressure measurements, two readings were taken with a mercury manometer just before and after two readings with the automated machine in a stable sitting condition. Comparison of these blood pressure determinations in 302 adults showed DBP readings from the automated device were

Table 5. Na-Li countertransport laboratory in Utah

A. Procedure specifications
    1. Laboratory RBC concentration of 7%
    2. Lithium-loading time of three hours
    3. Supernatant [Li$^+$] measured at 29, 40, 60 minutes
    4. Slopes from three points at each time
    5. Temperature maintained at 37.0 ± 1.0° C
    6. Five washes
B. Reproducibility
    1. Within 53 subjects, two to four tests each, 9.2% coefficient of variation
    2. For 10 samples, simultaneously tested, Utah 11% lower than Boston*
    3. Retested RBCs after freezing:
       1 day, 5% increase
       9 days, 2% decrease
       26 days, 42% decrease
       (much hemolysis, marked lithium 'leak')

---

* This difference was not statistically significant.

118

consistently 5 mm lower than those from ordinary auscultation with the mercury manometer. All blood pressure results of this analyses were adjusted for this difference by adding 5 mm to the fourth-phase DBP obtained from the infrasound device. This difference is not surprising, since the automated device uses a sensitive microphone with an automatically adjusted amplifier and detects sounds below the audible frequency range. This feature allows the device to obtain good diastolic readings in small children, which is not possible with ordinary auscultation. Getting accurate blood pressures from small children is important in these pedigree studies.

RESULTS

Diastolic blood pressure and countertransport

In Table 6, subjects are classified into three groups according to their history of blood pressure diagnosis or treatment. Subjects in Group 1 were on drug treatment for high blood pressure (HBP). The second group is labeled borderline blood pressure (BBP). Subjects in this group had been told by a physician that their blood pressure has been high at times, but they have not been given consistent long-term treatment. None of them were on drug treatment at the time of this study. Subjects in the third group were classified as normal blood pressure (NBP) and had never been told by a physician that their blood pressure was elevated.

Table 6. Possibilities for better Rx and Dx

Groups	N	Sitting DBP > 90	Standing DBP > 95*
1. HBP on RX	30	33%	13%
2. BBP by Hx	39	26%	13%
3. NBP by Hx	233	6%	8%

* This column indicates percent of subjects with *sitting* DBP < 90 mm Hg, but *standing* DPB > 95 mm Hg.

Rx = drug treatment
Dx = diagnosis
DBP = diastolic blood pressure
HBP = high blood pressure
BBP = borderline blood pressure
NBP = normal blood pressure
Hx = history

In Table 6, the average fourth-phase DBP for each group was derived from six measurements in the sitting position for each subject. A substantial proportion of treated and border- line hypertensives showed diastolic pressures in excess of 90 mm Hg. Approximately half of these elevated DBPs exceeded 95 mm Hg. Previously undetected hypertension was found in 6% of the remaining 233 adults. Standing DBP (two readings after two and four minutes standing) showed an average value 5 mm higher than the average sitting blood pressure in these 302 adults. Some individuals with normal sitting blood pressures showed an exaggerated increase in DBP upon standing.

The frequency of such individuals (DBP <90 mm Hg sitting, but >95 mm Hg standing) is indicated in Table 6. A higher frequency among known hypertensives suggests that standing blood pressure measurements could possibly become a method for detecting a form of clinically significant hypertension that is undetected by the usual sitting blood pressure evaluation. Careful studies are needed to evaluate the risk of atherosclerotic disease in such individuals.

Significantly higher SLC was found in hypertensives as shown in Table 7. Significantly higher SLC was also found in borderline hypertensives (as defined previously). Woman with a history of pregnancy-induced hypertension (PIH), who were normotensive at the time of screening, did not have higher SLC values

Table 7. SLC and BP in 302 Utah adults

Subjects	N	$\bar{X}$ Age	SLC		$\bar{X}$ DBP	
			$\bar{X}$	400+	Sit	Stand
1. HBP on Rx	30	50	315**	27%	87**	89**
2. BBP no Rx	39	44	299*	18%	80*	86*
3. Hx of PIH	11	33	265	9%	72	84
4. Normal BP	222	22	263	9%	74	80
Ages 45–82	51	56	267	10%	78	82
Ages 18–44	171	28	262	8%	73	80

* P<.01
** P<.001 vs. all normotensives

SLC = sodium lithium countertransport (μmol/RBC/h)
BP = blood pressure
N = number of subjects
$\bar{X}$ = mean
DBP = diastolic blood pressure
HBP on Rx = high blood pressure by history on treatment now
BBP no Rx = history of possible hypertension or borderline but not on treatment now
Hx of PIH = history of pregnancy-induced hypertension (normal BP when screened)

120

as compared with other normotensive adults. Values above 400 μmol/L RBC/h were found in 27% of hypertensives, 18% of borderline hypertensives, and 8 to 10% of normotensives.

It should be remembered that the normotensive patients in this study are members of hypertension-prone pedigrees. Since most hypertensives in this study do not have SLC values above 400, it would seem that either a lower borderline is required for an abnormal test or many hypertensives in our pedigrees did not have hypertension related to countertransport. It is also possible that facticiously low SLC values could have resulted from confounding variables such as drug treatments or disease status.

Mean DBPs were significantly higher in treated hypertensives and borderline hypertensives as compared with normotensives. It would be important to determine if these differences in blood pressures between treated hypertensives and normotensives are also associated with a residual increase in disease risk for hypertensives that could be potentially lowered if more aggressive treatment were to produce blood pressure levels equivalent to those seen in normotensives.

The drugs taken by the treated hypertensives are summarized in Table 8 together with the SLC values for those patients. While no distinct pattern is obvious, it seems possible that some of these antihypertensive medications could

Table 8. SLC values of hypertensives on medications

Medications	SLC Values				
1. Thiazides	530	450	333	330	235
	267	220	170	140	
2. Methyldopa	340 (1)	290 (5)			
3. Propranolol	500 (8)	420 (1, 9)	310	205	
4. Triamterine	380 (1)	320 (1)	287 (1)	150 (12)	
5. Chlorthalidone	440 (10)	395 (9)	320 (12)	290 (2)	210
6. Rauwolfia	398 (1)	190 (1)			
7. Spironolactone	281 (1)	254	140		
8. Furosemide	500 (3)				
9. Prazosin	420 (1, 3)	395 (5)			
10. Digoxin	440 (5)				
11. Zaroxolyn	265				
12. Metoprolol	358 (1)	320 (5)	150 (1, 4)		

Individual values for sodium-lithium countertransport (SLC) are listed for 30 subjects taking antihypertensive medications. The value of SLC is listed twice for patients on two medications except thiazides.

Numbers in parentheses indicate the number on this list of the other drug taken simultaneously. SLC values are sorted from highest to lowest to demonstrate the full range of values observed for subjects taking each medication.

influence SLC values. Several of the hypertensive subjects listed in Table 8 have quite low SLC values. The same variations of high and low values are also seen among the untreated borderline hypertensive subjects.

'Pondering the pedigrees' – visual inspection

Pedigree diagrams have been constructed and analyzed for 181 subjects in four pedigrees illustrated in Figures 1–4. Kindred 500 is displayed in Figure 1. The founding sibship contains 11 individuals labeled with the letters A–K. Five brothers and one sister had early heart attacks (D, E, G, H, I, K). Five of these six affected individuals had high blood pressure, as did two additional siblings.

In this pedigree, hypertension seems to have a severe level of onset at an early age. Person D had hypertension diagnosed at age 32 with DBPs above 110 mm Hg and had his first myocardial infarction at age 35. Brothers K and J had DBPs of 110 and 120 mm Hg, respectively, when first diagnosed at ages 38 and 45. It is interesting to note that none of these men had their hypertension detected and treated more than 4 years before the first myocardial infarction. Several of their offspring with borderline hypertension are currently being followed without treatment. It seems possible that more aggressive blood pressure treatment might be indicated in a setting such as this where the consequences seem to be so grave.

After screening 92 members of this high-risk pedigree, the only common risk factor found for coronary heart disease (CHD) was early, severe hypertension. The only individual (I) who had a heart attack without known hypertension did not have his blood pressure checked from age 20 until he had his first heart attack at age 42. It is possible that he had hypertension which was not manifest after his myocardial infarction due to decreased function of the left ventricle. This individual's son was known to have hypertension at age 25. For those affected siblings and descendants who have been screened, blood cholesterol levels were low normal, HDL was normal, and no diabetes was detected; none of those screened individuals with early myocardial infarction were cigarette smokers.

Visual inspection of SLC values in Kindred 500, including three generations (25 sets of parents with their offspring and 20 sibships with two or more siblings), fails to provide striking evidence for an obvious genetic mechanism.

Kindred 221 is illustrated in Figure 2. The founding mother had hypertension and an early cerebrovascular accident (CVA). Of six offsprings in Generation II, three have hypertension, all taking medication. In Generation III, one 30-year-old male with hypertension is being treated with dietary sodium restriction.

Persons A and B have informative matings with contrasting high, medium, and low values. All but one of the offspring have values that are intermediate. When offspring values approximate the midparent average values, a polygenic model is often suggested. Certain major gene models, such as additive or codominant models, could also be compatible with this finding.

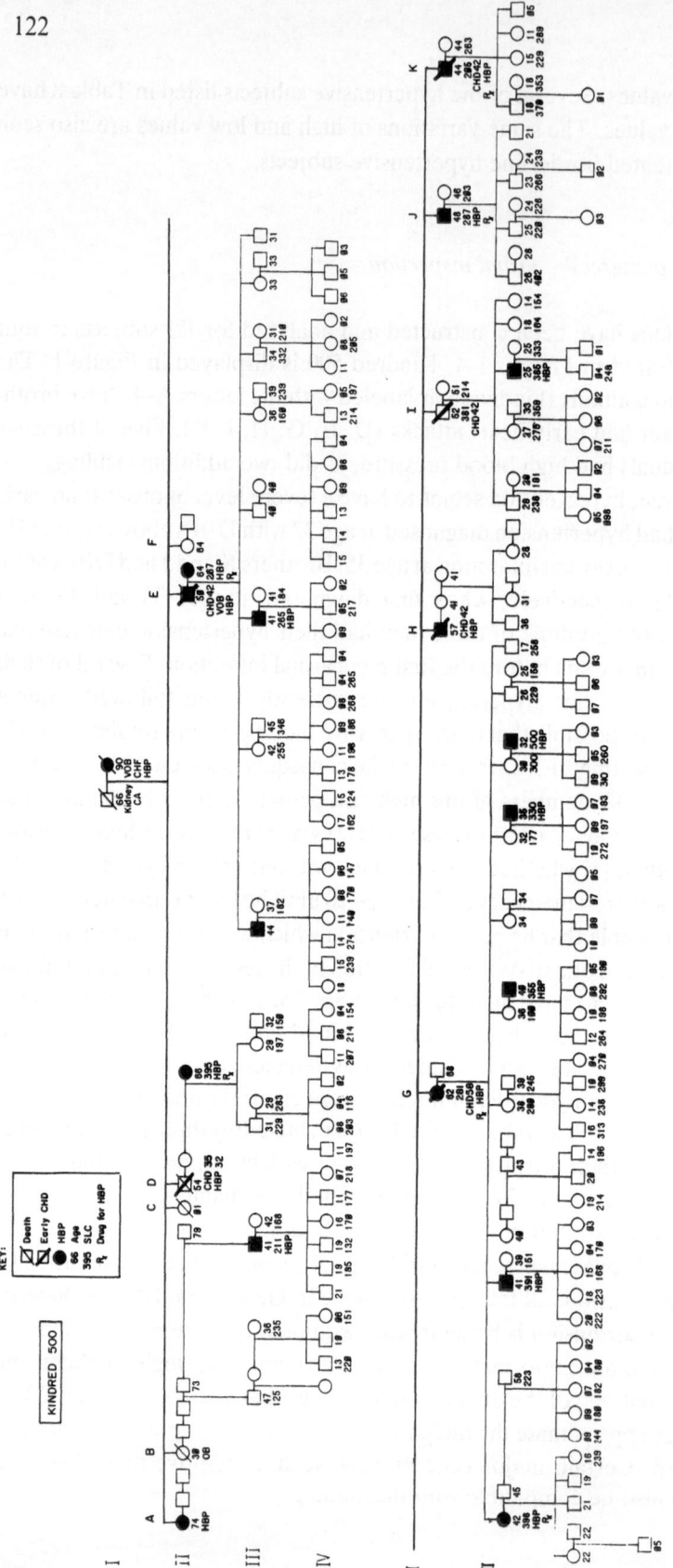

Figure 1. Computer-drawn pedigree diagram for Kindred 500. The letters A–K index the members of a single sibship. As indicated in the key, symbols notate deaths, early coronary heart disease (CHD), high blood pressure (HBP), the current age if living, or age at death. Other conditions are cancer (CA), obstetrical death (OB), very obese (VOB), congestive heart failure (CHF), and drug treatment for hypertension (Rx). A three-digit number below the age indicates the subject's value for sodium-lithium countertransport (SLC) as described in the text.

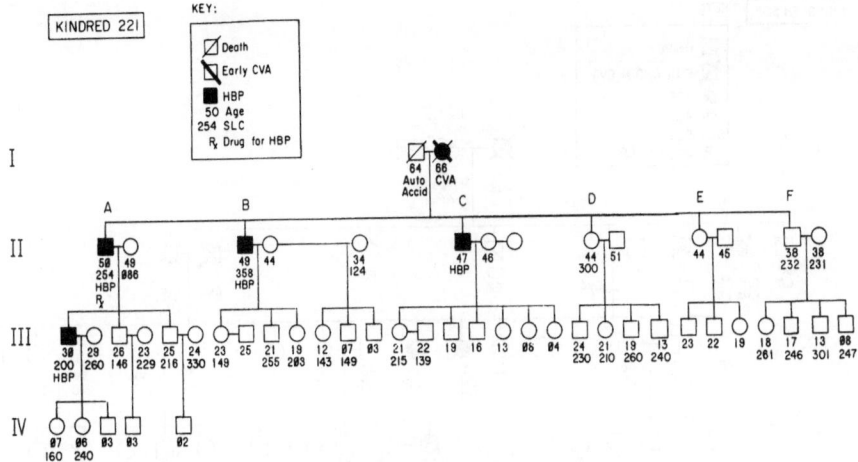

Figure 2. Computer-drawn pedigree diagram for Kindred 221. CVa = cerebrovascular accident. Other abbreviations as in Fig. 1.

Kindred 501 (Figure 3) shows an early stroke death in Generation I (founding mother), an early coronary in her daughter, and medicated hypertension in her grandson. His somewhat high value and his wife's very low value are associated with very low values in four children and average values in one. This could be related to a major gene for very low values or possibly lack of expression of high values in younger individuals.

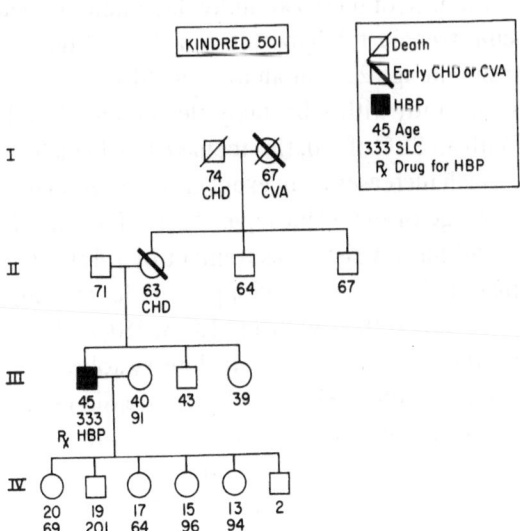

Figure 3. Pedigree diagram for Kindred 501. Abbreviations as in Fig. 1.

124

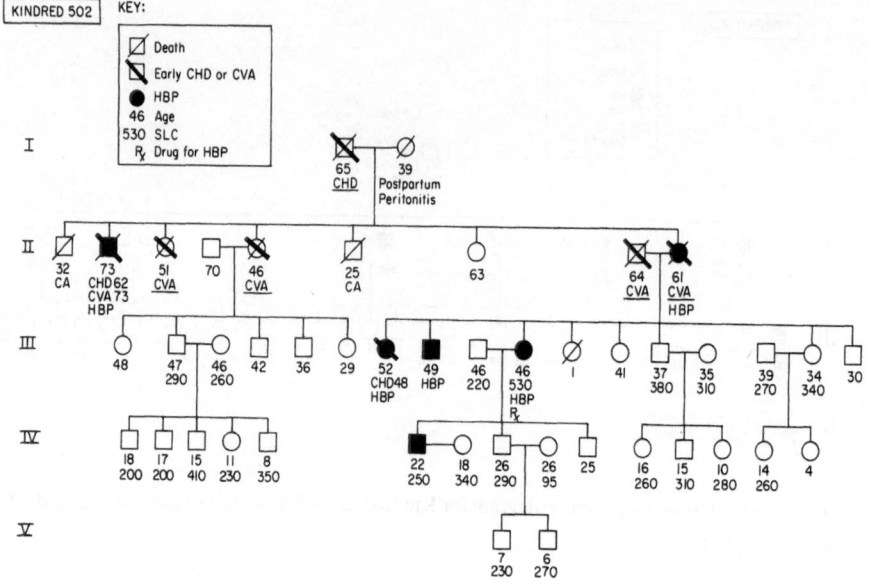

Figure 4. Pedigree diagram for Kindred 502. Abbreviations as in Fig. 1.

In Kindred 502 (Figure 4), the founding father died of early coronary disease and four of his seven children died of early strokes. The last daughter and her husband both died of early strokes. Three of their seven adult offspring have hypertension, and one daughter suffers from angina since age 48. Her 49-year-old hypertensive brother, also has some chest pains. Some kidney problems seem to have been suspected for each of these two individuals and for their mother. Their sister at age 46, being treated for hypertension, has a high SLC; her son has borderline hypertension at age 22, but an average SLC.

The only youth in our study with a distinctly elevated SLC is a 15-year-old male in Generation IV. With an SLC of 410, this teenage boy has a fourth-phase sitting DBP of 73 mm Hg, which increases in an exaggerated fashion to 87 mm Hg in the standing position (average of two values over four minutes). He is six feet tall, weighs 222 pounds, and has a wrist measurement of 7.4 cm (large frame). This height and weight places him above the 95th percentile, as compared with other men his age. His 8-year-old brother, with an SLC of 350, is also tall and heavy for his age (93rd percentile) but has relatively low systolic and diastolic blood pressures (below 20th percentile). His blood pressure did increase considerably under the psychological threat of blood drawing and after two minutes of isometric handgrip exercise. His DBP was 89 and 92 mm Hg in these two settings, compared with a resting DBP of 48 mm Hg.

The parents of these two young men have relatively average SLC values, and both are overweight. The father is 85 pounds above ideal weight, and the mother is 47 pounds above ideal weight. The father has a large frame like his son (wrist, 7.4 cm), is 5 feet 7 inches tall, and weighs 242 pounds. The mother is 5 feet 6 inches tall and weighs 187 pounds. It is interesting to note that the 15-year-old son is already 5 inches taller than his tallest parent.

Formal (mathematical) pedigree analysis

In an attempt to test for genetic heterogeneity, the first large pedigree (Kindred 500) consisting of 92 members was compared with a combined group of the remaining three pedigrees consisting of 46 members and with the 43 spouses from all four pedigrees. The frequency distribution of subjects by SLC levels within those groups and subdivided by youth, normotensive adults, and hypertensive adults is presented in Figure 5. The middle of seven categories of SLC levels is shaded in dark contrast to allow visual comparison between groups.

Half of the hypertensive adults were in the upper three categories of SLC levels, and the other half were in the average and lower categories. Most of the

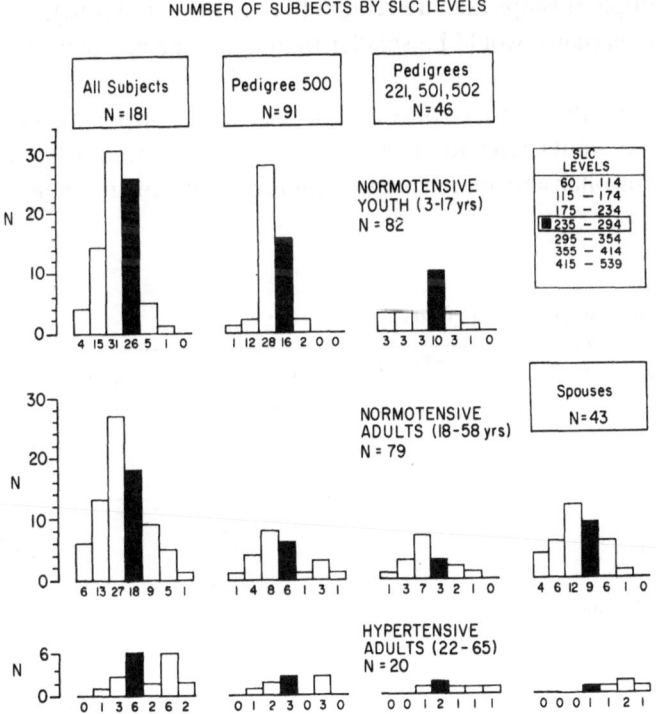

NUMBER OF SUBJECTS BY SLC LEVELS

Figure 5. The frequency distribution of subjects by sodium-lithium countertransport (SLC) divided into seven levels. To facilitate visual comparison of distributions, the middle level of each group is shaded.

average and low values came from Kindred 500, whereas both spouses and members of the other three pedigrees showed a larger proportion of hypertensives with values in the higher categories. Normotensive youth seemed to show fewer high values than normotensive adults. Three fourths of these youth, however, were from pedigree 500; this may be a phenomenon specific only to this pedigree.

The correlation of SLC values between pairs of relatives is summarized in Table 9, with separate results for Kindred 500 versus the other three combined as a group. Again, an interesting contrast is seen between these two groups. Mild, positive correlations are generally seen in Kindred 500, while strong positive correlations are seen in the others.

Since these sib-sib and parent-offspring pairs were derived from the same pedigrees, they are related rather than independent pairs. This lack of independence could produce correlation coefficients quite different from those that would be obtained from independent pairs of siblings or parents with their offspring. If there is strong, familial aggregation of a factor, one would generally expect the correlation coefficient to be falsely depressed and the spouse-spouse correlation to be inverse even if no association existed between spouses.

The correlation coefficient is a reflection of the ratio of variance between test pairs compared to the variance within test pairs. Sampling from a single pedigree produces multiple sibships that are related to each other (cousins), and thus the between-pairs variance would be smaller than that expected between independent sibships.

In like manner, the spouse-spouse correlation for spouse pairs sampled from a single pedigree would tend to show a false inverse association if the trait is genetically controlled and not related to common spouse environment or assorta-

Table 9. Correlations of SLC in Utah families

Relative pairs	Correlation Coefficients	
	Pedigree 500 (N = 114)	Other Pedigrees (N = 67)
1. Parent – son	.13 (60)	.26 (40)
2. Parent – daughter	.12 (85)	.36 (27)
3. Midparent – son	.18 (26)	.44 (18)
4. Midparent – daughter	.21 (37)	.69 (12)
5. Sibling – sibling	.08 (20)	.60 (13
6. Spouse – spouse	−.13 (20)	−.32 (11)

Pearson correlation coefficients for number of pairs is indicated in parentheses after each r-value and for parent-offspring and spouse-spouse comparison. Intraclass correlation for number of sibships is indicated in parentheses after r-values for sib-sib correlation.

tive mating. Since the members of the spouse pair are not related to each other, they would tend to have a large within-pair variance. Yet, because members of multiple spouse pairs are brothers and sisters from a given pedigree, the between-pair variance would be even smaller than the within-pair variance. As shown in Table 6, this phenomenon was observed for both groups. In this setting of spouse pairs drawn from the same pedigrees, one would expect a highly genetic trait to show a strong, inverse correlation between spouses. Thus, a higher inverse correlation between spouses in the second group is consistent with higher correlation among blood relatives when compared with the first group.

Table 10 presents the results of maximum-likelihood pedigree analysis of SLC in these two groups of Utah pedigrees. This methodology is an extension of segregation analysis and uses an iterative approach to determine which of several specified genetic models best fits the observed data [7]. For Pedigree 500, none of the models fit better than the sporadic model. For the group of three combined pedigrees, the pure polygenic model fits the data very well with an estimated heritability of 63%. The next best-fitting models are the mixed recessive polygenic and the pure recessive model. Dominant and codominant (additive) models show no significant fit to these data.

It would appear from both pedigree analysis and correlation analysis that there are some distinct differences between Kindred 500 and the other three pedigrees tested. These differences could represent genetic heterogeneity or could be the result of confounding variables, such as drugs or cardiovascular diseases, which were more prominent among the screened members of Pedigree 500 as compared with the other three pedigrees.

Table 10. Results of maximum-likelihood predigree analysis of SLC in Utah pedigrees

Genetic Models	Adjusted log likelihood differences*	
	pedigree 50	pedigree 221, 501, 502
Sporadic	0	0
Dominant	0	0.1
Recessive	0.3	1.2
Codominant	0	0
Polygenic	0	2.4
Mixed polygenic:		
+Dominant	0	0
+Recessive	0	1.3
+Codominant	0	0
Heritability estimate (under best model)	0	.63

* Differences in log likelihoods between tested and sporadic models after subtracting the difference in number of parameters estimated during maximization.

DISCUSSION

Better diagnosis and treatment of hypertension

The serious medical consequences of hypertension, even when it is partially treated, are well illustrated by the high rate of early coronary and cerebrovascular diseases in these high-risk pedigrees. Several of these affected individuals were treated for hypertension before the onset of their early heart attacks or strokes. This strongly suggests the need for earlier diagnosis and more aggressive treatment in some patients to prevent these serious complications. The rate of elevated DBPs among treated hypertensives and borderline hypertensives, as well as a significant rate among persons with no history of known hypertension, supports this philosophy.

Can the sensitivity and specificity of diagnosing initial or inadequately treated hypertension be improved by using additional blood pressure measures and other information? In other words, could some persons with unhealthy blood pressure elevations fail to be diagnosed or adequately treated using only the customary sitting blood pressure measurements? Might hypertension detection and monitoring be more precise with the use of additional blood pressure measurements such as during standing, bicycle or treadmill exercise, isometric handgrip exercise, or during normal daily activities using a portable blood pressure monitor with electronic recorder?

It has been suggested that ambulatory blood pressure (BP) during ordinary daily activities is most relevant for predicting cardiovascular risks in an individual subject [8]. In reported studies using intra-arterial cannulation, mean ambulatory BP in 25 suspected hypertensives correlated much better with DBP during bicycle exercise ($r = .83$) than during resting clinic measurements ($r = .46$) [9]. In another study of 54 hypertensive subjects with similar elevation of clinic BP, ambulatory BP from an arterial cannulation identified two distinct subgroups. Almost half of the subjects who did not show the expected 10-mm decrease in ambulatory BP compared with clinic BP had 64% end-organ damage (15/22), compared with 19% (6/32) in the other group. Mean exercise BP was also significantly higher in the first group [10].

Taking a careful family history can reveal individuals in need of such special attention. In addition, the average age of detection of high blood pressure within a given pedigree may indicate the need for careful blood pressure monitoring in early adult years.

It might also be useful if data could be obtained to weigh the risks and benefits of using a DBP of 85 mm Hg as the target instead of 90 mm Hg. This could reduce the number of treated hypertensives with pressures between 90 and 95 mm Hg and might have some benefits for those lowered from 90 to 85 mm Hg. Data from the Framingham study show that the rate of stroke in the 16 years following blood pressure measurement is approximately two- to threefold higher among men and women whose DBP is in the interval 85–89 mm Hg as compared with the previous interval of 75–84 mm Hg and is approximately equivalent to the rate among individuals in the level of 90–99 mm Hg [1]. Among men, the CHD rate within 16 years following blood pressure measurement was approximately 50% higher than men whose blood pressure was in the previous interval (75–84 mm Hg) and only somewhat less than the rate in men whose DBP was 90–99 mm Hg. While these data are limited because of relatively small sample size (19 CVAs and 42 CHDs), they at least provide some motivation for further examination of other data. If special tests such as erythrocyte cation transport become reliable tools for identifying those predisposed to hypertension, they could play an important role in facilitating earlier diagnosis and treatment of hypertension.

Variables associated with SLC

In a previous analysis, SLC was tested for correlation with 52 other variables collected in the first 181 individuals [11]. As in this analysis, SLC was significantly higher in hypertensives than in normotensives. Normotensive males had significantly higher values than females (average difference, 40 μmol/L RBC/h). This sex differential was found in children, teenagers, and adults who were normotensive. It has not been found in the Utah hypertensives tested thus far, but the sample size is much smaller. Plasma cholesterol showed a significant positive correlation with SLC, while plasma sodium showed an inverse correlation.

Abdominal girth, weight, wrist circumference, and age all showed a positive correlation with SLC in males and an inverse correlation with SLC in females. Adult females showed especially strong inverse correlation with these variables. When females under age 18 were subdivided into two groups before and after onset of menarche, postmenarcheal females showed inverse correlations between these variables and SLC similar to those seen in adult women, whereas premenarcheal girls showed positive correlations of these variables with SLC similar to those seen in men and boys. This strongly suggests that hormonal factors may influence SLC.

An additional study of pregnant women in Utah showed their SLC values to be markedly higher than nonpregnant females of the same age [12]. Follow-up of pregnant women after delivery suggests that approximately 3 months are required for SLC values to drop back into the range of nonpregnant women. This suggests that SLC is a characteristic built into the membranes of red blood cells during erythropoiesis. This also suggests that the effect of any particular drug, disease, or other condition on SLC could be accurately ascertained only if red blood cells are obtained either after 3 to 4 months of exposure to the condition (the life cycle of erythrocytes) or when the subjects have been free of that condition for at least the same period of time. It will be very useful to obtain data on subjects before and after treatment with contraceptive medications, antihypertensives, and a variety of other medications that could potentially affect SLC. Current results in Utah also indicate that SLC values are very low in erythrocytes obtained from cord blood at delivery [12].

Gaining a clear understanding of the effect of potential confounding variables is important for future studies. To clearly understand the genetic relationship of SLC will require careful correction or elimination of these confounders. Since all of the analyses in this study were performed in raw, unadjusted SLC values, the analyses should be considered preliminary and interpreted only to the degree that confounding influences are absent or insignificant in their effects. In a few preliminary analyses, we have adjusted SLC values for the effects of sex and plasma cholesterol and performed tests for familial correlation, genetic transmission, and multiple regression for the variables associated with SLC. In these preliminary analyses, there was no significant change in the results from adjusting for these two major variables. We have not, however, been able to perform these adjustments for the pregnant women, which would be interesting since pregnancy is associated with an approximately 50% rise in cholesterol level.

Genetics

If the results of these preliminary analyses are not confounded by treatment or other variables, current results would indicate that SLC is a polygenic trait with approximately 60% heritability in some pedigrees. Results would also indicate some genetic heterogeneity with lack of strong genetic control in some other pedigrees. This contrast between pedigrees was evident both in maximum-likelihood pedigree analysis and a test of correlation between pairs of relatives.

Several other studies of SLC have indicated that levels are higher in individuals with a positive family history for hypertension than in those without such a family history. That type of analysis could not be done effectively in this sample, since essentially all normotensive subjects in this study were from hypertension-prone pedigrees with the exception of the spouses. In other words, essentially all of these sujects had a positive family history for hypertension.

Need for standardized methodology

Careful collection and analysis of data are required to produce a uniform and reliable understanding of cation transport tests and their relationships to blood pressure and hypertension. Just as laboratory procedures must be carefully standardized to obtain reproducible and comparable results [13, 14], so should the clinical procedures such as blood pressure measurements and collection of questionnaire items be standardized to allow comparable contrasts or comparisons of data from different studies. In comparing SLC data from our study with results in

Boston, Europe, and elsewhere in the world, it appears that our data here in Utah are quite comparable to those obtained in Italy, but contrary to results in Boston and some other studies, especially with respect to hypertensives. To help determine whether such differences are attributable to differences in the population, it is very important to carefully characterize the exact nature of the patients studied. Their ancestral origins (Northern European, African, Mediterranean, Oriental, etc.) should be carefully determined and recorded. Questions regarding use of birth-control pills, pregnancy status, and perhaps even time of the menstrual cycle should be recorded. The family history of hypertension and associated disease should be carefully collected. This should include the careful enumeration of all individuals within specified degrees of relationship, identification of those individuals affected with specific disorders, and the age at onset of medical disorders such as hypertension.

When possible, several blood pressure measurements in a variety of circumstances should be taken to provide a stable mean. As a minimum, blood pressure should be measured in the lying, sitting, and standing positions. Other tests such as blood pressure after isometric grip exercise, bicycle exercise, and ambulatory blood pressures would be helpful.

The statistical analyses of data should also be standardized. Determinations of average SLC values and correlations of SLC values with other variables should be carried out in age- and sex-specific groups. Where possible, further stratifications should be carried out.

Genetic analyses are perhaps the most difficult to carry out in a standardized and reproducible fashion. It is useful and informative to visually inspect pedigrees. However, this is still a subjective process and cannot be considered a final method for genetic analyses. Correlations between parents and offspring, siblings, and spouses can be easily carried out and would be useful as a rough index of familial aggregation of cation transport. Definitive genetic analyses should include, wherever possible, maximum-likelihood pedigree analysis in which specific genetic models are compared. To omit this important step in determining the genetic characteristics of a carefully measured variable, such as SLC, would be analogous to performing the laboratory examination without appropriate attention to the temperature of the water bath or the length of the lithium-loading time.

Just as the expertise and technology in performing laboratory determinations requires a fastidious and careful approach, maximum-likelihood pedigree analysis is a complicated procedure requiring both genetic and computer expertise. There are several academic centers where the knowledge and computer expertise are available to perform these analyses. Investigators who are collecting cation transport and associated data, which deserve careful genetic analyses, should find competent genetic analysts to help them carry out such tests.

With careful standardization at all levels of data collection and analysis, with extensive communication between investigators pursuing the same interests, and with continued interchange in conferences such as this one, an in-depth understanding of the genetic, environmental, pathophysiological, and biochemical factors associated with hypertension should expand rapidly. Prompt clinical benefits should accrue in at least a subset of those afflicted with this disorder.

SUMMARY

Preliminary analyses of sodium-lithium countertransport and blood pressure among 384 subjects, aged 3 to 82, from hypertension-prone pedigrees in Utah are presented. Mean sodium-lithium countertransport (SLC) was significantly higher in hypertensives and subjects with borderline blood pressure as compared with normotensives. There was considerable overlap of values, with some hypertensives having low values and some normotensives having high values.

Positive correlations were observed for SLC values among siblings and parents with offspring but not between spouses. In three pedigrees, SLC appeared to be a polygenic trait with substantial heritability. In another large pedigree, correlations within sibships and parent-offspring pairs were much lower, and SLC did not fit any genetic models better than the sporadic model.

Mean SLC values in normotensives in Utah are similar to those found elsewhere. Mean SLC values in Utah hypertensives are similar to European results but lower than those reported for hypertensives in Boston. The reason for these differences is not clear. They could be due to confounding factors such as medications, or methods of selecting study subjects, or different population characteristics such as ancestral origins and gene pools.

An examination of the age at treatment of hypertension and onset of early coronary disease and stroke in these pedigrees suggests that hypertension needs to be detected earlier or treated more vigorously to prevent severe complications. Results of standing blood pressure measurements presented in this report suggest that some individuals who do not meet current sitting blood pressure criteria for hypertension may have ambulatory blood pressures in a range that promotes atherosclerosis. Further studies should be done to determine how to improve the sensitivity and accuracy for diagnosing clinically significant hypertension. Studies are also needed to decide if more aggressive treatment should be instituted to help prevent or delay the occurrence of early atherosclerotic problems in such high-risk pedigrees.

ACKNOWLEDGMENTS

Supported by a research grant from the National Heart, Blood and Lung Institute (HL 2485502), a research career development award to Dr. Williams (HL 00379-05), and the development fund of the University of Utah Pathology Department.

Acknowledgment to Art Ruby and Dorothy Hudman, R.N., for administering the screening clinic; to Mitzy Canessa, Ph.D., (Physiology Department, Harvard Medical School) for extensive help in developing the laboratory assay in Utah; and to Alta Price, M.D., Wendy Sprowell, Wayne Henschel, and Michael Lynch who helped carry out the laboratory determinations.

REFERENCES

1. Shurtleff D: The Framingham Study. Section 26, 16-year follow-up, Tables 1-2-A and 8-2-B. Washington, DC, Government Printing Office, 1970.
2. Hypertension Detection and Follow-up Program Cooperative Group: Five-year findings of the HDFP. I. Reduction in mortality of persons with high blood pressure, including mild hypertension. JAMA 242:2562, 1979.
3. The Management Committee: The Australian therapeutic trial in mild hypertension. Lancet 1:1261, 1980.
4. Williams RR: The role of genes in coronary atherosclerosis, in Hurst JW (editor): Update IV. The Heart. New York, McGraw-Hill, 1979, p 89.
5. Williams RR, Hopkins PN: Salt, hypertension, and genetic environmental interactions, in Sing CF, Skolnick M (eds): Genetic Analysis of Common Diseases: Applications to Predictive Factors in Coronary Disease. New York, Alan R. Liss, 1979, p 183.
6. Karlin S, Carmelli D, Williams RR: Index measures for assessing the mode of inheritance of continuously distributed traits: I. Theory and justifications. Theor Popul Biol 16:81, 1979.
7. Hasstedt SJ, Cartwright PE: Pedigree Analysis Package. University of Utah, Dept of Medical Biophysics and Computing, Technical Report No. 13, 1979.
8. Perloff D, Sokolow M: The representative blood pressure: Usefulness of office, basal, home and ambulatory readings. Cardiovasc Med 3:665, 1978.
9. Millar-Craig MW, Balasubramanian V, Mann S, et al.: Use of graded exercise testing in assessing the hypertensive patient. Clin Cardiol 3:236, 1980.
10. Floras JS, Hassan MQ, Sever PS, et al.: Cuff and ambulatory blood pressure in subjects with essential hypertension. Lancet 2:107, 1981.
11. Williams RR, Hunt SC, Kuida H, et al.: Sodium-lithium countertransport in hypertension-prone pedigrees. Unpublished observations.
12. Worley RJ, Pead G, Zelenkov K, et al.: Increased sodium-lithium countertransport in erythrocytes of pregnant women. N Engl J Med 307:412, 1982.
13. Smith JB, Ash KO, Hentschel WM, et al.: A kinetic expression for sodium-lithium countertransport in human red cells. Clin Chim Acta 122:337, 1982.
14. Smith JB, Price AL, Williams RR, et al.: A reproducible sodium-lithium countertransport assay: The outcome of changing key laboratory parameters. Clin Chim Acta 122:327, 1982.

DISCUSSION

Discussants: Erdmann, Williams, Funder, Hoffman, Meyer, Garay, Tosteson, MacGregor

Erdmann: I did not see whether all of the people you screened for sodium-lithium countertransport had drugs or not. Did you sort that out?

Williams: Yes, I reported the results for the treated and the untreated hypertensives (Table 7). They had very similar mean countertransport with high and low values in both groups. Both treated and untreated hypertensives had significantly higher mean flux than normotensives.

Funder: Your incubation time for loading the cells with lithium is 3 hr. You can reduce that to 20 min by performing the loading in a 150 mM LiHCO₃ medium thanks to the increased influx of lithium as LiCO₃ through the anion transport system.

Williams: Thank you. With our sample size, that could save me a lot of money.

Hoffman: What is the reproducibility of the sodium-lithium countertransport? Have you done that many times on one patient?

Williams: Yes, as I reported in Table 5, we have repeated two to four examinations on 52 individuals, and the coefficient of variation is 9.3 percent. We also ran duplicate samples of 10 individuals in Utah and Boston, and they agree with an 11 percent variation between the two.

Meyer: In one of your first slides, you said that you had also measured intracellular sodium concentration. I would like to know what sort of results you had.

Williams: That's an interesting question. Let me say that actually most of our analyses are very preliminary now. We have briefly looked at that and there was a complication. We have tried two procedures for determining intracellular sodium: using centrifuged cells before washing and after our washing procedure. We have two intracellular sodiums – the post-wash intracellular sodium and the pre-wash. The pre-wash is much higher and may affect plasma trapping. The post-wash intracellular sodium seems closer to the truth. It also looks like a polygenic trait and, believe it or not, in our first analysis the estimate of heritability was something like 99 percent for the post-wash intracellular sodium. Post-wash intracellular sodium also correlated inversely with sodium-lithium countertransport. The pre-wash intracellular sodium was less interesting and doesn't show significant correlations or genetic control.

Garay: We observed changes in co-transport during pregnancy. These changes appear with a 3-month lag. Have you observed it for the countertransport?

Williams: We have observed the same phenomenon for countertransport.

Garay: In pregnant females we observed a decrease in the maximal rate of co-transport. Regarding countertransport, are the changes in the maximal rate or in the affinity?

Williams: That's a good question. Since I'm not the laboratory person I don't know the answer to that.

Tosteson: They're all maximum rates, the internal lithium is . . .

Garay: Yes, but is there any change in affinity for internal lithium during pregnancy?

Tosteson: I don't know.

Williams: We haven't studied that. All of ours were done by the Canessa method, so all we're looking at is the maximum rate at similar relatively high lithium-loading levels.

Tosteson: Does anybody else have information on the affinity in pregnancy?

Williams: We do not. Countertransport increases in some pregnant women, but not in all. Some subjects stay at the same level. All tests were done at about the same lithium-loading level.

Garay: Does anybody have information about countertransport affinity for lithium in hypertensives?

Tosteson: Not that I know of, no systematic data.

MacGregor: I may have missed it, but I didn't gather how you define borderline hypertensives. If I'm right, their mean diastolic pressure was 80 mm Hg. Is that correct?

Williams: They were subjects who said a physician had told them that they had high blood pressure, but were not currently on medical treatment. Using six sitting measurements, their mean diastolic blood pressure was 80, which was significantly higher than the mean of 74 found in those with no history of hypertension.

MacGregor: So that over half of them actually had diastolics below 80. It seems to me we're redefining definitions. I wonder if you'd like to comment on that.

Williams: Yes, I would really like to. As I said at the beginning, I think that diagnosing hypertension using our current criterion of a sitting blood pressure consistently over 90 is both insensitive and nonspecific. I think there are probably some people who meet those criteria who don't have clinically significant hypertension. But from these pedigrees, I'm also convinced there are people who don't meet those criteria who are hypertensive. To answer your question specifically, there *are* individuals whose diastolic blood pressure goes from below 90 sitting to 110 standing. And then some of these individuals, when we have them do an isometric grip test, show a rise in blood pressure from 100/60 up to 180/120. We are just now starting to measure blood pressures during exercise and doing 24-hour ambulatory monitoring. My plea is that we try to examine a wide variety of blood pressure measurements – standing, sitting, during exercise, ambulatory – and really try to define hypertension more accurately. I'm worried about the false positives and the false negatives. But in the high-risk pedigrees I am studying, I am especially worried about false negatives – persons with harmful blood pressure not detected by current casual sitting criteria who may develop heart attacks in their 40s or strokes in their 50s like their ancestors, if their high blood pressures are not controlled.

CATION TRANSPORT ABNORMALITIES IN HUMAN AND RAT ESSENTIAL HYPERTENSION

Daniele Cusi, Cristina Barlassina, Patrizia Ferrari, Mara Ferrandi and Giuseppe Bianchi

INTRODUCTION

From the pioneering observations of Dahl and associates [1] on the positive correlation between the prevalence of hypertension and salt intake in different populations, several investigators have attempted to find a relationship between abnormal sodium metabolism and essential hypertension.

Sodium content has been reported to be increased in the arterial walls [2], leukocytes [3], and lymphocytes [4] of essential hypertensives. Some controversy exists about the level of sodium content of the erythrocytes (RBC). Sodium has been reported to be both higher [5, 6] and equal in essential hypertensive patients [7, 8] and even lower in some of their relatives [9].

More recently, much attention has been given to the study of the ouabain-resistant pathways of sodium transport in the RBC. RBC Na-K outward co-transport has been reported to be both slower [10, 11] and faster [12] and RBC Na-Li countertransport to be faster [13, 11] in different populations of essential hypertensive patients. These transport systems are positively correlated: i.e., the subjects with high Na-K co-transport also have high Na-Li countertransport, independent of their blood pressures, but for each value of Na-K co-transport the hypertensives have faster Na-Li countertransport [14].

The purpose of this paper is to report the most recent results obtained in our laboratory on RBC composition and cation fluxes, both in the genetically hypertensive MHS rats and in essential hypertensive humans, in order to unveil possible analogies or discrepancies between the two species.

RAT STUDIES

The study of the characteristics of the genetic forms of hypertension that develop spontaneously in some rat strains has been considered an important tool for understanding the pathogenesis of human essential hypertension. The rats of the Milano hypertensive strain (MHS) develop a spontaneous type of hypertension one month after birth [15]. Previous studies from our laboratory clearly demonstrated that hypertension could be crosstransplanted with the kidney even before the development of the disease, thus suggesting that the kidney was the main organ responsible for the development of the disease [16, 17].

Methods

Early hypertensive MHS male rat and their respective normotensive controls (MNS) of the same age and weight (28–31 days; 90–105 g) were used. Blood was drawn through a cannula that had been inserted through the left carotid artery under halothane anesthesia given 3–4 hours earlier.

Intra-erythrocyte cation concentration

Duplicate samples of 500 μl of blood were collected from the cannula into a heparinized syringe and immediately transferred into a plastic tube containing an ice-cold solution of $MgCl_2$ 110 mM and TRIS-MOPS buffer (pH 7.35, 4° C) 5 mM. The osmolarity of this solution was kept constant at 301–299 mosm/kg with further $MgCl_2$ or bidistilled water. The cells were washed twice with 100 vol of this solution. The cell suspension was then centrifuged at 12,000 g for 1 minute. In one of the duplicate samples, 0.50 μCi/ml of ^{125}I albumin was added before this last centrifugation in order to determine the percentage of extracellular water trapped in this last procedure. From the other tube the supernatant was again discarded, and approximately 25 μl of packed RBC (the exact volume determined gravimetrically) were added to 4 ml of bidistilled water in quadruplicate; this procedure was carried out at 4° C and did not take more than 20 minutes. Intracellular Na and K concentrations were determined by atomic absorption photometry (Perkin Elmer 400 S), with the appropriate dilutions, in order to work within the rectilinear range of the instrument.

Intracellular hemoglobin concentration

This was determined at the same time as the intracellular Na and K concentrations were measured and consisted of spectrophotometric determination of cyanmethemoglobin.

RBC volume

This was measured with a C 1000 Channalizer® coupled with a Coulter Counter®. The volumes were determined from the peak of the distribution curve. Lattice particles of 4.8 μm diameter were used as standard. The Isoton® used in the experiment was rendered iso-osmotic (300–298 mosm/kg) by adding bidistilled water. In summary, immediately after drawing, 200 μl of blood were transferred into prewarmed (37° C), diluted Isoton® solution and processed as usual by the

Coulter Counter®. All the hydraulic apparatus had been previously washed and equilibrated with the diluted Isoton®, in order to avoid differences in the electric signal amplitude due to differences in electric conductivity at the first readings.

Na effluxes determination

We followed the method described in [14], modified by using fresh cells without PCMBS loading. The solution for the determination of the ouabain-resistant sodium effluxes contained ouabain 5 mM and the solution for the determination of the sodium passive permeability contained ouabain 5 mM and bumetanide 0.1 mM. In fact preliminary, as yet unpublished, experiments have shown that bumetanide is about 500 times more effective, on a molar basis, than furosemide in inhibiting Na-K co-transport in human RBC and that a component of the ouabain-resistant Na efflux is inhibited by 0.1 mM bumetanide in rat RBC. On the basis of these observations, we assume that the ouabain-resistant, bumetanide-sensitive sodium efflux in rat RBC may be considered an expression of the Na-K co-transport. Due to the very fast cation fluxes in rodent RBC, the times for the sampling were 0, 5, 10, and 15 minutes for the total sodium effluxes and 0, 10, 20, and 30 minutes for the ouabain-resistant sodium effluxes. The haematocrit in the flux solutions was about 2%.

HUMAN STUDIES

Methods

Na-K co-transport at high intracellular sodium

This was measured according to the method previously cited (14) in order to work at an intracellular sodium concentration of about 30 mM.

Kinetic study of the Na-K co-transport

For the kinetic study, two different loading solutions were prepared: the Na-loading solution contained NaCl 130 mM, $NaPo_4$ buffer (pH 7.4, 4°C) 10 mM, TRIS-EGTA buffer (pH 7.4, 4°C) 10 mM, PCMBS* 0.02 mM; the K-loading solution contained KCl 130 mM, KPO_4 buffer (pH 7.4, 4°C) 10 mM, TRIS-EGTA buffer (pH 7.4, 4°C) 10 mM, PCMBS 0.02 mM. The cells were incubated for 20 hours at 4°C in loading solutions consisting of different mixtures of the Na and K loading solutions, in order to obtain final intracellular sodium concentrations

---

* 2,5 -p- chloromercuribenzenesulphonate (Na salt). SIGMA Chemical Company, St. Louis, Mo.

ranging from 4–5 mM to 45–50 mM. The remaining intracellular cation was K. The loading solutions were renewed after 6 h.

Na-Li countertransport

This was measured according to Canessa et al, (13), with minor modifications.

Statistical methods

For statistical analysis of the mean values, Student's t test was used when the distribution of the values was normal. When this was not the case, nonparametric Wilcoxon's test was used.

RESULTS

Rat studies

11 male MHS rats and 10 male MNS rats were used for the Na, K, and hemoglobin concentration determination and for RBC volumes. 13 male MHS rats and 14 male MNS rats were used for the Na effluxes determinations. The data are summarized in Table 1. Early hypertensive MHS rats have less intracellular sodium, smaller cell volume, and faster sodium extrusion by the Na-K co-transport as compared with their normotensive controls.

Table 1. Na efflux determination

	Body Weight (g)	Cell Volume (μ^3)	Hb (g/dL RBC)	$[Na]_i$ (mmol/L RBC)	$[K]_i$ (mmol/L RBC)
MHS	97.5 ± 0.92	42.3 ± 0.72	30.7 ± 0.49	2.34 ± 0.06	101.26 ± 2.5
p	n.s.	<0.001	n.s.	<0.02	n.s.
MNS	98.3 ± 2.3	47.3 ± 0.53	31.3 ± 0.35	2.57 ± 0.16	97.94 ± 2.68

Rate constants of Na extrusion (per hour)

	Na Pump	Na-K Cotransport	Passive Permeability
MHS	0.998 ± 0.05	0.044 ± 0.0065	0.136 ± 0.013
p	n.s.	<0.02	n.s.
MNS	0.926 ± 0.07	0.024 ± 0.0041	0.169 ± 0.017

Parameters measured in the RBC of early hypertensive MHS and their normotensive controls, MNS (mean values ± SEM). For statistical analysis. Student's t test was used.

Human studies

Na-K co-transport was measured in 64 essential hypertensive patients and in 38 matched normotensive controls. The mean value of Na-K co-transport is lower in essential hypertensives (essential hypertensives 342.9 ± 25.8; normotensives $422.6 \pm 23.8 \, \mu mol \cdot L \, RBC \cdot h$ mean value $\pm$ SEM; p<0.01); in Figure 1a, the frequency distribution as a function of the Na-K co-transport is reported. The distribution for the normotensives seems to be normal with a mode between 400 and 450, while for the hypertensives it seems to be bimodal, with a first mode at about 250 and the second one at about 650 $\mu mol \cdot L \, RBC \cdot h$ of sodium extrusion. The skewness test is significant (p<0.05) for a positive skewness of the distribution of the Na-K co-transport values ($g_1 = +0.659$). Although the data were not enough to attain statistical significance for the bimodality of the distribution, additional evidence that the distribution is bimodal may be found in Figure 1b, where the cumulative distribution of the Na-K co-transport values is plotted on a log probit scale. The change in the slope occured at a value of Na-K co-transport of about 550 $\mu mol \cdot L \, RBC \cdot h$. Six (16%) of the normotensives and 14 (22%) of the hypertensives had Na-K co-transport above this limit. The kinetic study was performed in 9 hypertensives with high Na-K co-transport, 7 with low Na-K co-transport, and 9 normotensives. Figure 2a shows the three curves obtained for the sodium extrusion by the Na-K co-transport as a function of intracellular sodium. The same data are expressed as percentage of the maximal attained rate in figure 2b. In this case, the curves for the high and low Na-K co-transport are totally superimposable. The K_m values for sodium extrusion are identical in the

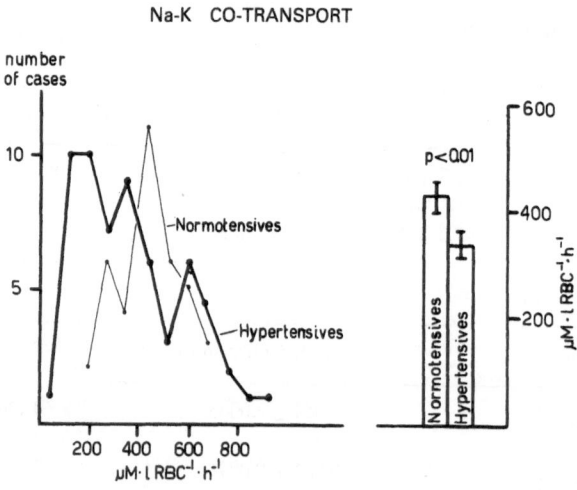

Na-K CO-TRANSPORT

Figure 1a. Frequency distribution of the Na-K co-transport values for hypertensives and normotensives. The mean values $\pm$ S.E.M. are reported on the right side.

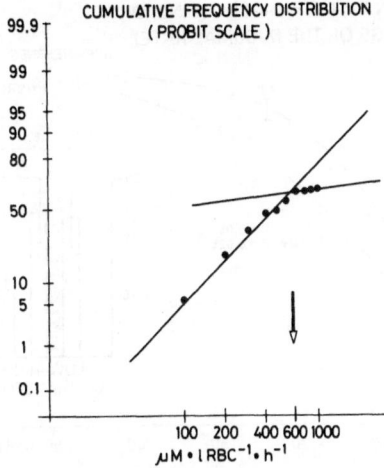

Figure 1b. Relative cumulative frequency as a function of the Na-K co-transport values plotted on a log probit scale. The arrow indicates the apparent notc on the frequency distribution, thus suggesting the bimodality of the distribution.

two groups of hypertensives (high Na-K co-transport 23.16 ± 5.04, low Na-K co-transport 24.57 ± 5.08 mM internal Na) and significantly higher ($p<0.05$) than the value for the normotensives (13.23 ± 1.93).

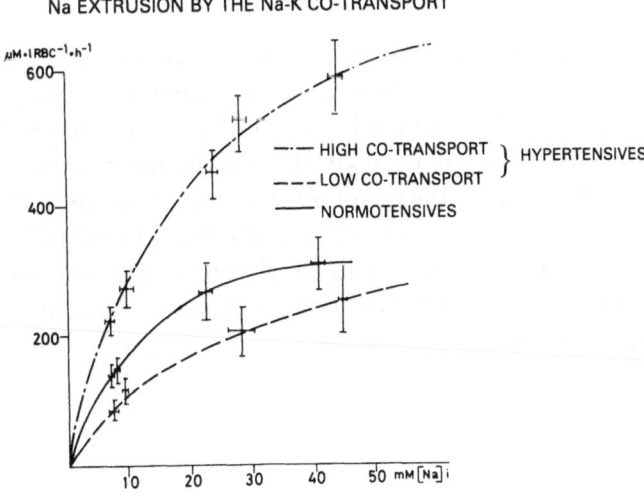

Figure 2a. Na extrusion by the Na-K co-transport as a function of intracellular sodium for the normotensives and the low and high co-transport hypertensives. The vertical and horizontal bars indicate the standard errors from the mean.

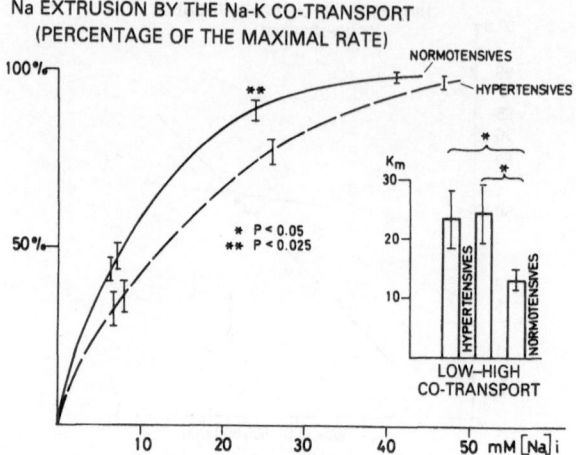

Na EXTRUSION BY THE Na-K CO-TRANSPORT
(PERCENTAGE OF THE MAXIMAL RATE)

Figure 2b. The Na extrusion by the Na-K co-transport is plotted as a percentage of the maximum attained rate. There is only one curve for the hypertensives, since the curves for the high and the low Na-K co-transport are superimposable. This is also confirmed on the right side of the figure, where the Km values are indicated.

Na-Li countertransport was measured simultaneously to Na-K co-transport in the same 64 essential hypertensive patients and in the 38 normotensive controls. The mean value of Na-Li countertransport was higher in the essential hypertensives (343 ± 22.5 vs 235 ± 17.9; $p > 0.01$). The frequency distribution of the values seems to be normal both for the essential hypertensive patients and for the controls.

Since the two transport systems were measured simultaneously in the same individuals, it was possible to study if they were somehow correlated. Na-K co-transport is highly significantly correlated to Na-Li countertransport both in the hypertensives ($r = 0.59$, $p < 0.001$) and in the normotensives ($r = 0.70$, $p > 0.001$). The slopes of the regression lines are not different (0.42 vs 0.45), but the intercepts on the y-axis are significantly different ($p > 0.01$), thus indicating that the regression lines are roughly parallel and that for any given value of Na-K co-transport the essential hypertensives tend to have faster Na-Li countertransport than the normotensives.

DISCUSSION

The main results of this study are: (1) Early hypertensive HS rats have faster RBC outward sodium extrusion by the Na-K co-transport, less intracellular sodium, and smaller cell volume. (2) The mean value of Na-K co-transport is lower in human essential hypertensives than in normotensive subjects. The frequency distribution curve of the values for the essential hypertensives seems to be bimodal, with values below and above the normal ones, even if the number of cases studied is too small for appropriate statistical analysis. The mean value for Na-Li countertransport is greater in the essential hypertensives, and the frequency distribution curves seem to be unimodal both for the hypertensives and the controls. (3) In two subgroups of hypertensives, one with high and the other with low Na-K co-transport values, the K_m values for Na extrusion by the Na-K co-transport are similar and significantly higher than that of the controls.

The finding of an identical K_m in the two groups of hypertensives with high and low rates of Na-K co-transport may suggest that in the patients with high Na-K co-transport an increased number of the hypothetical carriers compensates for the diminished apparent affinity for intracellular sodium. It is to be noted that, when compared with the normotensive controls, the group of patients with a high rate of Na-K co-transport at high intracellular sodium concentration also show an increased rate within the range of physiological intracellular sodium concentrations (Fig. 2a). However, this finding may be due to the relatively low Na-K co-transport values that were obtained in this particular small sample of normotensives.

All these data are difficult to interpret if we do not recall that essential hypertension is probably a multifactorial disease where different environmental and genetic factors operate simultaneously [18]. The picture may be somewhat simpler when dealing with genetically hypertensive rats. In fact, in the Milan strain, preliminary data suggest that the blood pressure differences between MHS and MNS may be due to two pairs of alleles [19]. Our finding of a faster bumetanide-sensitive sodium efflux in a $MgCl_2$-sucrose medium and of a faster sodium extrusion by the Na-K co-transport in a proportion of essential hypertensive subjects suggests a common pathogenetic mechanism. At present we can only speculate on the basis of what we have learned in the last years on the comparison of the prehypertensive stage in MHS and in humans (Table 2). We have previously defined as being in the prehypertensive stage those young normotensive subjects with both hypertensive parents [20], on the assumption that about 50% of them will develop hypertension later in their life [21], and we have compared them as a prehypertensive MHS group. The similarities are many: They both have a greater fraction of cardiac output going to the kidney, faster glomerular filtration rate, lower plasma renin activity, similar cardiac output, and peripheral resistances as compared with their appropriate controls [22, 23]. The finding of a faster glomerular filtration rate, together with normal sodium balance, implies that the overall renal tubular sodium reabsorption must be increased. The increase in tubular sodium reabsorption may occur through paracellular or transcellular pathways. If we admit that the latter is the pathway involved, then the data on the glomerular filtration rate may be taken as evidence

Table 2. Differences from appropriate controls of prehypertensive MHS and humans

	MHS rats	Humans
RBF (% of CO)	↑ (x)	↑
24-h Urinary output	↑	↑
Renal Na excretion (after loading)	↑	↑
Kidney pressor effect (after transplantation)	↑	↑ ?
GFR	↑ ? (o)	↑ (+)
Plasma renin	↓	↓
Urine kallikrein	↓	↓
Plasma aldosterone	=	=
Plasma Na and K	=	=
CO	= (x)	=
Erythrocytes Na Concentration	↓	↓ or = or ↑
Net erythrocyte cells membrane Na transport	↑	↑ ?

↓ or ↑, lower or higher in prehypertensive
(?) Indicates a trend and not a definitive result.
(x) Measured in anesthetized rats.
(o) Expressed per unit of kidney weight.
(+) Expressed per unit of body surface.
Reprinted from Bianchi and Barlassina (23), with modifications.

that in both tubular and RBC of MHS, the transport across their cell membrane is faster than in those of the MNS. The same explanation may be hypothesized for the subgroup of patients with high Na-K co-transport.

REFERENCES

1. Dahl LK, Love RA: Relation of sodium chloride intake to essential hypertension in humans. Fed Proc 13:426–431, 1954.
2. Tobian L Jr, Binon T: Tissue cations and water in arterial hypertension. Circulation 5:754–758, 1952.
3. Edmonson RPS, Hilton PJ, Thomas RD, et al.: Abnormal leucocyte composition and sodium transport in essential hypertension. Lancet 1: 1003–1006, 1975.
4. Ambrosioni E, Costa FV, Montebugnoli L, et al.: Intralymphocytic sodium concentration: A sensitive index to identify young subjects at risk of hypertension. Clin Exp Hypertens 3:675–691, 1981.
5. Losse H, Zumkley H, Wehmeyer H: Untersuchungen über den elektrolyt und wassergehalt von erythrozyten bei arterieller hypertonie. Z Kreislauff 51:43–50, 1962.
6. Wessel F: Sodium metabolism of RBC in hypertensive patients, in Zumkley H, Losse H (editors): Intracellular Electrolytes and Arterial Hypertension. International Symposium, Münster. Stuttgart, G Thieme Verlag, 1980, pp 221–227.
7. Burck HC: Die elektrolytkonzentration in menschlichen erythrozyten. Med Habil Schrift Tübingen, 1971.

8. Wambach G, Helber A, Bönner G, et al.: Natrium-Kalium-ATPase-Aktivität in erythrozytenghost und elektrolytkonzentrationen in erythrozyten von patienten mit essentieller hypertonie. Verh Dtsch Ges Inn Med 84:800–813, 1978.

9. Wessel F: Genetic aspects of sodium metabolism in RBC, in Zumkley H, Losse H (editors): Intracellular Electrolytes and Arterial Hypertension. Internal Symposium, Münster. Stuttgart, G Thieme Verlag, 1980, pp 221–227.

10. Garay RP, Dagher G, Pernollet MG, et al.: Inherited defect in a Na^+,K^+-co-transport system in erythrocytes from essential hypertensive patients. Nature 284:281–283, 1980.

11. Cusi D, Barlassina C, Ferrandi M, et al.: Relationship between altered Na^+-K^+ co-transport and Na^+-Li^+ countertransport in the red blood cells of 'essential' hypertensive patients. Clin Sci, in press.

12. Adragna N, Tosteson DC, Canessa M: Simultaneous measurement of Li-Na countertransport and Na-K co-transport in red cells of patients with essential hypertension. Clin Sci, in press.

13. Canessa M, Adragna N, Solomon H, et al.: Increased Na-Li countertransport in red cells of patients with essential hypertension. N Engl J Med 302:772–778, 1980.

14. Cusi D, Barlassina C, Ferrandi M, et al.: Familial aggregation of cation transport abnormalities and essential hypertension. Clin Exp Hypertens 3(4):871–884, 1981.

15. Bianchi G, Fox U, Imbasciati E: The development of a new strain of spontaneously hypertensive rats. Life Sci 14:339–347, 1974.

16. Bianchi G, Fox U, Di Francesco GF, et al.: The hypertensive role of the kidney in spontaneously hypertensive rats. Clin Sci Mol Med 45 (suppl 1):135s–139s, 1973.

17. Bianchi G, Fox U, Di Francesco GF, et al.: Blood pressure changes produced by kidney cross-transplantation between spontaneously hypertensive rats and normotensive rats. Clin Sci Mol Med 47:435–448, 1974.

18. Pickering G: High Blood Pressure, ed 2. London, Churchill, XXXX, pp 274–290.

19. Bianchi G, Cusi D, Ferrari P, et al.: Renal mechanisms in the pathogenesis of essential hypertension, in Laragh JH, et al. (editors): Frontiers in Hypertension Research. New York, Springer-Verlag, 1981, pp 169–172.

20. Bianchi G, Cusi D, Gatti M, et al.: A renal abnormality as a possible cause of 'essential' hypertension. Lancet X:173–175, 1979.

21. Ayman D: Heredity in arteriolar (essential) hypertension: A clinical study of blood pressure of 1524 members of 277 families. Arch Intern Med 53: 792–802, 1934.

22. Bianchi G, Cusi D, Barlassina C, et al.: The renal function pattern of young normotensive subjects who are predisposed to develop 'essential' hypertension. Unpublished observations.

23. Bianchi G, Barlassina C: Renal function in essential hypertension, in Genest J, et al. (editors): Hypertension: Physiopathology and Treatment, ed 2. New York, McGraw-Hill, 1982.

DISCUSSION

Discussants: Meyer, Cusi, Tosteson, Hoffman.

Meyer: I fully agree with most of your conclusions. Now the point I would like to ask you and also Dr. Williams is whether you presented data obtained in the same patient. In other words, do you find this correlation in one patient with a constantly high countertransport and a low co-transport, or do you have random distribution?

Cusi: Well, I'm not sure I understood. We generally run in the assay one blood whose transport value we know, and we accept the assay if we confirm that value. I don't have the numbers of the variation coefficient in intra-assay and within different assays, but the variation is very small.

Meyer: My question was, do the patients who have an increased V_{max} of the countertransport also have reduced co-transport? Are they the same persons?

Cusi: The V_{max} was calculated on very few people – just seven and nine. We have a quasi-V_{max} at 30 millimolar sodium intracellular – that is not V_{max} but approximates it. And the hypertensives with high values also have high countertransport values, while the normotensives with the same values have lower countertransport values. In other words, we never observed a hypertensive subject having both systems simultaneously abnormal (i.e., high Na-Li countertransport and low Na-K co-transport).

Tosteson: All right, we won't try and press on that any further. He's interested in whether you did the analyses in the same subjects.

Cusi: We did the analyses in the same subjects and we constantly got the same results in males. In females, the problem is different, because mentrual period does affect the co-transport. We didn't perform a systematic study on the countertransport. Some females have fluctuation in the co-transport values with menstrual periods, but in some males, the assay was repeated at least 20 times, and the value of the Na-K co-transport is constant.

Tosteson: Right. I think you and Dr. Meyer should get together afterwards to talk on this point.

Hoffman: The increase in red cell sodium that occurred on the continued washing – what temperature did you wash at?

Cusi: 4° C.

Hoffman: And at what speed?

Cusi: Not very high speed – about $1500 \times g$ for 10 to 15 min – because the rat cells are fragile and lyse very easily.

Hoffman: We have found that when the cells are centrifuged, or experience temperatures below 10° C, they become a little leaky to sodium, so that if you did the same experiment keeping the temperature above 10° C, I think you'd find that the cell sodium stayed relatively constant with multiple washings.

Cusi: Yes, that may be the case. But we have been washing without sodium; so I can't explain the increase in intracellular sodium. We have been washing the cells with magnesium chloride.

Hoffman: Then, since the cell sodium went up, they must have shrunk.

Cusi: Yes, that's the most reasonable explanation.

THE SODIUM/LITHIUM EXCHANGE MECHANISM IN ESSENTIAL HYPERTENSION: IS IT A SODIUM/PROTON EXCHANGER?

JØRGEN FUNDER, JENS OTTO WIETH, HENRICK ÆRENLUND JENSEN AND KARSTEN KLAAS IBSEN

INTRODUCTION

Since Canessa et al. [1] presented their findings suggesting that there may be an increased sodium-lithium countertransport in red cell membranes from patients with essential hypertension, there has been considerable interest in this cation exchange system, which can mediate sodium-lithium exchange and sodium-sodium exchange in a strictly coupled 1:1 transmembrane exchange process.

Besides obvious implications for diagnostic and genetic studies of the disease, a generalized change of a specialized membrane-transport function may have paramount importance for the exploration of the ill-understood pathogenesis of essential hypertension, if the transport mechanism plays a role for the regulation of vascular smooth muscle tone.

The present communication first summarizes the results of an investigation of Na-Li countertransport in a group of Danish patients and normal persons [2]. Next we present the result of an experimental study designed to delineate the physiological function of the transport system, which is unlikely to be sodium-lithium or sodium-sodium exchange diffusion. These experiments were carried out with bovine red cells, which have a transport capacity for sodium-sodium or sodium-lithium exchange diffusion exceeding that of the human red cell membrane by a factor of 10 to 50 [3–5]. We demonstrate that hydrogen ions compete with sodium for binding to the transport system. This observation forms the basis for considering whether this exchange diffusion system in red cells is in fact identical with a sodium-proton exchange system, which has been found to be essential for regulation of intracellular pH in many cell types [6].

LITHIUM PATHWAYS THROUGH THE HUMAN RED CELL MEMBRANE

At least five pathways for lithium have been demonstrated in the human erythrocyte membrane.

1. The active ATP-dependent sodium-potassium transport system, which mediates lithium influx at the K^+ site and lithium efflux at the Na^+ site. This active lithium transport is only seen at very low concentrations of extracellular po-

tassium and intracellular sodium and is completely inhibited by ouabain [7].

2. Passive lithium transport by the anion exchange mechanism. This lithium flux, seen in the presence of bicarbonate/carbonate ions, is ascribed by the transport of the anion $LiCO_3^-$ through the anion exchange system [8] and is completely abolished by the specific inhibitors of the anion exchange system [9].

3. Passive lithium transport by the sodium-potassium co-transport system. This furosemide-sensitive transport system, which mediates a coupled transport of potassium and sodium, is able to mediate a co-transport of lithium and potassium at high-lithium and low-sodium concentrations in the cell [10].

4. Sodium-sodium or sodium-lithium exchange diffusion. The transport system mediates a tightly coupled 1:1 exchange of sodium or of sodium for lithium across the membrane [11, 12]. Exchange diffusion is stopped when exchangeable cations (lithium or sodium) are removed from the trans-side of the membrane, as when lithium efflux takes place into sodium-free potassium-, choline- or magnesium chloride media.

5. Lithium leak. After blocking the four pathways listed above, a small lithium transport is still present, presumably representing electrodiffusion of lithium ions through the cell membrane. This flux is proportional to the lithium concentration gradient across the membrane and cannot be blocked by any known inhibitor.

DETERMINATION OF LITHIUM-SODIUM EXCHANGE DIFFUSION

Red cells were loaded with lithium in a 150 mM lithium bicarbonate medium at pH 7.4 and 38° C for 15 minutes, resulting in an intracellular lithium concentration of 7 mmol/L cells (range 5–10), corresponding to about 10 mmol/L cell water. The short incubation time suffices because lithium influx is increased 10 to 15 times to about 25 mmol (L/cells/h) when chloride is replaced by bicarbonate in the cell suspension [9]. After loading, the cells were washed five times with large volumes of a KCl medium to remove all the bicarbonate ions and the extracellular lithium ions, and the cells were used for determinations of lithium efflux into media containing either KCl or NaCl. Lithium efflux into the potassium medium exclusively occurs through the leak pathway 5 under the experimental condition used. This leak flux mmol Li^+/L/cells/h increases linearly with the intracellular lithium concentration and is described by the equation

$$J^{leak} = k \times (Li_i^+)$$

where (Li_i^+) is the intracellular lithium concentration (mmol/cells) and k/h is the rate constant of the leak efflux, which is of the order of magnitude 0.03/h in human red cells. Lithium efflux into the sodium medium includes two components: the leak flux just described, and the exchange of lithium for sodium through the exchange diffusion pathway 4. This exchange diffusion or countertransport of lithium for sodium displays saturation kinetics with a half maximum flux at an intracellular lithium concentration of about 1 mmol/L cells [3]. Saturation of the exchange diffusion pathway is attained when intracellular lithium concentration is above 5 mmol/L cells. The sodium-sensitive lithium exchange diffusion is calculated as the difference between the leak flux 5 and the sum of the fluxes through the leak plus the exchange pathways 4 + 5.

METHODOLOGICAL CONSIDERATIONS

It is clear that the evaluation of the capacity of the lithium-sodium countertransport in hypertension is made difficult by the small sizes of the clinical materials presented so far. We have therefore examined whether it is possible to store red cells before flux determinations in order to examine larger series of cell samples. Our results indicate that cells can be stored at 4°C in a medium containing 155 mM KCl and 10 mM glucose for at least four days without any change of the sodium-lithium exchange capacity [2].

Differences between results of the present study and that of Canessa et al. [1] do not seem to be related to the use of KCl or $MgCl_2$ media for the determination of the leak efflux in the two studies, since we were not able to demonstrate any significant differences between the lithium leak into media containing KCl, $MgCl_2$, or choline chloride [2].

SODIUM-LITHIUM EXCHANGE DIFFUSION IN ERYTHROCYTES FROM ADULTS

The capacity of the exchange system was compared in patient and control groups (Table 1):

Patients were 14 women and 17 men aged 27 to 74 years with mild to moderate essential hypertension, the diastolic blood pressure being above 105 mm Hg before treatment. Secondary hypertension was excluded by laboratory investigations including excretory urograms and/or isotope renography. Eight of the patients were untreated; 23 of the patients were treated, 7 with a thiazide only, 16 with a thiazide and a beta blocker, and in 6 or these patients the treatment also included a vasodilatator.

A control group of 10 women and 16 men aged from 18 to 88 years with normal blood pressure included both normal persons and patients admitted to the medical department. Diabetics and patients treated with hormones or cardiovascular drugs were excluded. In this group, 24 persons had no family history of hypertension. A family history could not be obtained for two of the normal men, but their sodium-lithium fluxes were within one SD of the normal mean value.

Table 1 shows that the mean values of exchange diffusion flux in red blood cells from the hypertensive males were 0.7 mmol/L cells/h and 0.4 mmol/L cells/h in

Table 1. Lithium efflux into KCl and NaCl media and the lithium-sodium countertransport in erythrocytes from patients with essential hypertension and from normal persons (mean and range). The sodium-lithium countertransport in red cells from hypertensive males was significantly increased compared to countertransport in red cells from in red blood cells from normotensive males (P <0.005). (From Ibsen et al. [27])

	No.	Age	Lithium efflux in Potassium Medium mmol/L cells/h	Lithium Efflux in Sodium Medium mmol/L cells/h	Exchange Diffusion mmol/L cells/h
Males					
Essential hypertensive	17	47.5 (30–67)	0.20 (0.12–0.46)	0.88 (0.52–2.01)	0.68 (0.35–1.55)
Normotensive	16	49.5 (18–88)	0.22 (0.12–0.39)	0.64 (0.51–0.88)	0.42 (0.30–0.64)
Females					
Essential hypertensive	14	51.5 (27–74)	0.17 (0.09–0.34)	0.58 (0.31–0.95)	0.41 (0.20–0.61)
Normotensive	10	43.5 (19–69)	0.21 (0.14–0.34)	0.55 (0.44–0.79)	0.34 (0.14–0.56)

Table 2. Lithium efflux into KCl and NaCl media and the lithium-sodium countertransport in red blood cells from children with and without a possible disposition to essential hypertension. No significant difference was found between the lithium-sodium countertransport fluxes in red cells from the two groups. (From Ibsen et al.) [2]

	Sex	No.	Age	Lithium Efflux in Potassium Medium mmol/L cells/h	Lithium Efflux in Sodium Medium mmol/L cells/h	Exchange Diffusion mmol/L cells/h
Normotensive children with one hypertensive parent	♂ ♀	9	13.0 (10–18)	0.22 (0.11–0.30)	0.57 (0.43–0.68)	0.35 (0.18–0.46)
Normotensive children with normotensive parents	♂ ♀	14	13.0 (7–17)	0.27 (0.19–0.37)	0.57 (0.36–0.80)	0.30 (0.16–0.52)

cells from normotensive males. The difference of 0.3 mmol/L cells/h is statistically significant (P<0.005, calculated by the unpaired Student's t-test). No significant difference was found between the mean values from the hypertensive and normotensive females, the mean values being 0.4 and 0.3 mmol/L cells/h, (P>0.2). Subdivision of the material with respect to severity of hypertension, graded by doses and number of drugs needed to normalize the blood pressure, did not disclose any further significant correlation between the magnitude of sodium-lithium exchange diffusion and the hypertensive state.

SODIUM-LITHIUM EXCHANGE DIFFUSION IN ERYTHROCYTES FROM CHILDREN

Two groups of children were examined:

One group consisted of four girls and five boys having one parent suffering from essential hypertension, thus being potentially disposed to the disease. At the time of the investigation, all the children had normal blood pressure, considering their age and sex.

A second group consisted of five girls and nine boys with normal blood pressure and with no family history of hypertension. No medication was given to any of the children in the two groups. Table 2 shows that the mean values and the ranges of sodium-lithium exchange diffusion in red blood cells from children without known disposition to hypertension were almost identical with the values from the children with a possible genetic disposition from a hypertensive parent, (0.05< P<0.1). No difference was found in the exchange flux values in erythrocytes from boys and girls.

CLINICAL IMPLICATIONS

The mean values of the countertransport fluxes in cells from normal persons were 50 to 80% higher than the values found by Canessa et al. [1], and a significant difference between patients and normal persons was found only in the male group (P<0.005). It is clear from the present study that measurement of sodium-lithium countertransport is not a unique test for the identification of approximately 9% of the Western population that ultimately will develop essential hypertension [14]. However, it must be taken into account that the diagnosis of essential hypertension is unlikely to represent a well-defined entity of disease with a singular etiology. It may be that there exists a subgroup of patients – predominantly male – with essential hypertension characterized by an increased capacity of the lithium-sodium exchange diffusion mechanism. The problem of whether this altered membrane function may play a role in the pathogenesis of the disease is considered in the following section, describing the interaction of hydrogen ions with the function of the sodium-exchange diffusion system.

EXPERIMENTAL INVESTIGATIONS ON BOVINE RED CELLS

Bovine red cells are characterized by a low capacity of the ouabain-sensitive active transport of sodium and potassium, and by a vivid sodium-sodium exchange diffusion [3]. The present study was carried out on ox red cells with intracellular sodium and potassium concentrations of approximately 70 and 25 mmol/L cells. The qualitative features of the sodium-lithium exchange system in the bovine red cells have previously been found to be similar to that of human red cells [4, 5], whereas the transport capacity is considerably larger, facilitating studies of the exchange mechanism.

In the search for a physiological role of the sodium-exchange diffusion system in cells other than erythrocytes, we have turned our attention to the possible role of calcium ions and of protons as exchange partners for sodium. Blaustein [15] has presented an attractive hypothesis according to which an increased intracellular calcium concentration causes contraction of vascular smooth muscle cells. If the sodium-exchange system could function as a sodium-calcium exchanger, the hyperactivity in essential hypertension might be envisioned as a compensatory mechanism, driving out calcium ions of the smooth muscle cells by the inward movement of sodium ions. However, all attempts to demonstrate an interaction of calcium with the sodium exchange system have been negative. We have previously found that calcium influx into beef red cells cannot be driven by an outwardly directed sodium gradient and that extracellular calcium is not an inhibitor of sodium-lithium exchange [4]. In addition, Table 3 shows that the efflux of sodium from bovine red cells into an isotonic magnesium chloride medium is not increased by the substitution of 10 mM magnesium with calcium. This is in contrast to the large exchange diffusion induced by extracellular sodium [3], or lithium [4, 5]. The investigation of Duhm and Becker [5] showed that the exchange system was distinct from the furosemide-sensitive, ouabain-resistant sodium transport system, the Na-K co-transport system discovered by Wiley & Cooper [16]. Transport of sodium through this system has been found to depend

Table 3. Sodium efflux from bovine red cells into sodium-free media containing 140 mM KCl, 70 mM $MgCl_2$, or 60 mM $MgCl_2$ + 10 mM $CaCl_2$. Efflux of sodium was not enhanced in the presence of 10 mM calcium, demonstrating that the ouabain-insensitive sodium exchange system is not able to use calcium as exchange partner for sodium. Sucrose was used to maintain isotonicity in the divalent cation-containing media. Experiments performed as described in Fig. 1.

Medium mM		Sodium efflux mmol/L cells/h	
KCl	140	0.68	0.84
$MgCl_2$	70	0.46	0.59
$CaCl_2$	10		
$MgCl^2$	60	0.50	0.55

Table 4. Sodium transport through the exchange diffusion pathway in bovine red cells in the presence of 140 mM NaCl or NaNO₃. The results demonstrate the independence of the presence of chloride. Experiments performed as described in Fig. 1. (Mean values, SE = 0.3, n = 4).

Medium mM		Sodium efflux mmol/L cells/h	
		pH 7.4	pH 7.9
NaCl	140	13.7	14.4
NaNO₃	140	14.7	12.3

on the presence of chloride [17, 18]. The results of Table 4 demonstrate that the sodium exchange between beef red cells and a 140-mM sodium medium is not affected by the complete substitution of chloride with nitrate.

We next determined the concentration dependence of the sodium self-exchange between beef red cells and media containing from 10 to 140 mM sodium chloride (substituting NaCl isotonically with KCl). The results shown in Figure 1 confirmed that the magnitude of the sodium exchange fluxes from the cells with

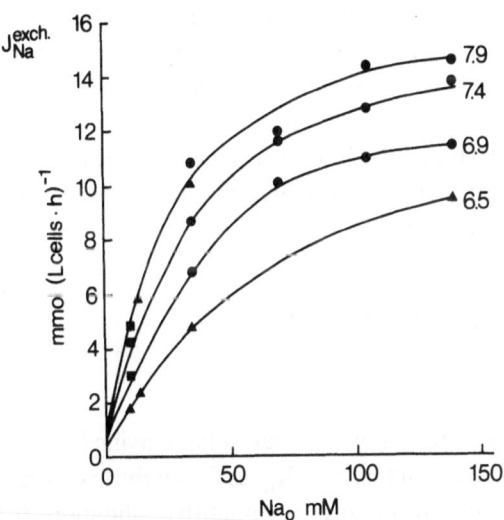

Figure 1. Sodium-sodium exchange diffusion in bovine red cells as a function of the extracellular sodium concentration determined at four pH values between 6.5. and 7.9. Exchange fluxes, corrected for sodium leak efflux, were calculated from measurements of ^{22}Na efflux at 38° C into media containing 10 to 140 mM sodium chloride, maintaining isotonicity by substituting NaCl with KCl. The media were buffered with TRIS 5 mM and potassium phosphate 5 mM and contained ouabain 10^{-4} M. Red blood cells from the same ox were used in all experiments. The cells contained 70 mmol sodium and 25 mmol potassium per L cells. One to four flux measurements were done at each experimental condition, coefficient of variation 5%. The curves were drawn by hand.

154

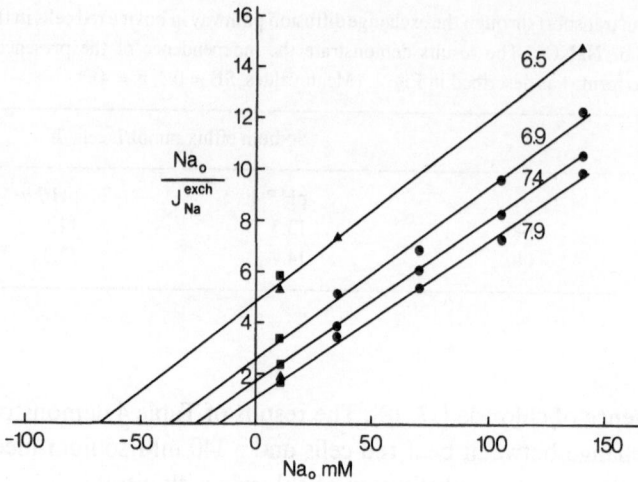

Figure 2. Dixon plot of the reciprocal values for the exchange diffusion flux of sodium *vs* the external hydrogen ion concentration at four different concentrations of external sodium (mM). The x and y coordinates of the point of common crossing of the lines correspond to $-K_{H+}$ and J_{max}, respectively.

an intracellular sodium concentration of 70 mmol/L cells is a function of both extracellular sodium and hydrogen ion concentrations [3].

The inhibitor constant for the hydrogen ions (K_{H+}) was determined from the Dixon plot in Figure 2. The intersection of the four lines in the second quadrant of the coordinate system shows that inhibition is competitive or mixed [19]. Distinction between these two types of inhibition can be made by means of a plot of Na_o/J_{Na}^{exch} against Na_o (Fig. 3) using the rate equations derived by Cornish-Bowden [19]. In the case of mixed inhibition:

$$\frac{Na_o}{J_{Na}^{exch}} = \frac{K_m^{app}}{J_{max}} + \frac{Na_o}{J_{max}} (1 + \frac{H_o}{K'_{H+}}) Na_o \qquad (1a)$$

where K_m^{app} is the concentration of external sodium giving half maximal flux at a given pH, J_{max} is the maximum flux, and K'_{H+} is the inhibitor constant for hydrogen ions causing the deviation from purely competitive inhibition. If $K'_{H+} \to \infty$, the inhibition is competitive, and the equation is reduced to the relation given by Hanes [20]:

$$\frac{Na_o}{J_{Na}^{exch}} = \frac{K_m^{app}}{J_{max}} + \frac{1}{J_{max}} Na_o \qquad (1b)$$

The interception with the ordinate is given by the first term and the slope of the

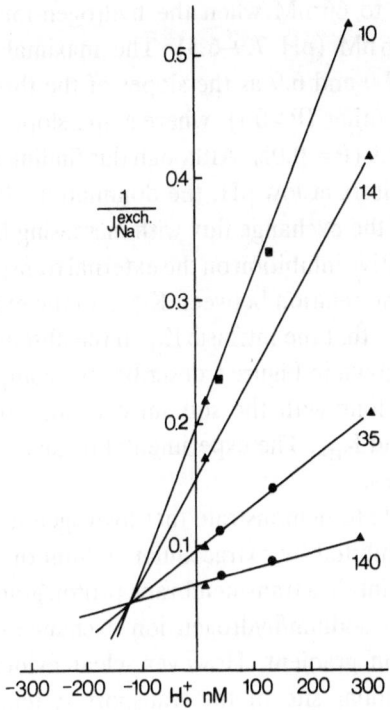

Figure 3. Data from Fig. 1 plotted according to Hanes (20). Abcissa: extracellular sodium concentration (Na_o mM); ordinate: Na_o divided by the sodium exchange flux (mmol/L cells/h). The reciprocal slope of the straight lines represents the maximum fluxes, J_{max}, and the extrapolation of the lines to the abcissa indicates the negative values of the apparent concentration of sodium for half maximal flux, K_m^{app}, at the four different pH values. The values are given in Table 5.

line by the second term in both equations. In a case of competitive inhibition, the lines will be parallel with a slope of $1/J_{max}$, wherecas mixed inhibition will make the lines converge towards the ordinate because the slope is proportional to Na_o (cf. eq. 1a). The values for K_m^{app} and J_{max} calculated from eq. 1b are given in Table 5.

Table 5. Values for the maximum exchange flux of sodium (J_{max}) and the variation of the apparent half-saturation constant for sodium (K_m^{app}) in the range 7.9–6.5, corresponding to a variation in hydrogen ion concentration from 13 to 316 nM. Values calculated from the data of Fig. 1, using eq. 1b.

pH	J_{max} mmol/L cells/h	K_m^{app} mM
7.9	16.1	16.6
7.4	15.9	27.1
6.9	14.5	36.0
6.5	13.8	65.8

K_m^{app} increases from 17 to 66 mM when the hydrogen-ion concentration is increased from 13 to 316 nM (pH 7.9–6.5). The maximal exchange fluxes are identical between pH 7.9 and 6.9 as the slopes of the three lines do not differ significantly from each other (P>0.1), whereas the slope of the line at pH 6.5 differs from that at pH 7.9 (P = 0.01). Although this finding indicates that protons may act as mixed inhibitors at low pH, the dominating effect of the protons in causing the decrease of the exchange flux with increasing hydrogen-ion concentration is due to competitive inhibition on the external transport site. The diagram of Figure 4, depicting the relation between K_m^{app} and the extracellular hydrogen-ion concentration, shows that the intrinsic K_{Na} in the absence of protons is about 17 mM. The equation shown in Figure 5 describes the competitive interaction of extracellular hydrogen ions with the sodium exchange flux by means of the parameters J_{max}, K_{Na}, and K_{H^+}. The experimental results are in good agreement with the predicted values.

We have not been able to demonstrate that hydrogen-ion influx from an acid KCl medium can be inhibited by extracellular sodium or lithium ions; neither have we been able to maintain a transmembrane proton gradient sufficiently long to determine whether a sodium/hydrogen ion exchange can be driven by an inwardly directed proton gradient. However, clear evidence for an effect of protons on the intracellular site of the transport system has been found in experiments showing that sodium exchange diffusion is inhibited when intracellular pH is lowered to 6.3, maintaining an extracellular pH of 7.9 (Table 6).

So far our investigation has demonstrated a competitive interaction of protons with the sodium-exchange diffusion system of bovine red cells. The physiological

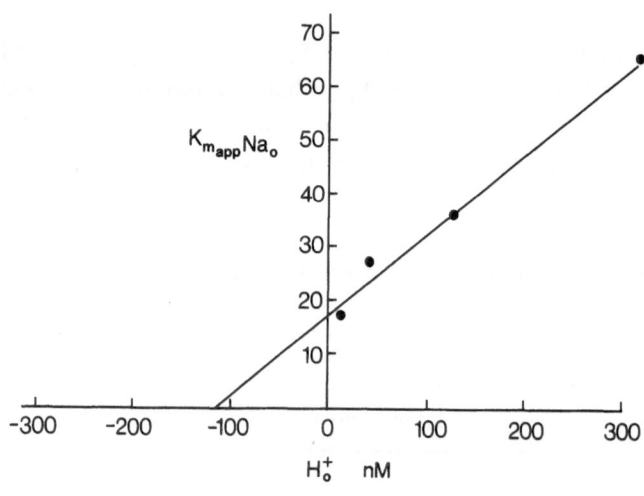

Figure 4. Variation of the apparent half-saturation constant for external sodium as a function of extracellular hydrogen-ion concentration. The intercept of the line with the ordinate (17 mM) gives the intrinsic half-saturation constant K_{Na} in the absence of protons (r = 0.99).

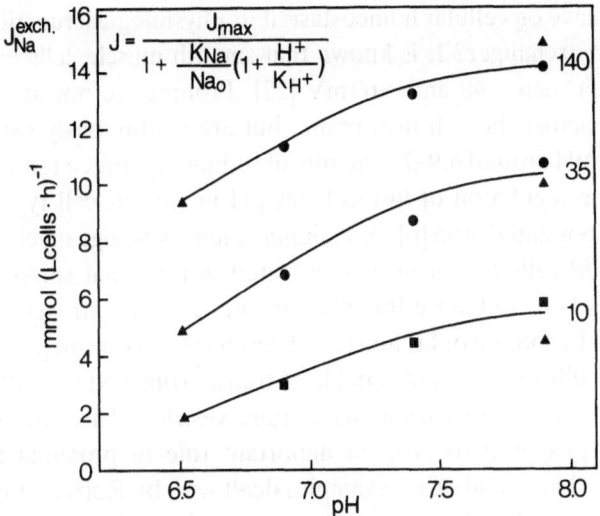

Figure 5. The curves drawn represent the relation between the exchange diffusion of sodium and the hydrogen ion concentration at three concentrations of extracellular sodium calculated from the equation given in the figure. Values for the constants are given in the text. The signatures represent experimental flux values obtained with red cells from the same cow. Experimental conditions as described in Fig. 1.

significance of these findings suggests that the sodium exchange pathway may in fact be a Na^+/H^+ exchanger, which is also able to transport Li^+, whereas the affinity for potassium, magnesium, and calcium is negligible.

SODIUM/PROTON EXCHANGE AND HYPERTENSION

The question is which physiological effects might a hyperactive sodium exchange

Table 6. Sodium efflux from bovine red cells with intracellular pH of 7.7. or 6.3 into 140 mM NaCl media with pH 7.9. The reduction of sodium exchange flux from the cells with low pH indicates that the intracellular site of the exchange system is inhibited by protons. Transport of protons through the membrane was reduced by inhibition of CO_2/HCO_3^- recycling with DIDS (4,4'-diisothiocyanostilbene-2,2'-disulfonate) (Cabantchick and Rothstein [2]). Experiments performed as described in Fig. 1.

pH erythrocytes	Sodium efflux mmol/L cells/h pH medium	
	7.9	
7.7	13.8	
6.3	10.2	8.7

158

mechanism have on cellular homeostasis if its physiological function is to operate as a Na^+/H^+ exchanger? It is known that smooth muscle cells have membrane potentials between -40 and $-60\,mV$ [22]. Protons are not at electrochemical equilibrium across the cell membrane, but are continuously extruded to keep intracellular pH around 6.9–7. The role of sodium/hydrogen ion-exchange mechanisms in the regulation of intracellular pH in various cell types has been reviewed by Roos and Boron [6]. A sodium/sodium exchange mechanism similar to that in ox red cells has been demonstrated in intestinal smooth muscle from guinea pig, where sodium efflux was enhanced when extracellular magnesium was replaced by sodium or lithium [23]. Kinsella and Aronson [24] have identified an exchange diffusion system capable of transporting sodium, lithium, and protons in rabbit renal microvillus membrane vesicles. This alleged Na^+/H^+ exchange was proposed to play an important role in proximal tubule urinary acidification. These and other examples dealt with by Roos and Boron [6] show that an exchange diffusion mechanism, specific for sodium, lithium, and hydrogen ions is found in many cell types.

According to the hypothesis of Blaustein [15], muscular tone of the resistance vessels is regulated by intracellular calcium. The concentration of intracellular calcium, in turn, depends on intracellular sodium concentration, because calcium removal from the cell is energized by the transmembrane electrochemical sodium gradient. A decrease of this gradient will thus tend to increase vascular tone, no matter by which mechanism the decreased gradient is established. One such mechanism is the sodium/proton exchange system. An increased activity of this mechanism will simultaneously increase the sodium influx and the removal of intracellular hydrogen ions. The increased intracellular sodium concentration may secondarily increase intracellular calcium concentration by slowing down the sodium-driven calcium extrusion. It is evident that the sodium-gradient hypothesis leaves the door open for a polymorphic pathogenesis of essential hypertension, because the pathological condition is evoked by increased activity of any transport system mediating sodium influx or by decreased activity of any transport mechanism performing sodium extrusion.

Finally, it must be considered whether an increased sodium/proton exchange can affect the tone of vascular smooth muscle by increasing the intracellular pH, as it may be the case in cerebral vessels, where an intracellular alkalosis caused by hypocapnia causes vascular contraction in contrast to the vasodilation that accompanies hypercapnemia as described by Schmidt [25] and Kety and Schmidt [26].

ACKNOWLEDGMENTS

We wish to thank veterinarian surgeon Dr. Ib Christiansen, Institute for Animal Reproduction, The Royal Veterinary and Agricultural University, Copenhagen,

Denmark, for supplying the bovine blood used in this study. The technical assistance of Mona Nielsen is gratefully acknowledged.

REFERENCES

1. Canessa M, Adragna RA, Bize I, et al.: Increased sodium-lithium countertranssport in red cells of patients with essential hypertension. N Engl J Med 302:772, 1980.
2. Ibsen KK, Jensen HA, Wieth JO, et al.: Essential hypertension. Sodium-lithium counter-transport in erythrocytes from patients and from children having one hypertensive parent. Hypertension 4, in press.
3. Motais R: Sodium movements in high-sodium beef red cells: Properties of an ouabain-insensitive exchange diffusion. J Physiol (Lond) 233:395, 1973.
4. Funder J, Wieth JO: Coupled lithium-sodium exchange in bovine red blood cells, in Straub RW, Bolis L (editors): Cell Membrane Receptors for Drugs and Hormones: A Multidisciplinary Approach. New York, Raven Press, 1978.
5. Duhm J, Becker B: Studies on lithium transport across the red cell membrane. V. On the nature of the Na^+-dependent Li^+ countertransport system of mammalian erythrocytes. J Membr Biol 51:263, 1979.
6. Roos A, Boron WF: Intracellular pH. Physiol Rev 61:296, 1981.
7. Rodland KD, Dunham PB: Kinetics of lithium efflux through the (Na,K)-pump of human erythrocytes. Biochim Biophys Acta 602:376, 1980.
8. Wieth JO: Effects of monovalent cations on sodium permeability of human red cells. Acta Physiol Scand 79:76, 1970.
9. Funder J, Tosteson DC, Wieth JO: Effects of bicarbonate on lithium transport in human red cells. J Gen Physiol 71:721, 1978.
10. Canessa M, Adragna RA, Bize I, et al.: Ouabain-insensitive cation transport in the red cells of normotensive and hypertensive subjects, in Zumkley H, Losse H (eds): Intracellular Electrolytes and Arterial Hypertension. Stuttgart, Georg Thieme Verlag, 1980, p 239.
11. Haas M, Schooler J, Tosteson DC: Coupling of lithium to sodium transport in human red cells. Nature 258:425, 1975.
12. Duhm J, Eisenried F, Becker BF, et al.: Studies on the lithium transport across the red cell membrane. I. Li^+ uphill transport by the Na^+-dependent Li^+ countertransport system of human erythrocytes. Pflugers Arch 364:147, 1976.
13. Duhm J, Becker BF: Studies on the lithium transport across the red cell membrane. IV. Interindividual variations in the Na^+-dependent Li^+ countertransport system of human erythrocytes. Pflugers Arch 370:211, 1977.
14. Relman AS: Mild hypertension: No more benign neglect. N Engl J Med 302:293, 1980.
15. Blaustein MP: Sodium ions, calcium ions, blood pressure regulation, and hypertension: A reassessment and a hypothesis. Am J Physiol 232:C165, 1977.
16. Wiley JS, Cooper RA: A furosemide-sensitive co-transport of Na + K in human red blood cell. J Clin Invest 53:745, 1974.
17. Dunham PB, Stewart GW, Ellory JC: Chloride-activated passive potassium transport in human erythrocytes. Proc Natl Acad Sci USA 77:1711, 1980.
18. Ellory JC, Stewart GW: The human erythrocyte Cl-dependent Na K co-transport system as a model for studying the action of loop diuretics. Br J Pharmacol, in press.
19. Cornish-Bowden A: A simple graphical method for determining the inhibition constants of mixed, uncompetitive and noncompetitive inhibitors. Biochem J 137:143, 1974.
20. Hanes CS: Studies on plant amylases. I. The effect of starch concentration upon the velocity of hydrolysis by the amylase of germinated barley. Biochem J 26:1406, 1932.

21. Cabantchik ZI, Rothstein A: Membrane proteins related to anion permeability of human red blood cell. I. Localization of disulfonic stilbene binding sites in proteins involved in permeation. J Membr Biol 15:207, 1974.

22. Jones AW: Content and fluxes of electrolytes, in Bohr D, Somlyo AP, Sparks HV Jr (editors): Handbook of Physiology, The Cardiovascular System. Vol II: Vascular Smooth Muscle. Bethesda, MD, American Physiological Society, 1980, p 253.

23. Brading AF: Sodium/sodium exchange in the smooth muscle of the guinea pig taenia coli. J Physiol (Lond) 251:79, 1975.

24. Kinsella JL, Aronson PS: Properties of the Na^+-H^+ exchanger in renal microvillus membrane vesicles. Am J Physiol 238:F461, 1980.

25. Schmidt CF: The influence of cerebral blood-flow on respiration. I. The respiratory responses to changes in cerebral blood-flow. Am J Physiol 84:202, 1982.

26. Kety SS, Schmidt CF: The effect of altered arterial tensions of carbon dioxide and oxygen on cerebral blood flow and cerebral oxygen consumption of normal young men. J Clin Invest 27:484, 1948.

DISCUSSION

Discussants: Hoffman, Funder, Abboud, Mulvani, Tosteson, Meyer

Hoffman: I'm wondering: Is that sodium-hydrogen exchange in the ox red cell amiloride-sensitive?

Funder: Amiloride does not inhibit the sodium/sodium exchange diffusion in bovine red cells even at a concentration of 5×10^{-3} and a pH of 7.4 in a 140-mM NaCl medium. If sodium/proton exchange is performed by the same system, this exchange will presumably be amiloride-insensitive, too.

Hoffman: Have you been able to turn the system around and measure a change in the medium pH induced by a sodium gradient?

Funder: Our attempts to demonstrate a net flux of hydrogen ion driven by a sodium gradient have been negative so far.

Abboud: I wonder to what extent the different results from the different laboratories could be ascribed to differences in sodium intake by the patients or differences in the way *in vitro* tests were performed? Could such factors influence the effects of pH and sodium on these transport systems? I wonder also whether circulating catecholamines have anything to do with these systems?

Funder: I do not know of any investigation correlating the sodium intake with the capacity of the lithium/sodium countertransport system. The differing results from different laboratories could, of course, be due to methodological differences, but could as well be due to, e.g., environmental factors. I don't know of any investigation of possible effects of catecholamines on lithium/sodium countertransport.

Mulvani: You raised the possibility that there is an increase in cellular sodium and said that on the sodium-calcium exchange hypothesis this would cause an increase in vasoconstriction. As I will be pointing out later on, I don't think the evidence for the hypothesis is overwhelming, and I think we ought to be cautious in accepting that hypothesis at present.

Tosteson: About the possible role of catecholamines: It's well known that in systems that have catecholamine receptors, for example bird red cells, the co-transport system is markedly activated by norepinephrine. Furthermore, there is a K-K exchange process in bird red cell membranes that's markedly activated by catecholamines. Thus, although it's not been well studied yet in many catecholamine-sensitive tissues in humans, it could be expected that this co-transport system would be activated in human cells that are sensitive to these hormones. So there is the possibility that some of the differences in the experimental results are related to one or more regulatory systems.

Funder: We know that some patients, with bipolar affective illness, have a low capacity of the transport system. Now we have found a group of hypertensive patients with a high capacity of the transport system. Does anyone know whether there is a lack of coincidence of hypertension and bipolar mental disease? If the same transport system is involved in hypertension and bipolar disease, patients with the affective disorder should be protected towards hypertension.

Hoffman: Since there is no response to your question, I suppose no one has found the correlation.

Meyer: No, I have no answer – obviously. But I think it's always very difficult to establish a correlation between infrequent diseases and very frequent ones like hypertension. The coincidence between two diseases can appear only if both diseases are very infrequent and if they are found in the same individual, which is not the case for both affective disorders and high blood pressure.

OUABAIN-SENSITIVE AND -INSENSITIVE CATION TRANSPORT IN IN NORMOTENSIVES AND HYPERTENSIVES IN HYPOKALEMIC STATES

ERLAND ERDMANN AND URSULA SCHMIDINGER

INTRODUCTION

Several years ago, it was reported that red blood cells of patients with essential hypertension contain an increased sodium concentration [1]. It could be demonstrated that the passive Na^+ influx into these erythrocytes was augmented in contrast to other types of hypertension [2]. Recently, results of a new test have been published by Garay and Meyer [3] showing abnormal net Na^+ and K^+ fluxes in erythrocytes of essential hypertensive patients. In Na^+-loaded/K^+-depleted red cells of these patients, a constant increase in net K^+ influx and a reduced ratio of Na^+/K^+ net fluxes were observed; this was not seen in hypertensives of renal origin. Wambach et al [4] reported an increased Na^+/K^+-ATPase activity in erythrocyte ghosts of patients with essential hypertension. In our earlier studies [5], we could not confirm these findings. We did, however, measure an increased number of ^3H-ouabain binding sites and of Na^+/K^+-ATPase activity in erythrocytes of patients with hypokalemia due to chronic diuretic treatment. Canessa et al [6] reported an increased sodium-lithium countertransport in red cells of patients with essential hypertension, apparently without overlap with normotensive people.

If these findings could be confirmed, we would be able to use a simple, noninvasive laboratory test to diagnose essential hypertension and possibly to avoid the onset of essential hypertension in the offspring by suitable treatment. With this in mind, we intended to investigate in the same persons (normotensives, essential hypertensives, and renal hypertensives) the Na^+/K^+ net fluxes, the number of Na^+/K^+-ATPase molecules, and the Na^+/Li^+ countertransport of the erythrocytes. When analyzing the obtained data, we found that there were abnormalities in Na^+/K^+ fluxes, especially in red cells of patients receiving diuretic treatment. We therefore included patients with hypokalemia due to chronic use or abuse of diuretics resulting in low serum potassium levels.

METHODS

Patients

Twentyeight normotensive volunteers (16 men and 12 women, aged 20–68 years, average 38) with blood pressures ≤140/90 mm Hg and without a history of high blood pressure were investigated. Six of these had at least one parent with essential hypertension (N ⊕). The remaining were without hypertensive family members (N ⊖).

Nineteen patients with secondary hypertension (11 men, 8 women; aged 19–72, average 47) were investigated. The clinical diagnoses were: 7 renal artery stenosis, 7 glomerulonephritis, 3 chronic pyelonephritis, 1 renin-producing tumor, 1 pheocromocytoma. Four of these patients had received kidney transplantation. All patients had blood pressures above 160/95 (mean 195/110) mm Hg.

Thirty-six patients suffered from essential hypertension. This diagnosis was believed when there was no other known cause of hypertension as evidenced by thorough clinical investigation (with renal angiography, etc.). Twenty men and 16 women (aged 21–83, mean 52 years) with blood pressures above 145/95 mm Hg (mean 185/105 mm Hg) were investigated. Since it was considered unethical to stop anthihypertensive treatment in these patients, drugs (β-blockers, vasodilators, and diuretics) were continued. There were 6 patients in the group of essential hypertension who had not been treated before this investigation.

Nine patients (1 man, 8 women; aged 28–74, mean 43 years) without hypertension were investigated because of serum potassium levels below 3.5 mmol/L (2.2–3.4; mean 3.0) due to chronic diuretic use or abuse (mainly furosemide or benzothiadiazides).

Blood was taken from a cubital vein, usually 20 ml; 500 U.S.P. heparin was added (Thrombophob®, Nordmark-Werke, Uetersen, Germany). The red cells were separated by means of centrifugation at 3000 × g for 10 minutes at 4°C, and plasma and buffy coat removed by suction.

Determination of sodium-lithium countertransport was carried out exactly as reported by Canessa et al [6].

Determination of net Na^+ and K^+ fluxes were carried out as described by Garay and Meyer [3] and by Garay et al [7] with 0.02 mM PCMB.

Determination of ^3H-ouabain binding sites was carried out as described earlier [5].

RESULTS

The erythrocyte Na^+ and K^+ concentrations in the different conditions are shown in Table 1. Due to a wide overlap of cation concentrations in the four times choline-washed red cells and the low number of patients, the differences were not significant.

Table 1. Intra-erythrocyte Na⁺ and K⁺ concentrations. $\bar{X} \pm SD$

	Age (years)	RR syst. (mm Hg)	RR diast. (mm Hg)	Erythrocyte Na⁺ (mmol/L$_e$)	K⁺ (mmol/L$_e$)	n
N⊖	32 ± 10	121 ± 5	75 ± 7	9.3 ± 2.1	96.9 ± 3.9	9
N⊕	30 ± 8	126 ± 13	78 ± 7	7.4 ± 0.7	96.4 ± 5.4	6
Essential hypertension	52 ± 16	185 ± 28	105 ± 15	8.3 ± 2.5	94.5 ± 5.8	21
Secondary hypertension	44 ± 16	195 ± 18	110 ± 9	8.5 ± 2.6	98.2 ± 5.9	9
Hypokalemia	39 ± 10	122 ± 27	72 ± 5	6.6 ± 0.9	94.9 ± 7.4	4

Net Na⁺ and K⁺ flux determinations (Fig. 1)

Using the method of Garay and Meyer [3, 7], we determined similar net Na⁺ efflux values (3.47 vs. 3.3 mmol/L$_e$) but higher net K⁺ influx values (2.74 vs. 1.4 mmol/L$_e$) in normotensives (N ⊖). The Na⁺/K⁺ flux ratios were significantly different ($P < 0.05$) from the normotensives (N ⊖) only in the hypokalemic group (Table 2), not in the essential hypertension group. Thus, we cannot confirm the work of Garay and Meyer [3, 7]. The apparent stimulation of the net K⁺ influx in hypokalemic states might be due to increased active Na⁺/K⁺ transport as evidenced by an increased number of Na⁺/K⁺-ATPase molecules, as reported previously [5, 8].

We did not find any significant differences in Na⁺ or K⁺ flux nor in the Na⁺/K⁺ flux ratios when analyzing separately patients without medication, high or low creatinine, with renal transplants, etc.

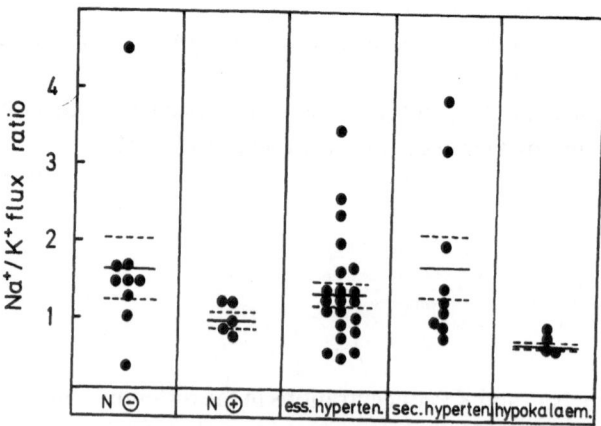

Figure 1. Na⁺/K⁺ flux ratios in erythrocytes. $\bar{X} \pm SEM$.

Table 2. Net Na$^+$ and K$^+$ fluxes of the erythrocytes. $\bar{X} \pm$ SD

	Net Na$^+$ efflux	Net K$^+$ influx	Na$^+$/K$^+$ flux ratio	n
N $\ominus$	3.47 $\pm$ 1.0	2.74 $\pm$ 0.9	1.59 $\pm$ 1.1	9
N $\oplus$	3.21 $\pm$ 0.4	3.59 $\pm$ 1.1	0.94 $\pm$ 0.2	5
Essential hypertension	3.89 $\pm$ 1.08	3.54 $\pm$ 1.4	1.31 $\pm$ 0.7	21
Secondary hypertension	4.13 $\pm$ 0.8	3.15 $\pm$ 1.3	1.69 $\pm$ 1.1	9
Hypokalemia	3.85 $\pm$ 1.1	5.6 $\pm$ 1.4	0.69 $\pm$ 0.1	4

Na$^+$/Li$^+$ countertransport determination

Table 3 gives the values of the Li$^+$ efflux of the Li$^+$-loaded erythrocytes into the Na$^+$ or Mg^{++} medium. Again, we cannot find a significant difference between normotensives (N $\ominus$) and hypertensives. There is a striking difference between these and the red cells of the hypokalemic patients (P<0.002). Our data thus do not confirm the data of Canessa et al [6]. Looking for a possible explanation, we investigated more closely those patients who were taking antihypertensive diuretic drugs. Table 4 clearly demonstrates that diuretic treatment (furosemide, chlorothiazides) do cause a significant alteration of the Na$^+$/Li$^+$ countertransport in the red cells, if serum potassium is low.

Table 3. Na$^+$/Li$^+$ countertransport of the erythrocytes. $\bar{X} \pm$ SD.

	Li$^+$ efflux in Na$^+$ medium	Li$^+$ efflux in Mg^{++} medium	Na$^+$/Li$^+$ countertransport	n
N $\ominus$	0.53 $\pm$ 0.10 ($\pm$0.02)	0.21 $\pm$ 0.08 ($\pm$0.02)	0.32 $\pm$ 0.10 ($\pm$0.02)	19
N $\oplus$	0.46 $\pm$ 0.10 ($\pm$0.04)	0.17 $\pm$ 0.08 ($\pm$0.04)	0.29 $\pm$ 0.08 ($\pm$0.04)	6
Essential hypertension	0.57 $\pm$ 0.20 ($\pm$0.04)	0.20 $\pm$ 0.06 ($\pm$0.01)	0.37 $\pm$ 0.10 ($\pm$0.02)	33
secondary hypertension	0.60 $\pm$ 0.20 ($\pm$0.05)	0.21 $\pm$ 0.06 ($\pm$0.01)	0.39 $\pm$ 0.10 ($\pm$0.02)	18
Hypokalemia	0.90 $\pm$ 0.20 ($\pm$0.07)	0.26 $\pm$ 0.10 ($\pm$0.04)	0.64 $\pm$ 0.20 ($\pm$0.07)	8

The patients with essential hypertension in our group did not have low serum potassium. Their Na$^+$/Li$^+$ countertransport values overlap considerably with those of normotensives (Fig 2).

Table 4. Influence of diuretics on Na⁺/Li⁺ countertransport of the erythrocytes. $\bar{X} \pm$ SEM

	Li⁺ efflux (mmol/L$_e$h)	Na⁺/Li⁺ counter-transport (mmol/L$_e$/h)	n
N ⊖	0.53 ± 0.02	0.32 ± 0.02	19
without diuretics K⁺ > 3.5	0.42 ± 0.04	0.25 ± 0.04	4
with diuretics K⁺ > 3.5	0.58 ± 0.04	0.37 ± 0.03	8
with diuretics K⁺ < 3.5	0.76 ± 0.09	0.51 ± 0.07	6
with diuretics K⁺ > 3.5 creatinine 1.4	0.55 ± 0.05	0.35 ± 0.04	8
with diuretics, (kidney transplant)	0.63 ± 0.09	0.41 ± 0.04	4
without drugs	0.63 ± 0.05	0.42 ± 0.04	6
with antihypertensive drugs (β-blockers, etc.)	0.54 ± 0.05	0.35 ± 0.05	9
with diuretics K⁺ > 3.5	0.58 ± 0.06	0.39 ± 0.05	12
with diuretics + antihypertensive drugs K⁺ > 3.5 creatinine > 1.4	0.46 ± 0.04	0.28 ± 0.04	4
hypokalemia	0.90 ± 0.07	0.64 ± 0.07	8

(The first five data rows are grouped under "Secondary hypertension"; the rows from "without drugs" through "with diuretics + antihypertensive drugs" are grouped under "Essential hypertension".)

Na⁺/K⁺-ATPase molecules per erythrocyte

It is accepted that the maximal number of ³H-ouabain binding sites reflects the number of Na⁺/K⁺-ATPase molecules [5, 9]. When measuring the ouabain binding sites in red cells of the different groups (Table 5), we found significant differences only in those of hypokalemic patients (P<0.025). Similar findings have been reported in detail earlier [5, 10]. We did show then that the number of

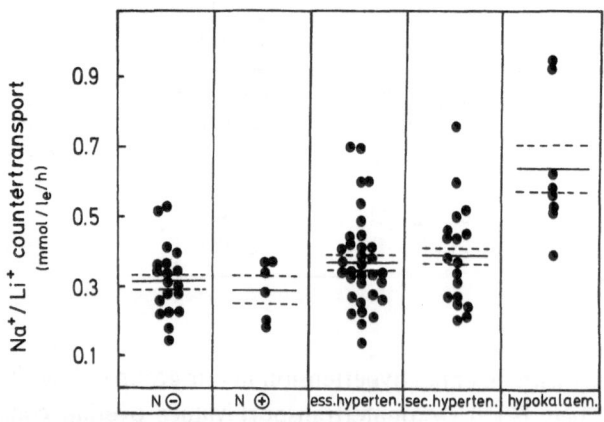

Figure 2. Na⁺/Li⁺ countertransport in the erythrocytes. $\bar{X} \pm$ SEM

Table 5. Number of ^{3}H-ouabain binding sites of the erythrocytes. $\bar{X} \pm SD$.

	N $\ominus$	N $\oplus$	essential hypertension	secondary hypertension	Hypokalemia
Number of ^{3}H-ouabain binding sites per erythrocyte $\bar{X} \pm SD$	393 ± 114	515 ± 327	465 ± 217	427 ± 220	813 ± 278
	$n = 13$	$n = 4$	$n = 30$	$n = 15$	$n = 7$

ouabain binding sites decreases again after correction of serum potassium levels. However this takes some 100–120 days, approximately the life span of the erythrocytes. Furthermore, there was an increase of ouabain binding sites when diuretics were taken, even before serum potassium levels decreased.

DISCUSSION

Our measurements of net Na$^+$/ and K$^+$ fluxes or Na$^+$/Li$^+$ countertransport in erythrocytes of normotensive or hypertensive patients were not significantly different. Thus, we cannot confirm the results given by Garay and Meyer [3], Garay et al. [7], or by Canessa et al. [6]. We did not find increased Na$^+$/ K$^+$-ATPase activity in red cells of patients with essential hypertension [5] as reported by Wambach et al. [4]. Therefore, at least in our patients, we cannot detect a constant cation transport abnormality in erythrocytes in essential hypertension.

We did disclose an increased Na$^+$/Li$^+$ countertransport in red cells of patients with hypokalemia due to diuretic drugs (Table 3). Hypertensive patients with diuretic treatment resulting in low serum potassium levels show the same abnormality (Table 4).

Discontinuing the diuretics for 2 weeks did not change the Na$^+$ Li$^+$ countertransport values significantly (data not shown) in two patients. Two patients took potassium-sparing diuretics (spironolactone). Their erythrocytes had normal Na$^+$/Li$^+$ countertransport values and normal ouabain binding sites.

The increase in ouabain binding sites in erythrocytes of hypokalemic patients has been reported earlier by us [5, 10] and in rat erythrocytes by Chan and Sanslone [11]. Apparently, low extracellular potassium stimulates the de novo synthesis of the Na$^+$/K$^+$ pump in red cells during erythropoiesis. Thus, erythrocytes maintain their intracellular Na$^+$ and K$^+$, although serum K$^+$ is low (see Table 1). This has been discussed in detail elsewhere [8]. A connection between the active Na$^+$/K$^+$ transport system and Na$^+$/Li$^+$ countertransport has not been reported to our knowledge. Direct or indirect connections are possible. Hypokalemia might stimulate both systems. The nature of the Na^+/Li^+ countertransport system is not quite clear yet, however. Further investigations in that respect are necessary.

We do not know whether the reported high Na^+/K^+-ATPase activity [4] or the increased Na^+/Li^+ countertransport [6] was due to chronic diuretic treatment, even though the drugs in their study were left out 6 days to 2 weeks prior to the investigation. We think, however, that the reported laboratory tests, at least in our hands, are not suited to distinguish between essential hypertension and secondary hypertension.

ACKNOWLEDGEMENT

Supported by the Deutsche Forschungsgemeinschaft (Er 65/2).

REFERENCES

1. Losse H, Wehmeyer H, Wessels F: Der Wasser- und Elektrolytgehalt von Erythrozyten bei arterieller Hypertonie. Klin Wochenschr 38:393, 1960.
2. Wessels F, Junge-Hülsing G, Losse J: Untersuchungen zur Natriumpermeabilität der Erythrozyten bei Normo- und Hypertonikern mit familiärer Hochdruckbelastung. Z Kreislaufforsch 56:374, 1967.
3. Garay RP, Meyer P: A new test showing abnormal net Na^+ and K^+ fluxes in erythrocytes of essential hypertensive patients. Lancet I:349–353, 1979.
4. Wambach G, Helber A, Bönner G, et al.: Natrium-Kalium-Adenosintriphosphatase-Aktivität in Erythozytenghosts von Patienten mit essentieller Hypertonie. Klin Wochenschr 57:169–172, 1979.
5. Erdmann E, Werdan K, Hegelberger T, et al.: Determination of the number of $(Na^+ + K^+)$-ATPase molecules, their enzymatic activity and the active Na^+/K^+-transport of human erythrocytes in Hypokalaemia and in hypertension, in Zumkley H, Losse H (editors): Intracellular Electrolytes and Arterial Hypertension. Stuttgart, Georg Thieme Verlag, 1980, pp 164–170.
6. Canessa M, Adragna N, Solomon HS, et al.: Increased sodium-lithium countertransport in red cells of patients with essential hypertension. N Engl J Med 302:772–776, 1980.
7. Garay RP, Elghozi JL, Dagher G, et al.: Laboratory distinction between essential and secondary hypertension by measurement of erythrocyte cation fluxes. N Engl J Med 302:769–771, 1980.
8. Erdmann E, Krawietz W, Koch M: Cardiac glycoside receptors in disease: The number of ouabain binding sites in human erythrocytes subject to regulation, in Skou JC, Nørby JG (editors): Na,K-ATPase, Structure and Kinetics. New York, Academic Press, 1979, pp 518–524.
9. Erdmann E, Hasse W: Quantitative aspects of ouabain binding to human erythrocyte and cardiac membrane. J Physiol 251:671–682, 1975.
10. Erdmann E, Krawietz W: Increased number of ouabain binding sites in human erythrocyte membranes in chronic hypokalaemia. Acta Biol Med Ger 36:879–883, 1977.
11. Chan PC, Sanslone WR: The influence of a low potassium diet on rat erythrocyte membrane adenosine triphosphatase. Arch Biochem Biophys 134:48–52, 1969.

DISCUSSION

Discussants: Haddy, Erdmann, MacGregor, Tobian, Langer, Tosteson, Folkow

Haddy: Your sodium-potassium ATPase measurements were not different in the essential hypertensives from those in the normotensives.

Erdmann: Right.

Haddy: Have you tried segregating them according to their renin status? That is, would the renin patients have a different sodium-potassium ATPase activity than the normal or the high?

Erdmann: Unfortunately, we have not. I could go back to my data because we have renin values of several patients, but I don't know the answer.

MacGregor: I think the observations are fascinating. How many of these receptors are already occupied by an endogenous ouabain-like substance? It might be that when you give a diuretic, you lose sodium, and you'll have less of this endogenous inhibitor around. That might be an explanation of the results with the hypokalemia, rather than the hypokalemia itself.

Erdmann: I have no answer to this, since I do not know of a real endogenous glycoside.

Tobian; When you give a diuretic, your body sodium goes down, so instead of putting out natriuretic hormone, you'd have less natriuretic hormone. You were talking about the binding sites. That would suggest an up-regulation of sites, and you did show more binding sites. This, then, could explain at least part of the data, but not the countertransport and co-transport, and they all seem to be part of the same picture.

Erdmann: I have up till now always considered the steeper potassium gradient as responsible for the increased number of sodium pumps.

Langer: How would you propose that the increase in V_{max} for ouabain binding comes about? What would be the mechanism?

Erdmann; As the time that they disappear agrees just about with the life span of erythrocytes, I think it must happen during erythropoiesis. That to me is very obvious.

Langer: O.K. So when you talk about chronic hypokalemia, the question is, how chronic does it have to be because of the half-life of your red blood cells?

Erdmann: We have looked at several patients who were chronically dialyzed, and with dialyzation you can take away potassium quite well. We have had several patients dialyzed quite strictly for potassium, and we did not see an increase in binding sites. So I think you need more than months, but I have not measured this.

MacGregor: I get a feeling that you are suggesting that in some of the published studies patients were on diuretics. Would someone like to comment on that?

Erdmann: I would not say that. What I think is much more interesting is that there seems to be regulation.

170

MacGregor: In patients with idiopathic edema, it is very difficult to know if patients are taking diuretics or not.

Erdmann: And that is the problem. Most of these women lie.

Folkow: May I ask Dr. Tosteson to give his final comments on this very interesting field?

Tosteson: I take the podium with great hesitancy with that kind of charge. This does represent a sort of watershed in the program. We have until now heard a number of papers that deal with the possible relationship between the transport of sodium and potassium ions across membranes and hypertension of unknown pathogenesis. On Saturday afternoon we shall take a very careful look at the possibility that there is inhibition of the sodium-potassium pump by a circulating inhibitor that somehow could be involved in the pathogenesis of hypertension. After what I thought were excellent introductory and comprehensive lectures by Drs. Yamori and Postnov that called to our attention the complexity of the syndrome, and the many possibilities that are still open in pathogenesis, we discussed the theme of ouabain-insensitive sodium and potassium transport in red cells, and the possible relationship to hypertension. We talked both about spontaneous hypertension in rats and also substantially about observations that have been made on human red cells.

I'd like to tell you where I am in my understanding of the story in human red cells. What we can say for certain about relationships between ouabain-insensitive pathways for sodium movements in human red cells and so-called essential hypertension is not very much. Perhaps a way of beginning to summarize would be to answer the questions that Dr. Abboud put: Are the differences in observations in different laboratories due to differences in ways that measurements are made, or are they due to differences in the red cells on which the measurements are made? I think the answer has to be both. There are a number of different methods that have been used and are being used that were reported today, and I think that at least some of the differences that have been reported are probably referable to differences in methods.

But I think we can also say that such methodological differences cannot account for all of the differences in the results. There certainly are differences in the red cells. In general, I think that we have to say that we do not understand the basis for these individual differences in the human population in these ouabain-insensitive modalities of sodium movement.

I think the evidence presented this afternoon shows in a rather compelling way that there is reason to believe that genetic factors are present and play a significant role. There also may very well be environmental factors, though they have not yet been clearly identified.

Some suggestions – for example, differences in hormonal status in female subjects – seem to be correlated with differences in red cell co-transport. But I think we must be very aware that much needs to be done to define more precisely what those environmental factors are. I think the point that was brought out by Dr. Burke, that some of the complexity may be in itself genetic in origin, is something that we should bear in mind as we proceed.

In my view the connections between individual differences in ouabain-insensitive sodium movements in red cells and increased peripheral resistance in essential hypertension are completely obscure. I hope that we'll learn something about pathways toward greater understanding in that direction from the part of the program on which we will be embarking in a few minutes. To my mind, the message that comes through very clearly is that hypertension comes trippingly off the tongue but clearly is a term that conveys many meanings of which we are only now coming to see the multiplicity.

Perhaps the place to draw a lesson would be from what we've learned about diabetes mellitus in the last 10 or 15 years. It's quite clear that an elevated blood sugar can be produced in a number of different ways. I think it seems quite obvious that the syndrome of so-called essential hypertension probably can be arrived at through a number of different pathogenic pathways. Perhaps we are now in the early phases of being able to discern ways of distinguishing between these different pathways. I think getting on to identifying informational macromolecules that can be associated with the different transport pathways with reasonable certainty is an important step to take in that direction. Perhaps that's enough by way of not very satisfactory summing up. I look forward now to having a look at some investigations that deal more directly with factors that are involved in regulating peripheral vascular resistance.

PRESYNAPTIC α-AUTORECEPTORS: PHARMACOLOGICAL PROPERTIES AND PHYSIOLOGICAL FUNCTION

K. Starke, A. Steppeler, and W. Auch-Schwelk

INTRODUCTION

The view that α-adrenoceptors can be divided into two major subgroups sprang mainly from studies on the pre- and postsynaptic α-receptors at junctions between postganglionic sympathetic neurons and muscle cells [1, 2]. The terms α_1 and α_2 were loosely suggested [3], then used to refer to post- and presynaptic α-receptors [4], and finally generalized [5, 6].

A subclassification of receptors is useful only to the degree that drugs are available to interact selectively with the one or the other subtype. Yohimbine was the first α_2-selective antagonist to be detected [7]. In this paper we summarize a comparison of the effects of some diastereomers of yohimbine at α_1- and α_2-adrenoceptors. The tissue selected was the main pulmonary artery of the rabbit. Although differences between the pre- and postsynaptic α-receptors of the rabbit heart and the cat spleen initially pointed to a heterogeneity of α-receptors [1, 2], the postsynaptic α-receptors of the rabbit pulmonary artery have become the α_1 prototypes, and the presynaptic α-receptors of the sympathetic neurons innervating the artery, the α_2 prototypes [5, 6].

Presynaptic α-receptors of noradrenergic fibers are sometimes called autoreceptors under the assumption that they are physiological sites of action of the transmitter noradrenaline itself. However, such a physiological function has recently been questioned [8–11]. In the second part of the present paper, we describe experiments in which this problem was re-investigated.

PHARMACOLOGICAL PROPERTIES

One type of experiment that we used to study the effects of yohimbine diastereomers on pre- and postsynaptic α-adrenoceptors is illustrated in Figures 1 and 2. Spiral strips of the rabbit pulmonary artery were pre-incubated with ^{3}H-noradrenaline $3\,\mu$M for 60 minutes and then superfused with ^{3}H-noradrenaline-free medium for 210 minutes. The superfusion fluid contained propranolol, cocaine, and corticosterone in order to block β-adrenoceptors and the neuronal and extraneuronal uptake of noradrenaline, respectively. The sympa-

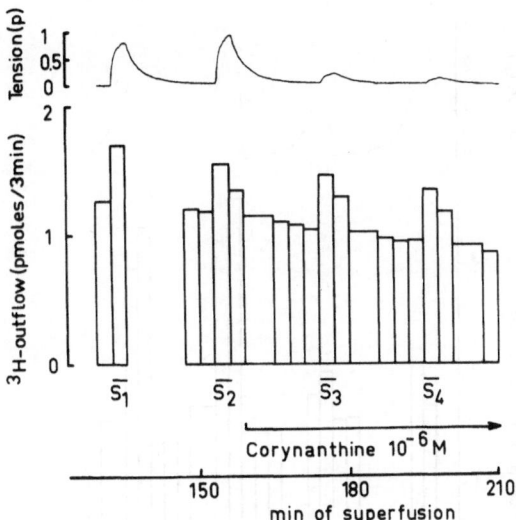

Figure 1. Effect of corynanthine on a pulmonary artery strip pre-incubated with ^{3}H-noradrenaline. After pre-incubation, the strip was superfused with medium containing propranolol 4 μM, cocaine 30 μM, and corticosterone 40 μM. The superfusate was collected in 3- or 6-min samples. The strip was stimulated four times for 3 min each at 2 Hz (S$_1$–S$_4$).

thetic axons at the adventitio-medial border were stimulated by short (0.3 msec) transmural electrical pulses, delivered at intervals of 21 minutes for 3 minutes each at a frequency of 2 Hz and supramaximal current strength (200 mA). The basal outflow of tritiated compounds consists mainly of deaminated metabolites of ^{3}H-noradrenaline and is due to leakage of the transmitter from the storage granules into the axoplasm, where it is catabolized by monoamine oxidase. The increase in tritium outflow caused by electrical stimulation, in contrast, consists mainly of ^{3}H-noradrenaline released by action potentials into the extracellular space. The stimulation-evoked overflow is, therefore, abolished in calcium-free medium or by tetrodotoxin [13]. With uptake mechanisms largely paralyzed, changes in the evoked overflow of tritium reflect changes in the release of ^{3}H-noradrenaline from the interior of the neurons. The principle features of the preparation were originally described by Su and Bevan [14].

As shown in Figure 1, corynanthine – a yohimbane derivative differing from yohimbine only in the configuration at C$_{(16)}$ which carries the methoxycarbonyl group – almost abolished the contractile response to stimulation. On the other hand, the stimulation-evoked overflow of tritium, i.e. the release of noradrenaline, was not changed. At the concentration used, corynanthine apparently blocked the postsynaptic α_1-adrenoceptors but had no detectable effect on the presynaptic α_2-adrenoceptors. In marked contrast, rauwolscine, an alloyohimbane derivative differing from yohimbine in the configuration at two asymmetric carbon atoms, increased the release of noradrenaline and increased rather than

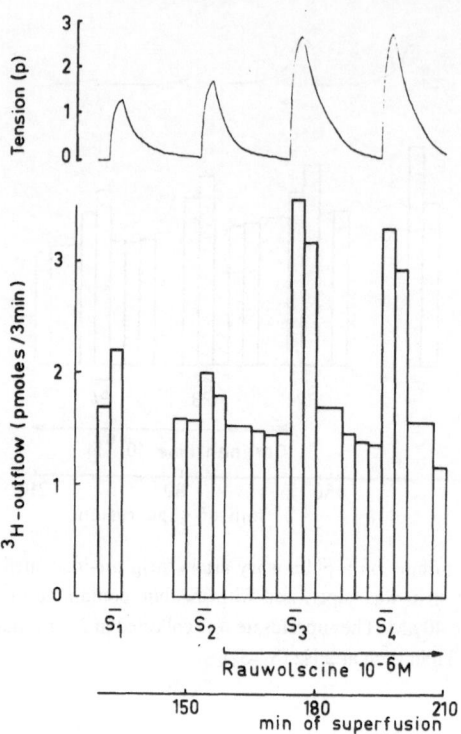

Figure 2. Effect of rauwolscine on a pulmonary artery strip pre-incubated with ^{3}H-noradrenaline. For details, see legend to *Figure 1*. From Weitzell et al. [12].

reduced the contractile response (Fig. 2). This pattern resembles that found with yohimbine [7]. At the concentration used, rauwolscine apparently blocked the presynaptic α_2-adrenoceptor and, hence, interrupted the self-inhibition of noradrenaline release, but had no major effect postsynaptically, so that the excess noradrenaline released could trigger an excess postsynaptic response.

In another series of experiments, the affinities of the diastereomers for the postsynaptic α_1-receptors were determined more directly by the antagonism against the contractile effect of exogenous noradrenaline. Under proper conditions, this yields the apparent dissociation constant K_B of the antagonist-postsynaptic α-receptor complex. A comparison of the presynaptic potency, as revealed by the effect on the stimulation-evoked overflow of tritium, with the K_B values, confirmed the α_2-preference of rauwolscine and yohimbine and the α_1-preference of corynanthine.

Three further diastereomers were studied: β-yohimbine – a yohimbane derivative differing from yohimbine only in the configuration at $C_{(17)}$, which carries the hydroxy group – behaved like yohimbine and rauwolscine. Pseudoyohimbine and 3-epi-α-yohimbine, compounds in which the nucleus of the molecule is highly angular because of a 3α-configuration, exerted a different pattern of effects. These drugs were only weak antagonists at both pre- and postsynaptic α-receptors, but at low concentrations accelerated the basal outflow of tritium due to a selective increase in the outflow of ^{3}H-3,4-dihydroxyphenylglycol. The effect resembled that of reserpine which is a chemically similar indole alkaloid with a 3α-configuration.

Figure 3 shows the place that the yohimbine diastereomers (except the reserpine-like compounds) occupy in the series of antagonists that we studied in the pulmonary artery. For each drug, the ratio of postsynaptic potency over presynaptic potency is indicated. Corynanthine has the second-highest preference for the postsynaptic α$_1$-adrenoceptor, being surpassed only by prazosin [15]. Yohimbine, β-yohimbine, and rauwolscine are the compounds that are most selective for the presynaptic α$_2$-adrenoceptor.

Why recommend arcane alkaloids when more common antagonists (Fig. 3) are available? First, of course, because of their superior selectivity. Second, being diastereomers, they share many physicochemical properties; for instance, they have similar lipid solubility [16]. Since we reported on the selectivity of the diastereomers, they have been employed repeatedly for the differentiation of α-receptor subtypes, in particular those compounds that are commercially available – namely yohimbine, rauwolscine, and corynanthine. With these three alkaloids, we have shown that the presynaptic α-autoreceptors of rat and rabbit brain are α$_2$ [17, 18], that the hindleg vasculature of the rabbit contains postsynap-

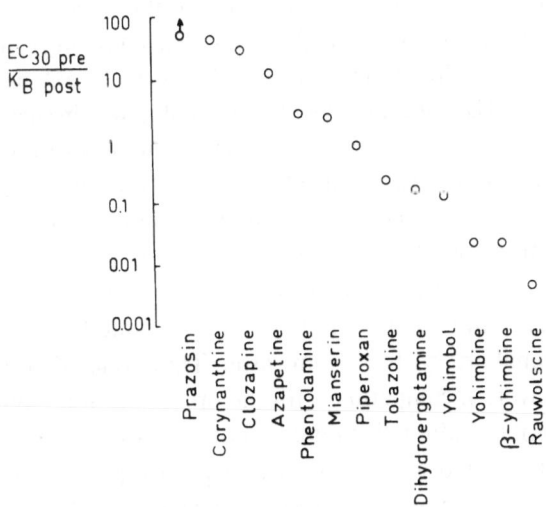

Figure 3. Relative pre- and postsynaptic effects of α-adrenoceptor antagonists in the pulmonary artery of the rabbit. EC$_{30\,pre}$, concentration that increased the evoked overflow of tritium by 30% (in experiments analogous to those of Figs. 1 and 2). K$_{B\,post}$, apparent dissociation constant of the antagonist-postsynaptic α-receptor complex.

tic, smooth muscle α_2-adrenoceptors [19], and that the smooth muscle α-adrenoceptors of the rabbit isolated aorta and pulmonary artery are purely α_1 [20]. By use of yohimbine, rauwolscine, and corynanthine, it has been shown that the smooth muscle α-receptors of guinea-pig aorta are α_1, whereas the α-receptors of the cholinergic neurons of the ileum and the trachea of the guinea pig are α_2 [21]. In pithed rats and in anesthetized dogs, the isomers display essentially the same selectivities as *in vitro* [22, 23]. The alkaloids have also been employed in radioligand-binding experiments. They have helped to identify the ^{3}H-clonidine binding site in homogenates from rat brain cortex as an α_2-receptor and the ^{3}H-WB 4101 binding site as an α_1-receptor [24] and to establish that ^{3}H-clonidine binds selectively to α_2-receptors in membranes from the guinea-pig ileum [25]. Finally, yohimbine and rauwolscine have been prepared in tritiated form for the labelling of α_2-receptors with radioactive antagonists [26, 27].

PHYSIOLOGICAL FUNCTION

The existence of presynaptic α-adrenoceptors at noradrenergic neurons can hardly be denied. As pointed out above, they were the α_2 prototypes and have led to the discovery of this subspecies of receptor in numerous tissues and with numerous techniques. It would be surprising if the prototype were a phantom.

The question as to whether the presynaptic α-adrenoceptors are autoreceptors – meaning that, apart from exogenous drugs, endogenous noradrenaline has access to the receptors and inhibits further release of noradrenaline – is more difficult to answer. The main evidence for a physiological role is, of course, the effect of antagonists as illustrated in Figure 2, which is strongly suggestive of the interruption of an ongoing α-adrenergic inhibition. As shown by extensive tables compiled in review articles [28, 29], the effect has been obtained in such a variety of tissues and with so many antagonists, that negative findings (no increase in release by an antagonist) should be scrutinized for possible reasons. In Gillespie's words [29]: 'On examination of the experimental conditions these (negative findings) serve mainly to prove the rule that α-antagonists increase overflow.' Kalsner [8–10] and Chan and Kalsner [11] recently confirmed the release-enhancing effect of phenoxybenzamine in ^{3}H-noradrenaline-pretreated vasa deferentia from guinea pigs and renal artery strips from cattle. They concluded, however, that their observations were incompatible with the operation of a physiological α-adrenergic inhibition of noradrenaline release. For instance, when the guinea-pig vas deferens was stimulated with trains of four pulses, phenoxybenzamine caused similar facilitation, independently of whether the interval between pulses was 0.07, 0.2, or 1 sec, although at the shorter intervals the perineuronal concentration of noradrenaline and, hence, the degree of feedback inhibition should have been greater [9]. Phenoxybenzamine increased even the release evoked by a single pulse when there should have been very little perineuronal noradrenaline

[8]. Yet, although these effects of phenoxybenzamine may indeed *not* have been due to the blockade of α-autoreceptors, as suggested by the authors, the relevance of their findings for the question of a physiological auto-inhibition is doubtful. Phenoxybenzamine is a notoriously nonspecific drug. In all four papers quoted above, it was used only at one very high concentration, namely 33 μM, and in each study it accelerated the basal outflow of tritium. The latter effect is well-known, unrelated to α-receptor blockade, and presumably due to interference with the vesicular storage of noradrenaline in a manner akin to what reserpine does [30]. It may be pertinent that the ability to increase the stimulation-evoked, exocytotic release of noradrenaline is an inherent property of reserpine-like drugs [31]. Hence, a reserpine-like action may be one mechanism by which phenoxybenzamine 33 μM increases action potential-evoked release of noradrenaline. This component, of course, will not obey predictions made for an α-adrenolytic mechanism and renders phenoxybenzamine 33 μM a priori little suited for probing the autoreceptor hypothesis in this manner [31, 32].

The critical studies of Kalsner and his colleagues prompted us to carry out similar experiments choosing what we thought might be more appropriate conditions. Isolated ear arteries from rabbits were pre-incubated with ^{3}H-noradrenaline 0.5 μM for 60 minutes and then perfused-superfused with ^{3}H-noradrenaline-free medium for 231 minutes as described by Allen et al [33]. ^{3}H-noradrenaline in the perfusate was determined after column chromatography [34]. The protocol is illustrated in Figure 4. Two cycles of electrical stimulation were applied to the arteries, each cycle consisting of three trains of pulses with train intervals of 11 minutes. The three trains were applied either in the (ascending) order of 10 shocks at 0.2 Hz, 10 shocks at 2 Hz, 100 shocks at 2 Hz or in the reverse (descending) order. The first cycle began after 153 minutes, and the second after 206 minutes of perfusion. In the two cycles of a particular artery, the order of pulse trains was the same, and in each experimental group, half of the arteries were stimulated in ascending order and the other half in descending order.

As shown in Figure 4, stimulation with 10 shocks at 0.2 Hz elicited only a small overflow of ^{3}H-noradrenaline. When the same number of pulses was given at 2 Hz, the overflow was higher, and with 100 pulses at 2 Hz, it was pronounced. In control experiments (upper panel of Fig. 4), responses in the second cycle were similar to those in the first cycle. Yohimbine 1 μM, added during the second cycle, changed neither the basal outflow of ^{3}H-noradrenaline nor the overflow elicited by 10 shocks at 0.2 or 2 Hz, but seemed to increase the overflow elicited by 100 shocks at 2 Hz (lower panel of Fig. 4).

For further evaluation, the stimulation-evoked overflow (after subtraction of the basal outflow) was expressed as percent of the tritium content of the tissue at the onset of the respective stimulation period. The overflow during the first cycle averaged $0.0042 \pm 0.0006\%$ for 10 shocks at 0.2 Hz, $0.017 \pm 0.002\%$ for 10 shocks at 2 Hz, and $0.17 \pm \& 0.02\%$ for 100 shocks at 2 Hz (means $\pm$ S.E.; n = 28). Ratios

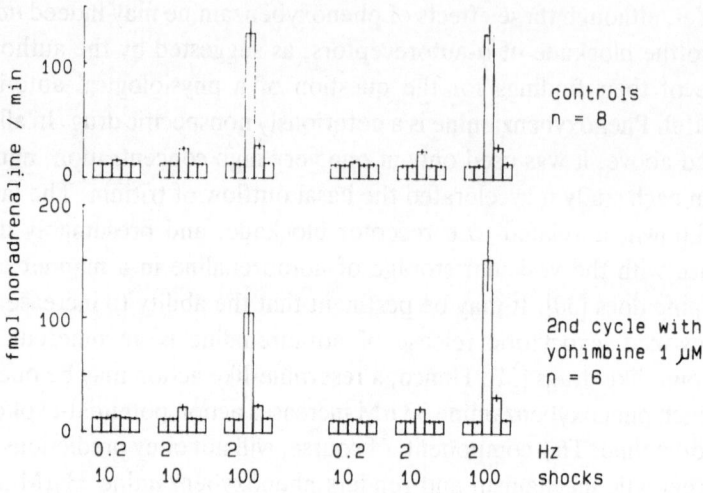

Figure 4. Effect of yohimbine on the outflow of ^{3}H-noradrenaline from ear arteries pre-incubated with ^{3}H-noradrenaline. After pre-incubation, the arteries were perfused with fresh medium. Two cycles of stimulation consisting of three trains of pulses each were administered to each artery. Stimulation parameters are indicated below the columns. The perfusate was collected in 1-min samples for 2 min before and 3 min after the onset of each train. Columns indicate the outflow of ^{3}H-noradrenaline in these five 1-min samples per pulse train. In the experiments represented in the lower panel, yohimbine was present from 25 min before the second cycle onwards. Means $\pm$ S.E.

between responses (as percent of tissue tritium) during the second cycle and the corresponding responses during the first cycle are shown in Figure 5. Because the overflow elicited by 10 pulses at 0.2 Hz was so small, the scatter of the ratios was large. Cocaine increased the overflow at all stimulation parameters. Clonidine caused a marked decrease except for 10 shocks at 0.2 Hz, presumably because of the scatter of the latter values. Yohimbine did not change the overflow evoked by 10 pulses at 0.2 or 2 Hz, but significantly increased the overflow evoked by 100 pulses at 2 Hz.

In another series, cocaine 10 μM was added throughout the 231 minutes of perfusion. With ^{3}H-noradrenaline reuptake inhibited, the stimulation-evoked overflow in the first cycle was augmented to $0.018 \pm 0.003\%$ for 10 shocks at 0.2 Hz, to $0.071 \pm 0.009\%$ for 10 shocks at 2 Hz, and to $0.48 \pm 0.08\%$ for 100 shocks at 2 Hz (n = 16). As shown in Figure 6, the scatter of the ratios second cycle/first cycle was now acceptable even for 10 shocks at 0.2 Hz. Again, yohimbine failed to increase the overflow evoked by 10 shocks at 0.2 Hz (there was actually a slight decrease) or 10 shocks at 2 Hz, but significantly increased the overflow evoked by 100 shocks at 2 Hz.

These results indicate that the effect of low concentrations of an α_2-antagonist on the release of noradrenaline does depend on the stimulation conditions. Apparently, facilitation occurs only when the stimulation is strong enough to

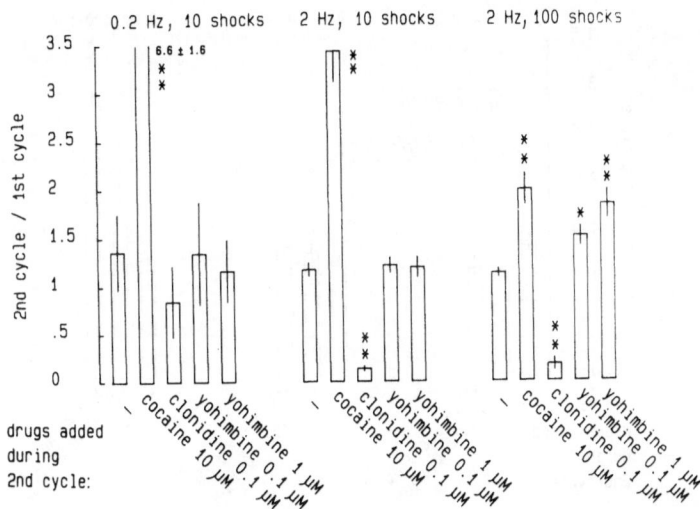

Figure 5. Effects of cocaine, clonidine, and yohimbine on the stimulation-evoked overflow of ^{3}H-noradrenaline from ear arteries pre-incubated with ^{3}H-noradrenaline. The experimental protocol is illustrated in Fig. 4. Ordinate, ratio between the overflow obtained in the second cycle and the corresponding overflow in the first cycle. Drugs were added 25 min before the second cycle and kept for the rest of the experiment. Means $\pm$ S.E. of 8 (controls), 4 (cocaine), 4 (clonidine), 6 (yohimbine 0.1 μM), and 6 (yohimbine 1 μM) experiments. Significant differences from controls: * $P < 0.05$; ‡ $P < 0.001$.

produce a marked release and, hence, a relatively high perineuronal concentration of noradrenaline. The lack of an effect of yohimbine on the overflow elicited by 10 shocks at 0.2 Hz in the absence of cocaine (Fig. 5) might have been due to the large variability. However, this explanation does not hold true for the lack of an effect on the response to 10 shocks at 2 Hz or to 10 shocks at 0.2 Hz in the presence of cocaine, when the variability was small and even the α-adrenergic inhibition caused by clonidine was readily demonstrable. Yohimbine did not enhance the evoked overflow of ^{3}H-noradrenaline by blocking its reuptake, because cocaine produced an antirely different pattern of changes (Fig. 5), and because the effect of yohimbine persisted in the presence of cocaine (Fig. 6).

Our findings are in general agreement with those of Markiewicz et al. [35] in the mouse vas deferens, of Constantine (personal communication) in the rabbit pulmonary artery, and of McCulloch et al. [36] and Story et al. [37] in guinea-pig atria, all suggesting that α$_2$-antagonists require a certain minimal perineuronal concentration of noradrenaline to facilitate the release of the transmitter. Story et al. [37] have pointed out that, in addition, a certain minimal time over which the neurons are stimulated (>1.5 sec in their experiments) is necessary for facilitation to become manifest; the auto-inhibition may take some time to develop, because the mechanism beyond the presynaptic α$_2$-receptor, perhaps the inhibition of adenylate cyclase, is relatively slow. This may be relevant for our experiments.

180

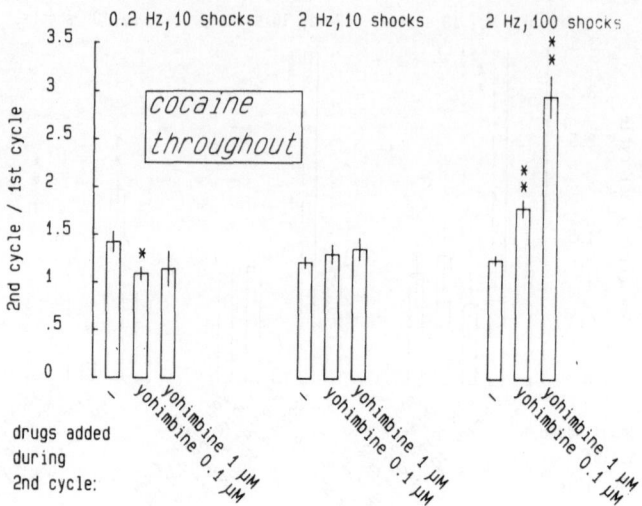

Figure 6. Effect of yohimbine on the stimulation-evoked overflow of ³H-noradrenaline from ear arteries pre-incubated with ³H-noradrenaline and then perfused with medium containing 10 μM cocaine. The experimental protocol is illustrated in Fig. 4. Ordinate, ratio between the overflow obtained in the second cycle and the corresponding overflow in the first cycle. Yohimbine was added 25 min before the second cycle and kept for the rest of the experiment. Means ± S.E. of 6 (controls), 6 (yohimbine 0.1 μM), and 4 (yohimbine 1μM) experiments. Significant differences from controls: * $P<0.05$; ‡ $P<0.001$.

Yohimbine increased the release of ³H-noradrenaline evoked by 100 pulses at 2 Hz in the absence of cocaine (which amounted to 0.17% of tissue tritium released over 49.5 sec), but did not increase the release evoked by 10 pulses at 2 Hz in the presence of cocaine (which amounted to 0.071% of tissue tritium released over 4.5 sec), although the perineuronal concentration of noradrenaline was probably higher in the latter case. Possibly, under our conditions, 4.5 sec was too short an interval for auto-inhibition to develop.

Together with independent evidence not discussed here (see 28, 29, 32, 38–40) the properties of the α-adrenolytic enhancement of noradrenaline release support the view that the presynaptic α₂-receptors of noradrenergic neurons are indeed autoreceptors and mediate a physiological auto-inhibition of the release of noradrenaline.

SUMMARY

Yohimbine and some diastereomeric alkaloids were used to compare pharmacologically the presynaptic α-adrenoceptors at the sympathetic neurons of the rabbit pulmonary artery with the postsynaptic α-receptors of this tissue. The presynaptic receptors (which are α₂) were selectively blocked by yohimbine and rauwolscine, and the postsynaptic receptors (which are α_1) by corynanthine. The diastereomers are good tools for the differentiation of α-adrenoceptor subtypes. Properties of the increase by yohimbine of the release of noradrenaline were studied in ear arteries from rabbits. Yohimbine failed to enhance action potential-evoked release of the transmitter when this release was small. A certain minimal perineuronal concentration of noradrenaline seemed to be necessary for the increase to become manifest. The results support the view that blockade of physiologically active presynaptic α-autoreceptors is the mechanism through which α-antagonists facilitate the release of noradrenaline.

REFERENCES

1. Starke K: Alpha sympathomimetic inhibition of adrenergic and cholinergic transmission in the rabbit heart. Naunyn Schmiedebergs Arch Pharmacol 274:18–45, 1972.
2. Langer SZ: The regulation of transmitter release elicited by nerve stimulation through a presynaptic feed-back mechanism, in Usdin E, Snyder SH (editors): Frontiers in Catecholamine Research. New York, Pergamon Press, 1973, pp 543–549.
3. Delbarre B, Schmitt H: A further attempt to characterize sedative receptors activated by clonidine in chickens and mice. Eur J Pharmacol 22:355–359, 1973.
4. Langer SZ: Presynaptic regulation of catecholamine release. Biochem Pharmacol 23:1793–1800, 1974.
5. Berthelsen S, Pettinger WA: A functional basis for classification of α-adrenergic receptors. Life Sci 21:595–606, 1977.
6. Starke K: α-Adrenoceptor subclassification. Rev Physiol Biochem Pharmacol 88:199–236, 1981.
7. Starke K, Borowski E, Endo T: Preferential blockade of presynaptic α-adrenoceptors by yohimbine. Eur J Pharmacol 34:385–388, 1975.
8. Kalsner S: Single pulse stimulation of guinea-pig vas deferens and the presynaptic receptor hypothesis. Br J Pharmacol 66:343–349, 1979.
9. Kalsner S: Adrenergic presynaptic receptors: Examination of a hypothesis in guinea pig vas deferens. Can J Physiol Pharmacol 57:717–724, 1979.
10. Kalsner S: Limitations of presynaptic adrenoceptor theory: The characteristics of the effects of noradrenaline and phenoxybenzamine on stimulation-induced efflux of [^{3}H]noradrenaline in vas deferens. J Pharmacol Exp Ther 212:232–239, 1980.
11. Chan CC, Kalsner S: An examination of the negative feedback function of presynaptic adrenoceptors in a vascular tissue. Br J Pharmacol 67:401–407, 1979.
12. Weitzell R, Tanaka T, Starke K: Pre- and postsynaptic effects of yohimbine stereoisomers on noradrenergic transmission in the pulmonary artery of the rabbit. Naunyn Schmiedebergs Arch Pharmacol 308:127–136, 1979.
13. Endo T, Starke K, Bangerter A, et al.: Presynaptic receptor systems on the noradrenergic neurones of the rabbit pulmonary artery. Naunyn Schmiedebergs Arch Pharmacol 296:229–247, 1977.
14. Su C, Bevan JA: The release of H³-norepinephrine in arterial strips studied by the technique of superfusion and transmural stimulation. J Pharmacol Exp Ther 172:62–68, 1970.
15. Cambridge D, Davey MJ, Massingham R: Prazosin, a selective antagonist of post-synaptic α-adrenoceptors. Br J Pharmacol 59:514P–515P, 1977.
16. Lambert GA, Lang WJ, Friedman E, et al.: Pharmacological and biochemical properties of isomeric yohimbine alkaloids. Eur J Pharmacol 49:39–48, 1978.
17. Hedler L, Stamm G, Weitzell R, et al.: Functional characterization of central α-adrenoceptors by

182

yohimbine diastereomers. Eur J Pharmacol 70:43–52, 1981.

18. Reichenbacher D, Reimann W, Starke K: Functional in vitro characterization of presynaptic α-adrenoceptors in the brain cortex of rabbits. Naunyn Schmiedebergs Arch Pharmacol (in press).

19. Madjar H, Docherty JR, Starke K: An examination of pre- and postsynaptic α-adrenoceptors in the autoperfused rabbit hindlimb. J Cardiovasc Pharmacol 2:619–627, 1980.

20. Docherty JR, Starke K: Postsynaptic α-adrenoceptor subtypes in rabbit blood vessels and rat anococcygeus muscle studied in vitro. J Cardiovasc Pharmacol 3:854–866, 1981.

21. Grundstrom N, Andersson RGG, Wikberg JES: Prejunctional $alpha_2$ adrenoceptors inhibit contraction of tracheal smooth muscle by inhibiting cholinergic neurotransmission. Life Sci 28:2981–2986, 1981.

22. Timmermans PBMWM, van Meel JCA, van Zwieten PA: Evaluation of the selectivity of α-adrenoceptor blocking drugs for postsynaptic α_1- and α_2-adrenoceptors in a simple animal model. J Auton Pharmacol 1:53–60, 1980.

23. Shepperson NB, Duval N, Massingham R, et al.: Pre- and postsynaptic alpha adrenoceptor selectivity studies with yohimbine and its two diastereoisomers rauwolscine and corynanthine in the anesthetized dog. J Pharmacol Exp Ther 219:540–546, 1981.

24. Tanaka T, Starke K: Antagonist/agonist-preferring α-adrenoceptors or α_1/α_2adrenoceptors? Eur J Pharmacol 63:191–194, 1980.

25. Tanaka T, Starke K: Binding of ^{3}H-clonidine to an α-adrenoceptor in membranes of guinea-pig ileum. Naunyn Schmiedebergs Arch Pharmacol 309:207–215, 1979.

26. Lavin TN, Hoffman BB, Lefkowitz RJ: Determination of subtype selectivity of alpha-adrenergic antagonists. Comparison of selective and nonselective radioligands. Mol Pharmacol 20:28–34, 1981.

27. Perry SD, U'Prichard DC: [^{3}H] Rauwolscine (α-yohimbine): A specific antagonist radioligand for brain α_2-adrenergic receptors. Eur J Pharmacol 76:461–464, 1981.

28. Starke K: Regulation of noradrenaline release by presynaptic receptor systems. Rev Physiol Biochem Pharmacol 77:1–124, 1977.

29. Gillespie JS: Presynaptic receptors in the autonomic nervous system, in Szekeres L (editor): Handbook of Experimental Pharmacology. Berlin, Springer, 1980, vol 54/I, pp 353–425.

30. Adler-Graschinsky E, Langer SZ, Rubio MC: Metabolism of norepinephrine released by phenoxybenzamine in isolated guinea-pig atria. J Pharmacol Exp Ther 180:286–301, 1972.

31. Cubeddu LX, Weiner N: Release of norepinephrine and dopamine-β-hydroxylase by nerve stimulation. V. Enhanced release associated with a granular effect of a benzoquinolizine derivate with reserpine-like properties. J Pharmacol Exp Ther 193:757–774, 1975.

32. Starke K: Presynaptic receptors. Ann Rev Pharmacol Toxicol 21:7–30, 1981.

33. Allen GS, Rand MJ, Story DF: Techniques for studying adrenergic transmitter release in an isolated perfused artery. Cardiovasc Res 7:423–428, 1973.

34. Graefe KH, Stefano FJE, Langer SZ: Preferential metabolism of (-)-^{3}H-norepinephrine through the deaminated glycol in the rat vas deferens. Biochem Pharmacol 22:1147–1160, 1973.

35. Markiewicz M, Marshall I, Nasmyth PA: Lack of feedback via presynaptic α-adrenoceptors by noradrenaline released by a single pulse. Br J Pharmacol 69:343P–344P, 1980.

36. McCulloch MW, Rand MJ, Story DF, et al.: Prejunctional α-adrenoceptors subserve a physiological role in cardiac noradrenergic transmission. J Auton Pharmacol 1:407–412, 1981.

37. Story DF, McCulloch MW, Rand MJ, et al.: Conditions required for the inhibitory feedback loop in noradrenergic transmission. Nature 293:62–65, 1981.

38. Starke K: Critical evaluation of the evidence for presynaptic autoinhibition of transmitter secretion, in Stjarne L, Hedqvist P, Lagercrantz H, et al. (editors): Chemical Neurotransmission 75 Years. London, Academic Press, 1981, pp 189–200.

39. Rand MJ, McCulloch MW, Story DF: Catecholamine receptors on nerve terminals, in Szekeres L (editor): Handbook of Experimental Pharmacology. Berlin, Springer, 1980, vol 54/I, pp 223–266.

40. Langer SZ: Presynaptic regulation of the release of catecholamines. Pharmacol Rev 32:337–362, 1981.

DISCUSSION

Discussants: Folkow, Starke, Langer, Brody, Abboud, Tosteson, Blaustein

Folkow: Maybe I can start the discussion with a question which relates to the situation in hypertension and membrane characteristics. As you know, investigators like Vanhoutte et al. have presented evidence to indicate that in SHR the amount of released adrenergic transmitter seems to be enhanced, at least in early life. Tomorrow, I will discuss some preliminary findings in another renal model suggesting the same thing. Interferences like the presence of the ouabain-like natriuetic hormone, or addition of ouabain itself which alters the membrane equilibrium, may well affect the transmitter release, as earlier discussed by Haddy, and Overback et al. We have in isolated microarteries some preliminary findings that might go in this direction concerning SHR. Now, with the methods you have available for analysis, it might be possible to clear up whether it is the 'primary' quantal release of transmitter that then is increased and/or it is an interference with the presynaptic α_2-receptors, so that they inhibit the release less efficiently and thereby cause a net increase of transmitter release per stimulus. Could you conceive of using the techniques that you are working with to be used with respect to the SHR neuroeffector junctions in order to trace what is going on? I think it's highly important to know if the CNS monoaminergic neurons and their transmitter release is similarly altered, as seems to be the case with the adrenergic nerve endings in vascular walls.

Starke: Yes, I think these methods can be used and have been used to study changes in presynaptic adrenoceptors in hypertension. In fact, there seem to be changes in presynaptic receptors in certain types of hypertension. For instance, presynaptic angiotensin receptors may be hypersensitive in hypertension. Angiotensin, by an action of angiotensin receptors on nerve terminals, facilitates noradrenaline release. When these receptors are hypersensitive, this would go into the right direction. More noradrenaline would be released. There may also be changes in presynaptic β-adrenoceptors in hypertension. But, not only the receptor mechanisms themselves may be changed. In addition, there may be more adrenaline than normally available at presynaptic β-receptors to facilitate the release of noradrenaline in hypertension. That would be a second mechanism. Not only the receptor mechanisms may be changed, there may also be a new input to the receptors. As regards ouabain-like substances, it has indeed been shown that ouabain facilitates the release of noradrenaline; this is independent of the receptors for endogenous ligands that I have talked about today.

Folkow: Would you think it's possible to use adrenal medullary cells as models, since they should be easier to handle than neurons, and to apply the techniques we have heard about this morning concerning their cell membrane and CA release?

Starke: Yes, that has been done with rather divergent results. It has been claimed that adrenal medullary cells contain α-adrenoceptors which, when activated, depress catecholamine release. But there is also maybe stronger evidence to the contrary. So my impression is that adrenal medullary cells are sufficiently different from noradrenergic nerve terminals to make them doubtful models for the investigation of presynaptic-receptor mechanisms.

Langer: In the experiments with yohimbine you showed that, depending on the frequency and the length of stimulation, you can either fail to modify or facilitate the release of norepinephrine by nerve stimulation. Could you tell us something about the end-organ responses which may be a meaningful parameter in these experiments, or were the concentrations of yohimbine too high so that they block both presynaptic α_2 and postsynaptic α_1-receptors as well?

Starke: Well, as to the 0.2 Hz, 10 shock experiments, the vasoconstrictor responses were too small to tell us anything. But, as to the stronger stimulation parameters, we got postsynaptic vasoconstrictor responses which reflected the presynaptic events. Whether we used yohimbine 0.1 micromolar or 1 micromolar, we got an increase in the postsynaptic response to stimulation. This was consonant with the presynaptic effects.

Brody: I wonder why you might not argue from your data with yohimbine that you fail to support the concept of presynaptic inhibition as a physiological mechanism? Since you do not get any facilitation at lower frequencies, is it not possible, therefore, that there isn't much reuptake at those frequencies and that termination of transmitter action is by some other mechanism?

Starke: But Dr. Folkow told us that our sympathetic fibers are normally firing at 1 or 2 Hz and not at 0.2 Hz. We got no facilitation with 0.2 Hz and with 2 Hz given only for 4.5 seconds, but did get facilitation with 2 Hz given for 50 seconds. I would expect that normally when the neurons are firing at an irregular frequency, there is an average firing rate of approximately one or two per second, and this would be the range for a feedback inhibition to occur. Moreover, even if there were no feedback inhibition in the resting state, there might be feedback inhibition when the neurons are firing more frequently when we are excited. In my opinion the data do show that at physiological frequencies of stimulation there is feedback inhibition.

Brody: Dr. Kathy Berechek in our laboratory has recently done some experiments demonstrating that epinephrine derived from the adrenal medulla can be taken up by the sympathetic nerve terminals and play an important neurotransmitter function.[1] I wonder if you or anybody else have any evidence about the possibility that vasomotor effects of epinephrine may be mediated through interactions with the α_1- and α_2-adrenoceptors pre- and postsynaptically.

Starke: Let me answer the question as to the presynaptic receptors. There is good evidence to demonstrate the existence of presynaptic β-adrenoceptors and that low concentrations of adrenaline mainly activate presynaptic β-adrenoceptors, so that we get facilitation of release. When you apply higher concentrations, then only the α-adrenergic effect of adrenaline comes into play. We are at present studying the effects of adrenaline infused into rabbits *in vivo,* and there again, when we use low concentrations of adrenaline, what we get is not a depression of release but facilitation because of the β-effect. The α-effect appears to be more on the pharmacological side; the β-effect may be more on the physiological side.

Abboud: Do you have any idea about the relative importance of the several mechanisms that facilitate release or affect norepinephrine concentration and its reuptake – for example, cocaine, ouabain – the inhibition of presynaptic α_2, or the relative contributions to the amounts released during sympathetic stimulation? Give us some idea about that.

Starke: When, by release, we understand the passage of the transmitter from the interior of the neurons into the extracellular space, then the only thing that modifies this so-defined release is presynaptic receptors or maybe ouabain. But ouabain is not an endogenous compound. So what remains are the presynaptic receptors, only they modify the release.

---

1. Berecek KH, Brody MJ: Evidence for a neurotransmitter role for epinephrine derived from the adrenal medulla. Am. J Physiol. 242: H593–H601, 1982.

Abboud: If we assume that ouabain acts through an inhibition of the sodium-potassium pump, then there may be endogenous factors that may modify that pump. I want you to give me some idea about these in your system, but maybe you haven't done the experiment. I would like to know if somebody has done the experiment in which ouabain has been compared to a presynaptic α_2-inhibition with respect to the amount of norepinephrine released.

Starke: Ouabain has been studied mainly for its effect on the evoked release of noradrenaline. And, indeed, if you apply ouabain at rather high concentrations – say 10^{-7} to 10^{-6} – then you do get some facilitation of release, but I have no idea what that means for physiology. Physiologically, what modifies or what controls the release of noradrenaline is the frequency of the firing of the neurons and the work of presynaptic receptor mechanisms, such as α-adrenoceptors and β-adrenoceptors.

Folkow: Dr. Tosteson indicated today that the ionic transport system might be particularly important for cells that have adrenergic innervation and receptors. Is that what you're going to comment upon now Dr. Tosteson?

Tosteson: I was going to ask a different question. It is true that the co-transport system is stimulated by noradrenaline, but it seems to be a β-receptor. What is the thinking about the mechanism by which the combination of the receptor with its agonist inhibits the release of noradrenaline-containing vesicles or, at least, noradrenaline into the extracellular space?

Starke: Talking of α-adrenoceptors, the only thing which we can be sure about is that it is only calcium-dependent modes of release that are modified. There are also calcium-independent modes of release, such as release evoked by indirectly-acting amines, and these are not modified. What is modified is the calcium-dependent release evoked by action potentials of high potassium. Now, what is between the receptor and the calcium-dependent release we do not know, we can only speculate. It has been speculated that, as in other α_2-adrenoceptors, an inhibition of adenylate cyclase is the mechanism by which activation of the receptor leads to inhibition of release or, the other way around, activation of adenylate cyclase should then facilitate the release of noradrenaline. However, we do not know in which direction CAMP levels in nerve terminals are modified when an α_2-agonist is added. It's only extrapolation from other systems.

Blaustein: I would like to come back to the question that Dr. Brody asked concerning whether or not the feedback mechanism plays a role physiologically. Is there any evidence about what rauwolscine or yohimbine actually do in a more intact preparation or *in vivo?* Do they elevate the blood pressure at least transiently?

Starke: Yes, exactly. Yohimbine and rauwolscine increase the blood pressure in most unanesthetized animals. We do not know, however, whether this effect reflects interruption of an ongoing presynaptic feedback mechanism. I can give you one other piece of evidence. Dr. Majewsky and I are investigating the effects of these alkaloids on the release of noradrenaline in anesthetized rabbits *in vivo,* and we eliminate any effects of the alkaloids on the disposition of noradrenaline by measuring simultaneously the clearance rate of ^{3}H-noradrenaline from the blood plasma. What we see is that rauwolscine and yohimbine markedly increase noradrenaline levels. (These are anesthetized animals and you get a decrease in blood pressure by the alkaloids.) The α-antagonist prazosin, at equally hypotensive doses, causes only a marginal increase in this *in vivo* release of noradrenaline. So – not only is there an increase in blood pressure in unanesthetized animals caused by rauwolscine and yohimbine, but there is also an increase of the *in vivo* release of noradrenaline which is not shared by the α_1-antagonist, indicating that the same things also are going on *in vivo.*

Folkow: A short comment concerning feedback interfering and the rate of discharge. Actually, the sympathetic discharge often comes in more or less pulse-synchronous bursts, perhaps three or four impulses in rapid sequence followed by a brief pause – particularly evident in man, who is after all *the* important subject. This pattern of firing is nicely illustrated in the excellent studies by Wallin et al. in Uppsala, Sweden. This may well influence the innervated effector cells in a somewhat different way than if the same number of impulses/minute is evenly spread.

Langer: I would also like to come back to the question of Mike Brody on this physiological significance in favor of the conclusions of Dr. Starke. It is precisely the fact that under the low-frequency stimulation, the .2-Hz stimulation during a short time, the postsynaptic end-organ effector responses were negligible, and only when stimulation was carried out at 2 Hz for 100 pulses was the postsynaptic response clearly measured. The latter postsynpatic response was in fact enhanced by the concentration of rauwolscine, which increased transmitter release. That, to my way of understanding, would support rather than be against the physiological role of α_2-adrenoceptors in modulating norepinephrine release.

THE EFFECTS OF DIDS AND ANION SUBSTITUTION ON AORTIC ^{36}CL TURNOVER IN ALDOSTERONE-INDUCED HYPERTENSIVE RATS

ELLEN T. GARWITZ AND ALLAN W. JONES

INTRODUCTION

Previous reports from our laboratory have indicated an increased exchange of Na, K, and Cl in blood vessels from DOCA- and aldosterone-hypertensive rats [1–3]. The steady-state efflux of ^{24}Na, ^{42}K, and ^{36}Cl in aorta from steroid-induced hypertensive rats is significantly elevated over that in vessels from control animals. Increases in the efflux of ^{42}K and ^{36}Cl have been assumed to result from an increase in the passive permeability of the vascular smooth muscle membrane to these ions. Equating the active component (K-dependent) of the sodium efflux to the passive influx, a similar increase in passive membrane permeability to sodium is evident [4]. These findings suggest that a relatively nonspecific increase in membrane permeability to small ions accompanies the development of mineralocorticoid-dependent hypertension in the rat.

It was the objective of the present study to delineate more precisely the changes in chloride turnover in vessels from aldosterone-hypertensive rats. There is evidence that a component of the chloride efflux in vascular smooth muscle is mediated by a Cl-Cl exchange mechanism. Villamil et al. [5] reported that in dog carotid artery, replacement of Cl⁻ with nitrate or methylsulfate significantly decreased the rate constant of the slowly exchanging ^{36}Cl fraction. However, Casteels [6] was unable to demonstrate any effect of anion substitution (propionate, nitrate, benzenesulphonate) on the ^{36}Cl efflux from *taenia coli* of the guinea pig. It is therefore not certain whether Cl-Cl exchange is operative in all types of smooth muscle. In the present study, the effects of Cl free solution were determined on the efflux of ^{36}Cl in aorta from aldosterone-hypertensive rats. The anion exchange blocker DIDS (4-4′-di-isothiocyanostilbene-2, 2′-disulphonic acid) was also used to evaluate the extent to which the chloride efflux is mediated by Cl-Cl exchange diffusion. This compound has been shown to specifically inhibit anion exchange in erythrocytes by binding to the Band III protein, which mediates anion exchange in these cells [7]. This approach was taken in an effort to determine whether the elevation in ^{36}Cl efflux in vessels from hypertensives resulted from an increase in the 'leak' flux component and to what extent an increase in Cl-Cl exchange diffusion might be involved.

METHODS

Male Sprague-Dawley rats (150–200 g) were unilaterally nephrectomized under ether anesthesia. An osmotic mini-pump (Alza Corp.) containing d-aldosterone dissolved in polyethylene glycol was implanted subcutaneously in the treated animals. Aldosterone was infused at a rate of 0.25 μg/h. Rats in the control group received a pump containing the vehicle only. The control animals were given a 1% wt/vol NaCl solution as drinking fluid. Treated rats were given a supplement of KCl (0.3% wt/vol) in the NaCl solution to maintain body weight. Systolic blood pressure was determined weekly by a tail-cuff technique.

On the morning of the experiment, the animals were sacrificed and the thoracic aorta was quickly removed. Loose connective tissue was stripped from the vessels which were slit lengthwise and then cut transversely into three pieces. The strips were mounted on stainless-steel holders and incubated at 37° C with the isotope. Two of the strips were incubated in normal Krebs solution containing ^{36}Cl (for washout into normal Krebs and propionate-substituted Krebs). The remaining aortic strip was incubated with ^{36}Cl in Krebs solution containing 0.1 mM DIDS (Polysciences Inc.), and these were subsequently washed out into 0.1 mM DIDS-containing medium. The normal Krebs solution had the following millimolar composition: Na^+, 146.2; K^+, 5.0; Mg^{2+}, 1.2; Ca^{2+}, 2.5; Cl^-, 143.9; HCO_3^-, 13.5; $H_2PO_4^-$, 1.2; and glucose, 11.4. Propionate-substituted Krebs had the same milli-molar composition of Na^+, K^+, HCO_3^-, $H_2PO_4^-$, Mg^{2+}, Ca^{2+} and glucose as normal Krebs, in addition to 141.5 $CH_3CH_2O_2^-$ (propionate) and 2.4 mM CH_2OH (CH-OH)$_4 \cdot COO^-$ (gluconate). All solutions were gassed with a 97% O–3% CO_2 mixture at 37° C to obtain a pH of 7.4.

After a 3-hour incubation with ^{36}Cl, the tissues were removed from the isotope, and the efflux experiments were begun. These procedures had been described in detail previously [8, 9]. In brief, the strips were passed through a series of tubes containing nonradioactive solution. The activity in the tubes and the vessels was counted on a liquid scintillation counter. Washout curves were calculated by sequentially adding the tissue and the tube counts in reverse order. These counts were then normalized in terms of percent initial activity. A digital computer was used to process the data. The fraction exchanged per minute for each washout period was computed, which under steady-state conditions represents the rate constant (k/min). Cellular chloride turnover was estimated as the turnover rate between 3 and 5 min washout. At this time, the rapidly exchanging extracellular ^{36}Cl has been cleared, and enough counts remain in the slowly exchanging cellular fraction (about 8% of the total counts) to insure accurate counting procedures.

RESULTS

Systolic blood pressure in the aldosterone-infused rats was significantly elevated

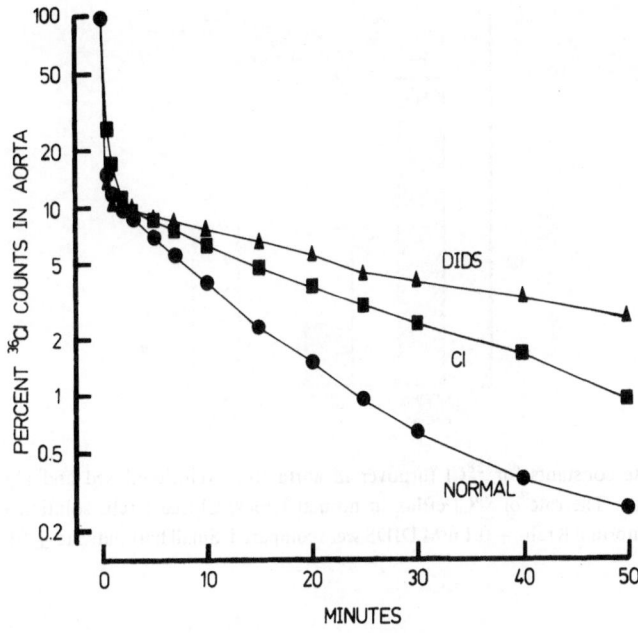

Figure 1. ³⁶Cl efflux in aortic strips from a vehicle-infused rat. Washout into normal Krebs (●), propionate-substituted Krebs (■), and normal Krebs solution containing 0.1 mM DIDS (▲). The points of each curve are joined by straight lines.

over that in the control animals (199 ± 6.5 vs. 119 ± 3 mm Hg; P<0.001), after four weeks of treatment. The rate of ³⁶Cl efflux in vessels from these two groups was compared in normal Krebs, propionate-Krebs and DIDS-containing Krebs solution. Figure 1 shows the effects of these solutions on the ³⁶Cl efflux in the aorta from a control animal. A significant slowing of the efflux occurred in propionate-substituted Krebs solution. Washout into DIDS-containing Krebs solution resulted in an even greater slowing of the ³⁶Cl efflux.

A summary of the effects of these solutions on the ³⁶Cl efflux from both aldosterone and control groups is presented in Figure 2. The total Cl efflux was significantly increased in aortas from the aldosterone-treated rats (0.246 ± 0.017 vs. 0.128 ± 0.003/min; P>0.001). Substitution of propionate for Cl⁻ resulted in a significant reduction of the efflux in both the vehicle-infused and aldosterone-treated rats. The rate constants for ³⁶Cl turnover in propionate-Krebs were however still significantly higher in the aldosterone-treated group (0.111 ± 0.006 vs. 0.060 ± 0.002/min; P<0.001). A similar effect was observed in aortas loaded and washed out into DIDS-containing Krebs solution (0.059 ± 0.012 vs. 0.033 ± 0.002 min; P<0.05).

The concentrations of slowly exchanging ³⁶Cl were estimated by extrapolation from the efflux curves and estimates of cell water, obtained as previously described [10]. There was no significant difference in cellular chloride concentration

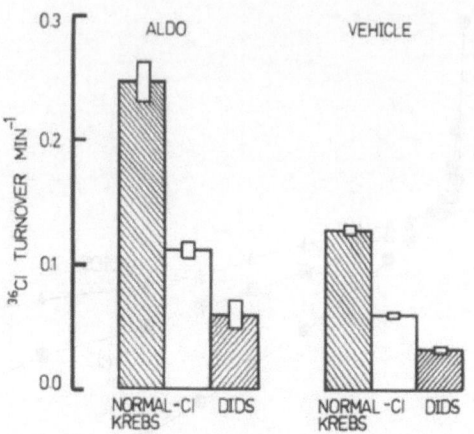

Figure 2. Rate constants for ³⁶Cl turnover in aorta from vehicle-infused and aldosterone-treated (0.25 μg/h) rats. The rate of ³⁶Cl efflux in normal Krebs, Cl-free Krebs solution (propionate-substituted), and normal Krebs + 0.1 mM DIDS were compared. Small bars indicate ± SEM for six to nine rats.

in aortas from the vehicle- and aldosterone-treated groups washed out into normal Krebs solution (57.0 ± 1.6 vs. 57.7 ± 3.1 mmole/kg cell H_2O, respectively). Pre-incubation in DIDS-containing Krebs solution slightly increased cellular chloride concentrations, but these increases were not statistically significant (vehicle, 61.6 ± 3.3 mmol/kg cell H_2O; aldosterone, 66.7 ± 5.2 mmole/kg cell H_2O).

DISCUSSION

These results indicate that a significant component of the chloride efflux in rat aorta is mediated by a Cl exchange diffusional mechanism. Complete chloride substitution with propionate reduced ³⁶Cl efflux by 52–55% in both control and aldosterone groups. DIDS reduced Cl effluxes to about 25% of the steady-state level. The elevated ³⁶Cl turnover in aorta from the aldosterone-hypertensive rats appears therefore to result from a proportional (two-fold) increase in both exchange diffusional and leak fluxes. This latter observation is consistent with the permeability hypothesis [1, 8, 11]. The earlier estimates for chloride permeability ($P_{Cl} = 5.8 \times 10^{-8}$ cm/sec in control rat aorta) were based on total steady-state effluxes, however, and may be too high by a factor of two to four times. Based on the present study, $P_{Cl} \leq P_K$ in vascular smooth muscle from control and aldosterone hypertensives. The absolute values are doubled in mineralocorticoid hypertension, which is indicative of increased membrane leakiness to ions [11].

It is not certain at this time why a greater percentage of the Cl efflux is inhibited by DIDS as compared with Cl substitution. To our knowledge, DIDS has not been previously applied to vascular smooth muscle. Although the specificity of DIDS as an inhibitor of anion exchange in RBC is good [7], it may in addition act on Cl leak or channel sites in vascular smooth muscle, thus resulting in an underestimate for the Cl leak under physiological conditions. On the other hand, our experiments with Cl substitution may not have completely blocked the exchange diffusional efflux of ^{36}Cl, in that HCO_3 remained in the incubation media. The leak estimated under these conditions may be too high. It is planned to repeat these experiments in Cl- and HCO_3-free solutions.

The cellular concentration of Cl as estimated from the slowly exchanging component was little altered in the aldosterone-hypertensive group. This confirms earlier observations on DOCA rats [1, 11]. Three-hour incubation in DIDS caused only a slight rise in cell Cl, and this was not statistically significant. The high Cl concentration in vascular smooth muscle is thought to result from an active influx mechanism [11] but little information is available concerning its characteristics. From this study, it appears that the relatively high cell Cl established by such a process is not blocked by DIDS. This study also confirms our earlier finding in relation to cellular Na regulation during mineralocorticoid hypertension [4]. Increased leakiness of the membrane is balanced by an increase in active transport such that a constant cell concentration is maintained. In terms of altered vascular function, the permeability effects predominate over those of altered ionic concentrations.

REFERENCES

1. Jones AW: Functional changes in vascular smooth muscle associated with experimental hypertension, in Bevan JA, Burnstock G, Johansson B (editors): Vascular Neuroeffector Mechanisms. Basel, Karger, 1976, p 182.
2. Jones A, Garwitz E, Mertens MS, et al.: Aldosterone-induced hypertension in rats, abstracted. Physiologist 22:64, 1979.
3. Garwitz ET, Jones AW, Freeman RH: Aldosterone infusion into the rat and dose-dependent changes in blood pressure and arterial ionic transport, abstracted. Fed Proc 40:527, 1981.
4. Jones AW: Kinetics of active sodium transport in aortas from control and deoxycorticosterone hypertensive rats. Hypertension 3:631, 1981.
5. Villamil MF, Rettori V, Yeyati N, et al.: Chloride exchange and distribution in the isolated arterial wall. Am J Physiol 215:833, 1968.
6. Casteels R: The distribution of chloride ions in the smooth muscle cells of the guinea pig's taenia coli. J Physiol 214:225, 1971.
7. Cabantchik ZI, Knauf PA, Rothstein A: The anion transport system of the red blood cell – the role of membrane protein evaluated by the use of 'probes.' Biochem Biophys Acta 515:239, 1978.
8. Jones AW: Reactivity of ion fluxes in rat aorta during hypertension and circulatory control. Fed Proc 33:133, 1974.
9. Jones AW: Altered ion transport in vascular smooth muscle from spontaneously hypertensive rats: Influence of aldosterone, norepinephrine and angiotensin. Circ Res 33:563, 1973.
10. Jones AW, Hart RG: Altered ion transport in aortic smooth muscle during deoxycoraticosterone

acetate hypertension in the rat. Circ Res 37:333, 1975.
11. Jones AW: Ionic dysfunction and hypertension, Altura B (editor): Advances in Microcirculation. Basel, Karger, vol 11, in press.

DISCUSSION

Discussants: Haeusler, Jones, Bohr, Overbeck, Sambhi, Tosteson, Haddy, Blaustein

Haeusler: This question is related to the increase in ionic permeabilities in vascular muscle of DOCA-salt hypertensive rats. Under the assumption that the cellular ion concentrations do not differ very much in normotensive and DOCA-salt hypertensive rats, what is the value for the diffusion potential in the latter, calculated from the altered ionic permeabilities?

Jones: Well, the diffusional potential that would result from that wouldn't change very much, and the permeabilities are altered by roughly the same percentage, so the diffusional potential is within several millivolts. Now, if the membrane resistance is decreased by a factor of two then that may have some effect on the electrogenic pump potential. But in general, the diffusional potentials we've calculated are not much different.

Haeusler: I remember a paper in which a very low resting membrane potential, approximately 20 mV, was recorded for vascular smooth muscle from DOCA-salt hypertensive rats. Apparently, this finding was never confirmed.

Jones: A bit of a concern with these tissue is that with this increased leak they seem to be more prone to traumatic damage. If something goes wrong in the lab, it's usually the hypertensive vessels that show the problems rather than the controls – so I'm a little concerned about tissue handling with micro-electrode work. You've got to have very good electrodes to get any cells to start with and I think anybody doing it would have to be rather careful to make sure that the cells were stable and in good condition when they impaled them and made their recordings.

Bohr: Is it an accepted general principle that if you get more sodium inside a cell it will induce the production of more pump sites?

Jones: At the moment that is not well demonstrated one way or the other. People are just demonstrating receptors for aldosterone in these cells and there may be some direct effect or potential effect of aldosterone that will induce protein synthesis. Whether that is going to cause synthesis of sodium pump sites, I don't know.

Bohr: My question is broader than just vascular smooth muscle.

Jones: Is it related to control by areas of the brain?

Bohr: Well, that too, of course but I have the impression that the renal mechanism has shifted over from a direct aldosterone induction of pump synthesis to an indirect one in which aldosterone induces more 'leak sites' which let in more sodium, and this induces pump site synthesis.

Jones: It would be a nice idea to test in these preparations. I have little information about the relation between cell sodium and direct synthesis of transport sites.

Haeusler: You have shown that in DOCA-salt hypertensive rats the norepinephrine-induced potassium efflux occurred at lower transmitter concentrations than in normotensive rats. However, if one looked at the magnitude of the efflux, it appeared to be smaller in DOCA-salt hypertensive rats. Would you like the comment on this?

Jones: The maximum increase in efflux that can be induced by maximal doses of norepinephrine are less in the hypertensives than in the controls. It's almost as if there's an upper limit on what can happen. In other words, the baseline of the hypertensives is elevated, so when one adds an agonist and increases membrane movement of ions, the rate constants seem to peak out at 0.035/min, and one just can't get things to move much more quickly than that. The controls are starting at a lower baseline; they have an extra capacity. I don't know if that's true, but that's phenomenologically what we do see: with maximum doses of norepinephrine, very often the controls and the hypertensives show just about the same rates. But at low doses, and when we normalize the data, of course, the shift is very dramatic.

Haeusler: Do you by any chance know whether this increase in efflux is calcium-dependent?

Jones: We've never really tried that. When we take away calcium, the potassium efflux increases and approaches a maximum of 0.045/min. Some years ago we did try a test dose of norepinephrine after an hour in calcium-free solution and lost the response, but the problem was that the basal rate was as high if not higher than it was in the presence of norepinephrine under control conditions. So I think, in these preparations, taking away calcium has a very large effect in increasing the membrane leakage to potassium. Indeed, the channels which are opened by N-epinephrine may be the same ones which open when calcium is removed.

Overbeck: I'm interested in hearing again how you explain the higher V_{max} in the DOCA hypertensive rats.

Jones: The interpretation is based on the observations that the half-saturation and the Hill coefficient aren't much different, and the V_{max} is elevated. This is consistent with the presence of more transport sites. These appear to result from increased synthesis. How does aldosterone influence this? We know we have to give salt to these animals to get these responses. If we just infuse aldosterone with tap water to drink we really don't observe very much, and we don't observe very much hypertension either. So the sodium load is an important component. The idea I like best is that there are aldosterone receptors which are indeed being activated, but salt must be a co-factor in order to get the synthetic processes going. There first may be an increased leak to ions. The leak itself then may take over and aldosterone may not directly be involved with pump synthesis.

This whole area of what controls the biosynthetic processes in smooth muscles is critical – not just for this question but for many problems related to atherosclerosis and dedifferentiation of cell growth, repair and so on. A lot of other tissues don't show the changes that a smooth muscle can undergo in response to changes in its environment.

Sambhi: If aldosterone increases the number of pump sites, why doesn't it do it in secondary aldosteronism states. You said that you tried some models of renal hypertension and didn't see any changes. Have you tried it under those conditions where aldosterone was quite high?

Jones: We didn't measure plasma aldosterones on renal hypertensive rats – I'm not sure how high they were. We have seen changes with ACTH infusion where plasma aldosterone is high, in animals with adrenals, but again, we had to let the animal drink saline to do this.

Tosteson: Dr. Bohr's results with pigs with volume-expanded hypertension showed that there were two categories, some that seem to get the hypertension because they have increased cardiac output, some because they have an increased vascular resistance. Is there any evidence of that sort of thing in the preparation that you've been studying? To what extent are these changes in transport in smooth muscle related to the development of the hypertension? Is hypertension in these animals primarily cardiac in origin, in which case these findings are interesting not only insofar as they might inform what's going on in the heart muscle? Or is there evidence that there is some sort of vascular change which is important in the hypertension? Now a quite different sort of question: Are cation fluxes influenced by DIDS?

Jones: We haven't done that yet on these preparations. In the rabbit carotid there are sodium potassium and chloride fluxes that are all furosemide-sensitive but we haven't done the DIDS component. I don't know if these animals' volumes expanded and have an alternate cardiac output. There has been some assumption some years ago that DOCA animals are volume expanded, but I'm not sure if that's held up. Dr. Haddy, have you measured volumes in these animals?

Haddy: No, not in this model

Jones: The renal hypertensive model did not induce changes in ion fluxes even though the pressures were equally high, so I don't think a cardiac output-induced pressure could alter vascular ion transport secondarily. Dr. Bohr, are the pigs' volumes expanded?

Bohr: No.

Jones: We're doing some fluxes on pigs but I've been rather remiss in not keeping up with the data; some of them show some changes and some don't.

Tosteson: Your working hypothesis is that there's an increased vascular resistance, that resistance vessels are somehow contracted in this preparation and your're looking at that.

Jones: Yes.

Haddy: With respect to the number of pump sites, do you know of anybody who has measured ouabain-binding in blood vessels of rats with DOCA-salt hypertension?

Jones: It would be difficult because one has to use such high concentrations to block the pump. I would think the nonspecific uptake would be a rather difficult and formidable problem. There are a few examples in the rabbit, but not in relation to hypertension.

Blaustein: To return to the question that was raised earlier about the role of aldosterone in increasing the number of sodium pumps, the question is whether this effect is primary or secondary. There clearly appears to be evidence for an increase in sodium pumps, but I think the mechanism is very controversial. It looks like it may not necessarily be due to an increase in intracellular sodium, at least in the epithelial models that have been looked at, although even there it's been controversial. But you didn't see an obvious elevation in cell sodium in the tissue of DOCA-treated animals.

Jones: That's under *in vitro* conditions, which I have emphasized several times. Possibly a pump inhibitor that blocks the pump 15 or 20 percent in the animal may chronically raise cell sodium. When the inhibitor is washed away, the full active pumping system is unmasked, so what is observed may not be exactly what was going on in the animal.

Blaustein: One other thing that I wanted to mention that you did emphasize very carefully: the effect of changes in tone or changes in the amount of catecholamine present. This must influence the permeabilities, which clearly must be very important when you take the tissue out and look at it *in vitro,* rather than looking at it *in situ.*

Jones: Yes. The rat aorta, by the way, has very few nerves. That's another reason we have used it. Rabbit vessels are well innervated.

FUNCTION OF THE SODIUM PUMP IN VASCULAR SMOOTH MUSCLE IN HYPERTENSION

HENRY W. OVERBECK

INTRODUCTION

Considerable evidence, dating back to the observation of Tobian and Binion in 1952 [1], suggests that there may be abnormalities in the function of the sarcolemmal sodium pump in vascular smooth muscle in hypertension. In 1974, Hendrickx and Casteels demonstrated that an electrogenic sodium pump, activated by levels of $[K^+]_0$ and inhibited by cardiac glycosides, exists in vascular tissue [2]. At approximately the same time, we reported attenuated arteriolar dilator responses to small local increases in plasma K^+ in animals with certain types of experimental hypertension (3,4) and also in certain patients with essential hypertension (5) (Fig. 1). This attenuation suggested inhibition of the sodium pump of the vascular membrane, perhaps by a digitalis-like substance. It is noteworthy that we conducted these investigation *in vivo,* where we observed arteriolar, rather than conduit artery, function and where the effects of a circulating inhibitor would likely be detected. It is also noteworthy that the attenuated responses appeared to be specific for K^+. Thus, we attributed three abnormal responses to functional, rather than structural, abnormalities in the resistance vessels. In 1972, on the basis of this evidence, we proposed the hypothesis that a decreased sarcolemmal sodium-pump activity may underlie the arteriolar vasoconstriction in certain forms of experimental hypertension [3, 4]. In 1974, we extended this hypothesis to essential hypertension in man [5].

To further test this hypothesis, we next modified methods developed by Brody and Akera so that we might measure ^{86}Rb uptake by vascular muscle *in vitro* as an additional index of pump activity [6]. Using these techniques, we demonstrated (Fig. 2) highly significant decreases in ouabain-sensitive ^{86}Rb uptake in both arteries and veins from dogs with chronic one-kidney perinephritic hypertension. This observation added strong evidence to the hypothesis. We proposed at that time that the defect might be attributable to a blood-borne pump inhibitor and that vasoconstriction would be initiated either by effects on membrane voltage-dependent Ca^{2+} channels or on transmembrane Ca^{2+}-Na^+ exchange.

Dahl and his co-investigators had suggested in 1969 [7] that a humoral factor, with both natriuretic and pressor properties, might be involved in the mechanisms of hypertension. Haddy and Overbeck in 1976 [8] expanded this suggestion,

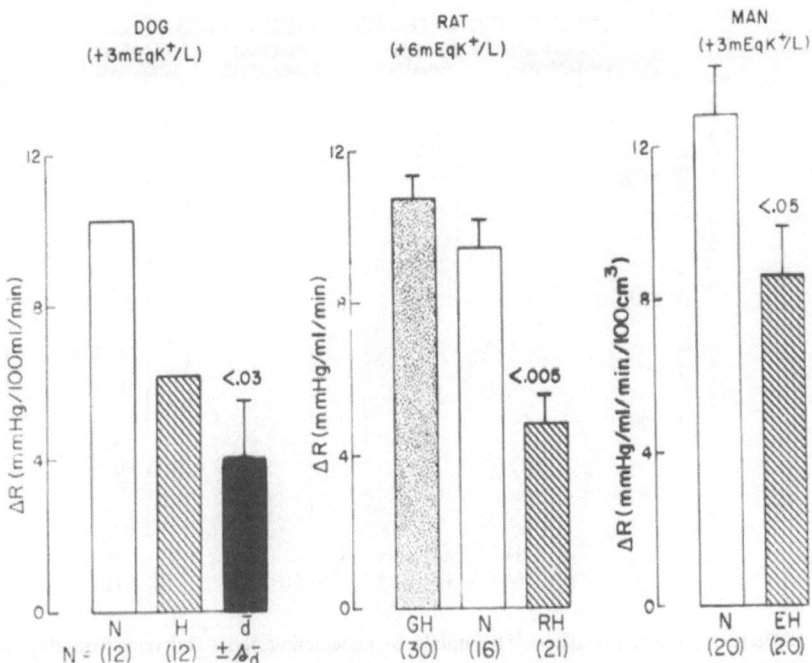

Figure 1. Attenuated K⁺-vasodilation in hypertensive dogs (chronic 1-kidney perinephritic), rats (chronic two-kidney Goldblatt), and humans (essential). Isotonic KCl solution infused into brachial (dog, human) or femoral (rat) artery to raise limb arterial plasma [K⁺] by 3–6 mEq/L, while perfusion pressure and flow monitored. Means (adjusted for covariance effects of initial limb resistance) ± SEM and N (numbers of observations) provided. N represents normotensive controls, H represents perinephritic hypertensive dogs, GH represents genetic (New Zealand) hypertensive rats, RH represents Goldblatt hypertensive rats, EH represents essential hypertensive men. *P* values for comparison of means calculated by analysis of covariance.

proposing that the putative natriuretic hormone, released in response to volume expansion in experimental and human essential hypertension, might be this hypertensinogenic factor operating by inhibiting membrane sodium-pump activity in cardiovascular muscle. Since 1976, a number of investigators have provided evidence relevant to this hypothesis, seeking humoral factors an using several *in vitro* techniques to assess sodium-pump activty in vascular smooth muscle in hypertension. (For the purposes of this review, we exclude studies of erythrocytes or leukocytes).

In vitro evidence from most [9–18], but not all [19–22], of these laboratories appears not to support the hypothesis, in that increases, rather than decreases, in vascular sodium-pump activity were observed. These increases were usually explained by the invesigators as compensatory responses a 'primary' increase in membrane Na⁺ 'leakiness.'

It is noteworthy that all of this work has been done in rats, a species notably insensitive to cardiac glycosides, because the glucoside rapidly dissociates from

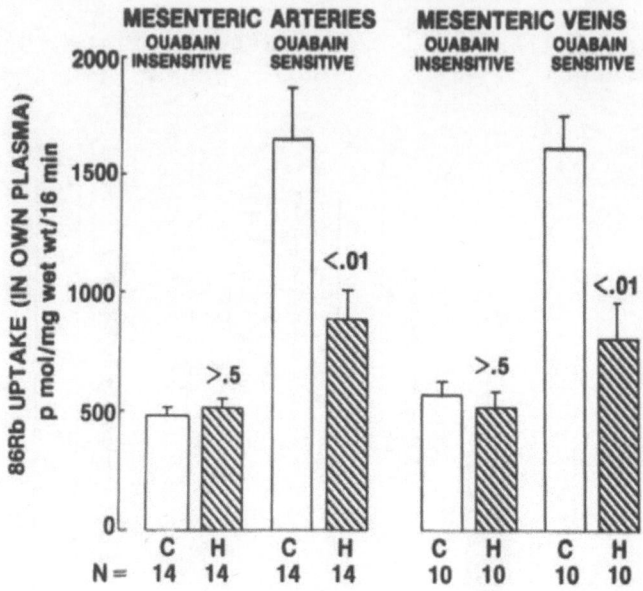

Figure 2. Decreased ouabain-sensitive ^{86}Rb uptake by mesenteric arteries and veins from dogs with chronic on-kidney perinephritic hypertension. Incubation *in vitro* in Krebs-Henseleit solution. Clear bars represent values in control normotesive, and cross-hatched bars represent values in perinephritic hypertensive dogs. Means ± SEM and N values provided. *P* values calculated by unpaired Student's *t* test.

the pump molecule [23]. Thus, it has been suggested by others that failure to observe pump inhibition in rat vascular tissue studied *in vitro* (or in vascular beds perfused with artifical solution [16–18]) may indicate that the circulating inhibitor is no longer bound to the pump molecule by the time the measurements are made. However, this explanation would not answer why increases in pump activity are observed, rather than no change. We, therefore, inquired further into the mechanisms of the increased pump activity observed *in vitro* experiments in rats, remaining mindful of the ample evidence for *in vivo* pump inhibition and for circulating inhibitor substances.

METHODS AND RESULTS

Work from Dahl's laboratory suggested a hypertensinogenic humoral factor in his strain of salt-sensitive rats [7], and work from Tobian's laboratory suggested volume expansion in this model [24]. Therefore, we chose first to investigate vascular pump activity in Dahl salt-sensitive (S) and resistant (R) rats. We documented increases in plasma volume in the S rats on high salt [25]. The significantly increased ouabain-sensitive ^{86}Rb uptakes we observed in freshly excised and rapidly processed tail artery and aorta in this model of volume-expanded experimental hypertension are presented in Figure 3 and have been confirmed by Haddy's laboratory [26]. It is noteworthy that tail artery sodium-pump activity was elevated equally in Dahl S rats on low- or high-salt diets, but plasma volume was increased only in the latter. The S rats were hypertensive on both diets (though more so on high salt).

We next studied rats with chronic one- and two-kidney Goldblatt hypertension, documenting that plasma renin activity was elevated only in the latter [27]. Again (Fig. 4) we observed only significant increases in sodium-pump activity in freshly excised arteries. It was noteworthy, in this regard, that the magnitude of these increases was similar in the two forms of Goldblatt hypertension. Because techniques used by the two laboratories were almost identical, it is difficult to explain the contrasting observation by Haddy's laboratory of decreased tail artery pump activity in rats with one-kidney Goldblatt hypertension [21] (or DOCA-salt hypertension [19], see below).

Ouabain-sensitive ^{86}Rb uptake by segments of vessels *in vitro* is expressed in terms of unit tissue weight. Thus, among other explanations, observed increases

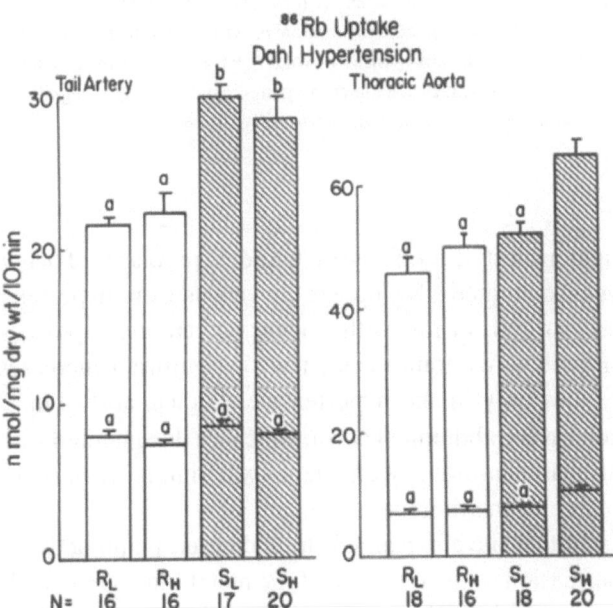

Figure 3. Increased total and ouabain-sensitive ^{86}Rb uptakes by tail arteries and thoracic aortas from Dahl S rats. Incubation *in vitro* in Krebs-Henseleit solution. R rats represented by clear bars, S rats by cross-hatched bars. Subscript L indicates low (0.4%) and H indicates high (8%) NaCl diet fed for 4–6 weeks. N values provided. Larger bars indicate means ± SEM of total ^{86}Rb uptakes, smaller enclosed bars indicate ouabain-insensitive ^{86}Rb uptakes. Bars sharing superscript letters are *not* significantly different ($p > 0.05$) by analysis of variance. Significant differences for total uptakes reflect similar differences in ouabain-sensitive uptakes.

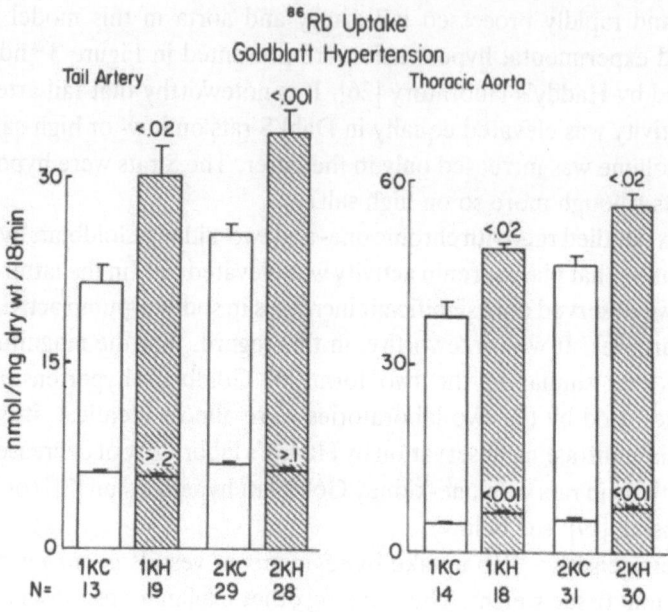

Figure 4. Increased ^{86}Rb uptakes by tail artery and thoracic aorta from chronic one-kidney (1KH) and chronic two-kidney (2KH) Goldblatt hypertensive (cross-hatched bars) and appropriate normotensive control (1KC and 2KC, clear bars) rats. Incubation *in vitro* in Krebs-Henseleit solution. N values provided. Larger bars indicate means ± SEM of total ^{86}Rb uptakes, smaller enclosed bars indicate ouabain-insensitive uptakes. P values calculated by paired Student's *t* test. Significant differences for total uptakes reflect similar differences in ouabain-sensitive uptakes.

in uptake might reflect the effects of tissue hyperplasia. To investigate this possibility, we also studied ^{86}Rb uptake by vessels from hypertensive and normotensive vascular beds of rats with chronic coarctation hypertension [28]. As indicated in Figure 5, we found evidence for significant increases in vascular pump activity, not only in the hypertensive thoracic aorta but also equal or greater increases in the abdominal aorta, which we documented was not exposed to elevated intravascular pressure and hence was unlikely to have hyperplasia, at least to the degree of the thoracic aorta.

Other investigators have explained the increased pump activity observed in vessels in hypertension as the response of the membrane pump to elevated levels of intracellular sodium [9]. We also investigated this possibility, by using lithium substitution procedures similar to those developed by Friedman [29] to assess total cellular-sodium contents in the arterial tissue. Aortas from rats with coarctation hypertension had levels of cellular sodium similar to those of aortas from control normotensive rats. Similarly, in rats with DOCA-salt, and one-kidney Grollman hypertension, the increases we observed in ouabain-sensitive ^{86}Rb uptake by arteries (see below) were not associated with elevated levels of total

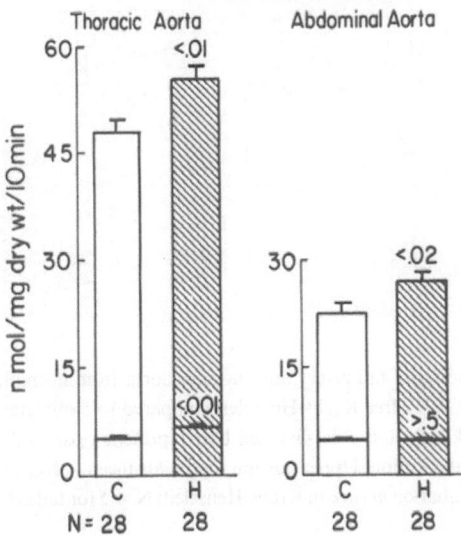

Figure 5. Increased ^{86}Rb uptakes by thoracic aorta and abdominal aorta of rats with chronic co-arctation hypertension (cross-hatched bars) and sham-coarcted normotensive controls (clear bars). Incubation *in vitro* in Krebs-Henseleit solution. N values provided. Bars and P values as in Figure 4.

cell sodium. We further reasoned that if higher levels of intracellular sodium in tissue from hypertensives did explain their increased pump activity, then one should be able to duplicate this increased activity by subjecting tissue from normotensive rats to sodium-loading procedures. Thus, excised aortas from control normotensive rats (Dahl R rats and normotensive Sprague-Dawley rats) underwent prolonged (60-minute) exposure to K^+-free Krebs-Henseleit solution at 37° before ^{86}Rb uptake was measured. It may be seen from Figure 6 that, although the prolonged sodium-loading procedures significantly increased cell sodium in arteries from normotensive Dahl R rats (over levels produced by our standard 5-minute loading procedures), these loading procedures failed to increase ouabain-sensitive ^{86}Rb uptake by these vessels; uptake levels remained lower than those by vessels from hypertensive S rats [25].

We devised an additional experiment to study in more detail the relationship of cell sodium to pump activity in vascular smooth muscle in hypertension [30]. We varied cell sodium over a wide range in both normotensive and hypertensive vessels *in vitro,* by use of incubating solutions with varying sodium content and by use of the sodium ionophore, monensin, which increases the passive permeability of the sarcolemma to Na^+. We studied rats with chronic DOCA-salt hypertension; one-kidney, one-figure-eight (Grollman) hypertension; and appropriate normotensive control rats. Thoracic aortas and tail arteries were excised from

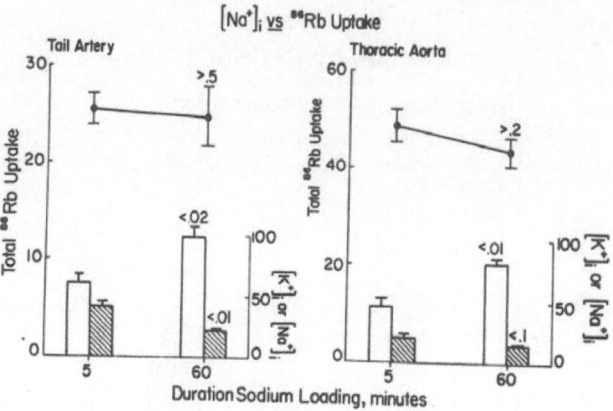

Figure 6. Cellular sodium loading of tail artery and thoracic aorta from normotensive Dahl R rats. Effects of 60-min loading in 37° K$^+$-free Krebs-Henseleit compared to 5-min standard loading at 0°. Clear bars represent total cell Na$^+$, and cross-hatched bars represent vessel wall K$^+$ (mean ± SEM; N = 9) measured by lithium substitution. Upper portion represents mean ± SEM of total ^{86}Rb uptake (nmole/mg dry wt/10 min). Incubation *in vitro* in Krebs-Henseleit; N = 5 for tail artery, N = 6 for aorta.

these rats. ^{86}Rb uptakes were measured immediately in some freshly dissected tail arteries and aortas, whereas other aortas were stored overnight at 4° and, the next morning, equilibrated at 37° for 3 hours in aerated Krebs-Henseleit solution to restore cell-ion contents toward normal levels before ^{86}Rb uptakes were measured. In some cases, the ^{86}Rb incubating solution also contained monensin, 10 μg/ml, to increase cell sodium, or 20 mM Na$^+$ (sucrose substitution) to decrease cell sodium. After 15 minutes of ^{86}Rb uptake in these solutions (in the presence or absence of 1 mM ouabain), the aortic segments were immediately immersed for 40 minutes in a 4° solution of LiCl to substitute Li$^+$ for extracellular Na$^+$. The segments were then dried, weighed, and acid-extracted. Aliquots were counted for ^{86}Rb and analyzed by atomic-absorption spectroscopy for Na$^+$. Thus, in the same segment of artery, we were able to assess both total cell sodium and tissue Rb uptake.

Table 1 presents the findings in DOCA-salt and Grollman hypertension. In freshly excised aorta (and tail artery) from rats with chronic DOCA-salt hypertension, we found elevated levels of ouabain-sensitive ^{86}Rb uptake that could not be explained on the basis of differences in total cell sodium. Similarly, in equilibrated aortas with low levels of cell sodium and in equilibrated tissue exposed to monensin with intermediate levels of cell sodium, we again found higher ^{86}Rb uptakes in the hypertensive tissue that could not be explained on the basis of higher levels of cell sodium. Our findings in chronic Grollman hypertension were similar. Ouabain-sensitive ^{86}Rb uptake was elevated in the hypertensive tissue, whether tissue Na$^+$ was low, following incubation in low Na$^+$ medium; high,

Table 1. Findings in DOCA-salt and Grollman hypertension

Treatment	Group (N)	Total Aortic Cell Na$^+$ (nmol/kg)	Ouabain-Sensitive ^{86}Rb Uptake by Aorta (nmol/15 min/mg)
Equilibrated	Control (12)	13.6 $\pm$ 0.8	4.6 $\pm$ 0.1
	Doca-salt (20)	12.9 $\pm$ 1.0	10.1 $\pm$ 1.4*
Equilibrated plus monesin	Control (14)	25.7 $\pm$ 2.0	17.2 $\pm$ 1.3
	Doca-salt (14)	24.1 $\pm$ 1.6	22.1 $\pm$ 2.0*
Fresh tissue	Control (10)	54.2 $\pm$ 2.3	32.4 $\pm$ 3.8
	DOCA-salt (7)	58.2 $\pm$ 2.6	45.3 $\pm$ 3.8*
20 mM na$^+$ solution	Control (5)	7.2 $\pm$ 0.9	1.4 $\pm$ 0.4
	1-kidney Grollman (5)	7.0 $\pm$ 0.9	2.9 $\pm$ 0.1*
150 mM Na$^+$ solution	Control (15)	14.7 $\pm$ 1.0	4.4 $\pm$ 0.6
	1-kidney Grollman (18)	12.8 $\pm$ 0.7	7.3 $\pm$ 1.3*
150 mM Na$^+$ solution plus monensin	Control (14)	25.5 $\pm$ 1.9	12.5 $\pm$ 1.9
	1-kidney Grollman (10)	24.4 $\pm$ 2.6	20.9 $\pm$ 2.1*

* $p < 0.05$ by Student's t test comparison of hypertensive and control values. 'Equilibrated' refers to overnight-stored aortas equilibrated in Krebs-Henseleit solution for 3 h before ^{86}Rb uptake. '20 mM Na$^+$ solution' refers to Krebs-Henseleit in which Na$^+$ was 20 mM and sucrose substituted to maintain osmolality. Monensin added to incubation media at 10 μg/ml. Control rats were uninephrectomized and drinking either .9% NaCl-.2% KCl (DOCA-salt controls) or tap water (Grollman controls).

following exposure to monensin; or intermediate, following incubation in normal Krebs-Henseleit.

Figure 7 presents individual ouabain-sensitive ^{86}Rb uptakes in tissue from rats with DOCA-salt hypertension and pooled data from normotensive control rats (which did not differ) plotted against individual levels of tissue Na$^+$ content. These are the same data summarized in Table 1. Curve fitting indicates a sigmoid relation, with a clear difference between hypertensive and normotensive tissues. For any level of total cell sodium, ouabain-sensitive ^{86}Rb uptake is significantly greater in the tissue from the hypertensive rats. Furthermore, maximal ^{86}Rb uptake is greater (P<0.05) in hypertensive than in normotensive tissue.

DISCUSSION

The outstanding findings of our studies, as well as other studies, of membrane sodium-pump activity in vascular smooth muscle in hypertension are the following: 1) *In vivo* studies in several species provide evidence for decreased pump activity. 2) Evidence from *in vitro* studies of vessels from hypertensive rats is conflicting; however, most evidence indicates that pump activity is increased, rather than decreased. 3) Evidence from our laboratory indicates that these

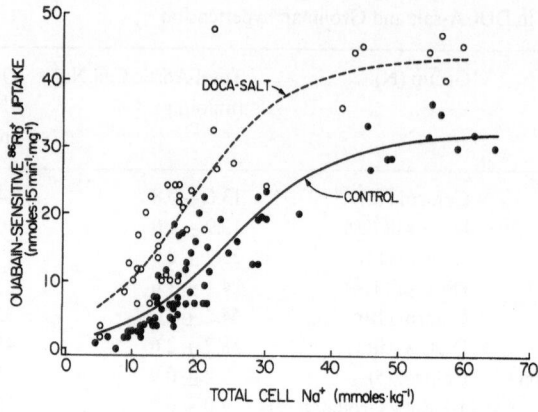

Figure 7. Sigmoid relation between total cell Na$^+$ and ouabain-sensitive ^{86}Rb uptake in thoracic aortas (means of same data presented in Table 1). Values for rats with chronic one-kidney DOCA-salt hypertension and pooled one-kidney normotensive control rats represented as open and closed circles, respectively. Curves computer-generated for sigmoid relation according to equation: Rb uptake = K/1 + exp[-(A · total cell Na$^+$ + B)]), where K = maximal Rb uptake, A = rate o change of upslope of curve, and B = intercept of curve on vertical axis. R^2 for curve in DOCA-salt rats = 0.94; R^2 for curve in normotensive control rats = 0.95. Derived values for normotensive control rats are: K = 31.9 ± 1.7, A = 0.13 ± 0.02, B = −3.14 ± 0.32. Derived values for DOCA-salt hypertensive rats are: K = 43.2 ± 2.6 (P<0.001), A = 0.13 ± 0.03 (P>0.05), B = −2.47 ± 0.41 (P>0.05).

increases observed in rat tissue *in vitro* may not be related to volume expansion, to activity of the renin-angiotensin-aldosterone system, or to tissue hyperplasia/ hypertrophy. 4) Evidence from our laboratory suggests that the increases also may not be directly attributable to elevated total cell sodium.

In our laboratories, *in vivo* studies of blood-perfused vascular beds in animals with experimental renal hypertension [3, 4] and in patients with essential hypertension [5], as presented in Figure 1, have uniformly provided evidence suggesting decreased activity of the membrane sodium pump in vascular smooth muscle. The unique value of these studies lies in their potential to detect the effects of blood-borne inhibitors on the smooth muscle cells of arterioles. Because the attenuated responses to local intra-arterial infusions of K$^+$ were specific, and because the effects of differences in baseline vascular resistances were considered in data interpretation, it is unlikely that the attenuated responses are attributable to structural, rather than functional, abnormalities in the vessel wall. Instead, the hypertensives' responses resembled the attenuation of K$^+$-induced vasodilation produced by ouabain [2]. It is especially noteworthy that in rats with two-kidney Goldblatt hypertension, our *in vivo* studies [4] provided evidence for pump inhibition; in contrast, our *in vitro* studies [27] indicated increased pump activity.

Clearly, in hypertensive rats, even in presumably volume-expanded forms of hypertension (e.g., DOCA- salt, one-kidney Goldblatt, Dahl salt- sesitive), most *in vitro* studies [9–15] of vascular muscle (and studies of solution-perfused vascular beds [16–18]) have provided evidence for increases, rather that decreases, in pump activity. Although many of these studies were conducted in tissue several hours after excision [9–15], even in our freshly excised tissue [25, 27, 28] or in vascular beds perfused with artificial solutions [16–18], evidence for increased, rather than decreased, pump activity is observed. Because such increases are seen in solution-perfused vascular beds, it is unlikely that differences between *in vivo* and *in vitro* studies are attributable to differences between resistance and conduit arteries. Furthermore, the increases observed in rat arteries studied *in vitro* contrasts with the decreased pump activity in similar *in vitro* studies of vessels from hypertensive dogs (Fig. 2), a species considerably more sensitive to digitalis.

We documented increases in levels of plasma renin activity in the rats with two-kidney, but not in rats with one-kidney, Goldblatt hypertension [27]. These observations, together with the increase in plasma volume we documented only in the Dahl S rats on high salt [25], tend to dissociate the elevations we observed in vascular sodium pump activity from function of the renin-angiotensin-aldosterone system and from volume-expansion. (However, it is possible that further investigation may associate the increased pump activity with some function of renin-angiotension-aldosterone and/or volume expansion. For example, these pump abnormalities may characterize 'volume-dependent' forms of hypertension [31], where elevated mean systemic pressure reflects a disproportion between plasma volume and vascular capacitance. Or they may be associated with abnormalities in central volume or in a volume-sensing function, for example, left atrial stretching.)

The increased pump activity we and most other laboratories have observed in *in vitro* studies of vascular muscle from hypertensive rats might reflect normal turnover of an increased number of pump molecules per unit tissue weight, due to growth of the smooth muscle cells. Tissue hypertrophy in hypertension would be expected to decrease pump activity per unit tissue weight by decreasing the ratio of sarcolemmal surface area to tissue volume. In contrast, hyperplasia of vascular smooth muscle in hypertension would increase the ratio of sarcolemmal area to tissue volume and therefore could explain increased pump activity per unit tissue weight. Our observation in rats with coarctation hypertension – that increases in pump activity of the normotensive abdominal aorta were at least equal to those of the hypertensive thoracic aorta – provides good evidence that hyperplasia does not account for the increases observed in pump activity in hypertension. This is because hyperplasia of the walls of the normotensive abdominal aorta in coarctation hypertension is considerably less than that in the hypertensive thoracic aorta [32, 33]. Our observations in coarctation hypertension also suggest that the increases in tissue pump activity are not attributable to other pressure-induced changes in the vascular wall.

The increased pump activity observed in *in vitro* studies in hypertensive rats might also reflect increased turnover of a normal number of pump molecules per unit tissue weight. It is unlikely that this increased turnover is related to increased $[K^+]_0$, because medium K^+ is held constant. Although other investigators have suggested that increased pump activity may be related to increases in $[Na^+]_1$, our data would also argue against this explanation. We found no significant increases in cell Na^+ in arterial tissue from rats with coarctation, DOCA-salt, or Grollman hypertension accompanying the increased pump activity. Furthermore, we observed that at each level of cell Na^+ over a wide range, pumping, including Na^+-induced maximal levels of pump activity, was greater in hypertensive tissue. A similar observation in rats with DOCA-salt hypertension has been made by Jones [15]. Finally, we were unable, by cell sodium loading (exposure to monensin or to K^+-free medium), to produce levels of pump activity in tissue from normotensive rats as great as those we observed in tissue from hypertensive rats. (However, there remains the unlikely possibility that our sodium-loading procedures did not fill an intracellular Na^+ compartment critical for the function of the membrane sodium pump.)

Influx of Na^+ into the smooth muscle cells increased with monesin exposure, mimicking the increased membrane Na^+ permeability that has been observed in hypertensive vascular smooth muscle [34]. Yet, for similar contents of cell sodium, monensin did not increase sodium pump activity over levels seen in untreated tissue. These data would argue that the increased pump activity of smooth muscle of hypertensive rats may not represent merely a response to increased 'leakiness' of the cell membrane, per se, with Na^+ efflux due to increased pump activity exactly matching the increased Na^+ influx, and total cell Na^+ remaining normal.

Although other agents present in the vascular wall – for example, prostaglandins [35] – might be involved, we favor the explanation that the increased pump activity of rat vascular muscle observed in vitro is attributable to the effects of increased numbers of pump molecules per unit sarcolemma. Others [9] have suggested that chronic increases in membrane Na^+ 'leakiness' might result in de novo synthesis of additional membrane pump molecules. We, however, feel it is also possible that in certain forms of hypertension, a circulating digitalis-like pump inhibitor might induce the formation of more pump molecules per unit sarcolemma. (Induction of membrane Na^+, K^+-ATPase in cardiovascular muscle by chronic digitalis treatment of animals has been reported [36].) This explanation would account for many observations, including in vivo evidence for pump inhibition and increasing evidence for a circulating pump inhibitor in hypertension [37, 38]. Thus, in vivo net pump activity would be depressed by the circulating inhibitor. In contrast, when the tissue from hypertensive rats is excised and studied in vitro (or perfused in situ with an artificial medium), the pump inhibitor would rapidly dissociate from the pump molecule, the increased pump activity then observed reflecting solely the effects of the additional induced pump molecules. This would also explain why both in vivo [3] and in vitro [6] studies provide evidence for pump inhibition in dogs, a species more sensitive to digitalis.

Our suggestion requires testing, for example, estimation of concentration of sarcolemmal pump molecules by tritiated ouabain binding. Such measurements have recently been made sucessfully in arterial tissue from rats (Wong, S.K., personal communication).

SUMMARY

Considerable evidence from *in vivo* studies in dogs, rats, and humans and from *in vitro* studies in dogs, supports the hypothesis that decreased activity of the sarcolemmal sodium pump in vascular smooth muscle may underlie the vasconstriction in certain forms of hypertension. However, most *in vitro* studies in hypertensive rats indicate increased, rather than decreased, vascular pump activity.

To investigate this latter observation and its underlying mechanisms, we measured ouabain-sensitive ^{86}Rb uptake in aortas and tail arteries excised from rats with several forms of experimental hypertension: Dahl salt-sensitive (S) rats; one- and two-kidney Goldblatt hypertension; coarctation hypertension; DOCA-salt hypertension; and one-kidney Grollman hypertension. We also used lithium-substitution methods to measure total cell Na^+ content in arteries.

In all cases, we found evidence for significant increases in vascular pump activity. We could not relate these increases to: 1) plasma volume expansion, because tail artery sodium-pump activity was elevated equally in Dahl S rats on low- or high-salt diets, but plasma volume was increased only in the latter; 2) activity of the renin-angiotensin-aldosterone system, because arterial pump activity was elevated equally in one- and two-kidney Goldblatt hypertension, but PRA was increased only in the latter; 3) vascular tissue hyperplasia/hypertrophy, because pump activity was increased equally in the thoracic and abdominal aortic tissue in coarctation hypertension, but intra-aortic pressure was elevated only in the former; or 4) increased Na^+ content in the vascular smooth muscle cells, because cell sodium was not elevated in arteries from the hypertensive rats, and maximally stimulated (by high levels of cell sodium) pump activity was greater in hypertensive tissue.

We conclude that the *in vivo* and *in vitro* data together are best explained by a circulating digitalis-like pump inhibitor that induces the formation of additional sarcolemmal pump molecules. Thus, *in vivo* net pump activity would be depressed; but when tissue from rats (a species notably insensitive to cardiac glycosides because of rapid dissociation from the pump molecule) is excised and studied *in vitro*, the pump inhibitor would rapidly dissociate, the increased pump activity then observed reflecting the effects of the additional induced pump molecules.

208

ACKNOWLEDGMENTS

The many co-investigators who participated in most of these studies are listed as co-authors in the designated references, which provide details of individual experiments.

REFERENCES

1. Tobian L Jr, Bibion JT: Tissue cations and water in arterial hypertension. Circulation 5:754–758, 1952.
2. Hendrickx H, Casteels R: Electrogenic sodium pump in arterial smooth muscle cells. Pflugers Arch 346:299–306, 1974.
3. Overbeck HW: Vascular responses to cations, osmolality and angiotensin in renal hypertensive dogs. Am J Physiol 223:1358–1364, 1972.
4. Overbeck HW, Clark DWJ: Vasodilator responses to K^+ in genetic hypertensive and in renal hypertensive rats. J Lab Clin Med 86:973–983, 1975.
5. Overbeck HW, Derifield RS, Pamnani MB, et al.: Attenuated vasodilator responses to K^+ in essential hypertensive men. J Clin Invest 53:678–686, 1974.
6. Overbeck HW, Pamnani MB, Akera T, et al.: Depressed function of a ouabain-sensitive sodium-potassium pump in blood vessels from renal hypertensive dogs. Circ Res 38 (suppl II):II-48–52, 1976.
7. Dahl LK, Knudsen KD, Iwai J: Humoral transmission of hypertension: Evidence from parabiosis. Circ Res 24/25 (suppl I):I-21–33, 1969.
8. Haddy FJ, Overbeck HW: The role of humoral agents in volume-expanded hypertension. Life Sci 19:935–948, 1976.
9. Friedman SM, Friedman CL: Cell permeability, sodium transport and the hypertensive process in the rat. Circ Res 39:433–441, 1975.
10. Hermsmeyer K: Electrogenesis of increased norepinephrine sensitivity of arterial vascular muscle in hypertension. Circ Res 38:362–367, 1976.
11. Webb RC, Bohr DF: Potassium relaxation of vascular smooth muscle from spontaneously hypertensive rats. Blood Vessels 16:71–79, 1979.
12. Friedman SM: Evidence for enhanced sodium transport in the tail artery of the spontaneously hypertensive rat. Hypertension 1:572–582, 1979.
13. Mulvany MJ, Nyborg N, Nilsson H: Effect of sodium-potassium-dependent ATPase inhibition on noradrenaline-activated calcium sensitivity of mesenteric resistance vessels in adult spontaneously hypertensive rats. Clin Sci 59:203s–205s, 1980.
14. Friedman SM, Nakashima SM: Evidence for enhanced Na transport in hypertension induced by DOCA in the rat. Can J Physiol Pharmacol 56:1029–1035, 1978.
15. Jones AW: Kinetics of active sodium transport in aortas from control and deoxycorticosterone hypertensive rats. Hypertension 3:631–640, 1981.
16. Göthberg G, Jandhyala B, Folkow B: Studies on the role of sodiumpotassium activated ATPase as determinant of vascular reactivity in Wistar-Kyoto and spontaneously hypertensive rats. Clin Sci 59:187s–189s, 1980.
17. Göthberg G, Jandhayala B, Folkow B: Influence of the Na-K-activated ATPase on resistance vessel reactivity in normotensive rats compared with rat models of primary and secondary hypertension. Acta Physiol Scand 109:4A, 1980.
18. Cohen DM, Borh DF: Renal vascular potassium relaxation in two-kidney one-clip hypertensive rats, abstracted. Physiologist 24:6, 1981.

19. Pamnani MB, Clough DL, Haddy FJ: Altered activity of the sodium potassium pump in arteries of rats with steroid hypertension. Clin Sci Mol Med 55:41s–43s, 1978.

20. Pamnani MB, Clough DL, Haddy FJ: Na+-K+ pump activity in tail arteries of spontaneously hypertensive rats. Jpn Heart J 20 (suppl I):228–230, 1979.

21. Pamnani MB, Clough DL, Huot S, et al.: Vascular Na+-K+ pump in various models of experimental hypertension, abstracted. Proc Int Soc Hypertens 101, 1980.

22. Songu-Mize E, Bealer SL, Caldwell RW: Effects of antero-ventral 3rd ventricular lesions on vascular 'Na-pump' activity, abstracted. Fed Proc 40:410, 1981.

23. Schwartz A, Lindenmayer GE, Allen JC: The sodium-potassium adenosine triphosphatase: Pharmacological, physiological and biochemical aspects. Pharmacol Rev 27:3–134, 1975.

24. Tobian L, Lange J, Azar S, et al.: Reduction of natriuretic capacity and renin release in isolated blood perfused kidneys of Dahl hypertension-prone rats. Circ Res 43 (suppl I):I-92–98, 1978.

25. Overbeck HW, Ku DD, Rapp JP: Sodium-pump activity in arteries of Dahl salt-sensitive rats. Hypertension 3:306–312, 1981.

26. Pamnani MB, Clough DL, Huot SJ, et al.: Vascular Na+-K+ pump activity in Dahl S and R rats. Proc Soc Exp Biol Med 165:440–444, 1980.

27. Overbeck HW, Grissette DE: Sodium-pump activity in arteries of rats with Goldblatt hypertension. Hypertension 4:132–139, 1982.

28. Overbeck HW, Bell DR, Grissette DE, et al.: Function of the sodium pump in arterial smooth muscle in hypertension – Role of pressure. Hypertension, in press.

29. Friedman SM, Mar M, Nakashima M: Lithium substitution analysis of Na and K phases in a small artery. Blood Vessels 11:55–64, 1974.

30. Brock TA, Smith JB, Overbeck HW: Relationship of vascular Na+-K+-pump activity to intracellular sodium in hypertensive rats. Hypertension, in press.

31. Coleman TG, Samar RE, Murphy WR: Autoregulation versus other vasoconstrictors in hypertension. A critical review. Hypertension 1:324–330, 1979.

32. Overbeck HW: Cardiovascular hypertrophy and 'waterlogging' in coarctation hypertension – Role of sympathoadrenergic influences and pressure. Hypertension 1:486–492, 1979.

33. Bevan RD: An autoradiographic and pathological study of cellular proliferation in rabbit arteries correlated with an increase in arterial pressure. Blood Vessels 13:100–128, 1976.

34. Jones AW, Hart RG: Altered ion transport in aortic smooth muscle during desoxycorticosterone acetate hypertension in the rat. Circ Res 37:333–341, 1975.

35. Lockette WE, Webb RC, Bohr DF: Prostaglandins and potassium relaxation in vascular smooth muscle of the rat. The role of Na-K ATPase. Circ Res 46:714–720, 1980.

36. Bluschke V, Bonn R, Greeff K: Increase in the (Na+,K+)-ATPase activity in heart muscle after chronic treatment with digoxin or potassium deficient diet. Eur J Pharmacol 37:189–191, 1976.

37. Gruber KA, Rudel LL, Bullock BC: Increased circulating levels of an endogenous digoxin-like factor in hypertensive non-human primates. Hypertension, in press.

38. De Wardener HE, MacGregor GA: Dahl's hypothesis that a saluretic substance may be responsible for the sustained rise in arterial pressure: Its possible role in essential hypertension. Kidney Int 18:1–9, 1980.

DISCUSSION

Discussants: Hoffman, Overbeck, Bohr, Jones, Mulvany, Ericman, Blaustein

Hoffman: In the studies where you have increased uptake of rubidium at high cell sodiums is there a net loss of sodium from the cells during ouabain-sensitive uptake of rubidium? Have you measured that? There could be other forms of ouabain-sensitive increases in rubidum uptake that did not lead to net movements of sodium, although they were mediated by the pump.

Overbeck: We used the lithium-substitution methods to look at total cell sodium immediately before and after the rubidium-uptake procedure in tissue from rats that had coarctation hypertension, and we didn't find decreases in the cell sodium that we were measuring. But I can't say what would happen with very high levels of intracellular sodium; we didn't look at that.

Bohr: I want to give you an example of pump activity in another species that is ouabain-sensitive. A pig has a tail that is usually about ten inches long, so Clinton Webb from time to time studies pigtail artery before and after DOCA implant. Within three days after DOCA implantation, about the time the pressure starts to go up, there's an increase in potassium relaxation which, as you know, is his index of sodium potassium ATPase activity. That was just an aside, but it is an animal that's ouabain-sensitive.

David Dawson, at the University of Michigan, looks at permeability of turtle colon epithelium and this sodium leak is increased by aldosterone and the pump activity increases in a matter of hours. The leak occurs immediately with the aldosterone. If he blocks the leak with amiloride, not letting sodium into the cell, then there's no subsequent increase in pump activity. Alan Jones has shown that these membranes really are leakier to sodium. I wonder if you're entirely comfortable that the pump loading is increased in response to the increased sodium coming in and so well matches this that you really don't see an increase in intracellular sodium content without having to involve the pump inhibitor.

Overbeck: I think that's still possible. However, I point out that we also had the data from chronic one-kidney, figure-of-eight hypertension. I don't believe there is evidence for increased permeability in that form of hypertension. Is that true, Dr. Jones?

Jones: We did a series of one-kidney renal hypertension and measured ^{42}K efflux. We did not see any changes. We did these at around 10 weeks. Of what duration were your figure-of-eight ligatures?

Overbeck: They had four weeks of hypertension levels above 150 systolic, but it was about six weeks after the figure-of-eight procedure in most rats.

Jones: Ours were about that range. Maybe we should go back and investigate it. Have you seen any changes with the Dahl rats? You commented about some increase there. It was a little bit of a teaser because it's on a wet-weight basis, and are you sure that is not due to hypertrophy of the tissue or do you think there really is an alteration in pump activity in the Dahl rat?

Overbeck: Our conclusions in the Dahl rat were identical whether we expressed the data in terms of wet weight or dry weight. So no, I don't think so.

Jones: Did you measure extracellular spaces and cell water?

Overbeck: No, we didn't do that.

Jones: In the DOCA animals, we measured a 30 percent expansion in cell contents per dry weight. It would be nice to have the cell waters per unit weight and divide that into the moles taken up per weight.

Mulvany: We have found that in small vessels from spontaneously hypertensive rats the media thickness is a greater proportion of the total wall thickness. Therefore, I think that unless you actually can be quite certain that the proportion of the wall containing cells is remaining the same, then you have a possible artifact creeping in there.

Overbeck: I think that's still possible. We've looked pretty carefully for growth of the abdominal aorta in coarcted hypertensive rats and Rosemary Bevan has looked at it in rabbits that had coarctation hypertension. There's really very little evidence for hyperplasia or hypertrophy of the abdominal aorta which we've documented remains normotensive by measuring conscious blood pressures for days and days. The blood pressure just doesn't go up. This is in the normotensive part of the aorta which is below the clip. Pressures there stay really perfectly normal, undistinguishable from pressures in sham-coarcted rats.

Ericman: Did you measure vanadate, because there you would have an inhibitor which under certain situations could stimulate active transport? It is vital, I think, to your hypothesis, that the intracellular sodium is not exchanged faster or the intracellular sodium concentration stays constant. Now if one measures the total sodium concentration, one can't pick it up, but how about sodium activity with sodium-sensitive electrodes? Did you think of that?

Overbeck: These are excellent suggestions which we have not done yet. We haven't measured vanadate and we haven't used sodium-sensitive electrodes. The question is raised whether there could be an intracellular compartment that we're not filling by our loading technique in the tissue from the normotensive rats. I think this is possible but I think it's rather unlikely because we got the total cell sodium up to 100 millimoles per kilogram and we still couldn't increase the pumping in a normotensive tissue to the levels we saw in the hypertensive tissue. So, although the sodium could be compartmentalized, I think that it is unlikely.

Blaustein: The preceding discussion has raised a number of interesting points. The problem concerns what happens if you look at changes in pump activity when the cells obviously must remain, on the average, in some kind of steady sodium balance. The question then is, do you have a change in leak? Is cell sodium elevated or is it depressed? Certainly, one of the observations that brought us to the hypothesis about a relationship between a circulating sodium-pump inhibitor and hypertension is the evidence in red and white blood cells for elevated cell sodium. Then, of course, the question comes up as to why cell sodium is elevated in those cells. And, is there increased or reduced pumping in those cells? I suspect we're going to hear more about that in the near future.

EVIDENCE AGAINST RAISED INTRACELLULAR SODIUM CAUSING MYOGENIC CONTRACTION IN RAT RESISTANCE VESSELS

M.J. MULVANY, C. AALKJAER, H. NILSSON, AND T. PETERSEN

INTRODUCTION

A number of recent findings have pointed to possible molecular mechanisms that could account for the long-suspected association between sodium intake and the development of essential hypertension.

First, various abnormalities in the sodium-extrusion mechanisms of erythrocytes from essential hypertensives have been shown [1, 2]. Second, the plasma of essential hypertensives appears to contain a natriuretic factor. Third, it has been demonstrated that certain large arterial vessels (e.g., rabbit aorta [3] and guinea-pig aorta [4], contract under conditions where their intracellular sodium concentration is raised. On the basis of such findings, it has been suggested [5, 6] that essential hypertension could be due to some alteration in sodium metabolism, which causes a general increase in intracellular sodium level. If increased intracellular sodium causes vasoconstriction, this would explain the increased peripheral resistance associated with essential hypertension.

However, this attractive and elegant theory has a weakness in that it has not yet been demonstrated conclusively that raised intracellular sodium causes constriction of the vessels actually involved in the control of peripheral resistance: the small arteries and arterioles. Although Lang and Blaustein [7] have provided evidence from perfusion experiments that this could be the case, the crucial evidence obtainable only from isolated resistance-vessel preparations has been lacking. In an attempt to answer some of these questions, we have therefore investigated the *in vitro* effect of raising intracellular sodium in rat resistance vessels with lumen diameters of about 150 μm, when mounted as ring preparations on a myograph [8]. As controls, larger rat arteries (aorta and tail artery) were also tested. Intracellular sodium was raised by inhibiting the Na, K-ATPase either with 1mM ouabain or K-free solutions. The results suggest that while raised intracellular sodium may cause contraction of larger vessels, it does not seem to have a vasoconstrictive effect in the smaller vessels. Indeed, under conditions where the intracellular sodium level is raised, the responses to noradrenaline are actually depressed.

METHODS

Segments of mesenteric and femoral 150-μm resistance vessels [9, 10] and of tail arteries (internal diameter ca. 600-μm) and thoracic aorta (internal diameter ca. 2 mm) were taken from adult (ca. 12 wk) Wistar-Kyoto rats. The segments were mounted as ring preparations on an isometric myograph [8] and set to normalized internal circumference L_1, as described previously [9].

The solutions used had the following compositions (in mmol/L). Physiological salt solution (PSS): NaCl, 119; KCl, 4.7; NaHCO$_3$, 25; CaCl$_2$, 2.5; KH$_2$PO$_4$, 1.18; MgSO$_4$, 1.17; ethylenediaminetetraacetic acid (EDTA), 0.026; glucose, 5.5. High-potassium solution (K-PSS): PSS in which KCl was substituted for NaCl on an equimolar basis. All solutions were bubbled with 5% CO$_2$ in O$_2$ and held at 37°C to give pH 7.4. Drugs used were ouabain (Merck) and phentolamine (CIBA).

In the pharmacological experiments, vessels were mounted on a double myograph and, where possible, it was arranged that a large vessel and a small vessel were tested simultaneously, so that they were exposed to exactly the same solutions. Intracellular recordings of membrane potential were made with vessels mounted on a single myograph, the arrangement permitting simultaneous measurements of vessel-wall tension and membrane potential [11]. Intracellular sodium content was estimated using a modification on the Li-substitution method of Friedman et al. [12]. With this method [13], intracellular sodium content was estimated from the washout curves of previously loaded ^{22}Na. Sodium contents were related to estimates of cell volume made at the start of each experiment from microscopic observation of each vessel when mounted on the myograph [14].

Results are presented at mean $\pm$ SE (n = number of vessels).

RESULTS

At the start of experiments, vessels were set to normalized internal circumference L_1 (see Methods). The corresponding internal diameters, L_1/π, were ca. 2 mm (aorta), 600 μm (tail arteries), and 150 μm (mesenteric and femoral resistance vessels). Vessels were then stimulated with K-PSS, the response to which is denoted as ΔT_K. The basal tension at L_1 corresponded to about 0.9 ΔT_K in the resistance vessels.

Mechanical effects of prolonged exposure to ouabain and K-free solutions

Resting vessels

The effects of exposing the four types of vessels studied in this investigation to

214

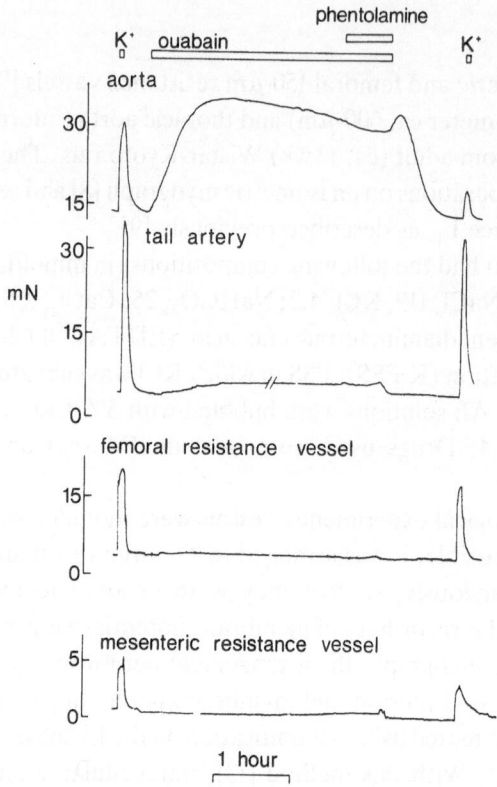

Figure 1. Records of effect of ouabain (1 mM) as shown by lower bar, on isometric wall tension (ordinate) in rat aorta, tail artery, femoral resistance vessel, and mesenteric resistance vessel, as indicated. At K⁺, vessels are exposed to K-PSS. For periods indicated by upper bars, phentolamine (1 μM) was added to the solutions. For further details, see Methods.

1 mM ouabain are shown in Figure 1, which shows typical records over a 3-hour period. Aortae responded to ouabain (n = 6) with a response equal to about 1.0 ΔT_K, which developed over about 20 minutes, and which was then maintained over the entire 3-hour period. Addition of the alpha-blocker, phentolamine (1 μM) during the final 30 minutes of this period had no effects on the ouabain response.

Tail arteries also responded to ouabain (n = 3), the tension increasing over about 1 hour by about 0.15 ΔT_K. Here, phentolamine had a small depressive effect on the ouabain response. Neither femoral (n = 2) nor mesenteric (n = 8) resistance vessels produced any large maintained tension in response to ouabain (tension after 3 hours was 0.06 ± 0.06 ΔT_k [n = 2, femoral], 0.06 ± 0.08 ΔT_K [n = 8, mesenteric]), although in some cases (7 out of 11 vessels) the femoral vessels developed an initial transient response to ouabain, peaking at about 0.1 ΔT_K, lasting about 20 minutes, which was not inhibitable by phentolamine.

The response to K-PSS after the 1-hour washout period in PSS following the exposure to ouabain was normally at least 50% of the K-PSS response at the start of the experiments.

Corresponding experiments with K-free solutions in the presence of phentolamine gave similar results in all vessels, except that the tail artery sometimes also developed an initial transient (ca. 15 minutes) response on withdrawal of potassium. In the absence of phentolamine, transient responses on withdrawal of potassium were also seen in both types of resistance vessels, but the aorta responses were little affected.

Activated mesenteric resistance vessels

The effect of 1 mM ouabain on the active responses of mesenteric resistance vessels to repetitive stimulation with noradrenaline (3 minutes every 8 minutes) is shown in Figure 2. Inclusion of ouabain caused an initial potentiation of the responses but thereafter a decline, such that after 2 hours the amplitude of the tonic part of the responses (measured after 3 minutes stimulation) was reduced by about 50%. Upon washout of ouabain, the responses fell initially even further, but then recovered within about 1 hour to a level higher than that seen at the start of the experiment. The initial phasic parts of the responses were much less affected by the ouabain treatment. Exactly similar results were obtained with

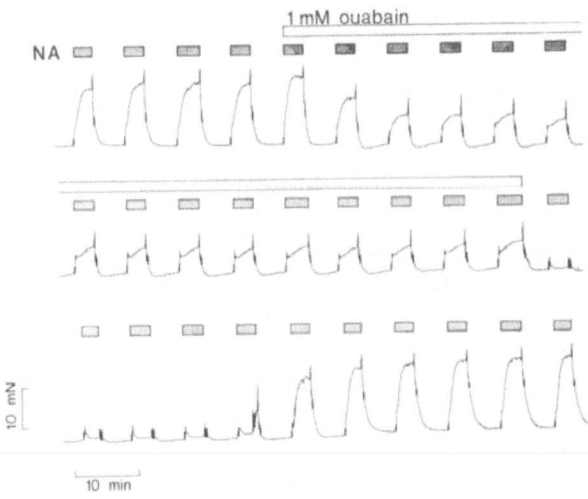

Figure 2. Effect of ouabain on responses of mesenteric resistance vessels to repetitive noradrenaline stimulation. Figure shows continuous record of vessel, which was stimulated every 8 minutes for 3 minutes with a submaximal dose (1 μM) of noradrenaline (dotted bars). The noradrenaline solutions contained 3 μM cocaine. Between stimulations, the bathing solution was PSS. For period indicated by open bar, the noradrenaline solutions and the PSS contained 1 mM ouabain. Vessel normalized internal diameter ($= L_1/\pi$) was 222 μm. Segment length was 1.77 mm. From Mulvany et al. [15].

three other mesenteric resistance vessels. In four other mesenteric resistance vessels, in which K-free solutions were used instead of ouabain, essentially similar results were also obtained.

Effect of ouabain on intracellular sodium content and membrane potential in mesenteric resistance vessels

The effect of ouabain on the intracellular sodium content of mesenteric resistance vessels in shown in Figure 3. Under control conditions in which vessels were held in PSS for up to 2 hours, the intracellular sodium concentration was estimated (see Methods) to be 13 ± 1 mmol/L cells (n = 22). In the corresponding experiments in which vessels were instead held in PSS containing 1 mM ouabain for 2 hours, the sodium content was found to be 63 ± 5 mmol/L cells (n = 8).

The membrane potential of the vessels in PSS was initially -54 ± 1 mV (n = 13). As previously, ouabain had no effect on the wall tension but produced first a transient depolarization, followed by a continuous gradual depolarization reaching -45 ± 2 mV (n = 13) after 30 minutes. Reintroduction of PSS then caused repolarization to -57 ± 2 mV (n = 8) within 5 minutes. Further details of these experiments are presented elsewhere [15], where it is also shown that K-free solution had similar effects on the membrane potential.

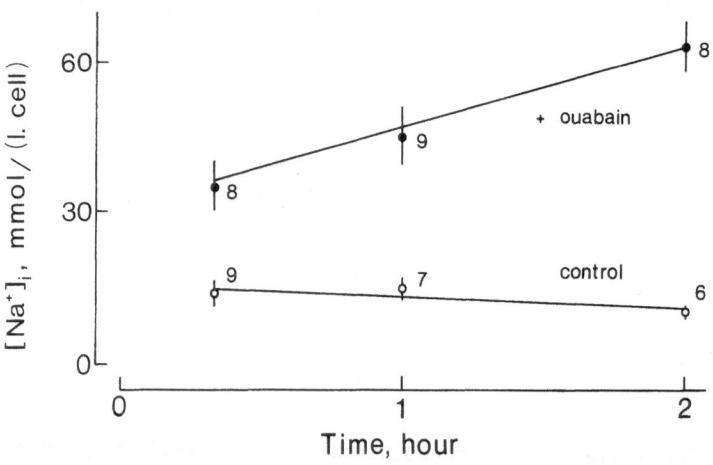

Figure 3. Effect of 1 mM ouabain on intracellular sodium content of rat mesenteric resistance vessels. Intracellular sodium contents of rat mesenteric resistance vessels estimated as described in Methods after being held in PSS (open symbols) or in PSS containing 1 mM ouabain (filled symbols) for the times indicated. The number beside each point shows number of vessels. Bars show SE.

Acute effect of ouabain on noradrenaline-activated mesenteric resistance vessels

Although as indicated above, prolonged exposure to ouabain causes a depression of the responses of mesenteric resistance vessels to noradrenaline, the acute effect of ouabain was to potentiate noradrenaline responses. This is illustrated by the records shown in Figure 4, which shows the effect on membrane potential and wall tension of adding 1 mM ouabain to a vessel already submaximally activated with noradrenaline. In such experiments (n = 5), the exposure to noradrenaline (ca. 1 μM) had caused the wall tension to increase and the membrane to depolarize to -37 ± 5 mV. Addition of ouabain caused within 3 minutes a further increase in wall tension of 0.14 ± 0.05 ΔT_K and a simultaneous depolarization (P<0.01) of 6.2 ± 1.2 mV.

In corresponding experiments, in which instead of adding ouabain, potassium was withdrawn from the solutions, similar changes in wall tension and membrane potential were seen.

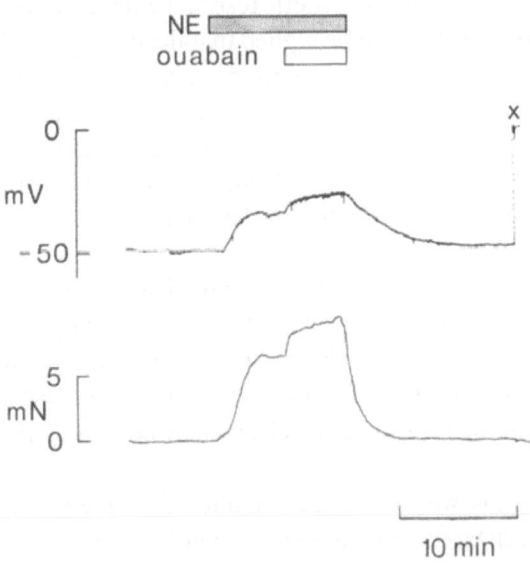

Figure 4. Acute electrophysiological responses of norepinephrine-activated mesenteric resistance vessels to ouabain. Upper records show membrane potential and lower records the simultaneously measured total wall force. Vessels were submaximally activated with norepinephrine as indicated by dotted bars. Open bar shows where 1 mM ouabain was added to suffusate (open bar); at X micro-electrode was withdrawn from vessel. Vessel normalized internal diameter ($= L_1 \leq \pi$) was 267 μm. Segment length was 1.57 mm. From Mulvany et al. [15].

DISCUSSION

The aim of the present investigations was to test the attractive hypothesis [5] that increased intracellular sodium can cause vasoconstriction of resistance vessels. The results, however, show that, in contrast to aorta and tail artery, the resistance vessels do not contract under conditions of ouabain-induced, increased intracellular sodium. Moreover, in the mesenteric resistance vessels, at least, the responses to noradrenaline are actually reduced following prolonged exposure to ouabain. On the other hand, we have shown that ouabain can have an acute potentiating effect on the response of activated vessels. This potentiating effect appears to occur too rapidly for it to be caused by any change in intracellular sodium, and we would suggest that it is probably due to the depolarizing effect of ouabain, which we have demonstrated. These results therefore suggest that increased intracellular sodium does not have a vasoconstrictive effect in the resistance vessels we have tested, and the results are therefore at variance with the hypothesis, although they do not of course disprove it.

The effect of ouabain, which we see in the resting aorta and tail artery preparations, as well as the acute potentiating effect of ouabain in the activated mesenteric resistance vessels is in general agreement with previous investigations of the action of this glycoside in isolated vascular smooth muscle. The lack of response of the resistance vessels to ouabain and the depressive effect of long-term exposure to ouabain of the mesenteric resistance vessels have not, however, been seen in other vessels. It might be argued that the discrepancy is due to some nonspecific effects of the high concentration of ouabain that we had to use, owing to the well-known insensitivity of rat Na, K-ATPase to ouabain.

However, since we have shown that such exposure to ouabain causes both an increase in intracellular sodium and membrane depolarization, it seems reasonable to conclude that the glycoside has in fact inhibited the Na, K-ATPase as expected. Moreover, the effects (or lack of effect) of ouabain were also seen with K-free solutions, another method of inhibiting the Na, K-ATPase. Lastly, since the larger vessels do respond to ouabain (and K-free solutions), it seems unlikely that the failure of the resistance vessels to respond is due to some inhibitory effect of the high ouabain concentration. Therefore, we believe that ouabain was having its expected actions in the resistance vessels, namely being a specific inhibitor of the Na, K-ATPase.

The 'resistance vessels' we have tested had internal diameters of about 150 μm and are therefore much larger than those often considered to produce the bulk of the precapillary vascular resistance. It might therefore be thought that our results are irrelevant to factors concerned with peripheral resistance. Those who have actually measured pressures in vessels of this size have found, however, that 30% or more of the precapillary vascular resistance lies in vessels proximal to those with lumen diameter 200 μm [16, 17]. Furthermore, we have evidence that the pharmacological properties of the vessels, with respect to noradrenaline and calcium, at least, do seem to reflect those of perfused vascular beds [14, 15, 18]. We therefore consider that the vessels we have examined do play an important role in the control of peripheral resistance, and may well provide useful information about the properties of the smaller resistance vessels.

If, however, the results from our resistance vessels are providing information about the vascular bed as a whole, then our results are somewhat surprising. It is, for example, a very common observation that injection of cardiac glycosides causes an increase in peripheral resistance [19]. Two explanations, not related to intracellular sodium levels, may be considered. First, the increase could be due to the glycosides causing release of catecholamines from the adrenergic nerve terminals [20]. Second, the response could be due to the depolarizing action of cardiac glycosides. Our experiments provide some support for both views. First, when the Na, K-ATPase was inhibited with K-free solutions, a phentolamine-inhibitable response was seen, indicating that under these conditions, at least, neural noradrenaline was being released. Second, we found that ouabain (and K-free solution) had an acute potentiating effect on the noradrenaline response, probably due to its depolarizing action: Since the vasculature is normally partially activated *in vivo,* a similar effect would be expected.

Thus, there is no direct contradiction between the data presented here and that presented elsewhere. We would, though, suggest that any myogenically-mediated vasoconstrictive action of cardiac glycosides could as well be due to their depolarizing action, rather than to their causing an increase in intracellular sodium.

In conclusion, the results of this investigation suggest to us that there are grounds for questioning whether raised intracellular sodium will cause contraction of resistance vessels. We therefore suggest that further investigations are necessary before it is accepted that raised intracellular sodium may play a role in the etiology of essential hypertension.

ACKNOWLEDGMENTS

We thank Jorgen Andresen for excellent technical assistance. This work was supported by the Danish Medical Research Council.

SUMMARY

We have examined effects of procedures which should inhibit Na, K-ATPase activity, and thereby increase intracellular sodium concentrations, in large and small arterial ring preparations from rats. Ouabain (1 mM) and K-free solution caused myogenic contraction of aorta and tail artery, but had no long-lasting myogenic effect on 150-μm mesenteric and femoral resistance vessels. In mesenteric resistance vessels, ouabain caused the intracellular sodium concentration to rise from ca. 13 mmol/L cells to ca. 63 mmol/L cells over 2 hours, as well as depolarization of the cell membranes. Acute exposure of noradrenaline-activated mesenteric resistance vessels to ouabain or K-free solutions caused potentiation of the responses and depolarization. However, prolonged exposure (30 minutes to 2 hours) reduced the responses of these vessels to repetitive noradrenaline stimulation. The results suggest that raised intracellular sodium is not in itself sufficient to cause or potentiate contraction of the resistance vessels we have tested. We conclude that further investigations are required before it can be accepted that raised intracellular sodium can in itself be a factor of importance in the etiology of hypertension.

REFERENCES

1. Canessa M, Adragna N, Solomon HS, et al.: Increased sodium-lithium countertransport in red cells of patients with essential hypertension. N Engl J Med 302:772-776, 1980.
2. Caray RP, Meyer P: A new test showing abnormal Na^+ and K^+ fluxes in erythrocytes of essential hypertensive patients. Lancent 1:349-353, 1979.
3. Reuter H, Blaustein MP, Haeusler G: Na-Ca exchange and tension development in arterial smooth muscle. Philos Trans R Soc Lond [Biol] 265:87-94, 1973.
4. Ozaki H, Karaki H, Urakawa N: Possible role of Na-Ca exchange mechanism in the concentrations induced in guinea-pig aorta by potassium free solution and ouabain. Arch Pharm 304:203-209, 1978.
5. Blaustein MP: Sodium ions, calcium ions, blood pressure regulation, and hypertension: A reassessment and a hypothesis. Am J Physiol 232:C165-C173, 1977.
6. Blaustein MP: Commentary. What is the link between vascular smooth muscle sodium pumps and hypertension? Clin Exp Hypertens 3:173-178, 1981.
7. Lang S, Blaustein MP: The role of the sodium pump in the control of vascular tone in the rat. Circ Res 46:463-470, 1980.
8. Mulvany MJ, Halpern W: Mechanical properties of vascular smooth muscle cells in situ. Nature 260:617-619, 1976.
9. Mulvany MJ, Halpern W: Contractile properties of small arterial resistance vessels in spontaneously hypertensive and normotensive rats. Circ Res 41:19-26, 1977.
10. Nilsson H, Mulvany MJ: Prolonged exposure to ouabain eliminates the greater noradrenaline-dependent calcium sensitivity of resistance vessels in spontaneously hypertensive rats. Hypertension 3:691-697, 1981.
11. Mulvany MJ, Nilsson H, Flatmann JA, et al.: Positive and negative inotropic effects of Na-K-ATPase inhibitors on rat mesenteric resistance vessels: An electrophysiological and pharmacological study. Circ Res (in press).
12. Friedman SM, Mar M, Nakashima M: Lithium-substitution analysis of Na and K phases in a small artery. Blood Vessels 11:55-64, 1974.
13. Aalkjaer C, Mulvany MJ: The intracellular-sodium content of mesenteric resistance vessels: Effect of exposure to ouabain, abstracted. Acta Physiol Scand (in press).
14. Mulvany MJ, Hansen PK, Aalkjaer C: Direct evidence that the greater contractility of resistance vessels in spontaneously hypertensive rats is associated with a narrower lumen, a thicker media and a greater number of smooth muscle cell layers. Circ Res 43:854-864, 1978.
15. Mulvany MJ, Korsgaard N, Nilsson H, et al.: The calcium sensitivity of resistance vessels is

increased in spontaneously hypertensive rats but not in renal hypertensive rats. Proceedings of the 4th International Meeting on Rats with Genetic Hypertension and Related Studies (in press).

16. Bohlen HG, Gore RW, Hutchins PM: Comparison of microvascular pressures in normal and spontaneously hypertensive rats. Microvasc Res 13:125-130, 1977.

17. Folkow B, Hallback M, Jones JV, et al.: Dependence of external calcium for noradrenaline contractility of resistance vessels in spontaneously hypertensive and renal hypertensive rats, as compared with normotensive controls. Acta Physiol Scand 101:84-97, 1977.

18. Mulvany MJ, Aalkjaer C, Christensen J: Changes in noradrenaline sensitivity and morphology of arterial resistance vessels during development of high blood pressure in spontaneously hypertensive rats. Hypertension 2:664-671, 1980.

19. Mason DT, Braunwald E: Studies on digitalis. X. Effects of ouabain on forearm vascular resistance and venous tone in normal subjects and in patients in heart failure. J Clin Invest 43:532-543, 1964.

20. Gillis RA, Quest JA: The role of the nervous system in the cardiovascular effects of digitalis. Pharmacol Rev 31:19-97, 1980.

DISCUSSION

Discussants: Blaustein, Mulvany, Bohr, Tobian, Funder, Haeusler

Blaustein: I'd like to discuss the possible role of other mechanisms versus the sodium-calcium exchange mechanism in regard to control of smooth muscle cell calcium. The diameter of these vessels in the state where they're actually looked at here is about 150 to 250 microns, whereas *in situ* they are 50 microns or less; thus, *in situ* there is considerable tone. As Dr. Mulvany pointed out, the evidence is that when you have some tone (i.e., when you introduce norepinephrine), you begin to see some effects on calcium flux, modifying the sodium pump activity or sodium distribution. What I would point out, therefore, is one very important factor: the condition (tone) of the system with regard to when the fluxes are tested.

An important point was mentioned by Dr. Overbeck, namely that under conditions where you raise vascular potassium concentration locally there is, in fact, relexation, when you appear to stimulate the sodium pump by raising extracellular potassium. Mason and Braunwald[1] looked at forearm vascular resistance in man. When they perfused with low concentrations of ouabain, they found that there's a peripheral effect that increases vascular resistance. In the rat-hindlimb preparation, we see increased vascular resistance when one does manipulations to inhibit the sodium pump (Lang and Blaustein[2]). So, I think that one has to be very careful about what the conditions are and how much the transport system is being stressed (e.g., how much tone there is). If there is a lot of tone, that may well mean that free calcium levels are elevated, cell sodium may be elevated, and that may contribute to a very different response than the one that's seen in the nearly fully relaxed vessel (e.g., when intracellular free Ca^{2+} is below the contraction threshold).

Mulvany: I'm certainly in agreement. I think it's very important that we realize that under *in vivo* conditions there is a tone. In the resting vessel we get a depolarization in response to ouabain but no contraction, whereas when its's activated then we do get a contraction, and this is probably due to the fact that there was a certain threshold for the potential to have an effect on the contractile ability of the vessels.

[1] Mason DT, Braunwald E: J Clin Invest 43:532-543, 1964.
[2] Lang S, Blaustein MP: Circ Res 46:463-470, 1980.

Blaustein: One thing that I wanted to point out is that I think we have some disagreement about the effect of potassium-free solution and the response to the presence of norepinephrine. Apparently, you get a contraction before you see any change in membrane potential.

Mulvany: I think that the first thing to be said is that these measurements of membrane potential are extremely difficult to make. We find that the effects of the potassium-free solution on the membrane potential are often smaller than those of ouabain, but I think this is partly due to the fact that this is a suffusion experiment where it takes several minutes for the potassium to come all the way down. The effects of the ouabain will be much quicker because we're infusing one millimole ouabain and we get up to a useful concentration much more quickly.

Blaustein: That's not the problem. I would agree that may be the proof of the pudding, namely, that you begin to lower potassium and you see an increase in tension before you see a change in membrane potential when you haven't really gotten the potassium down to zero. Certainly if you put in enough ouabain, it's easier to completely inhibit the pump than it is to really try to pull out all the potassium.

Bohr: The difference between the aorta and the little tubes I think is primarily that the aorta is virtually not innervated.

Mulvany: The small mesenteric vessels are heavily innervated. But, as I pointed out, we get the same results in the tail arteries, which are even more heavily innervated. The femoral vessels that we look at are less innervated, but again we get the same results.

Tobian: You didn't talk much about the differences between hypertensive and normotensive arteries studied in this way. Do you have any information that you want to share with us on that?

Mulvany: I have no information I want to show. We have had a brief look at intracellular sodium. The SHRs do show a slightly increased intracellular sodium but we're going to repeat that to be quite sure about it first. But it looks as though it may be about 30 percent up.

Funder: I wonder whether you have done any experiment changing pH in your preparation, and is it possible to use sodium microelectrodes to evaluate the sodium concentration?

Mulvany: It would certainly be a big advantage to be able to use a sodium-sensitive electrode. As far as the pH is concerned, we haven't done any systematic studies on this. I don't think any of these results are particularly dependent on the pH.

Haeusler: I was a bit surprised to see that during incubation with ouabain the contractile response to norepinephrine faded away. I had expected the opposite, namely, a more pronounced contraction in a preparation partially depolarized by ouabian. Have you any explanation for this result?

Mulvany: I entirely agree it's very unexpected and we've done a lot of studies to try and elucidate the possible cause. It does not seem to be due to the increased sodium: If we do this kind of experiment where first we incubate in ouabain, then put vessels into a sodium-free solution for half an hour and then carry on in normal sodium, the responses are completely unaffected. In the calcium dose-response experiments, the vessels become much less sensitive to calcium following ouabain exposure. It's as though the receptor-operated channels have become less permeable to calcium. I'd say this is not due to changes in the ionic content. Maybe it's due to some changes in cAMP levels. I don't know. But we're trying to elucidate the causes of it.

ROLE OF AN OUABAIN-LIKE HUMORAL AGENT AND THE SODIUM-POTASSIUM PUMP IN LOW-RENIN HYPERTENSION

FRANCIS J. HADDY

INTRODUCTION

It is now clear that the pathophysiology of hypertension in man varies from subject to subject. Renin and aldosterone levels, blood pressure response to angiotensin antagonists, converting-enzyme inhibitors and diuretics, and other measures indicate that angiotensin plays a preponderant role in some patients, while volume is more important in others. Laragh [1-3] feels that all naturally occurring human hypertensive diseases can be arranged in a pathophysiologic spectrum that ranges from a preponderant dependence on angiotensin to a preponderant dependence on effective blood volume. Malignant hypertension and primary aldosteronism are the clinical expressions of these polar extremes. Within the spectrum are the intermediate forms of hypertension exhibiting an inappropriate excess of one of these factors relative to the other, unilateral renovascular and high-renin essential hypertension at one end and low-renin essential hypertension at the other end.

Low-renin patients, whose high blood pressure appears to be associated with overfilling of the central circulation, often are hemodiluted relative to the high-renin patients and, in contrast to the latter subjects, fail to respond to antirenin drugs [2]. They do respond to diuretics, however [2].

The mechanism of the elevated pressure in low-renin patients is not clear. It does not appear to be related to the blood volume per se, since sudden increase in volume in normal subjects or animals does not immediately raise pressure (see references in [4]). It does raise pressure with time however, suggesting some indirect effect of the increase in volume.

It is this indirect mechanism that has occupied our research time in recent years. We have reproduced a number of models of low-renin hypertension in animals and examined indices of sodium-pump activity in their blood vessels, because it is known that they contain excess sodium [5] and that normal blood vessels respond to sodium-pump inhibition with constriction (see references in [6]). We have also examined the plasma for sodium-pump inhibiting activity. We here summarize our findings, as well as related findings of others.

EVIDENCE FOR SUPPRESSED SODIUM-PUMP ACTIVITY

We used ouabain-sensitive ^{86}rubidium uptake by freshly excised blood vessels and Na$^+$/K$^+$-ATPase activity of cardiac microsomes (mainly sarcolemma) as indices of Na$^+$/K$^+$ pump activity in four models of low-renin hypertension. These included one-kidney, one-wrapped hypertension in the dog and one-kidney, one-clip; one-kidney, DOCA-saline; and reduced renal mass-saline hypertension in the rat. Both indices were suppressed relative to those in appropriate normotensive control animals.

The ^{86}Rb-uptake technique was adapted to blood vessels by Pamnani [7]. The technique measures maximum capacity to pump rubidium, which is handled by the pump like potassium. Rubidium is used instead of potassium because its radioactive form has a lower energy emission and longer half-life than the radioactive form of potassium. The vessels were taken from the animal and immediately placed in a cold postassium-free solution to stop the Na$^+$/K$^+$ pump and load the cells with sodium. They were then placed in a warm solution containing nonradioactive rubidum to start up the pump. The solution also contained ^{86}Rb, and its uptake was measured 18 minutes later. This was examined both in the absence and presence of ouabain. The difference is the ouabain-sensitive ^{86}Rb uptake, which reflects active pumping of sodium and potassium. The uptake in the presence of ouabain, i.e., the ouabain-insensitive ^{86}Rb uptake, reflects distribution of ^{86}Rb in extracellular space and passive penetration into cells (determined by cell membrane permeability and surface area).

Ouabain-sensitive ^{86}Rb uptake was significantly reduced in the arteries of all four models after four weeks of hypertension, whereas ouabain-insensitive ^{86}Rb uptake was unaffected (except in the DOCA model where it was increased [7-11]). In the one-kidney, one-wrapped model, the defect was also present in mesenteric veins [7, 10], indicating that it does not result from elevated pressure. A time-course study in the reduced renal mass-saline model showed that the onset of the hypertension correlated with the onset of reduced pump activity [12].

Na$^+$/K$^+$-ATPase activity was measured in cardiac rather than vascular smooth muscle microsomes, because the methods for measurement in the latter are still rudimentary. Na$^+$/K$^+$-ATPase activity in cardiac microsomes of the rats was calculated as the difference between total ATPase activity (measured in the presence of potassium) and Mg^{++}-ATPase activity (measured in the absence of potassium and in the presence of ouabain). Na$^+$/K$^+$-ATPase activity was significantly reduced in all three rat models of low-renin hypertension, whereas Mg^{++}-ATPase activity was increased [13-15]. In the case of the one-kidney, one-clip model, the findings were the same in microsomes obtained from the right ventricle [16], again indicating that the defect is not secondary to elevated pressure.

The findings in the one-kidney, DOCA-saline model are of special interest because they suggest both increased permeability (increased ouabain-insensitive ^{86}Rb uptake) and decreased pump activity (decreased ouabain-sensitive ^{86}Rb uptake), precisely the combination that should raise intracellular sodium concentration to the highest level. Jones and Hart [17], Jones [18], Friedman and Nakashima [19], and Moura and Worcel [20] also find evidence for increased permeability to ions in this model. Songu-Mize et al. [21] recently confirmed our finding of decreased ouabain-sensitive ^{86}Rb uptake. On the other hand, Friedman and Nakashima [14], Jones [18], and Brock and Overbeck [22] find evidence for increased pump activity in the one-kidney, DOCA-saline model. Brock and Overbeck [22] also report increased pump activity in one-kidney, figure-eight hypertension, another low-renin model. However, all of these investigators interposed a long incubation period before measuring pump activity, a procedure which could have washed away a pump-suppressing substance (see below). We in fact find that the suppressed ouabain-sensitive ^{86}Rb uptake seen in fresh tail arteries taken from rats with one-kidney, DOCA-saline hypertension disappears during prolonged incubation [10].

RELATION TO VOLUME EXPANSION AND A HUMORAL AGENT

We were able to reproduce the changes in ouabain-sensitive ^{86}Rb uptake by simple rapid volume expansion; i.e., intravenous infusion of an iso-osmotic solution of sodium chloride in normal rats reduced ouabain-sensitive ^{86}Rb uptake by the tail artery relative to that in the normal sham-infused rat without affecting ouabain-insensitive ^{86}Rb uptake [10, 23] - exactly the changes observed in the models of low-renin hypertension. Furthermore, when we took plasma from these volume-expanded animals, boiled it, and applied the supernate to the rail artery taken from another rat [10, 23], we again reproduced the changes; i.e., we were able to transfer the defect to another animal via the plasma, suggesting that the pump defect in the expanded rat results from a humoral agent.

Since there is evidence that animals with low-renin hypertension are volume-expanded, this invited the search for similar plasma activity in the hypertensive animals. We therefore prepared a new series of dogs with one-kidney, one-wrapped hypertension and applied supernate of boiled plasma from these dogs and control, normotensive, sham-wrapped dogs to rat tail arteries. We found a reduction in ouabain-sensitive ^{86}Rb uptake without a change in ouabain-insensitive ^{86}Rb uptake [10, 11, 24], the same changes seen in the hypetensive animals' own blood vessels. We were able to produce the same result with plasma supernate from rats with one-kidney, one-clip and reduced renal mass-saline hypertension [11]. Songu-Mize et al. produced the same result with plasma from rats with one-kidney, DOCA-saline hypertension (personal communication). Thus, as in the saline-expanded rat, the pump suppression seen in the animal with low-renin hypertension appears to result from a ouabain-like humoral factor.

SOURCE OF THE OUABAIN-LIKE HOMORAL AGENT

Working with Dr. James Buggy, we showed that ouabain-sensitive ^{86}Rb uptake by the tail artery was higher in the volume-expanded rat with an anteroventral third ventricle (AV3V) lesion than in the volume-expanded rat with a sham AV3V lesion [11, 25]. This is the same lesion that prevents or ameliorates certain forms of low-renin hypertension in rats [26, 27] and eliminates the appearance of antinatriferic activity in plasma on volume expansion [28]. In very recent experiments [29], we showed that the AV3V lesion prevents 1) reduced renal mass-saline hypertension in the rat, 2) the appearance of the ouabain-like humoral agent in the plasma of these animals, and 3) the pump suppression in the tail artery of these rats. Thus, we think the AV3V area produces or influences the production of the ouabain-like humoral agent. Songu-Mize et al. reached the same conclusion because the AV3V lesion prevented both the hypertension and the pump suppression in the DOCA model[21].

MECHANISM OF THE VASCULAR ACTION OF THE OUABAIN-LIKE HUMORAL AGENT

Working with David Harder, we showed that the smooth muscle cell in tail arteries taken from rats with one-kidney, one-clip hypertension is depolarized relative to the cell in tail arteries taken from control animals [30]. The measurements were made some 90 minutes after placing the tail arteries in a modified Krebs solution, and the findings were not different whether or not the solution contained phentolamine and 6-hydroxydopamine. Furthermore, supernate of boiled plasma from the one-kidney, one-clip hypertensive animal quickly depolarized the smooth muscle cell in the tail artery taken from a normal rat [30]. The degree of depolarization was the same as produced by ouabain. These findings are compatible with the hypothesis that the humoral agent binds quickly but tightly to smooth muscle cells producing electrogenic pump suppression and hence depolarization. Since Ca^{++} permeability is sensitive to the membrane potential, this should result in calcium influx and vasoconstriction.

In vivo, the humoral agent could depolarize the smooth muscle cell both by direct and indirect actions, the former resulting from binding to the smooth muscle cell itself and the latter from binding to the sympathetic nerve endings. We previously suggested that the pump defect extends to the adrenergic nerve terminals in low-renin hypertension [6, 31, 32]. We suggested this because the literature indicates that: 1) neuronal norepinephrine uptake is inhibited by ouabain; 2) the blood vessels and heart of animals with low-renin hypertension are depleted of endogenous norepinephrine, less responsive to sympathetic nerve stimulation, and unable to normally take up and retain norepinephrine; 3) the retention and store of cardiac norepinephrine correlates negatively with the sodium intake in the rat, i.e., the higher the sodium intake, the lower the retention and store of norepinephrine and the higher the blood pressure; and 4) patients with at least one type of low-renin hypertension (primary aldosteronism) appear to have a functional sympathectomy, i.e., they have impaired cardio-vascular reflexes (see references in [6, 31, 32]).

A defective norepinephrine pump should initially increase the concentration of norepinephrine in the neuromuscular cleft, depolarize the smooth muscle cell, and thereby contribute to the hypertension. This might account for the findings of Takeshita and Mark [33] in the Dahl salt-sensitive rat where a high salt intake increases hindquarter vascular resistance in part via the sympathetic nervous system and enhances the resistance responses to sympathetic nerve stimulation (suggesting that a high salt intake facilitates the release or inhibits the reuptake of norepinephrine). It might also account for the observations of Dietz and colleagues [34] in stroke-prone, spontaneously hypertensive rats where a high dietary sodium intake impairs cardiac noradrenaline inactivation by the cocaine-dependent uptake mechanism in association with an accelerated rise in blood pressure.

Eventually, the norepinephrine pump defect, particularly if coupled with decreased synthesis and increased release, should lead to depletion of nor-epinephrine in the nerve terminal and in the neuromuscular cleft. This 'denerva-tion' should also produce depolarization. (The phenomenon of denervation supersensitivity is thought to result in part from depolarization subsequent to reduction in Na^+/K^+-ATPase and Na^+/K^+ pump activities, the former from reduction in the amount of the enzyme [35].) It should also impair reflex compen-sation for the direct stimulating action of the humoral agent on vascular smooth muscle. Both denervation depolarization and impaired reflex compensation could contribute to the hypertension. Thus, a norepinephrine pump defect could eventually account for the decreased endogenous norepinephrine content of blood vessels and heart; decreased catecholamine nerve fluorescence; decreased vascular response to sympathetic nerve stimulation; decreased capacity of the sympathetic nervous system to take up and retain norepinephrine that is seen in animals with low-renin hypertension (one-kidney, one-clip; one-kidney, DOCA-salt); and for the impaired cardiovascular reflexes seen in patients with primary aldosteronism (see references in [6, 31, 32]). It could also in part account for increased sensitivity to injected norepinephrine.

Freas and Muldoon [36] in fact find evidence for a factor in plasma from the normal dog that inhibits vascular norepinephrine uptake; i.e., the ability of the isolated saphenous vein to take up norepinephrine from Krebs-Ringers solution decreases when homologous plasma is added to the solution. It will be of interest to see whether this inhibitory activity of plasma increases with acute volume expansion or during the development of low-renin hypertension.

CAN SUPPRESSION OF THE NA$^{+/+}$ PUMP IN CARDIAC AND VASCULAR SMOOTH MUSCLE IN FACT RAISE BLOOD PRESSURE?

It has long been known that the cardiac glycosides, potent inhibitors of Na$^+$/K$^+$-ATPase and Na$^+$/K$^+$ pump activity, increase cardiac contractility, constrict blood vessels, and sensitize blood vessels to vasoconstrictor agents. It has more recently become clear that they also raise blood pressure in both animals [37] and man [38], provided the heart is normal and particularly if diuresis is not allowed to occur [39]. These are conditions met in the low-renin models of hypertension; the heart is initially normal and the kidneys are manipulated organically or functionally to make excretion of water and salt more difficult. The increase in blood pressure results entirely from a rise in total peripheral resistance [37, 38]. This again is similar to that in the low-renin models of hypertension. Vanadate, a naturally occuring Na$^+$/K$^+$-ATPase inhibitor, also raises blood pressure in normal animals, both on intravenous infusion [40] and during prolonged dietary administration [41].

NATURE OF THE OUABAIN-LIKE HUMORAL AGENT

In 1976 we [4] proposed that 'in the volume-expanded hypertension, there is a circulating agent that suppresses cardiovascular membrane Na$^+$/K$^+$-ATPase, resulting in reduced activity of the Na$^+$/K$^+$ pump and hence increased contractility of heart, arteries and veins. In blood vessels where electrogenicity of the pump is pronounced, the increased contractility may be secondary to depolarization.' In discussing the identity of the agent, we [4] said that 'natriuretic hormone should be considered. An agent that both activates the cardiovascular system and decreases tubular reabsorption of sodium is attractive on teleological grounds, because such actions would be the best way to rid the body of the extra salt and water (the increase in blood pressure would deliver more salt and water to the tubule where it would be rejected). The action of such an agent would explain why extracellular fluid volume may return toward normal values in the steady state. It would also explain the exaggerated natriuresis seen on salt loading in the hypertensive animal.' Natriuretic hormone also seemed to be a reasonable choice on the basis of the data available in the literature at the time. Its level rises with volume, it inhibits sodium-pump activity in the renal tubule, and 'in the animal with reduced renal mass, reduction of salt intake in direct proportion to the reduction in glomerular filtration rate eliminates assay evidence for the agent in the serum and also prevents the rise in blood pressure ... Volume expansion inhibits renal Na$^+$/K$^+$-ATPase and produces an agent in kidney and serum which inhibits Na$^+$/K$^+$-ATPase obtained from normal kidney.'

Shortly thereafter, Blaustein [42] also considered natriuretic hormone to be a good possibility, and we reaffirmed our belief in more extensive reviews [6, 32,

43]. Subsequent studies tend to strengthen this possibility. Both the humoral suppressor of the vascular sodium-potassium pump observed in our studies and natriuretic factor are heat-stable. The appearance of natriuretic hormone in the plasma of rats during acute volume expansion is blocked by an AV3V lesion [28]. As pointed out above, ouabain-sensitive ^{86}Rb uptake by the tail artery is higher, and plasma ouabain-like activity, assayed on the tail artery, is lower than in sham-lesioned animals [11, 25]. Natriuretic factor reduces short-circuit current in the toad bladder; so does plasma supernate from dogs with one-kidney, one-wrapped hypertension (Chen et al., unpublished observation). The humoral pump suppressor observed in our studies does not appear to be vasopressin or the natriuretic factor recently extracted from rat atria [44] because they fail to reproduce the effect of supernates of boiled plasma from hypertensive or volume-expanded animals when added to our assay system (tail artery from a normal rat) [45].

Release of natriuretic hormone may be related to distention of the pulmonary vascular bed. The evidence from water immersion in the seated position is of particular interest because this allows specific distention of the intrathoracic circulation for hours or even days [46]. Immersion to the neck evokes a number of volume-regulator responses, including diuresis and natriuresis. It appears that several neurohumoral systems are involved, including the ADH, the renin-angiotensin-aldosterone, and the natriuretic hormone systems. With respect to the latter, recent studies [46] disclose the presence of natriuretic hormone (rat biossay) in the urine of normal subjects undergoing immersion. Furthermore, a sodium-transport inhibitor (toad-bladder biossay) also has been found in the serum of normal subjects undergoing immersion. Therefore, the receptors for natriuretic hormone may be in the central circulation, in which case elevation of total blood volume would not be an absolute requirement for its release. In fact, enhance release could occur in the face of reduced total blood volume. Re-distribution of blood from the systemic to the pulmonary circuit has been reported in hypertension (just as occurs when a vasoconstrictor agent is infused into a normal animal). It should be noted that the blood pressure of the normal monkey gradually rises during a 40-minute period of immersion to the neck [47].

Natriuretic hormone is a small molecule (molecular weight <500) that is resistant to heat. Its chemical structure, however, is still unknown. De Wardener, who provided the first convincing biossay evidence for the presence of a circulating natriuretic factor in animals, has more recently concentrated the efforts of his laboratory [48, 49] on purifying and identifying a natriuretic factor found in human urine where it increases with increased sodium intake. On intravenous injection in the rat, the purified preparation has a rapid onset and short duration of action. Its characteristics include a molecular weight of less than 500, resistance to hydrolysis and proteolytic enzymes, and an absence of amino acids. It is a polar substance and appears to be a sugar attached to a ring structure. It binds to digoxin antibodies 10 times better than digoxin and inhibits Na^+/K^+-ATPase many times more than ouabain. It also stimulates glucose-6-phosphate dehydrogenase (G6PD) activity in kidney slices, which they believe also signifies a decrease in Na^+/K^+-ATPase activity.

An agent with similar activity and characteristics has been extracted from bovine hypothalamus by Haupert and Sancho [50]. This agent inhibits active sodium transport across anuran membranes, ouabain binding to frog urinary bladder, and Na^+/K^+-ATPase from kidney. It appears to be a low-molecular-weight, basic nonpeptide. Fishman [51] prepared a fraction of guinea pig brain containing a substance that blocks ouabain binding to Na^+/K^+-ATPase and inhibits uptake of ^{86}Rb into human erthrocytes. It has a low molecular weight and withstands acid hydrolysis. Lichtstein and Samueloy [52] extracted a ouabain-like compound from rat brain. It inhibits ouabain binding and Na^+/K^+-ATPase activity in rat brain synaptosomes. It has a low molecular weight, and its activity is not influenced by treatment with protease, trypsin, and other proteolytic enzymes.

On the other hand, Gruber and Buckalew [53] have purified an agent with natriuretic and antinatriferic activity from the plasma of salt-loaded dogs that appears to be a heat-stable, low-molecular-weight, acidic peptide. The same plasma extracts that contain natriuretic hormone also contain a factor that cross-reacts with antidigoxin antibodies and inhibits Na^+/K^+-ATPase [54]. These data suggest that natriuretic hormone is an endogenous digoxin-like substance, an 'endoxin,' and a potential vasoconstrictor. The same laboratory reported that plasma levels of 'endoxin' are elevated in subhuman primates with spontaneous and two-kidney, one-clip hypertension [55]. Of interest is the observation that intravenous injection of antidigoxin antibody lowers the blood pressure of rats with one-kidney, DOCA-saline hypertension (Kojima et al., personal communication).

It would be on interest to apply these partially pure preparations to the rat tail artery to see whether they reduce ouabain-sensitive ^{86}Rb uptake. It would also be of interest to inject them intravenously to see whether they raise blood pressure, particularly in an animal with impaired ability to excrete salt and water (as is the case in the low-renin models of hypertension considered above). Plasma extracts containing 'endoxin' taken from salt-loaded dogs apparently do sensitize the arteriole in the rat cremaster muscle to the vasoconstrictor action of norepinephrine [56] and apparently do slowly raise blood pressure on intravenous injection in the rat (Gruber et al., personal communication).

We [57] previously pointed out that the old and recent literature in fact suggests the presence of an unknown, slowly-acting pressor and sensitizing agent in the blood of animals with low-renin hypertension. The agent is a small molecule and, like natriuretic hormone and the humoral pump suppressor observed in our studies, it is heat-stable. The evidence for such an agent dates back to 1940 when Solandt et al. [58] cross-circulated blood between two dogs - one with one-kidney, one-clip hypertension and the other small and nephrectomized, and found that pressure rose in the small nephrectomized animal. The pressor response was delayed in onset, taking about one hour to appear. In 1953, Gordon et al. [59] circulated blood for 30 to 60 minutes between two rabbits, one with one-kidney, one-clip hypertension and the other salt-loaded but normotensive, and found that pressure increased in the normotensive salt-loaded assay rabbit. The response was delayed in onset and prolonged. The maximum increase in pressure was not reached until 2 to 3 hours after completion of the 30- to 60-minute cross-circulation.

In 1965, Hinke [60] noted that plasma from rats with one-kidney, DOCA-salt hypertension increased the vasoconstrictor response of an isolated, perfused rat tail artery to norepinephrine. Something in the plasma sensitized the vessel. In 1969, Dahl et al. [61] placed their salt-resistant rat in parabiosis with their salt-sensitive rat and found that in the resistant rat hypertension now also developed when both animals were fed salt or when one-kidney, one-clip hypertension was produced in the sensitive strain. Something crossed from one animal to the other. Almost as an afterthought, they speculated that a common pathogenic mechanism exists in both salt hypertension and renal hypertension and suggested that many of the apparent anomalies of the angiotensin-aldosterone system in hypertension could be explained if a sodium-excreting hormone were postulated that had the capacity of also inducing hypertension when produced by a hypertension-prone subject. They apparently never pursued this possibility. Since then a number of investigators have described pressor, sensitizing, and constrictor activity in blood from man and animals with low-renin hypertension (see references in [31, 32]; also see [62, 63]).

Obviously, the relation between this agent, natriuretic hormone, and the agent observed in our studies warrants further investigation.

SODIUM-POTASSIUM PUMP ACTIVITY IN HYPERTENSIVE MAN

There have been no studies of sodium-potassium pump activity in the heart and blood vessels of hypertensive humans, but increased sodium content in arterial wall [5] and studies of white and red cells suggest that a pump defect may exist in some hypertensive subjects (see references in [6]). Of particular interest is the observation that ouabain-sensitive ^{22}Na efflux from isolated leukocytes obtained from patients with uncomplicated essential hypertension is suppressed [64]. This defect is accompanied by increased intracellular sodium and water. It seems to be more pronounced in those subjects with low-renin hypertension [65]. The hypertension of preeclampsia is also associated with reduced ouabain-sensitive ^{22}Na efflux and elevated sodium in leukocytes [66]. The increase in leukocyte sodium content in black hypertensive Jamaicans reportedly is not associated with decreased sodium-pump activity [67]; the subjects were not categorized according to renin status.

Recent studies suggest the presence of a circulating ouabain-like agent. Poston et al. [68] found that white cells from normal subjects exhibit reduced ouabain-sensitive ^{22}Na efflux when incubated in plasma from hypertensive subjects. Furthermore, plasma from normal subjects on a high-salt diet has an increased ability to stimulate renal G6PD activity, which correlates inversely with Na$^+$/K$^+$-ATPase activity [48]. The same is apparently true of plasma from patients with essential hypertension [62]. Fitzgibbon et al. [69] found a negative correlation between ^{22}Na$^+$ efflux from red cells and the spontaneous dietary sodium intake in male patients with essential hypertension when the incubation media was the patients' plasma, but not when the cells were incubated in artificial medium. When plasma was the medium, the efflux rate from red cells from patients with essential hypertension was less than efflux rate from red cells from normotensive subjects when the spontaneous sodium intake exceeded 200 mmol/24 h. The ouabain-sensitivity of the abnormality was not indicated, but in another study the same investigators [70] induced changes in sodium intake in males with essential hypertension and again observed changes in ^{22}Na efflux. These changes were in the ouabain-sensitive component. Wessels and Zunkley [71] reported that the increased sodium influx characteristic of the red cells of hypertensive subjects is transmissable by the plasma of some patients with essential hypertension to the red blood cells of normotensive subjects. Noteworthy is the observation that natriuretic hormone is elevated in the plasma of subjects with primary aldosteronism [72].

If in fact there is a circulating Na$^+$/K$^+$-ATPase inhibitor in the plasma of hypertensive subjects, there should be evidence for altered norepinephrine metabolism. Esler and colleagues [73] found evidence for the existence of defective neuronal norepinephrine uptake in eight of 37 hypertensive patients. Greenberg et al. [74] found that peripheral venous plasma of both normotensive and hypertensive patients enhances tyramine-induced catecholamine release, indicating that hypertensive plasma is more active than normotensive plasma.

SUMMARY

The immediate mechanism of sodium-dependent, low-renin hypertension has been particularly obscure. Recent studies suggest that it results in part from the release of a ouabain-like factor, perhaps natriuretic hormone, from the brain. This humoral factor inhibits Na$^+$/K$^+$-ATPase, and hence the active pumping of sodium and potassium in the muscle cells of blood vessels and the heart, as well as in their adrenergic nerve endings. The pump suppression causes increased contractile activity and hence increased arterial blood pressure. In the muscle cells of the blood vessels, the increased contractile activity appears to be related to membrane depolarization. In this review, the evidence bearing on this hypothesis is brought up to date.

REFERENCES

1. Laragh JH: Vasoconstriction-volume analysis for understanding and treating hypertension: The use of renin and aldosterone profiles. Am J Med 55:261-274, 1973.
2. Laragh JH: Basic principles for the office evaluation and treatment of high blood pressure: Part II. Laboratory evaluation and treatment. Cardiovascular Reviews and Reports 2:1318-1338, 1981.
3. Laragh JH, Letcher RL, Pickering TG: Renin profiling for modern diagnosis and treatment of hypertension. JAMA 241:151-156, 1979.
4. Haddy FJ, Overbeck HW: The role of humoral factors in volume expanded hypertension. Life Sci 19:935-948, 1976.
5. Tobian L: Interrelationship of electrolytes, juxtaglomerular cells and hypertension. Physol Rev 40:280-312, 1960.
6. Haddy FJ, Pamnani M, Clough D: The sodium-potassium pump in volume expanded hypertension. Clin Exp Hypertens 1:295-336, 1978.
7. Overbeck HW, Pamnani MB, Akera T, et al.: Depressed function of a ouabain-sensitive sodium-potassium pump in blood vessels from renal hypertensive dogs. Circ Res 38 (Suppl 2):48-52, 1976.
8. Huot S, Pamnani M, Clough D, et al.: Depressed Na^+/K^+ pump activity in tail arteries of reduced renal mass hypertensive rats. Fed Proc 39:1188, 1980.
9. Pamnani MB, Clough DL, Haddy FJ: Altered activity of the sodium-potassium pump in arteries of rats with steroid hypertension. Clin Sci Mol Med 55:41s-43s, 1978.
10. Pamnani MB, Clough DL, Huot SJ, et al.: Sodium-potassium pump activity in experimental hypertension, in Vanhoutte PM, Leusen I (editors): Vasodilatation. New York, Raven Press, 1981, pp 391-403.
11. Pamnani M, Hunt S, Buggy J, et al.: Demonstration of a humoral inhibitor of the Na^+/K^+ pump in some models of experimental hypertension. Hypertension 3 (Suppl 2):96-101, 1981.
12. Muot SJ, Pamnani MB, Clough DL, et al.: Vascular Na^+/K^+ pump activity and development of reduced renal mass hypertension in rats. Physiologist 23:91, 1980.
13. Clough DL, Pamnani MB, Maddy FJ: Decreased Na,K-ATPase activity in left ventricular myocardium of rats with one-kidney DOCA-saline hypertension. Clin Res 26:361, 1978.
14. Clough D, Pamnani M, Muot S, et al.: Left ventricular Na, K-ATPase activity in rats with reduced renal mass hypertension and spontaneous hypertension. Physiologist 23:91, 1980.
15. Clough DL, Pamnani MB, Overbeck HW, et al.: Decreased myocardial Na,K ATPase in rats with one-kidney Goldblatt hypertension. Fed Proc 36:491, 1977.
16. Clough DL, Pamnani MB, Overbeck, et al.: Decreased Na,K-ATPase in right ventricular myocardium of rats with one-kidney Goldblatt hypertension. Physiologist 20:18, 1977.
17. Jones AW, Hart HG: Altered ion transport in aortic smooth muscle during deoxycorticosterone acetate hypertension in the rat. Circ Res 37:333-341, 1975.
18. Jones AW: Kinetics of active sodium transport in aortas from control and deoxycorticosterone hypertensive rats. Hypertension 3:631-640, 1981.
19. Friedman SM, Nakashima M: Evidence for enhanced Na transport in hypertension induced by DOCA in the rat. Can J Physiol Pharmacol 56:1029-1035, 1978.
20. Mours A, Worcel M: Antihypertensive action of aldosterone antagonists: RV 28318 and spironolactone. Effects on smooth muscle permeability to Na^+ and Rb^+. Proceedings of the 8th Scientific Meeting of the International Society of Hypertension, 1981, p 303.
21. Songu-Mize E, Bealer SL, Caldwell RW: The role of the central nervous system in vascular sodium pump activity and hypertension. Circulation 64:IV-190, 1981.
22. Brock TA, Overbeck HW: Elevated intracellular Na^+ may not explain increased sodium pump activity in arteries from hypertensive rats. Clin Res 29:832A, 1981.
23. Pamnani MB, Clough DL, Steffen RP, et al.: Depressed Na^+-K^+ pump activity in tail arteries

234

from acutely volume expanded rats. Physiologist 21:88, 1978.

24. Pamnani M, Huot S, Steffen R, et al.: Evidence for a homoral Na$^+$ transport inhibiting factor(s) in one-kidney, one-wrapped hypertensive dogs. Physiologist 23:91, 1980.

25. Pamnani M, Buggy J, Huot S, et al.: Vascular Na$^+$-K$^+$ pump activity in acutely saline loaded rats with anteroventral third ventricle (AV3V) lesions. Fed Proc 40:390, 1981.

26. Brody MJ, Fink GD, Buggy J: The role of the anteroventral third ventricle (AV3V) region in experimental hypertension. Circ Res 43 (Suppl 1):2-13, 1978.

27. Buggy J, Fink GD, Haywood JR, et al.: Interruption of the maintenance phase of established hypertension by ablation of the anteroventral third ventricle (AV3V) in rats. Clin Exp Hypertens 1:337-353, 1978.

28. Bealer S, Haywood JR, Johnson AK, et al.: Impaired natriuresis and secretion of natriuretic hormone in rats with lesions of the anteroventral 3rd ventricle. Fed Proc 38:1232, 1979.

29. Huot S, Buggy J, Jagusiak M, et al.: Anteroventral third ventricle (AV3V) lesions, vascular Na$^+$-K$^+$ pump activity and development of reduced renal mass (RRM) hypertension (HT) in rats. Fed Proc, in press.

30. Pamnani MB, Harder DR, Huot SJ, et al.: Vascular smooth muscle membrane potentials and the influence of a ouabain-like humoral factor in rats with one-kidney, one-clip hypertension. Physiologist 24:6, 1981.

31. Haddy FJ: Mechanism, prevention and therapy of sodium-dependent hypertension. Am J Med 69:746, 758, 1980.

32. Haddy FJ, Pamnani MB, Clough DL: Humoral factors and the sodiumpotassium pump in volume expanded hypertension. Life Sci 24:2105-2118, 1979.

33. Takeshita A, Mark AL: Neurogenic contribution to hindquarters vasoconstriction during high sodium intake in Dahl strain of genetically hypertensive rat. Circ Res 43 (Suppl 1):86-91, 1978.

34. Dietz R, Schomig A, Rascher W, et al.: Partial replacement of sodium by potassium in the diet restores impaired noradrenaline inactivation and lowers blood pressure in SHR-SP. Proceedings of the 8th Scientific Meeting of the International Society of Hypertension, 1981, p 107.

35. Wong SK, Westfall DP, Fedan JS, et al.: The involvement of the sodiumpotassium pump in postjunctional supersensitivity of the guinea-pig vas deferens as assessed by [^{3}H] ouabain binding. J Pharmacol Exp Ther 219:163-169, 1981.

36. Freas W, Muldoon SM: Effect of plasma on norepinephrine accumulation in the canine saphenous vein. Physiologist 24:32, 1981.

37. Vatner SF, Higgins CB, Franklin D, et al.: Effects of a digitalis glycoside on coronary and systemic dynamics in conscious dogs. Circ Res 28:470-479, 1971.

38. DeMots H, Rahimtoola SH, McAnulty JH, et al.: Effects of ouabain on coronary and systemic vascular resistance and myocardial oxygen consumption in patients without heart failure. Am J Cardiol 41:88-93, 1978.

39. Haddy FJ, Scott JB: Mechanism of the acute pressor action of hypokalemia, hypomagnesemia, and hypo-osmolality. Am Heart J 85:655-661, 1973.

40. Inciarte DJ, Steffen RP, Dobbins DE, et al.: Cardiovascular effects of vanadate in the dog. Am J Physiol 239:H47-H56, 1980.

41. Steffen RP, Pamnani MB, Clough DL, et al.: Effect of prolonged dietary administration of vanadate on blood pressure in the rat. Hypertension 3 (Suppl 1):173-178, 1981.

42. Blaustein M: Sodium ions, calcium ions, blood pressure regulation and hypertension: A reassessment and a hypothesis. Am J Physiol 232:C165-C173, 1977.

43. Haddy FJ, Pamnani MB, Clough DL: Role of a humoral factor in low renin hypertension, in Lichardus B, Schrier RW, Ponec J (editors): Hormonal Regulation of Sodium Excretion. New York, Elsevier/North-Holland Biomedical Press, 1980, pp 379-385.

44. Sonnenberg ATV, Borenstein HB, de Bold AJ: Rapid and potent natriuretic response to intravenous injection of atrial myocardial extract in rats. Physiologist 23:13, 1980.

45. Link WT, Pamnani MB, Huot SJ, et al.: Effect of atrial extract on vascular Na$^+$-K$^+$ pump activity.

Physiologist 24:59, 1981.

46. Epstein M: Renal effects of head-out immersion in man. Physiol Rev 58:529-581, 1978.

47. Peterson TV, Gilmore JP, Zucker IH: Initial renal responses of nonhuman primate to immersion and intravascular volume expansion. J Appl Physiol 48:243-248, 1980.

48. Alaghband-Zadeh L, Fenton S, Clarkson E, et al.: Preliminary studies for the possible detection in plasma of the small molecular weight urinary natriuretic material, in Lichardus B, Schrier RW, Ponec J (editors): Hormonal Regulation of Sodium Excretion. New York, Elsevier/North-Holland Biomedical Press, 1980, pp 341-348.

49. Clarkson EM, Young DR, Raw SM, et al.: Chemical properties, physiological action and further separation of a low molecular weight natriuretic substance in the urine of normal man, in Lichardus B, Schrier RW, Ponec J (editors): Hormonal Regulation of Sodium Excretion. New York, Elsevier/North-Holland Biomedical Press, 1980, pp 333-340.

50. Haupert GT Jr, Sancho J: Sodium transport inhibitor from bovine hypothalamus. Proc Natl Acad Sci USA 76:4658-4660, 1979.

51. Fishman MC: Endogenous digitalis-like activity in mammalian brain. Proc Natl Acad Sci USA 76:4661-4663, 1979.

52. Lichtstein D, Samuelov S: Endogenous ouabain-like activity in rat brain. Biochem Biophys Res Comm 96:1518-1523, 1980.

53. Gruber KA, Buckalew VM Jr: Further characterization and evidence for a precursor in the formation of plasma antinatriferic factor. Proc Soc Exp Biol Med 159:463-467, 1978.

54. Gruber KA, Whitaker JM, Buckalew VM Jr: Endogenous digitalis-like substance in plasma of volume-expanded dogs. Nature 287:743-745, 1980.

55. Gruber KA, Whitaker JM, Rudel LL, et al.: Increased levels of a digitalis-like factor (endoxin) in hypertension. Fed Proc 40:535, 1981.

56. Plunkett WC, Gruber KA, Hutchins PM, et al.: Vascular reactivity is increased by factors in plasma of volume expanded dogs. Clin Res 28:827, 1980.

57. Haddy FJ, Pamnani MB, Clough DL: Humoral factors and the sodium-potassium pump in volume expanded hypertension, in Worcel M et al. (editors): New Trends in Arterial Hypertension, INSERM Symposium No. 17. New York, Elsevier/North-Holland Biomedical Press, 1981, pp 189-199.

58. Solandt DY, Nassim R, Cowan CR: Hypertensive effect of blood from hypertensive dogs. Lancet 1:873-874, 1940.

59. Gordon DB, Drury DR, Shapiro S: The salt-fed animal as a test object for pressor substances in the blood of hypertensive animals. Am J Physiol 175:123-128, 1953.

60. Hinke JAM: In vitro demonstration of vascular hyper-responsiveness in experimental hypertension. Circ Res 17:359-371, 1965.

61. Dahl LK, Knudsen KD, Iwai J: Humoral transmission of hypertension: Evidence from parabiosis. Circ Res 24, 25 (Suppl 1):21-33, 1969.

62. MacGregor GA, Fenton S, Markandu ND, et al.: An increase in a circulating sodium transport inhibitor – the link between salt intake, abnormalities of sodium transport, and the development of high blood pressure in essential hypertension. Proceedings of the 8th Scientific Meeting of the International Society of Hypertension, 1981, p 263.

63. Simon GC: Long-term in vivo effects of circulating humoral factors from volume expanded renal hypertensive rats. Clin Res 29:722A, 1981.

64. Edmondson RPS, Thomas RD, Hilton PJ, et al.: Abnormal leukocyte composition and sodium transport in essential hypertension. Lancet 1:1003-1009, 1975.

65. Edmondson RPS, MacGregor GA: Leucocyte cation transport in essential hypertension. Its relationship to the renin angiotensin system, in Zunkley H, Losse H (editors): Intracellular Electrolytes and Arterial Hypertension. Stuttgart, Thieme, 1980, pp 187-193.

66. Forrester TE, Alleyne GA: Leukocyte electrolytes and sodium efflux rate constants in the hypertension of pre-eclampsia. Proceedings of the 7th Scientific Meeting of the International Society of Hypertension, 1980, p 35.

67. Forrester TE, Alleyne GA: Sodium, potassium, and rate constants for sodium efflux in leucocytes from hypertensive Jamaicans. Br Med J 283:5-7, 1981.

68. Poston L, Sewell RB, Wilkinson SP, et al.: Evidence for a circulating sodium transport inhibitor in essential hypertension. Br Med J 282:847-849, 1981.

69. Fitzgibbon WR, Morgon T, Myers JB, et al.: Evidence that the relationships between red cell $^{22}Na^+$ efflux and Na^+ intake is mediated by a humoral factor. Proceedings of the 8th Scientific Meeting of the International Society of Hypertension, 1981, p 131.

70. Myers JB, Fitzgibbon WR, Morgan TO: Effect of acute and chronic salt loading on ^{22}Na efflux in males with essential hypertension. Prodeedings of the 8th Scientific Meeting of the International Society of Hypertension, 1981, p 307.

71. Wessels F, Zunkley H: Sodium metabolism in red cells in hypertensive patients, in Zunkley H, Losse H (editors): Intracellular Electrolytes and Arterial Hypertension. Stuttgart, Thieme, 1980, pp 59-68.

72. Kramer HJ: Antinatriferic and natriuretic activities in human plasma following acute and chronic salt-loading, in Kramer HJ, Kruck F (editors): Natriuretic Hormone. New York, Springer-Verlag, 1978, pp 24-33.

73. Esler M, Jackman G, Bobik A, et al.: Norepinephrine kinetics in essential hypertension: Defective neural uptake of norepinephrine in some patients.

74. Greenberg S, Goldstein B, Wilson WR: Effects of plasma from hypertensive patients on the response to angiotensin and norepinephrine in dogs and rats. Clin Pharmacol Ther 15:337-343, 1974.

DISCUSSION

Discussants: Erdmann, Haddy, Langer, Blaustein, Overbeck

Erdmann: I think one of the unique features of properties of ouabain or digitalis is that it has positive inotropic action. If somebody uses the word ouabain-like substance or digitalis-like substance, I expect him to show in the contracting heart or papillary muscle, that it has positive inotropic properties, and if it cannot be shown, I think we should drop this expression.

Haddy: We use the term simply because it reduces ouabain-sensitive rubidium-86 uptake like ouabain. I think the only group that has studied the physiology of the factor is the Gruber-Buckalew group. They applied their factor to cremaster arterioles and looked at the responsiveness of those arterioles to norepinephrine; their factor increased the norepinephrine response. They've also very recently infused their purified factor intravenously into the normal rat. This is not a pentolinium blocked rat – it's not a rat that has its kidneys out – it's just a normal rat and they observed a small, slow rise in arterial blood pressure. That's the only group I know of that has had enough of the purified preparation to study its physiology.

Langer: If I understood correctly, your humoral factor is heat resistant.

Haddy: Right.

Langer: So it is different from the heat-sensitive humoral factor that would inhibit norepinephrine uptake.

Haddy: No, no. The factor that inhibits norepinephrine uptake is also heat stable.

Langer: But it's different from the one you have been talking about.

Haddy: I don't know whether it's different; all I know is that Freas and Muldoon have demonstrated that plasma from the normal dog, when applied to a saphenous vein from a normal dog inhibits norepinephrine uptake.

Langer: Yes, but does the supernatant of the whole plasma do the same?

Haddy: We haven't tested it.

Langer: Do you have a concentration-effect relationship when you dilute your factor or when you concentrate it?

Haddy: All the data shown was with a one-to-one dilution.

Langer: Because in such work, a concentration-effect relationship is essential, and if you don't have enough activity in your plasma, you may have to concentrate it by different means. This is a crucial element in your work.

Haddy: We appreciate what you're saying. One of the problems is that most of the models we're working with are rat models. They can give us only about 2 ml of supernate and Dr. Pamnani's assay of the supernate takes 2 ml. I think Dr. Pamnani will have to miniaturize his assay before we can get a good dose-response relationship.

Blaustein: At most, in the steady state, any cell with a 3:2 sodium-potassium pump ratio, according to calculations by Dr. Philip Asher[1], can maintain, at infinite membrane resistance, an electrogenic pump contribution to the membrane potential of about 10 millivolts. If you partially inhibit the pump, you may only get a few millivolts, perhaps three at most, under reasonable conditions of viability. Even under those circumstances, if you inhibit the pump, cell sodium will tend to go up so that the active sodium extrusion will again equal the leak influx. In the smooth muscle cell for example, one would then expect the pumped efflux of sodium to come back to its original level, and there would be no net change in electrogenic pumping. Under those circumstances, the contribution of membrane potential from the electrogenic pump (or the depolarization) might be only a very small amount. It will be caused by the change in the ion gradients, rather than by a change in the pumping itself. Now the other possibility, of course, is that the effects are occurring primarily on the nerve terminals, causing increased release and reduced reuptake of neurotransmitter. Under these circumstances you may get a larger membrane depolarization. Thus, one has to think about where the effects are occurring.

Haddy: The change in membrane potential is not nerve related, at least in this artery. The reason is that some of the experiments were done after treatment with 6-hydroxydopamine and phentolamine and the changes in those experiments were not different from those in the untreated. The only evidence I have that this is electrogenic depolarization is that ouabain produces the same change, i.e., we see depolarization, and that it's the same supernatant that reduces ouabain-sensitive rubidium-86 uptake.

Blaustein: With a very high concentration of ouabain, clearly, you can turn off the pumps, in which case you get two effects: one is the reduction in the pump current and the second is the secondary changes in the ion gradients, which can be very large. So, you can get a very big change in membrane potential. That's not likely to occur under reasonable physiological conditions where, over the long term, you'd expect to reach some new steady state (*slightly elevated*) of sodium concentration in the cell.

[1] Thomas RC: *Physiol Rev* 52:563-594, 1972.

Overbeck: I think these are very interesting results. However, I'm sure the group perceives that we didn't get the same results in fresh tissue in DOCA hypertension, and in Goldblatt hypertension. I have a question about the work that Dr. Harder did with you on membrane potential. He told me that in normotensive tissue treated with hypertensive supernates, the effect could be washed out within five minutes, but that he was never able to wash out the effect in hypertensive tissue.

Haddy: No, you misunderstood. It looked like it might wash out in about two hours in those experiments. But there weren't enough experiments to answer your question. The reason I said it looks like it binds tightly is because a depolarization was present 90 minutes after removing the arteries from the animal.

Tosteson: You mentioned these experiments with the anti-digoxin antibody producing hypotension only in hypertensive animals. How do you interpret that experiment in relation to your hypothesis?

Haddy: This was the study of Kojima et al. in which they prepared antibodies to digoxin, injected them intravenously in the DOCA salt model, and got a prompt fall in blood pressure which lasted for an hour, but no effect in the control animal. If the humoral agent binds to the anti-digoxin antibody, this would explain the effect.

Tosteson: But isn't that a rather disturbing result since no one is implying that this compound, whatever it might be, is really chemically very much like digoxin.

Haddy: Gruber and Buckalew have shown that their agent cross-reacts with anti-digoxin antibody, i.e., their natriuretic hormone cross-reacts with anti-digoxin antibodies.

AN INCREASE IN A CIRCULATING INHIBITOR OF Na+/K+-ATPase: THE LINK BETWEEN SODIUM AND VASCULAR TONE IN EXPERIMENTAL AND INHERITED HYPERTENSION?

G.A. MacGregor, and H.E. de Wardener

INTRODUCTION

The Chinese were the first to realize the relationship between salt intake and blood pressure. 'If large amounts of salt are taken, the pulse will stiffen or harden' (Huang Ti Nei Ching Su Wen, circa 200 B.C.). Nevertheless, it is not yet known how an increase in salt intake causes an increase in peripheral resistance, and thereby a rise in blood pressure. Dahl [1] was the first to propose that a hormone that increased sodium excretion might also cause a rise in blood pressure. The principal evidence that a circulating substance other than aldosterone modifies the urinary excretion of sodium comes from experiments in which the fluid volume of an animal, which has been given large amounts of salt-retaining steroids, is rapidly increased without diminishing its plasma protein concentration of packed cell volume. In these experiments, the presence of the natriuretic substance is simultaneously assayed, either by a denervated or isolated kidney perfused at a controllable pressure or by a recipient animal cross-circulated with the expanded donor animal [2].

Over the years, it has been repeatedly demonstrated what when the volume of body fluids are expanded, the plasma not only acquires natriuretic properties but it also develops an increased capacity to inhibit sodium transport and, in particular, Na+/K+-ATPase activity. Gonick et al. [3], using a plasma extract from the rat, demonstrated that the net inhibition of sodium transport found in the frog skin was probably due, at least in part, to inhibition of Na+/K+-ATPase. Gruber et al. [4], using a similar but more extensive extraction technique, obtained a fraction from dog plasma that also inhibits preparations of isolated membrane Na+/K+-ATPase, competes for digoxin with digoxin antibodies, and displaces ouabain from receptor sites. De Wardener et al. [5] measured the capacity of untreated human plasma to modify Na+/K+-ATPase activity directly, using a cytochemical technique to measure guinea pig renal Na+/K+-ATPase activity in intact cells. Dilutions of 1:20 to 1:500 on a high-sodium diet inhibited Na+/K+-ATPase activity approximately 25 times more than plasma from the same subjects on a low-sodium diet. As inhibition of Na+/K+-ATPase is associated with stimulation of glucose-6-phosphate dehydrogenase (G6PD), and the cytochemical technique used to measure G6PD activity in intact cells, in contrast to that for measuring Na^+K^+-ATPase activity, is easier and has been in use for several years, Fenton et al. [6] have developed an assay to measure the capacity of biological fluids to stimulate G6PD activity *in vitro* as a marker of their ability to inhibit Na^+/K^+-ATPase. It was found that the capacity of untreated plasma from normal subjects on a high-sodium diet was approximately 20 times greater than the plasma from the same subjects on a low-sodium diet.

It is possible that several substances are responsible for the change in the plasma's capacity to inhibit Na^+/K^+-ATPase. Most of the work that has been performed to investigate the nature of the natriuretic hormone has been carried out on the low-molecular-weight natriuretic material obtained from the urine. This substance inhibits Na^+/K^+-ATPase and stimulates G6PD [6]. It has a molecular weight below 500; it is very polar in that it is most soluble in water and insoluble in chloroform and ether; it is relatively resistant to acid hydrolysis; and it does not contain any amino acids [7]. The structure of the active material appears to consist of a sugar attached to a heterocyclic component containing nitrogen.

Theoretically, it is not unreasonable to assume that sodium balance should be controlled from a neural area closely related to that which regulates water balance, since both are eventually related to the regulation of blood volume. One of the afferent limbs that monitors blood volume and thus may control the secretion of natriuretic hormone is the intrathoracic blood volume, particularly the left auricular pressure. The overriding importance of the intrathoracic blood volume in causing a rise in urinary sodium excretion has been demonstrated by experiments in which a man in the sitting position is immersed in water [8]. This maneuver, which induces a sustained increase in the intrathoracic blood volume and in urinary sodium excretion, continues despite a gradual *decrease* in total blood volume. The intrathoracic blood volume of a man immersed while sitting in water is approximately 700 ml greater than when he is standing. One quarter of this volume is in the heart, and most of it is in the auricles. It is probable that it is the consequent rise in left auricular pressure that causes the natriuresis, for a rise in right auricular pressure causes an antinatriuresis. In support of the proposal that a rise in intrathoracic blood volume is associated with an increase in the concentration of a circulating sodium-transport inhibitor, Epstein et al. [9] demonstrated that natriuretic extracts prepared from urine excreted during the natriuresis of water immersion was significantly more natriuretic than extracts obtained from control urine.

The suggestion that a circulating natriuretic substance might raise the blood pressure was first put forward by Dahl et al. [1] to explain the results of an experiment in parabiotic rats, one of which was a salt-sensitive hypertensive rat and the other, a salt-resistant normotensive rat. They stated that 'many of the apparent anomalies of the angiotensin-aldosterone system in hypertension could be explained if a sodium-excreting hormone were postulated which had the capacity of also inducing hypertension when produced by a hypertensive-prone individual.' No notice was taken of this remarkable proposition, presumably because it was so contrary to the well-known observation that a diuretic, or a salt-losing state, causes the blood pressure to fall. The authors themselves never pursued their own suggestion.

THE RISE IN ARTERIAL PRESSURE IN ACQUIRED HYPERTENSION ASSOCIATED WITH RETEN-TION OF SODIUM

There is evidence in chronic renal failure in man and in certain experimental animal models – such as reduction of renal mass, removal of one kidney, and either wrapping the other in cellophane or placing a clip on the other renal artery, in all of which there is sodium retention – that there is a rise in the concentration of a circulating sodium-transport inhibitor [10]. It is known that the administration of mineralocorticoids raises the plasma concentration of a circulating sodium-transport inhibitor [11]. Bricker et al. [12] demonstrated the presence of a low-molecular-weight natriuretic sodium-transport inhibitor in uremic serum and urine. Haddy and Overbeck [10], whose primary interest is vasomotor tone and the control of blood pressure, were the first to propose that a rise in the concentration of a circulating sodium-transport inhibitor might be responsible for certain forms of induced hypertension in which there is sodium retention. They were first led to this conclusion by finding that the vasodilating properties of an intra-arterial infusion of potassium could be blocked by ouabain [13] and that the vasodilation induced by potassium was less pronounced in these various experimental models of hypertension than in control animals [14]. Additional evidence for an increase in the concentration of a circulating sodium-transport inhibitor has been obtained by Simon and Pamnani. Simon [15] found that serum obtained from dogs with perinephritic hypertension increased the uptake of sodium, potassium, and water in aortic smooth muscle cells in culture. More recently, Pamnani ct al. [16] have demonstrated that the ouabain-sensitive Rb uptake of segments of rat-tail artery from normal rats incubated in plasma from hypertensive uninephrectomized dogs, in which the other kidney had been wrapped in cellophane, was significantly lower than when incubated in plasma from a normotensive dog.

Evidence for a circulating vasoactive substance

Hinke [17] perfused the isolated tail artery of normotensive and hypertensive rats with blood from either other normotensive rats or hypertensive uninephrectomized rats given DOCA and a high intake of sodium. The blood from the hypertensive rat caused a significantly greater constriction of the tail arteries whether they had been obtained from normotensive or hypertensive rats.

Michelakis et al. [18] measured the effect of intravenous noradrenaline and angiotensin on the arterial pressure of assay rats before and after the intravenous administration of $20\,\mu l$ of plasma from normotensive dogs and hypertensive uninephrectomized dogs with a clip on the other renal artery. The rise in arterial pressure induced in the assay rat by noradrenaline and angiotensin was substantially greater after the injection of plasma from the hypertensive dogs. Similar results were obtained by Self et al. [19] when the plasma was obtained from rats made hypertensive with high sodium intakes.

Abnormalities of sodium transport in blood vessels

There are many claims that in experimental hypertension, there is not only a raised concentration of a circulating sodium-transport inhibitor, but also that the blood vessels have an impaired sodium transport. The ouabain-sensitive 86Rb uptake of mesenteric and tail arteries and the splanchnic veins is reduced, while microsomal Na^+/K^+-ATPase obtained from cardiac muscle is depressed [20]. In keeping with the reciprocal relation between Na^+/K^+-ATPase and G6PD activity mentioned above, Laing and Gardner [21] found an increase in G6PD activity in cardiac muscle from uninephrectomized DOCA salt-loaded dogs. In addition, there are several reports that in experimental hypertension the intracellular sodium content of the rat aorta and mesenteric artery is raised [22]. Nevertheless, some workers who have used different techniques have found that the Na^+/K^+-ATPase activity of the aorta and tail arteries is increased and the intracellular sodium is normal; in the conditions studied, the increase appeared to be due to an increased permeability [23].

Mechanism whereby a circulating sodium-transport inhibitor might increase the tone of smooth muscle

Haddy [24] has suggested that the circulating sodium-transport inhibitor reduces Na^+ pump current. This reduces the pump's contribution to the resting membrane potential. The consequential depolarization increases the influx of calcium, and this increases the intracellular concentration of free calcium. Blaustein [25], on the other hand, has proposed that a sodium-transport inhibitor would increase intracellular free calcium by its effect on the sodium-calcium exchange mechanism.

Possible sequence of events responsible for the rise in arterial pressure in experimental hypertension

A possible sequence for the rise in arterial pressure in the acquired or induced forms of hypertension associated with sodium retention is illustrated in Figure 1. The sodium retention, which is more marked as the sodium intake is increased, at first increases the total blood volume and thus, the intrathoracic blood volume. The latter increases the left auricular pressure, and the resulting afferent vagal stimulation stimulates the hypothalamus to secrete increased quantities of the circulating inhibitor of Na$^+$/K$^+$-ATPase. This increases the urinary sodium excretion and prevents a continuing accumulation of sodium. Inhibition of sodium transport raises the intracellular concentration of free calcium and thereby increases the tone of the arteries, veins, and heart muscle. The increase in tone of the arteries causes the arterial pressure to rise, whereas the increase in tone of the veins is the cause of the diminished compliance of the peripheral venous bed [26]. Therefore, it is probable that, as in the inherited forms of hypertension (see below), the decrease in venous compliance by redistributing blood from the periphery to the center is at first partly, and later perhaps wholly, responsible for a continuing increase in intrathoracic blood volume. This is particularly relevant in those animals in which, after an initial rise, the blood volume either returns to normal or is reduced below normal, though the arterial pressure remains raised.

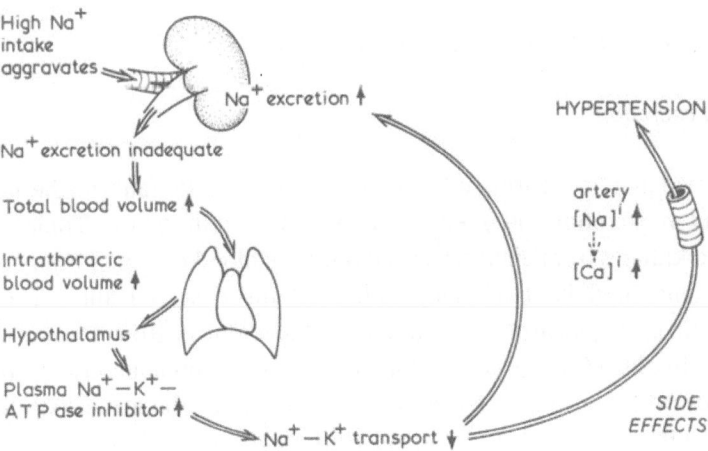

Figure 1. Origin of the rise in arterial pressure in acquired hypertension associated with renal sodium retention.

THE RELATION OF A CIRCULATING SODIUM-TRANSPORT INHIBITOR TO THE RISE IN
ARTERIAL PRESSURE IN INHERITED HYPERTENSION

Inherited hypertension of unknown cause in man is known as essential hypertension. In the rat, there are two forms of inherited hypertension of unknown cause.
In one, the rise in arterial pressure is contingent upon a large increase in sodium
intake, whereas the control normotensive strain is unaffected by such an increase
(the Dahl salt-sensitive and salt-resistant hypertensive rat). In the other form of
inherited rat hypertension, the rise in arterial pressure occurs on a normal sodium
intake (the spontaneously hypertensive rat).

Cross-transplantation experiments

Borst and Borst de Geus [27] were the first to propose that the underlying
abnormality in essential hypertenstion might be due to an impairment of the
kidney's control of sodium excretion. Convincing evidence to support this suggestion has come from cross-transplantation experiments in rats with inherited
hypertension. This difficult experiment has been performed in the Dahl salt-
sensitive hypertensive rat [28], in the Milan hypertensive strain [29], and in the
Okamoto spontaneously hypertensive rat [30]. In all three, the results have
demonstrated that the 'hypertension follows the kidney.' It is difficult to exagger-
ate the importance of this finding, for it implies that all the various abnormalities
that have been described in these three forms of hypertension in the rat must
either be secondary to a renal abnormality or they are unrelated to the mechanism
that causes the pressure to rise.

Evidence of a renal difficulty in excreting sodium

Sodium excretion

Direct evidence in an isolated kidney that the genetic fault in the kidney is a
difficulty in excreting sodium can only be obtained in the rat. Tobian et al. [31]
perfused kidneys from eight-week-old rats with blood obtained from normal rats
and demonstrated that the kidneys of the sodium-sensitive Dahl rat excreted less
sodium at each perfusion pressure than the kidneys from the normotensive
control. In the Milan [32] and the stroke-prone spontaneously hypertensive
strains of rat [33], there is a transient period ending about the sixth to seventh
week of life when the fractional excretion of sodium is lower, the cumulative
retention of sodium is greater, and the plasma renin activity is lower in the
hypertensive strain of rat than in the normotensive control rat. At the end of this
period, the blood pressure of the hypertensive strain rat has risen considerably.

Once the rat is adult, no difference in sodium excretion or plasma-renin activity can be discerned. In man, Grim et al. [34] studied normotensive monozygotic and dizygotic twins and have established the presence of 'strong heritable influences on the renal excretion of sodium which are most readily identified in the volume-expanded state.' Using a relatively slow infusion of saline (2 L in 4 h), they demonstrated that normotensive first-degree relatives of patients with essential hypertension excrete less sodium than control subjects.

Salt intake

The relation between sodium intake and the arterial pressure in both human populations and stock colony rats also suggests that the genetic abnormality in the kidney is a difficulty in excreting sodium. Gleiberman's (1971) [35] review of the available data in 27 populations shows that there is a significant correlation between the arterial pressure and the salt intake ($P<0.0005$). And that populations that consume less than 60 mEq/day of sodium have no rise of arterial pressure with age. In stock colony rats arterial pressure rises with age and increasing sodium intake [36].

Changes in blood volume

In the Dahl sodium-sensitive hypertensive rat, plasma renin activity is low, and in the young spontaneously hypertensive rat, there is a period of sodium retention and a fall in plasma renin activity [32, 33], suggesting a probable increase in blood volume. But thereafter, plasma renin activity returns to normal [32, 33], and the blood volume in the rats with inherited hypertension is either normal or low [37]. The blood volume in the adult individual with essential hypertension is also either normal or low [38]. But in both the rat [37] and the human forms [39] of inherited hypertension, there is diminished venous compliance and a rise in either the central blood volume or in the ratio of the intrathoracic to the total blood volume. The conclusion that an increased peripheral venous tone shifts blood from the periphery to the chest is supported by the finding that in essential hypertension, the pulmonary wedge pressure is increased (Safar and London, personal communication), and in the rat with inherited hypertension [40], the left auricular pressure is raised. It is possible, therefore, that the raised concentration of circulating sodium-transport inhibitor in essential hypertension and the decrease in Na^+/K^+-ATPase activity, which can be demonstrated in certain tissues in the hypertensive rat and man with essential hypertension, are due to the maintained distension of the intrathoracic vascular bed and, in particular, the raised left auricular pressure.

Exaggerated natriuresis

There is another abnormal phenomenon suggesting that though total blood volume may be normal or reduced, animals and individuals suffering from these two forms of hypertension behave as if their blood volume was raised. Both the spontaneously hypertensive rat and man with essential hypertension have an accelerated natriuresis upon being given a rapid intravenous infusion of saline (2 L in 1 h in man). The natriuresis is greatest in hypertensive patients in whom plasma renin activity is lowest [41]. In both the rat and man, the accelerated natriuresis is unrelated to changes in peritubular capillary hydrostatic or colloid osmotic pressure [42] and can be elicited early in life before the rise in arterial pressure [43]. The phenomenon of accelerated natriuresis is highly suggestive of a state in which there is a continuing need to oppose a persistent tendency to retain sodium. It occurs in primary aldosteronism and in normal subjects given aldosterone even when, as in essential hypertension, there is no measurable increase in extracellular fluid volume [44].

Evidence for a raised concentration of a circulating sodium-transport inhibitor

Poston et al. [45] were the first to demonstrate that the blood of patients with essential hypertension has an increased ability to inhibit sodium transport. They first confirmed that white cells obtained from hypertensive patients had an increased intracellular concentration of sodium and a reduced efflux-rate constant, due principally to a decrease in the ouabain-sensitive component of the efflux-rate constant [46]. They then incubated white cells from normotensive subjects in the serum of hypertensive patients. The normal white cells developed an impairment of sodium transport, which was similar to that found in the hypertensive patients' own white cells in that they now had a reduction in the ouabain-sensitive component of the efflux-rate constant. The efflux-rate constant of normotensive white cells incubated in the serum of another subject did not change. These results suggest that the serum of patients with essential hypertension contains an increased concentration of a substance with ouabain properties, i.e., an inhibitor of Na^+/K^+-ATPase. Ambrosioni et al. [47] have repeated these cross-incubation experiments using lymphocytes. They have found that the intracellular sodium concentration of lymphocytes from normotensive subjects increased after incubation in the plasma of hypertensive patients. Edmondson and MacGregor [48], using leukocytes, have observed that the sodium-efflux rate constant of white cells of hypertensive patients is inversely correlated to plasma renin activity. MacGregor et al. [49] have measured the plasma's capacity to stimulate G6PD activity in intact cells as a marker of its ability to inhibit Na^+/K^+-ATPase activity in hypertensive patients and 23 normotensive subjects. The ability of the plasma of the hypertensive patients to stimulate G6PD was significantly greater (P<0.001) than the plasma of the normotensive subjects. There was a significant correlation between the systolic pressure, the mean arterial pressure, the diastolic pressure, and the plasma's capacity to stimulate G6PD (P<0.001). In addition, the ability of the plasma from the seven hypertensive patients whose plasma renin activity was below normal to stimulate G6PD was significantly greater than the plasma from the other patients.

There is only one observation on the concentration of the circulating sodium-transport inhibitor in the inherited forms of hypertension in the rat. Poston et al. [50] have incubated microsomal fractions of Na^+/K^+-ATPase from the brain in serum from spontaneously hypertensive and control rats. They have found that after the age of six weeks, Na^+/K^+-ATPase activity of the microsomal fractions incubated in serum of the hypertensive rats was significantly lower than when incubated in control serum.

Evidence for circulating vasoactive substance

Michelakis et al. [18] injected 15-20 μl of plasma from hypertensive patients and normotensive subjects into bilateral nephrectomized rat under the influence of pentolinium. The plasma from hypertensive patients, particularly those with low plasma renin activity, increased the vascular reactivity of the rats to noradrenaline and angiotensin, whereas plasma from normotensive subjects did not have this effect. Bloom et al. [51] perfused the isolated rabbit femoral artery with plasma using a constant flow pump. The addition of noradrenaline to the plasma from hypertensive patients caused a greater rise in perfusion pressure than when it was added to plasma from normotensive subjects. Tobian et al. [52] have demonstrated that the blood of the salt-sensitive hypertensive rat causes a significant increase in vascular resistance of the cross-perfused hindquarters of the normotensive salt-resistant rat.

Campbell et al. [53] transplanted small segments of rat-tail artery into the anterior chamber of rats for a period of eight weeks. They found that when the arteries of 2-week-old spontaneously hypertensive rats were placed into the eye of normotensive control rats and vice versa, the membrane potential of the artery when excised eight weeks later was that appropriate to the host animal. In other words, the membrane potential of an artery from a spontaneously hypertensive rat placed into the eye of a normotensive rat had a normal membrane potential, whereas the membrane potential of an artery from a normotensive rat implanted into the eye of spontaneously hypertensive rats showed the same impairment as the hypertensive rat's own tail artery. This remarkable demonstration, that by some humoral mechanism a spontaneously hypertensive rat can impair the electrical properties (presumably by inhibiting sodium transport) of an artery through which no blood is flowing, could not be repeated using tail arteries from 12- to 16-week-old rats. This suggests that arterial smooth muscle cells are more sensitive to the humoral factor than mature cells. Greenberg et al. [54] have explored the cause of the increased reactivity, diminished passive extensibility, and increased thickness of the portal vein in the spontaneously hypertensive rat in experiments in which a hypertensive rat was parabiosed with a normotensive rat. The arterial pressure of the normotensive strain rat rose, but the portal venous pressure remained normal. Nevertheless, the portal vein of the normotensive-strain rat parabiosed to a spontaneously hypertensive rat acquired the properties of the portal vein of the spontaneously hypertensive rat; it became less distensible, developed medial hypertrophy, and its contractility when challenged with noradrenaline was greater.

Abnormalities of sodium transport in essential hypertension

Red cells

Abnormalities of sodium transport in the red cells of patients with essential hypertension have been described for many years [55]. Many parameters have been studied with a variety of different techniques, which sometimes makes comparison difficult or impossible. Some of the discrepancies in the results obtained by different workers are probably due to methodological differences. With one exception [56], there is agreement that the intracellular sodium concentration is raised [57], and some of these groups found an associated reduction in ouabain-sensitive sodium efflux-rate constant [58, 59, 60]. But, according to Garay et al. [61] and Wambach et al. [62], the ouabain-sensitive sodium efflux is normal, though Garay et al. found that net Na^+ extrusion is diminished [61]. Others, some of whom do not report their findings on the function of the ouabain-sensitive pump, have studied two components of the ouabain-insensitive sodium-transport mechanism. They report that the lithium-sodium or sodium-sodium countertransport is increased in Milan [63], Boston [56], Moscow [64], Leeds [60], and Paris [65], while Na^+/K^+ co-transport is decreased in Cologne [62], Milan [63], and Paris [65], normal in Amsterdam [66], and raised in Boston [65]. One group, who reported an increased intracellular sodium and a depressed ouabain-sensitive sodium-efflux rate constant, found that both these abnormalities were corrected by the administration of diuretics [58] and that the associated increase in lithium-sodium countertransport was not influenced by the diuretics [58]. There are two other reports that the high intracellular sodium concentration is reduced to normal by diuretics [67, 68]. Three groups find that the abnormalities they describe are also present in the red cells of the children of hypertensive parents [62, 63, 67]. Postnov et al. [64] claim that the red cell membranes have a diminished calcium-binding capacity.

White cells

The results of observations made on white cells are strikingly more uniform than those on the red cells. There is agreement that in both whole leukocyte fractions, and lymphocytes alone, the intracellular sodium concentration is raised [47, 69, 70, 71] and that the ouabain-sensitive sodium efflux-rate constant is decreased [69, 71]. There is also agreement that these abnormalities are reversed by the administration of diuretics [69, 70, 71, 72]. In addition, Ambrosioni et al. [47] found that the lymphocytes of children of hypertensive parents also have a higher intracellular-sodium concentration.

Vessels

Tobian and Binion [73] found the sodium and water content of renal arteries removed at post mortem from patients who had suffered from hypertension is raised. Overbeck et al. [74] found that the vasodilator response of forearm vessels to an intra-arterial infusion of potassium was less pronounced in a patient with essential hypertension than in a normotensive person. They suggested that this phenomenon might be due to a reduced Na^+/K^+-ATPase activity. It is of interest that the calcium-entry antagonists, nifedipine and verapamil, which are claimed to block the influx of calcium into the smooth muscle cell following depolarization, cause a much greater fall in blood pressure in patients with high blood pressure than those with normal blood pressure [75]. Work comparing the increase in forearm blood flow with interarterial verapamil has shown that verapamil causes a greater increase in forearm blood flow in patients with high blood pressure as compared to normotensive subjects, whereas there was an equal increase in blood flow with another vasodilator, nitroprusside [76], It would seem likely that this functional abnormality of the smooth muscle cell to calcium-entry antagonists in essential hypertension is related to an abnormality of calcium transport, possibly due to a raised concentration of the sodium transport inhibitor. The finding that the abnormal blood flow response to verapamil in the hypertensive patients was reversed by treatment with diuretics [77] supports this concept.

Inherited hypertension in the rat

Red cells

Five groups [78-82] have reported that the intracellular sodium concentration is raised in the spontaneously hypertensive rat, whereas Wessels and Samizadeh have found it to be low [83]. Mendonca et al. [84], however, found that though the intracellular sodium concentration is normal, it rises abnormally after the administration of sodium. Losse et al. using ion-selective electrodes, have found that both the intracellular sodium and calcium concentration are raised [78]. The reason for this increase in intracellular sodium is not clear. It has been shown that the red cell has an increased permeability [81, 82, 85] and diminished net sodium extrusion [86] but an increased sodium efflux [81, 86]. On the other hand, Berglund et al. [79] have found that there is an increased content of Na^+/K^+-ATPase. Lithium-sodium countertransport is normal [87].

White cells

Because of the small number of easily available leukocytes in a rat, Jones et al. have developed a method for the study of cation transport in rat thymocytes [88]. They have found that the intracellular sodium content of thymocytes obtained from the spontaneously hypertensive rat is positively related to the systolic pressure, whereas the sodium-efflux rate constant is negatively correlated with the systolic pressure. No increase in the permeability of the thymocytes to sodium was observed.

Vessels

The rubidium uptake of the rat-tail artery is either normal [89] or increased [90], and the vasodilatory responses to an arterial infusion of potassium is normal [91]. There is also evidence that Na^+/K^+-ATPase activity is increased or normal [92]. Nevertheless, smooth muscle from the aorta has a decreased ability for net accumulation of potassium and extrusion of sodium [93], and plasma membrane from smooth muscle has a lower calcium-binding ability [94].

Sequence of events in essential hypertension

In essential hypertension, it is proposed that the underlying genetic lesion is a renal difficulty in excreting sodium, which becomes more apparent as the sodium intake is increased. The difficulty in excreting sodium may initially cause an increase in total blood volume and therefore a rise in intrathoracic blood volume. This stimulates the hypothalmus to secrete an increased quantity of a circulating sodium-transport inhibitor, which potentially may inhibit sodium transport across all cell membranes. In the kidney, it adjusts sodium excretion so that sodium balance is normal, but normal balance is only achieved by a maintained rise in the circulating sodium-transport inhibitor. This persistent increase raises the tone and vascular reactivity of the smooth muscle of the arteries and veins; thus, arterial pressure rises and venous compliance is diminished. The increased venous tone is responsible for a shift of blood from the periphery to the center. This raises the intrathoracic pressure and perpetuates the stimulus for an increased secretion of sodium-transport inhibitor, even if the adjustment to sodium excretion has caused the total blood volume to return to normal or below normal. (See Figure 2.)

OTHER POSSIBLE CONSEQUENCES OF A RAISED CONCENTRATION OF A CIRCULATING INHIBITOR OF SODIUM TRANSPORT

Ouabain is known to directly inhibit the enzyme Na+/K+-ATPase. The endogenous circulating sodium-transport inhibitor also inhibits Na+/K+-ATPase, perhaps preferentially through a receptor on the cell wall. It is possible, therefore, to suggest from the known actions of ouabain some consequences of a rise in the concentration of the endogenous inhibitor of Na+/K+-ATPase in essential hypertension.

Plasma renin

A significant proportion of patients with essential hypertension have a low plasma renin activity. Those individuals with the lowest plasma renin activity have the highest concentrations of circulating sodium-transport inhibitor as judged by both the G6PD assay [49] and sodium-efflux rate constant of the patients' own white cells [48]. *In vitro* experiments on rat renal cortical slices, isolated glomeruli, and isolated perfused kidneys have demonstrated that either ouabain or raising the intracellular calcium in some other way dimishes renin secretion [95].

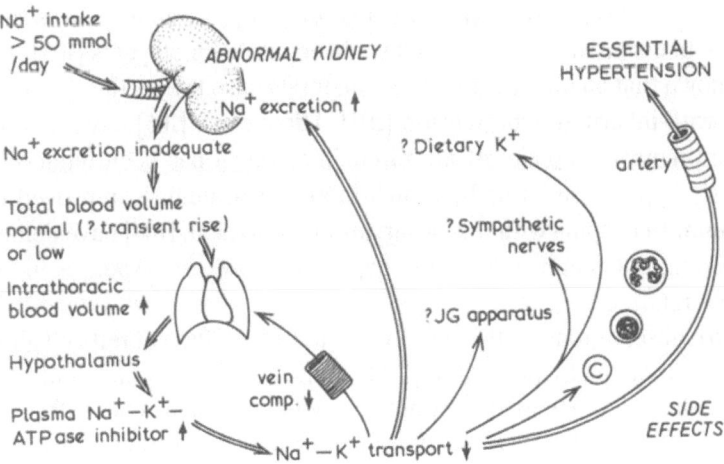

Figure 2. Origin of the rise in arterial pressure in inherited hypertension.

It is possible, therefore, that the low plasma renin activity in essential hypertension is in part due to the direct effect of the circulating sodium-transport inhibitor on the juxtaglomerular cells.

Sympathetic activity

There is evidence that as they develop hypertension, children of parents with established hypertension [96] and young rats of the spontaneously hypertensive strains have an increased sympathetic activity [97]. Falkner et al. [98] found that salt loading in children of hypertensive parents increases the evidence of sympathetic overactivity, while Schoming et al. [99] have demonstrated that in the normotensive control rat, a low-sodium diet lowers plasma noradrenaline and a high-sodium diet raises the plasma noradrenaline of a spontaneously hypertensive rat. *In vitro,* ouabain increases noradrenaline output from the nerve terminal [100] and diminishes the reuptake of noradrenaline [101], thus increasing the amount of noradrenaline available to react with the receptors on the effector cell membrane. In view of these findings, it is interesting that Dietz et al. [102] have recently shown that the nerve-terminal uptake of noradrenaline in an isolated perfused heart is markedly reduced when the heart is obtained from a spontaneously hypertensive rat that has been on a high-sodium intake. These observations are compatible with the concept that the increased sympathetic activity in essential hypertension and in the inherited forms of hypertension in the rat may be due to the raised concentration of circulating sodium-transport inhibitor.

Dietary potassium

Claims and demonstrations that the ingestion of potassium reduces the arterial pressure in essential hypertension have been made for 50 years [103]. It has also been shown that an increase in potassium intake also lowers the arterial pressure of rats with inherited hypertension [104]. Dietz et al. [105] have found that the impaired neuronal uptake of noradrenaline, which has been induced in spontaneously hypertensive rats by a high intake of sodium, is improved by giving potassium. In keeping with this observation, Goto et al. [104] have demonstrated that feeding potassium reduces the hyperactive pressor responses in Dahl salt-sensitive rats.

In vitro observations on the activity of Na^+/K^+-ATPase of red-cell ghosts show that it is stimulated by potassium [106]. In the absence of potassium, there is no activity, there is a steep rise in activity with potassium concentrations up to 5 mmol/L, and the activity is maximized at 10 mmol/L. In view of this finding, it is perhaps not surprising that potassium *increases* noradrenaline uptake into the nerve terminal, thereby having an opposite effect to ouabain [107]. Collectively, these observations suggest that the hypotensive effect of potassium and its ability to reduce sympathetic overactivity may be due to its counteracting the effect of the increased concentration of a circulating Na^+/K^+-ATPase inhibitor.

SUMMARY

In essential hypertension it is proposed that the underlying genetic lesion is a renal difficulty in excreting sodium, which becomes more apparent as the sodium intake increases. The difficulty in excreting sodium may initially cause an increase in total blood volume and therefore a rise in intrathoracid blood volume. This stimulates the hypothalamus to secrete an increased quantity of a circulating sodium-transport inhibitor, which potentially may inhibit sodium transport across all cell membranes. In the kidney it adjusts sodium excretion so that sodium balance is normal, but normal balance is only achieved by a maintained rise in the circulating sodium-transport inhibitor. This persistent increase raises the tone and vascular reactivity of the smooth muscle of the arteries and veins; thus, arterial pressure rises and venous compliance is diminished. The increased venous tone is responsible for a shift of blood from the periphery to the center. This raises the intrathoracic pressure and perpetuates the stimulus for an increased secretion of sodium-transport inhibitor, even if the adjustment to sodium excretion has caused the total blood volume to return to normal, or below normal.

REFERENCES

1. Dahl LK, Knudsen KD, Iwai J: Humoral transmission of hypertension. Evidence from para-biosis. Circ Res 14/15 (suppl 1):I-121-I-123, 1969.
2. De Wardener HE: Natriuretic hormone. Clin Sci Mol Med 53:1-8, 1977.
3. Gonick HC, Kramer IIJ, Paul W, et al.: Circulating inhibitor of sodium-potassium-activated adenosine triphosphatase after expansion of extra-cellular fluid volume in rats. Clin Sci Mol Med 53:329-334, 1977.
4. Gruber KA, Whitaker JM, Buckalew VM Jr: Endogenous digitalis-like substance in plasma of volume-expanded dogs. Nature 237:743-745, 1980.
5. De Wardener HE, MacGregor GA, Clarkson EM, et al.: Effect of sodium intake on the ability of human plasma to inhibit renal Na^+/K^+-adenosine triphosphatase in vitro. Lancet 1:411-412, 1981.
6. Fenton S, Clarkson EM, MacGregor GA, et al.: An assay of the capacity of biological fluids to stimulate renal glucose-6-phosphate dehyrogenase (G6PD) activity in vitro as a marker of their ability to inhibit sodium-potassium dependent adenosine triphosphatase (Na^+/K^+-ATPase) activity. J Endocrinol, in press.
7. Clarkson EM, Raw SM, de Wardener HE: Two natriuretic substances in extracts of urine from normal man when salt depleted and salt loaded. Kidney Int 10:381-394, 1976.
8. Epstein M: Cardiovascular and renal effects of head-out water immersion in man. Application of the model in the assessment of volume homeostasis. Circ Res 39:619-628, 1976.

9. Epstein M, Bricker NS, Bourgoignie JJ: Presence of a natriuretic factor in urine of normal men undergoing water immersion. Kidney Int 13:152-158, 1978.

10. Haddy FJ, Overbeck HW: The role of humoral agents in volume expanded hypertension. Life Sci 19:935-948, 1976.

11. Poston L, Wilkinson SP, Sewell R, et al.: Inhibition of leucocyte sodium transport during mineralocorticoid 'escape.' Clin Sci: 57:589, 1979.

12. Bricker NS, Klahr S, Puekerson M, et al.: In vitro assay for a humoral substance present during volume expansion and uraemia. Nature 219:1058-1059, 1968.

13. Chen WT, Brace RA, Scott JB, et al.: The mechanism of the vasodilator action of potassium. Proc Soc Exp Biol Med 140:820, 1972.

14. Overbeck HW: Vascular responses to cations, osmolality, and angiotensin in renal hypertensive dogs. Am J Physiol 223:1258-1264, 1972.

15. Simon G: Angiopathic serum factor in perinephritic hypertensive dogs. Hypertension 1:197-200, 1979.

16. Pamnani MB, Buggy J, Huot SJ, et al.: Studies on the role of a humoral sodium transport inhibitor and the anteroventral third ventricle (AV3V) in experimental low-renin hypertension. Clin Sci 61:57s-60s, 1981.

17. Hinke JAM: In vitro demonstration of vascular hyper-responsiveness in experimental hypertension. Circ Res 17:359-371, 1965.

18. Michelakis AM, Mizukoshi H, Huang C, et al.: Further studies on the existence of a sensitizing factor to pressor agents in hypertension. J Clin Endocrinol Metab 41:90-96, 1975.

19. Self LE, Battarbee HD, Gaar KA, et al.: A vasopressor potentiator for norepinephrine in hypertensive rats. Proc Soc Exp Biol Med 153:7-12, 1976.

20. Pamnani MB, Clough DL, Huot SJ, et al.: Vascular sodium-potassium activity in various models of experimental hypertension. Clin Sci 59:179s-181s, 1980.

21. Laing CP, Gardner DL: Cardiac metabolism in early rat hypertension: Quantitative enzyme histochemistry in the prenecrotic phase. Br J Exp Pathol 45:502-513, 1964.

22. Schoffeniels E: Ionic composition of arterial wall, in Symposium on Biochemistry of the Vascular Wall. Angiologica 6:65-88 (1-24), 1969.

23. Jones AW: Kinetics of active sodium transport in aortas from control and deoxycorticosterone hypertensive rats. Hypertension 3:631-640, 1981.

24. Haddy FJ: What is the link between vascular smooth muscle, sodium pump and hypertension? Clin Exp Hypertens 3(1):179-182, 1981.

25. Blaustein MP: Sodium ions, calcium ions, blood pressure regulation and hypertension: A reassessment and a hypothesis. Am J Physiol 232(3):C165-173, 1977.

26. Yamanoto J, Trippodo NC, McPhee AA, et al.: Decreased total venous capacity in Goldblatt hypertensive rats. Am J Physiol 240:H487-492, 1981.

27. Borst JGG, Borst de Geus A: Hypertension explained by Starling's theory of circulatory homeostasis. Lancet 1:677-682, 1963.

28. Dahl LK, Heine M: Primary role of renal homografts in setting chronic blood pressure levels in rats. Circ Res 36:692-696, 1975.

29. Bianchi G, Fox U, Di Francesco GF, et al.: Blood pressure changes produced by kidney cross transplantation between spontaneously hypertensive rats and normotensive rats. Clin Sci Mol Med 47:435-438, 1974.

30. Kawae K, Watanebe TX, Shiono K, et al.: Influence of blood pressure on renal isografts between spontaneously hypertensive and normotensive rats utilizing the F_1 hybrids. Jpn Heart J 20:886-894, 1979.

31. Tobian L, Lange J, Azer S, et al.: Reduction of natriuretic capacity and renin release in isolated, blood perfused kidneys of Dahl hypertensionprone rats. Circ Res 43:I-92-97, 1978.

32. Bianchi G, Baer PG, Fox U, et al.: The role of the kidney in the rat with genetic hypertension. Postgrad Med J 53 (suppl 2):123-135, 1977.

33. Dietz R, Schomig A, Haebara A, et al.: Studies on the pathogenesis of spontaneous hypertension of rats. Circ Res 43 (suppl 1):I-98-106, 1978.

34. Grim CE, Miller JZ, Luft FC, et al.: Genetic influences on renin, aldosterone, and the renal excretion of sodium, potassium following volume expansion and contraction in man. Hypertension I:583-590, 1979.

35. Gleibermann L: Blood pressure and dietary salt in human populations. Ecol Food Nutr 2:143-156, 1973.

36. Meneely GR, Tucker RG, Darby WJ, et al.: Chronic sodium toxicity: Hypertension, renal and vascular lesion. Am J Int Med 39:991-998, 1953.

37. Trippodo NC, Yamamoto J, Frolich ED: Whole body venous capacity and effective total tissue compliance in SHR. Hypertension 3:104-111, 1981.

38. Tarazi RC, Frolich ED, Dustan HP: Plasma volume in man with essential hypertension. N Engl J Med 278:762-765, 1968.

39. Safar ME, London GM, Levenson JA, et al.: Rapid dextran infusion in essential hypertension. Hypertension 1:615-623, 1979.

40. Noresson E, Rickstein SE, Thoren P: Left atrial pressure in normotensive and spontaneously hypertensive rats. Acta Physiol Scand 107:9-12, 1979.

41. Schalekamp MADH, Krauss XH, Schalekamp-Kuyken MPA, et al.: Studies on the mechanism of hypernatriuresis in essential hypertension in relation to measurements of plasma renin concentration, body fluid compartments and renal function. Clin Sci 41:219-231, 1971.

42. Willassen Y, Ofstad J: Renal sodium excretion and the peritubular capillary physical factors in essential hypertension. Hypertension 2:771-779, 1980.

43. Wiggens RC, Basar I, Slater JDH: Effect of arterial pressure and inheritance on the sodium excretory capacity of normal young men. Clin Sci Mol Med 54:639-647, 1978.

44. Rovner DR, Conn JW, Knoppf RF, et al.: Nature of renal escape from the sodium-retaining effect of aldosterone in primary aldosteronism and in normal subjects. J Clin Endocrinol Metab 25:53-64, 1965.

45. Poston L, Sewell RB, Wilkinson SP, et al.: Evidence for a circulating sodium transport inhibitor in essential hypertension. Br Med J 282:847-849, 1981.

46. Edmondson RPS, Thomas RD, Hilton PJ, et al.: Abnormal leucocyte composition and sodium transport in essential hypertension. Lancet I:1003-1005, 1975.

47. Ambrosioni E, Costa FV, Montebugnoli L, et al.: Increased intralymphocytic sodium content in essential hypertension: An index of impaired Na^+ cellular metabolism. Clin Sci 61:181-186, 1981.

48. Edmondson RPS, MacGregor GA: Leucocyte cation transport. Its relationship to the renin angiotensin system in essential hypertension. Br Med J 282:1267-1269, 1981.

49. MacGregor GA, Fenton S, Alaghband-Zadeh J, et al.: Evidence for a raised concentration of a circulating sodium transport inhibitor in essential hypertension. Br Med J 283:1355-1357, 1981.

50. Poston I, Jones RB, Hilton PJ: The effect of spontaneously hypertensive rat serum on rat brain Na^+/K^+-ATPase, an inverse correlation with age and blood pressure. Clin Sci 62:44-45, 1981.

51. Bloom DS, Stein MG, Rosendorff C: Effects of hypertensive plasma on the responses of isolated artery preparation to noradrenaline. Cardiovasc Res 10:268-274, 1976.

52. Tobian L, Pumper M, Johnson S, et al.: A circulating humoral pressor agent in Dahl S rats with NaCl hypertension. Clin Sci 57:3455-3475, 1979.

53. Campbell GR, Chamley-Campbell J, Short N, et al.: Effect of cross transplantation on normotensive and spontaneously hypertensive rat arterial muscle membrane. Hypertension 5:534-543, 1981.

54. Greenberg S, Gaines K, Sweatt D: Evidence for circulating factors as a cause of venous hypertrophy in spontaneously hypertensive rats. Am J Physiol 241:H421-430, 1981.

55. Losse H, Wehmeyer H, Wessels F: Der wasser und electrolytgehalt von erythrozyten bei arterieller hypertonie. Klin Wselir 38:393, 1960.

56. Canessa M, Adragna N, Solomon HS, et al.: Increased sodium-lithium countertransport in red cells of patients with essential hypertension. N Engl J Med 302:772-776, 1980.

57. Meyer P, Garay RP (editors): Genetic markers in essential hypertension. Clin Exp Hypertens 4(3), 1981.

58. Montari A, Borghi L, Canali M, et al.: Altered sodium efflux in red blood cells from essential hypertensive subjects, in Zumkley H, Losse H (editors): Intracellular Electrolytes and Arterial Hypertension. Stuttgart, Georg Thieme Verlag, 1980, pp 135-144.

59. Aderounmu A, Salako LA: Abnormal cation composition and transport in erythrocytes from hypertensive patients. Eur J Clin Invest 9:369-375, 1979.

60. Morgan T, Myers J, Fitzgibbon W: Sodium intake, blood pressure and red cell sodium efflux. Clin Exp Hypertens 3(4):641-653, 1981.

61. Garay RP, Dagher G, Pernollet MG, et al.: Inherited defect in a Na^+/K^+ co-transport system in erythrocytes from essential hypertension. Nature 284:281, 1980.

62. Wambach G, Haeber A, Bonner G, et al.: Natrium-kalium-adenosinetriphosphatase-aktiortat in erythrozytenghosts von patienten unit essentieller hypertonie. Klin Wochenschr 7:169, 1979.

63. Cusi D, Barlasina C, Ferrandi M, et al.: Familial aggregation of cation transport abnormalities and essential hypertension. Clin Exp Hypertens 3(4):871-874, 1981.

64. Postnow YV, Orlov SN, Shevchenko A, et al.: Altered sodium permeability, calcium binding and Na/K-ATPase activity in the red cell membrane in essential hypertension. Pflugers Arch 371:263-269, 1977.

65. Canessa M, Bize I, Solomon H, et al.: Na countertransport and co-transport in human red cells: Function, dysfunction and genes in essential hypertension. Clin Exp Hypertens 3(4):783-795, 1981.

66. Swarts HGP, Bonting SL, De Pont JJHM, et al.: Cation fluxes and (Na^+/K^+) activated ATPase activity in erythrocytes of patients with essential hypertension. Clin Exp Hypertens 3(4):831-849, 1981.

67. Wessels Von F, Zumkley H, Losse H: Untersuchungen zur frage des zusammenhanges zwischen kationepermeabilitat der erythrozyten und hochdruckdisposition. Z Kreislaufforsch 59:415-426, 1970.

68. Gessler Von U: Intra- und extrazellulare electrolytveranderungen bei essentieller hypertonie vor und nach behandlung. Z Kreislaufforsch 51:177-183, 1962.

69. Poston L, Jones RB, Richardson PJ, et al.: The effect of antihypertensive therapy on abnormal leucocyte transport in essential hypertension. Clin Exp Hypertens 3:693-701, 1981.

70. Arayoe MA, Khati IM, Yao LL, et al.: Leucocyte intracellular cations in hypertension: Effect of antihypertensive drugs. Am Heart J 96:731-738, 1978.

71. Thomas RD, Edmonson RPS, Hilton PJ, et al.: Abnormal sodium transport in leucocytes from patients with essential hypertension and the effect of treatment. Clin Sci Mol Med 48:169s-170s, 1975.

72. Ambrosioni E, Tartagni F, Montebugnoli L, et al.: Intralymphocytic sodium in hypertensive patients, in Zumkley H, Losse H (editors): Intracellular Electrolytes and Arterial Hypertension. Stuttgart, Georg Thieme Verlag, 1980, pp 78-86.

73. Tobian L, Binion JT: Tissue cations and water in arterial hypertension. Circulation 5:754-758, 1952.

74. Overbeck HW, Derifield RS, Pamnani MB, et al.: Attenuated vasodilator responses to K^+ in essential hypertensive man. J Clin Invest 53:678-686, 1974.

75. MacGregor GA, Markandu ND, Bayliss J, et al.: Circumstantial evidence that an abnormality of calcium transport may be important in essential hypertension. Clin Sci 60:6, 1981.

76. Robinson BF, Bayley S, Dobbs RJ: Response of forearm resistance vessels to verapamil and sodium nitroprusside in normal and hypertensive man: Evidence for a functional abnormality of vascular smooth muscle in primary hypertension. Clin Sci 60:7, 1981.

77. Robinson BF, Chiodini P, Dobbs RJ, et al.: On the mechanism of the abnormal response to verapamil and nitroprusside in the resistance vessels of men with primary hypertension. Clin Sci 62:32, 1981.

78. Losse H, Zidek W, Zumkley H, et al.: Intracellular Na$^+$ as a genetic marker of essential hypertension. Clin Exp Hypertens 3(4):627-640, 1981.

79. Berglund G, Sigstrom C, Lundins S, et al.: Intra-erythrocyte sodium and (Na$^+$/K$^+$-activated)-ATPase concentration and urinary aldosterone excretion in spontaneously hypertensive rats. Clin Sci 60:229-232, 1981.

80. Ben-Ishay D, Aviram A, Viskoper R: Increased erythrocytes sodium efflux in genetic hypertensive rats of the Hebrew University strain. Experientia 31:660-662, 1975.

81. Postnov YV, Orlov S, Gulak P, et al.: Altered permeability of the erythrocyte membrane for sodium, potassium in spontaneously hypertensive rats. Pflugers Arch 365:257-263, 1976.

82. Yamori Y, Nara YR, Ohtaka M: Ion permeability of erythrocyte membrane in spontaneously hypertensive rat. Jpn Heart J 18:604-605, 1977.

83. Wessels F, Samizadeh A: Sodium metabolism of RBC, aorta, heart and skeletal muscle in spontaneously hypertensive rat, in Zumkley H, Losse H (editors): Intracelllar Electrolytes and Arterial Hypertension. Stuttgart, Georg Thieme Verlag, 1980, pp 111-115.

84. Mendonca M de, Garay RP, Ben-Ishay D, et al.: Abnormal erythrocyte cation transport in primary hypertension. Clin Exp Hypertens 3(suppl I):I-179-183, 1981.

85. Friedman SM, Nakashima M, McIndoe RA, et al.: Increased erythrocyte permeability to Li$^+$ and Na$^+$ in the spontaneously hypertensive rat. Experientia 32:476, 1976.

86. Mendonca M de, Gichois M-L, Garay RP, et al.: Abnormal net sodium and potassium fluxes in erythrocytes of four varieties of genetically hypertensive rats, in Zumkley H, Losse H (editors): Intracellular Electrolytes and Arterial Hypertension. Stuttgart, Georg Thieme Verlag, 1980, pp 135-144.

87. Wiley JS, Clarke D, Hutchinson JS, et al.: Factors affecting the sodium permeability of rat erythrocytes. Clin Exp Hypertens 3(4):703-712, 1981.

88. Jones RB, Patrick J, Hilton PJ: Increased sodium content and altered sodium transport of spontaneously hypertensive rat. Clin Sci 61:313-316, 1981.

89. Pamnani MB, Clough DL, Huot SJ, et al.: Vascular Na$^+$/K$^+$ pump activity in Dahl S & R rats. Proc Soc Exp Biol Med 165:440-444, 1980.

90. Overbeck HW, Ku DD, Rapp JP: Sodium pump activity in arteries of Dahl salt-sensitive rats. Hypertension 3:306-312, 1981.

91. Overbeck HW, Clark DWJ: Vasodilator to K$^+$ in genetic hypertensive and in renal hypertensive rats. J Lab Clin Med 86:973-983, 1975.

92. Abel PW, Tropani A, Matsuki N, et al.: Unaltered membrane properties of arterial muscle in Dahl strain genetic hypertension. Am J Physiol 241:H244-247, 1981.

93. Jones AW: Altered ion transport in vascular smooth muscle from spontaneously hypertensive rat. Circ Res 33:563-572, 1973.

94. Postnov YV, Orlov SN: Alteration of membrane control over intracellular calcium in essential hypertension and in spontaneously hypertensive rats, in Zumkley H, Losse H (editors): Intracellular Electrolytes and Arterial Hypertension. Stuttgart, Georg Thieme Verlag, 1980, pp 144-151.

95. Churchill MC, Churchill PC: Separate and combined effects of ouabain and extracellular potassium on renin secretion from rat renal cortical slices. J Physiol 300:105-114, 1980.

96. Falkner B, Onesti G, Angalakos ET, et al.: Cardiovascular response to mental stress in normal adolescents with hypertensive parents. Hypertension 1:23-30, 1979.

97. Hallback M: Interaction of autonomic hypersensitivity and environmental stimuli: Importance for the development of spontaneously hypertensive rats, in Onesti G, Fernandes M, Kim K (editors): Regulation of Blood Pressure by Central Nervous System. New York, Grune & Stratton, 1976, p 129.

258

98. Falkner B, Onesti G, Angelakos E: Effect of salt loading on the cardiovascular response to stress in adolescents. Hypertension 3(suppl II):II-195-199, 1981.

99. Schoming A, Dietz R, Roseler W, et al.: Sympathetic vascular tone in spontaneous hypertension of rats. Klin Wochenschr 56 (suppl I):131, 1978.

100. Nakazato Y, Ohga A, Onoda Y: The effect of ouabain on noradrenaline output from peripheral adrenergic neurones of isolated guinea-pig vas deferens. J Physiol 278:45-54, 1978.

101. Leitz FH, Stefano FJE: Effect of ouabain and desipramine on the uptake and storage of epinephrine and neteraminol. Eur J Pharmacol 11:278-285, 1970.

102. Dietz R, Schoming A, Rascher W, et al.: Contribution of the sympathetic nervous system to the hypertensive effect of a high sodium diet in stroke prone spontaneously hypertensive rats (SHR-sp). Unpublished observations.

103. Addison WLT: The use of sodium chloride, potassium chloride, sodium bromide and potassium bromide in cases of arterial hypertension which are amenable to potassium chloride. Can Med Assoc J 18:281-285, 1928.

104. Goto A, Tobian L, Iwai J: Potassium feeding reduces hyperactive central nervous system pressor responses in Dahl salt sensitive rats. Hypertension 3 (suppl II):I-128-134, 1981.

105. Dietz R, Schoming A, Rascher W, et al.: Partial replacement of sodium by potassium in the diet restores impaired noradrenaline inactivation and lowers blood pressure in SHR-sp. Clin Sci 61 (suppl 7):69s-71s,1981.

106. Dunham ET, Glynn IM: Adenosine triphosphatase activity and the active movements of alkali metal ions. J Physiol 156:274-293, 1961.

107. Bagdanski DF, Blaszkowski TP, Tissari AM: Mechanism of biogenic amino transport and storage. Biochim Biophys Acta 211:521-532, 1970.

DISCUSSION

Discussants: Duhm, Mulvany, MacGregor, Brody, Erdmann, Overbeck, Haddy, Haeusler

Duhm: I noted that a 1:100 dilution of human plasma inhibited the sodium potassium pump of your kidney by 90 percent. I wonder why the pump in the human donor was not inhibited by 100 percent?

MacGregor: That's a good point. These cytochemical bioassays are exquisitely sensitive and I don't think I could answer your point directly because there may be differences in sensitivity of the guinea pig kidney compared to the human kidney. It does seem, based on the cytochemical bioassay, that human plasma is a potent inhibitor of guinea pig kidney sodium-potassium ATPase.

Mulvany: I think you gave the impression that the increased tone could only be accounted for on the basis of sodium-calcium exchange. I don't in any way want to claim that this theory is invalidated. But, I think it is also true that, should sodium-calcium exchange not be important you could still account for increased vasoconstriction since a sodium-potassium-ATPase inhibitor would probably cause a depolarization.

MacGregor: Yes. I agree entirely that there could be other mechanisms whereby an increase in intracellular sodium could increase peripheral resistance. I think the studies with the calcium antagonists possibly suggest that it might be secondary to a raised intracellular calcium.

Mulvany: If I could just come back to rats, we find that there appears to be an increased calcium sensitivity which could account for increased calcium permeability of the SHR vessels, and if that's the case, then I think one would expect the calcium antagonists to have a greater effect in the SHR than in the normotensive, and this could be the same in humans.

MacGregor: The other problem is that calcium antagonists partially block the action of vasoconstrictors such as norepinephrine and angiotensin II.

Brody: I'd like to comment on a human syndrome which might well be explored in this problem, that is the condition known as neurogenic hypernatremia. It is caused by hypothalamic tumors in the same region of the brain as the AV3V lesion is made in rats. There are remarkable similarities between the effect seen in man and rat. Like rats, the human subjects lack thirst and maintain chronic hypernatremia. I don't know whether they lack a natriuretic factor but AV3V-lesion rats do lack the normal ability to secrete a natriuretic factor in response to volume and sodium expansion.[1] Gruber and Buckalew made such measurements for us and were unable to detect such a factor in the lesioned rats that had an abnormal natriuretic response. The normal rats, which exhibited a brisk natriuresis, did have a detectable factor. So my specific suggestion for those who may be working in this area with human subjects is: if you run across subjects with hypothalamic tumors, they would represent an excellent human model to test for the actions of the proposed inhibitor.

Erdmann: Your hypothesis stands and falls on the presence of such an inhibitor. You said that it has a very high affinity to guinea pig kidney. I have measured this enzyme in the guinea pig kidney and it is not very susceptible to ouabain, it's more than ten times less susceptible than most human organs. So I think, as this is so important, you should tell us something more about your inhibitor. Is it boilable and still have effect and potency, does it have a positive ionotropic effect, as you have so often paralleled it to ouabain and, if it is in such high potency, shouldn't it have cardiac effects which are pronounced?

MacGregor: Professor de Wardener and Dr. Clarkman are working on the structure of urinary natriuretic extract. I would point out that the cytochemical bioassays are using intact cultured cells. I think that probably this inhibitor is working through a cell receptor, whereas ouabain directly inhibits the enzyme. I think it's very unlikely that a hormone would directly inhibit an enzyme. I'm not aware of any hormone that does that.

Overbeck: I noticed that your group feels that the low renin essential hypertensives most likely have this defect and you described this as a defect in genetic hypertension. My first question is, do you know of any evidence that would suggest that low renin essential hypertension is in fact, genetic, and my second question is, the nifedipine response that you've seen, is that more pronounced in essential hypertensives with low renin?

MacGregor: I can't directly answer the first question. It's been established for many years that hypertension is inherited. I'm not aware of any studies showing that low renin against normal renin is more or less inherited. In general terms, certainly our experience is that the higher the blood pressure and the longer the patient has had high blood pressure, excluding malignant hypertension, the lower the renin. On the whole, therefore, the low-renin patients are the more severe hypertensives. We're excluding high-renin and malignant patients. Now to answer your second question, yes, there is an inverse relationship between renin and response to nifedipine - in other words the lower the renin the greater the response - but there's a much better correlation with the blood pressure than the renin status.

Haddy: I'd like to come back to the influence of plasma on norepinephrine uptake into the nerve terminals. Dr. Freas and Dr. Muldoon have recently used the Vanhoutte preparation of the dog

---

[1] Bealer SL, Haywood JR, Gruber KA, et al.: Preoptic-hypothalamic periventricular lesions reduce natriuresis to volume expansion. *Amer. J. Physiol.* (in press).

saphenous vein and have shown that plasma from the normal anesthetized dog inhibits the uptake of norepinephrine into the nerve terminals. It's a heat-stable small molecular weight substance.

MacGregor: I think that's fascinating.

Haeusler: You are using a coupled assay for the determination of the hypothetical factor. In other words, you do not measure directly the inhibition of sodium-potassium ATPase but the increase in glucose-6-phosphate dehydrogenase activity. What are your control experiments to exclude that, for instance, the hypothetical factor disturbs the normally occurring coupling between ATPase and glucose-6-phosphate dehydrogenase activity?

MacGregor: What we have done is use simultaneous assays with ouabain and the purified natriuretic extract from the urine. When you add either the natriuretic extract or ouabain there is inhibition of sodium-potassium ATPase at the same time as there is a stimulation of glucose-6-phosphate de-hydrogenase. However, we are using an indirect assay and I agree that we should be cautious in our interpretation.

Abboud: Did you do the reverse experiment in the low renin hypertensive animal - take away salt and see whether the plasma factor would disappear or be reduced?

MacGregor: We did a few hypertensives initially on high and low sodium diet and there was a small reduction, with five days of a low sodium diet, in the ability of the plasma to stimulate glucose-6-phosphate dehydrogenase but it still remained very high. I think the mechanism causing a fall in blood pressure with reduction of sodium intake in essential hypertension is probably different from the mechanism whereby blood pressure is raised. Remember it takes many years for blood pressure to rise. If you put a patient on a low sodium diet, the blood pressure, is down within a few days, so that I think that's more related to a less reactive renin system.

THE ROLE OF SODIUM–CALCIUM EXCHANGE IN THE GENESIS OF ESSENTIAL HYPERTENSION

MORDECAI P. BLAUSTEIN

INTRODUCTION

The central role of sodium in the genesis of essential hypertension is well documented in the literature. A striking correlation between dietary sodium and the incidence of essential hypertension in various populations has long been recognized. Indeed, sodium restriction or the administration of a natriuretic agent frequently serves as appropriate and adequate therapy to control blood pressure in hypertensive individuals.

Objective evidence of defective sodium metabolism can often be obtained in the form of elevated intracellular sodium levels in patients with essential hypertension. This is most easily determined in red blood cells and white blood cells (see below).

The aforementioned considerations indicate why it is so important to understand the role of sodium as a causative agent in this disease, which is so prevalent in accultured societies such as those of the United States and Western European countries. Recently, a comprehensive hypothesis of the genesis of essential hypertension was enunciated [1-3]. This hypothesis provides a rational explanation for the role of sodium in the manifestation of the disease. In this article, I review the hypothesis, focusing on the possible peripheral vascular mechanisms that produce the increased vascular resistance in hypertension.

THREE KEY FACTORS IN ESSENTIAL HYPERTENSION

There appear to be three key factors in the genesis of essential hypertension [3]: a genetic factor, a humoral factor, and an environmental factor (namely, sodium). Superimposed on these factors is a poorly understood resetting of the circulatory reflex mechanisms that normally help to maintain the blood pressure within a limited dynamic range.

The inherited factor may be a defect in the body's ability to excrete a sodium load. Although such a defect remains to be identified in humans with the disease, the Dahl sodium-sensitive strain of rats may be an excellent model system in which to explore this possibility [3]. Chronic renal transplantation experiments have demonstrated that, in the Dahl rats, the primary defect appears to reside in the kidneys [4, 5]. Transplantation of kidneys from salt-sensitive to salt-resistant rats renders the latter salt-sensitive. Conversely, replacement of kidneys in a salt-sensitive rat with those from a salt-resistant rat renders the former insensitive to salt. These findings suggest that even if the genetic defect (e.g., a transport abnormality) is present in tissues other than the kidney, its presence must be inconsequential for the expression of hypertension. As discussed elsewhere in this symposium, at least two transport defects in erythrocytes (in furosemide-sensitive Na/K co-transport, and in Na-Li countertransport) have been described and could, perhaps, serve as genetic markers for essential hypertension. But, unless these defects contribute to reduced renal Na excretion, they may not be responsible for the expression of the hypertension. Indeed, a furosemide-sensitive Na/K/Cl co-transport at the apical (luminal) borders of renal tubular epithelial cells appears to participate in the resorption of Na and Cl. A defect in this transport system might be expected to *increase,* rather than decrease, Na excretion; moreover, furosemide may induce natriuresis by inhibiting this transport system. (Note, however, that it is not known whether or not the erythrocyte and renal Na/K co-transport systems are identical.)

With an inherited (renal) defect in sodium excretion, excessive sodium ingestion will tend to increase extracellular fluid volume. The normal homeostatic responses may then be reduced renin and aldosterone secretion and increased secretion of a hormone that promotes sodium excretion, namely, natriuretic hormone [6]. This could be the humoral factor first recognized by Dahl in his rat model of essential hypertension [7]. This hormone may inhibit sodium reabsorption by blocking sodium pumps at the peritubular (basolateral) borders of renal tubule cells [8]. Moreover, this could be the agent that greatly enhances excretion of a sodium load in patients with essential hypertension [9]. There is accumulating evidence [10, 11] to support the hypothesis [1, 12] that a circulating sodium transport inhibitor plays a central role in essential hypertension in humans.

Clearly, with a restricted sodium intake, the stimulus for secretion of a natriuretic agent is removed. A large sodium intake may be necessary to raise the level of natriuretic hormone above normal in hypertension-prone individuals who would, otherwise, be unable to excrete this salt load because of an inherited renal defect. (One possibility that should be mentioned in this context is that, perhaps, the receptors for the natriuretic hormone may be reduced or defective in individuals with the predisposition to develop essential hypertension; thus, more hormone than normal may be required to excrete a given salt load.)

One of the problems with this hypothesis is that hypertensive patients rarely exhibit overt fluid retention (and expanded extracellular fluid volume). However, the fact that many hypertensives have low plasma renin levels may, in fact, be further evidence that normal homeostatic mechanisms are effectively compensating to prevent net sodium and fluid retention.

Normally, Na retention is associated with the development of hypertension -

for example, in the deoxycorticosterone (DOCA) + salt model; DOCA with salt restriction does not lead to hypertension. However, there are some conditions in which marked Na retention is not associated with hypertension: one is so-called 'essential hypernatremia' in man [13], and another occurs in animals with lesions in the anteroventral hypothalamus adjacent to the third ventricle [14]. Indeed, most patients with essential hypernatremia appear to have intracranial lesions in the region of the hypothalamus [13]. Perhaps most relevant is the finding that the anteroventral hypothalamic lesions in rats can be used to treat or prevent Na-dependent hypertension (e.g., associated with renal lesions, DOCA treatment, or genetic defects, as in the Dahl rats) [14]. These observations may bear on the independent evidence that natriuretic hormone is secreted in the brain and probably in the hypothalamus [6].

NATRIURETIC HORMONE INHIBITS SODIUM TRANSPORT IN NONRENAL CELLS

Thirty years ago, Tobian and Binion [15] showed that the sodium content of arterial smooth muscle was elevated in hypertension. During the past twenty years, numerous investigators have documented the fact that the sodium concentration in erythrocytes and leucocytes is elevated in patients with essential hypertension [16-18]. Recently, Poston et al [11] demonstrated that blood plasma from hypertensive patients contains a substance that inhibits sodium transport in leukocytes from normal individuals; this could, of course, provide the explanation for the elevated sodium content in the various cells from hypertensive patients.

All of these studies are consistent with the idea that natriuretic hormone levels may be elevated in the plasma of hypertensive patients. This hormone may be the agent responsible for the high intracellular sodium concentrations in various types of cells, including vascular smooth muscle cells, in these individuals. Furthermore, it is important to stress the fact that the sodium-concentration gradient will be reduced in the cells that are affected because plasma sodium concentrations remain normal in these patients.

In chronic hypertension, the arterial walls are thickened. Although the smooth muscle cells often appear hypertrophied, there is also usually a substantial thickening of the connective tissue. This thickening is frequently referred to as 'waterlogging' because much Na and water may be retained in the extracellular matrix. As a result of this arterial wall thickening, there is a consequent narrowing of the lumen; this may be expected to cause increased peripheral vascular resistance. Therefore, a number of authors have suggested [19, 20] that waterlogging may be the primary defect in essential hypertension. However, although this defect may contribute to the hypertension, two factors indicate that it is probably a consequence and not a cause of the disease: 1) With effective therapy in some hypertensives, the blood pressure may revert to normal levels long before the pathologic changes recede; 2) The venous tissue of hypertensive individuals does not usually exhibit pathological (morphological) changes. Nevertheless, the venous tissue in these patients does exhibit increased contractility and reactivity.

NATRIURETIC HORMONE AND ITS RELATIONSHIP TO THE INCREASED PERIPHERAL VASCULAR RESISTANCE

If there is, indeed, a genetic renal defect and, as a consequence of excessive sodium intake, an elevated level of natriuretic hormone in the plasma of hypertensive patients, a fundamental question remains: How is this translated into the increased peripheral resistance that is the hallmark of hypertension? Two hypotheses have been put forth to explain this interrelationship between elevated natriuretic hormone levels and increased peripheral vascular resistance. According to the hypothesis of Haddy and Overbeck [12, 21, 22], the main manifestation of the circulating sodium-pump inhibitor may be a steady depolarization of the vascular smooth muscle cells. Vascular smooth muscle cells have voltage-regulated Ca channels [23, 24], and depolarization should enhance their permeability to calcium. As a result, calcium influx would increase because the large electrochemical gradient for calcium, across the plasma membrane, favors calcium entry; this causes the cytoplasmic calcium concentration to rise, thereby promoting muscle contraction. Haddy and Overbeck attribute the depolarization to inhibition of the electrogenic sodium pumps in the smooth muscle cells [25]. However, as pointed out elsewhere [26], the Haddy-Overbeck hypothesis is implausible on theoretical grounds. There can be no significant reduction in the electrogenic sodium pump's contribution to the resting-membrane potential in the steady state, when the pumps are only partially inhibited. This is due to the fact that, when the pumps are partially inhibited, the pumped sodium efflux (including the electrogenic component) must rise until the efflux again equals the leak influx. This will occur when the cell sodium concentration rises appropriately.

Additional evidence that is inconsistent with the Haddy-Overbeck hypothesis comes, in part, from the work of Haddy and his colleagues [27]. They found, and we have confirmed [2], that raising the extracellular potassium concentration from normal range (4-6 mM) to 12-15 mM induces a 'paradoxical' relaxation in vascular smooth muscle. It is 'paradoxical' because this increase in extracellular potassium should depolarize the arterial smooth muscle cells by about 5-6 mV [28] and might thereby activate the voltage-regulated calcium channels in the plasma membrane. The fact that relaxation, rather than contraction, occurs with this depolarization implies that the threshold voltage for activating the calcium channels is more than 5-6 mV positive to the resting potential. An explanation that fits the data better is that the increase in extracellular potassium stimulates the sodium pump and thereby reduces intracellular sodium; this will result in a decrease in intracellular calcium and will therefore promote vascular smooth muscle relaxation (see below).

The alternative hypothesis is that it is this rise in cytoplasmic sodium concentration, *per se,* that contributes to the increased peripheral vascular resistance [1, 2]. There are several possible ways in which this may occur, and each must be evaluated in turn.

One possibility is that the natriuretic hormone also inhibits sodium pumps in sympathetic neurons. In this case, the reduced sodium gradient across the plasma membrane of sympathetic nerve terminals may then contribute to the increased sympathetic tone that apparently plays a role in hypertension. This will result from the fact that, in nerve terminals, sodium and calcium transport are coupled by a counterflow transport mechanism; e.g., sodium ions enter in exchange for exiting calcium. Because of the operation of the Na-Ca exchange mechanism, which is diagrammed in Figure 1, the calcium-concentration gradient across the

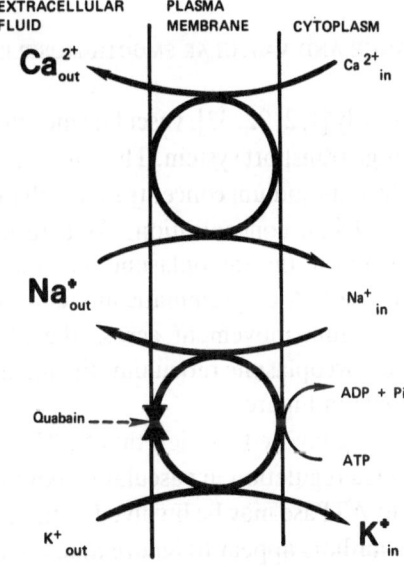

Figure 1. Diagram illustrating the parallel sodium pump (lower) and sodium-calcium exchange (upper) transport systems that function in the nerve terminals and in vascular smooth muscle. The sodium pump utilizes energy from ATP hydrolysis to accumulate potassium and extrude sodium, thereby maintaining a large electrochemical gradient for sodium. The energy from the latter gradient can then be used to power calcium extrusion via the sodium-calcium exchange mechanism. Because of this, the limiting calcium electrochemical gradient will depend upon the sodium gradient; the precise relationship will depend upon the Na:Ca stoichiometry (i.e., the number of sodium ions exchanged for each calcium). In many types of cells the stoichiometry appears to be about 3 Na:1 Ca, which would be sufficient to maintain the free intracellular calcium concentration in the physiological range [29, 30]. An interesting feature of these transport systems (see diagram and text) is that sardiotonic steroids, such as ouabain, selectively inhibit the sodium pump and do *not* directly affect the sodium-calcium exchange mechanism.

plasma membrane will be tightly linked to the sodium-concentration gradient. Therefore, a reduction in the sodium gradient - for example, as a result of a rise in cell sodium - will cause the cytoplasmic calcium concentration to rise as well [29]. Then, because neurotransmitter release is triggered by a rise in the cytoplasmic calcium concentration, we might expect both tonic (spontaneous) as well as depolarization-evoked catecholamine release to be enhanced. This increased transmitter release could be expected to activate the smooth muscle contraction to a greater extent than normal. Obviously, increased contraction of the smooth muscle in the walls of the small resistance vessels will directly increase peripheral vascular resistance. It even seems possible that these cellular mechanisms might contribute to enhanced central sympathetic nervous system activity, although the situation in the CNS must surely be much more complex.

These cannot be the only mechanisms, however, because there is considerable evidence that vascular smooth muscle reactivity (the contractile response to a given stimulus) is enhanced in patients with hypertension [31]. Thus, the smooth muscle itself must be altered.

SODIUM-CALCIUM EXCHANGE AND VASCULAR SMOOTH MUSCLE TONE

As we have shown previously [1, 2, 32, 33], vascular smooth muscle also possesses a sodium-calcium exchange transport system. Therefore, in this tissue, too, a rise in the cytoplasmic steady-state sodium concentration will produce a concomitant rise in the cytoplasmic calcium concentration. As a result, there will also be increased storage of calcium in the sarcoplasmic reticulum (i.e., both free and stored calcium levels will rise). A diagrammatic model of the cell that illustrates the main pathways of calcium movement across the plasma membrane and limiting membrane of the sarcoplasmic reticulum, the main intracellular calcium storage organelle, is shown in Figure 2.

A few authors [34, 35] have favored the view that Na/Ca exchange does not play an important role in cell Ca regulation in vascular smooth muscle, and favor the view that a Ca-dependent ATPase may be involved as the dominant Ca transport system. However, these authors appear to ignore much of the available data [1], including the observation that a portion of the Ca efflux is directly dependent on external Na [32]. Moreover, partial inhibition of the Na pump, with K reduction or ouabain addition, which should raise intracellular Na, sensitizes vascular smooth muscle to agonists such as norepinephrine. These data support the view that Na/Ca exchange plays an important role in the regulation of intracellular calcium in vascular smooth muscle.

In smooth muscle, as in other types of muscle, the immediate trigger for contraction is appropriate elevation of the cytoplasmic free (ionized) calcium concentration [35]. However, vascular smooth muscle is known to maintain constant tension or 'tone' [37]. Two possible mechanisms could account for this

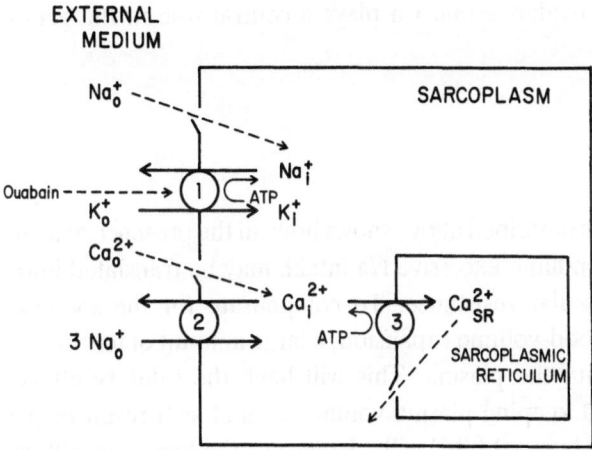

Figure 2. Diagram of vascular smooth muscle cell illustrating the mechanisms that appear to play a major role in the regulation of free cytoplasmic (sarcoplasm) calcium. 1. ATP-dependent, ouabain-sensitive, Na-K exchange pump. 2. Plasma membrane Na/Ca exchange mechanisms. 3. Sarcoplasmic reticulum ATP-dependent Ca pump. The route of calcium entry through the plasma membrane (shown as a gated pathway with rate coefficient k_2) can be inhibited by verapamil and nifedipine (see text). From Blaustein [1], with permission.

tone: 1) The steady-state free-calcium concentration may be maintained above contraction threshold, so that the muscle fibers are always partially contracted, or 2) There may be spontaneous, asynchronous activation of the smooth muscle fibers so that, at any given moment, at least some of the fibers are partially or completely contracted. With either mechanism, the increased cytoplasmic calcium that would result from the sodium-pump inhibition and the rise in cell sodium would be expected to increase vascular smooth muscle tone and contractility. As mentioned above, the increased tone is manifested as an increase in peripheral resistance and observed as an elevation of blood pressure. Vascular smooth muscle tension is a graded function of the calcium concentration [36]. Therefore, if the calcium concentration is constantly maintained above the contraction threshold, any increase in the calcium level will be immediately translated into an increase in tension. However, if the second explanation for tone (i.e., spontaneous, asynchronous activity) is correct, then the calcium that enters the cytoplasm from the extracellular fluid and/or the intracellular stores (sarcoplasmic reticulum) during depolarization will be superimposed on an elevated baseline. Moreover, if the stores are more fully saturated than normal, more Ca will be released from the intracellular stores in response to a given stimulus. The net result will be a higher free-Ca level and, therefore, greater tension than normal when the smooth muscle fibers are activated under these circumstances.

Agents that block calcium entry into vascular smooth muscle, such as verapamil and nifedipine [38], are often effective in treating hypertension. This may be additional evidence that Ca plays a central role in the genesis of essential hypertension.

SUMMARY

The hypothesis described above shows how, in the presence of an inherited defect in renal Na handling, excessive Na intake may be translated into an increase in peripheral vascular resistance. To compensate for the sodium overload and tendency to blood-volume expansion, a large amount of natriuretic hormone will be secreted into the plasma. This will have the salutary effect of promoting natriuresis and keeping plasma volume normal as a result of the inhibition of sodium pumps in renal tubal cells. However, the hormone will, as a side-effect, inhibit sodium pumps in other cells as well. Unfortunately, as a consequence of the inhibition of sodium pumps in vascular smooth muscle cells (and, perhaps, sympathetic-nerve terminals), the sodium concentration in these cells will rise. Then, as a result of sodium-calcium exchange, the calcium concentration in these cells will also increase. This rise in cell-Ca will be translated, either directly or indirectly, into an increase in vascular smooth muscle tone. Thus, peripheral vascular resistance and, therefore, blood pressure will increase.

Perhaps the most interesting feature of this hypothesis is that it lends itself directly to experimental testing and verification. Clearly, we should look for: 1) a specific inherited defect in renal tubular handling of sodium; 2) identification and isolation of the natriuretic hormone, and proof of its elevation in the plasma of patients with essential hypertension; 3) proof that the natriuretic hormone inhibits sodium pumps, including those in vascular smooth muscle cells; and, 4) more direct evidence that the sodium-calcium exchange-mechanism functions in vascular smooth muscle cells.

As outlined here, the hypothesis does not explain why the normal circulatory-reflex-control mechanisms can no longer maintain the blood pressure in the normal range when the vascular smooth muscle tone is increased. Clearly, the control mechanisms must be reset to a new, higher dynamic range of blood pressures. This may occur when the primary increase in peripheral vascular tone (due to Ca gain by the cells) prevents adequate reflex relaxation of the arterial smooth muscle by reduction of sympathetic discharge. Clearly, this aspect deserves further investigation.

ACKNOWLEDGMENTS

I thank Dr. J.M. Hamlyn for critical comments on the manuscript and Ms. M. Tate for preparing the typescript. Supported by NSF grant PCM-7911704 and a grant from the Muscular Dystrophy Association.

REFERENCES

1. Blaustein MP: Sodium ions, blood pressure regulation and hypertension: A reassessment and a hypothesis. Am J Physiol 232:C165-C173, 1977.
2. Blaustein MP: How does sodium cause hypertension? An hypothesis, in Zumkley H, Losse H (editors): Intracellular Electrolytes and Arterial Hypertension. Stuttgart, Georg Thieme Verlag, 1980, pp 151-157.
3. De Wardener HE, MacGregor GA: Dahl's hypothesis that a saluretic substance may be responsible for a sustained rise in arterial pressure: Its possible role in essential hypertension. Kidney Int 18:1-9, 1980.
4. Tobian L, Coffee K, McCrea P, et al: Comparison of the antihypertensive potency of kidneys from one strain of rats susceptible to salt hypertension and kidneys from another strain resistant to it, abstracted. J Clin Invest 45:1080, 1966.
5. Dahl LK, Heine M, Thompson K: Genetic influences of the kidney on blood pressure. Evidence from chronic homografts in rats with opposite predispositions to hypertension. Circ Res 34:94-101, 1974.
6. De Wardener HE: The control of sodium secretion. Am J Physiol 235:F163-F173, 1978.
7. Dahl LK, Knudsen DKD, Heine M, et al: Effects of chronic excess salt ingestion. Genetic influence on the development of salt hypertension in parabiotic rats: Evidence of a humoral factor. J Exp Med 126:687-699, 1967.
8. Fine LG, Bourgoignie JJ, Hwang KH: On the influence of natriuretic factor from patients with chronic uremia on the bioelectrical properties and sodium transport of the isolated mammalian collecting tubule. J Clin Invest 58:590-597, 1976.
9. Viskoper JR, Czaczkes JW, Schwartz N, et al.: Natriuretic activity of a substance isolated from human urine during excretion of a salt load. Comparison of hypertensive and normotensive subjects. Nephron 8:540-548, 1971.
10. Edmondson RP, MacGregor GA: Leucocyte cation transport in essential hypertension: Its relation to the renin-angiotensin system. Br Med J 282:1267-1269, 1981.
11. Poston L, Sewell RB, Wilkinson SP, et al.: Evidence of circulating sodium transport inhibitor in essential hypertension. Br Med J 282:847-849, 1981.
12. Haddy FJ, Overbeck HW: The role of humoral agents in volume expanded hypertension. Life Sci 19:935-948, 1976.
13. Ross EJ, Christie SBM: Hypernatremia. Medicine 48:441-473, 1969.
14. Brody MJ, Fink GD, Buggy J, et al.: The role of the anteroventral third ventricle (AV3V) region in experimental hypertension. Circ Res 43(suppl I):I2-I13, 1978.
15. Tobian L, Binion JT: Tissue cations and water in arterial hypertension. Circulation 5:754-758, 1952.
16. Losse H, Wehmeyer H, Wessels F: Der Wasser- und Elektrolytgehalt von Erythrozyten bei arterieller Hypertonie. Klin Wochenschr 38:393-395, 1960.
17. Von Gessler U: Intra- und extracellulare Elektrolytveranderungen bei essentieller Hypertonie vor und nach Behandlung. Z kreislaufforsch 51:177-183, 1962.
18. Edmondson RPS, Thomas RD, Hilton PJ, et al.: Abnormal leukocyte composition and sodium transport in essential hypertension. Lancet 1:1003-1005, 1975.
19. Folkow B, Hallbock M, Lundgren Y, et al.: Importance of adaptive changes in vascular design for establishment of primary hypertension studied in man and in spontaneously hypertensive rats. Circ Res 32/33(suppl 1):1-16, 1973.
20. Folkow B: Cardiovascular structural adaptation: Its role in the initiation and maintenance of primary hypertension. Glin Sci Mol Med 55(suppl 4):1-20, 1978.
21. Haddy FJ, Pamnani M, Clough D: The sodium-potassium pump in volume expanded hypertension. Clin Exp Hypertens 1:295-336, 1979.
22. Overbeck HT: The sodium pump in cardiovascular muscle in hypertension: Whose hypothesis?

270

Clin Exp Hypertens 1:551-556, 1979.

23. Fleckenstein A: Specific pharmacology of calcium in myocardium, cardiac pacemakers and vascular smooth muscle. Annu Rev Pharmacol Toxicol 17:149-166, 1977.

24. Johansson B, Somlyo AP: Electrophysiology and excitation-contraction coupling, in Bohr DF, Somlyo AP, Sparks HV (editors): Handbook of Physiology, Section 2. The Cardiovascular System, Volume II. Vascular Smooth Muscle. Bethesda, MD, American Physiological Society, 1980, pp 301-323.

25. Hendrickx H, Casteels R: Electrogenic sodium pump in arterial smooth muscle cells. Pflugers Arch 346:299-306, 1974.

26. Blaustein MP: What is the link between vascular smooth muscle sodium pumps and hypertension? Clin Exp Hypertens 3:173-178, 1981.

27. Chen WT, Brace RA, Schott JB, et al.: The mechanism of the vasodilator action of potassium. Proc Soc Exp Biol Med 140:820-824, 1972.

28. Casteels R, Kitamura K, Kuriyama H, et al.: Excitation-contraction coupling in the smooth muscle cells of the rabbit main pulmonary artery. J Physiol (Lond) 271:63-79, 1977.

29. Blaustein MP: The interrelationship between sodium and calcium fluxes across cell membranes. Rev Physiol Biochem Pharmacol 70:33-82, 1974.

30. Blaustein MP, Nelson MT, Sodium-calcium exchange: Its role in the regulation of cell calcium, in Carafoli E (editor): Calcium Transport Across Biological Membranes. New York, Academic Press, 1982.

31. Mendelowitz M: Vascular reactivity in systemic arterial hypertension. Am Heart J 85:252-259, 1973.

32. Reuter H, Blaustein MP, Haeusler G: Na-Ca exchange and tension development in arterial smooth muscle. Philos Trans R Soc Lond (Biol) 265:87-94, 1973.

33. Lang S, Blaustein MP: The role of the sodium pump in the control of vascular tone. Circ Res 46:463-470, 1980.

34. Droogmans G, Casteels R: Sodium and calcium interactions in vascular smooth muscle cells of the rabbit ear artery. J Gen Physiol 74:57-70, 1979.

35. Van Breemen C, Aaronson P, Loutzenhiser R: Sodium-calcium interactions in mammalian smooth muscle. Pharmacol Rev 30:167-208, 1979.

36. Filo RS, Bohr DF, Ruegg JC: Glycerinated skeletal and smooth muscle. Calcium and magnesium dependence. Science 147:1581-1583, 1965.

37. Uchida E, Bohr DF: Myogenic tone in isolated perfused resistance vessels. Occurrence among vascular beds and along vascular trees. Circ Res 25:549-555, 1969.

38. Lederballe-Pedersen O, Mikkelsen E, Korneruf HJ, et al.: Effects of nifedipine on blood pressure, regional hemodynamics, plasma renin activity, and plasma catecholamines in patients with arterial hypertension. Acta Med Scand (suppl) 625:65, 1978.

DISCUSSION

Discussants: Langer, Blaustein, Mulvany, Jones

Langer: You showed that the plasma from a low-renin hypertensive patient potentiated the response to norepinephrine in an isolated rabbit blood vessel. Would you see the same effect if cocaine were present under the conditions of your experiment, and have you tried to see whether another agonist like angiotensin that contracts vascular smooth muscle would be equally potentiated?

Blaustein: I don't know whether the experiment with cocaine has been done yet, but we're certainly planning to. It's been done with other agonists. For example, the response to angiotensin II is also potentiated after treatment with hypertensive plasma - so I think it is not a question of reuptake.

Mulvany: It would be very nice if we could demonstrate that the small vessels raised the intracellular sodium that caused contraction and that would tie everything up, but the important thing is what actually happens to small vessels. As far as your results with the aorta are concerned, clearly, we have no argument about them: There certainly seems to be a sodium-calcium exchange mechanism. As regards your indications that there could be a neurogenic effect, we wouldn't disagree there, either. The response of our resistance vessels in potassium-free solution was phentolamine-dependent, and therefore, norepinephrine was probably being released from the nerves. However, as regards your perfusion experiments, I would question whether the intracellular sodium has risen in the low potassium experiments that you describe. Using a perfusion system it must take a certain amount of time for the potassium concentration to change, but the changes that you're seeing are occurring within one minute. Do you have any evidence to support the idea that the intracellular sodium could have changed sufficiently in that time to produce the sort of effects that you're seeing?

Blaustein: We don't have any evidence, but certainly the cells are very small and changes in sodium pump rate would be expected to have a fairly rapid change in cell sodium, but again the effects may be synergistic. That's one of the very interesting features, that may occur, not only one the smooth muscle cells, but also on the small nerve terminals. However, I should point out that, in most experiments, the aortic strips were treated with plasma for several minutes before the agonists were applied.

Mulvany: Clearly, it would be important for someone to try and measure the intracellular sodium and see whether it is changing quickly or not.

Blaustein: The measurement of intracellular sodium with electrodes has been done in cardiac muscle. When you change extracellular sodium, for example, or inhibit the sodium pump, the changes are very rapid and those cells are much larger than the vascular smooth muscle cells. If you change extracellular sodium, you do see changes in intracellular sodium within seconds.

Mulvany: When you used 11.8 millimole external potassium, you got a relaxation, and you then referred to electrophysiological data that was made on large vessels.

Blaustein: Rabbit ear artery.

Mulvany: It is my recollection that Dr. Hermsmeyer has measured membrane potential as a function of extracellular potassium in rat-tail artery, and I believe the curve was shifted somewhat to the right compared to the data you showed.

Blaustein: It would be ideal to do these experiments with small blood vessels. Certainly the best way to do them would be *in situ* with flowing blood.

Mulvany: And the last point is that your perfusion experiments were done in the presence of plasma. You had dog red cells present in the perfusate.

Blaustein: There were dog red cells in order to raise the oxygen tension. We used them because we wanted cells with low potassium concentrations, so that if we had a slight hemolysis, we wouldn't raise the potassium too much.

Mulvany: You said that this effect induced a small increase in perfusion pressure. In other words, we're dealing with a situation where there is tone already present.

Blaustein: Absolutely. And if there was no tone we did have preparations where we could see virtually nothing and as soon as we raised tone with norepinephrine we began to see an effect with changing potassium concentration.

Jones: We did attempt some years ago to look at the role of sodium-calcium exchange. I felt it might play a role in cell-volume regulation, because when one puts ouabain on the teniae coli or other smooth muscles, the ion gradients dissipate and yet there's only about a 10 percent swelling. If one then reduces calcium one can show quite a large amount of swelling and the one idea I had was that perhaps there is a sodium-calcium exchange with calcium going in and moving three sodium or two sodium out that would work osmotically. The cells did not accumulate much calcium nor remain contracted. What roles do other Ca transport systems play, and what is the relative importance of those and Na-Ca exchange?

Blaustein: The observations that you have just mentioned fit with those of Deitman and Ellis[1] in cardiac muscle. They obtained evidence for an exchange of entering calcium for exiting sodium.[2] In addition, there is certainly evidence that there's another calcium transport system that I haven't discussed, namely the calcium ATPase. There are two calcium ATPases, one is certainly in sarcoplasmic reticulum, and that could play some role in relaxing cells that have gained a lot of calcium if they're not continuing to gain calcium. On the other hand, there's evidence for a calcium ATPase in plasma membranes of many cells. The key question is: What are the relative roles of the two kinds of transport systems in the plasma membrane for controlling cell calcium? That's been a very difficult question to answer. In some cells, where you can look at even moderate perturbations in the sodium distribution, there is a concomitant change in cell calcium, as predicted by the sodium-calcium exchange model (see Blaustein and Nelson[3]; Shem and Fozzard[4]). The way to tell what's happening would be to have a calcium electrode and a sodium electrode in the cells. The evidence in cardiac muscle is that when you make small changes in the sodium gradient the calcium gradient goes along, but the evidence just isn't there for smooth muscle. I tried to describe some effects with moderate changes in the sodium gradient, or what we think would produce changes in the sodium gradient, that appeared to have a dominant effect because they alter the contraction as an indirect measure of the level of calcium in the cell. And clearly these are all indirect effects and we need much more direct experimentation.

[1] Deitman, Ellis: *J. Physiol* 277:437-453, 1978.
[2] Baker PF, et al.: *J Physiol* 200:431-458, 1969.
[3] Blaustein MP, Nelson MT: In *Membrane Transport of Calcium:* E Carfoli, editor, London, Academic Press, 1982, pp. 217-236.
[4] Shen SS, Fozzard: *J Gen Physiol,* in press.

II. NEURAL CONTROL OF BLOOD PRESSURE

INTRODUCTION: NEURAL CONTROL

F. Abboud

Exciting new concepts have emerged in the last decade, implicating the sympathetic nervous system in the pathogenesis and maintenance of arterial pressure in many different types of hypertension.

1. One concept relates to the fact that the sympathetic nervous system does not only cause hypertension through the vasoconstrictor influence of the released neurotransmitter, but may contribute to a chronic hypertensive state, through a trophic influence on vascular smooth muscle favoring hypertrophy, or through an effect on vascular membranes inducing electrical events which may facilitate depolarization and augment contraction.

2. Another important concept relates to the increasing appreciation of the complexity of the determinants of a sympathetic vasoconstrictor response. Three main components regulate reflex sympathetic responses:

a. An *afferent* component, with input from various receptors throughout the vascular system and various parts of the body such as skeletal muscle and viscerae, may modulate vasomotor and cardiac neurons in the brain stem. Defects in the sensitivity of arterial baroreceptors, cardiac sensory afferents or, as suggested more recently, of renal afferents as well as somatic afferents could play a determining role in the rate of firing of central neurons and the sympathetic response.

b. The *central* neurons which form the 'central substrate' of sympathetic drive and include not only neurons in the brain stem but in the forebrain and higher centers. This area of exploration has been immensely complex but of great importance. The role of hypothalamic regions in maintaining the arterial blood pressure in various models of hypertension, ranging from genetic to renal hypertension, underlines the almost ubiquitous involvement of the sympathetic nervous system in any type of hypertension regardless of the initiating cause.

Not only specific regions in the brain are being mapped out for their effects on sympathetic drive, but also the identification of various neuropeptides and monoamines as transmitters or facilitators of transmission is a major area of investigation where the available information is almost at a primitive level.

c. The *efferent* arm of the reflex is a third component. The role of various presynaptic receptors in regulating the amount of neurotransmitter released during stimulation is now defined with more specificity. Defects in the pre- and postsynaptic receptors in different models of hypertension are being identified, and the complexity and scope of the different types of receptors which can modulate norepinephrine release is of great magnitude. The responsiveness of vascular muscle to the released norepinephrine may be linked to a genetic defect in vascular muscle membranes related to cation transport, which in turn determines the electrical events preceding contraction.

3. A third important concept linking the sympathetic nervous system and hypertension has to do with the fact that the sympathetic nervous system is implicated in not only 'neurogenic hypertension' but in genetic types of hypertension as well as in renal hypertension.

In the various genetic types of hypertension, for example, the Dahl salt-sensitive strain or the SHR, there appears to be a greater degree of sympathetic drive, particularly under stressful psychological influences or during salt loading. In the Dahl salt-sensitive strain, the administration of salt increases sympathetic drive. A parallel phenomenon may exist in borderline hypertensive humans who are salt sensitive, but not in normotensive humans. Whether the exaggerated sympathetic response in the genetic hypertensives exposed to an increased salt intake represents the release of a depolarizing 'natriuretic factor' is another challenging area for future investigation.

Similarly, in renal hypertension the sympathetic influence is predominant. The link between the kidney and the central nervous system may be through the central action of angiotensin or through visceral sensory afferents within the kidney itself, which may function as baroreceptors in concert with or following the resetting of the arterial or cardiac receptors. Another renal connection to the sympathetic nervous system may be through the release of a vasodepressor humoral substance from the kidney exposed to a sudden rise in pressure. This substance, which may be analogous to the renomedullary depressor lipids, inhibits sympathetic discharge through an effect on the peripheral or central nervous system, and certainly requires further exploration.

The Symposium on Neural Control of Blood Pressure explores some of the recent advances in the three concepts highlighted above. It will be evident from the presentations that the involvement of the sympathetic system is critical in almost any type of hypertension and that the involvement may be linked directly to genetic, renal as well as neurogenic hypertensive states.

EVIDENCE FOR THE PARTICIPATION OF SPECIFIC HYPO-THALAMIC PATHWAYS IN THE PATHOGENESIS OF HYPERTENSION

MICHAEL J. BRODY, DIANE K. HARTLE, R. WALLACE LIND AND ALAN KIM JOHNSON

INTRODUCTION

Previous studies from our laboratories have demonstrated that a small region of anterior hypothalamus plays a critical role in the development and maintenance of a number of different forms of experimental hypertension [1]. These studies focused on the tissue immediately surrounding the most anterior and ventral portions of the third cerebral ventricle. This tissue, referred to as the AV3V region, was first identified as the site of action for the dipsogenic action of angiotensin administered into the ventricular system. Subsequent studies, which demonstrated that the same neural substrates were critical for the centrally mediated pressor effects of angiotensin, led us to examine the influence of lesion of the AV3V region on the development of renin- and nonrenin-dependent forms of renal hypertension, as well as other forms of hypertension with different etiologies. These studies indicated that one- and two-kidney models of renal hypertension, deoxycorticosterone-salt hypertension, neurogenic hypertension produced by lesions of the nucleus tractus solitarius, and hypertension in Dahl salt-sensitive rats could all be prevented or attenuated by AV3V lesions [2].

We have been interested in the neural pathways that are responsible for mediating the central contribution to the development of hypertension. Several earlier studies have focused on the functional neuroanatomy of pathways originating in the AV3V region. Based on the study by Swanson et al. [3], we examined the effects of lesions in the ventromedial hypothalamus-median eminence region [4] and central gray [5] on regional hemodynamic responses elicited by electrical activation of the AV3V region. Ventromedial hypothalamic lesions attenuated the muscle vasodilation and splanchnic vasoconstriction produced by AV3V stimulation. In studies carried out in animals with chronic lesions of the same area, the pressor response to centrally administered angiotensin was abolished, as was the development of renal hypertension [6]. Central gray lesions also attenuated the cardiovascular effects produced by AV3V stimulation. These results provided functional evidence that pathways carrying vasomotor information from the AV3V region descend through midline periventricular sites in the hypothalamus and mesencephalon.

The purpose of recent studies to be reviewed in this paper was to determine the intrahypothalamic distribution of pathways activated within the AV3V region by chemical and electrical stimulation. The findings indicate that separate pathways mediate the vasomotor responses elicited by electrical and chemical stimulation and that these pathways probably play different functional roles in the expression of several diverse forms of experimental hypertension. A detailed summary of some of these results is found elsewhere [7].

METHODS

Studies were carried out on rats receiving lesions or knife cuts in the rostral hypothalamus. After recovery from surgery required for placement of these lesions, the rats were instrumented for recording arterial pressure in the conscious state using indwelling catheters. The animals also received lateral ventricular cannulas for cerebroventricular administration of angiotensin, carbachol, and hypertonic sodium chloride. In other studies, animals with specific knife cuts were prepared with stimulating electrodes in the AV3V region and were studied under anesthesia for the regional hemodynamic effects of electrical stimulation of this area. Hindquarter, mesenteric, and renal blood flows were recorded using miniaturized pulsed Doppler flow probes according to techniques described elsewhere [8]. The location of lesions and knife cuts was verified in each animal by standard histological techniques. Overlap analysis of these lesions was used to define critical areas of tissue needed for various responses.

RESULTS AND DISCUSSION

Pressor responses produced by central administration of angiotensin were employed initially to determine the anterior hypothalamic pathways critical for the effects of this peptide. Pressor responses to angiotensin were abolished by lesions that included tissue running bilaterally along the lamina terminalis from the organum vasculosum of the lamina terminalis dorsally to the anterior commissure. More caudal lesions near the margin of the preoptic and anterior hypothalamic areas also abolished the pressor response. These data suggested that a pathway necessary for the centrally mediated pressor effect of angiotensin projects along the lamina terminalis and then descends through anterior hypothalamus rostral to the paraventricular nuclei. Knife cuts made horizontally through the proposed descending part of the projections also abolished the responses to angiotensin. Furthermore, these knife cuts attenuated the pressor effect of angiotensin administered intravenously [9].

This anterior hypothalamic knife cut, which attenuates the responses to angiotensin administered either centrally or peripherally, was examined for its effect on several models of experimental hypertension. Of the different models, only renin-dependent hypertension, produced by suprarenal aortic ligation, was attenuated. The one-kidney Grollman model of hypertension, DOCA-salt hypertension, and a neurogenic form of hypertension produced by sinoaortic deafferentation were unaffected by the knife cut. These data suggested that an anterior hypothalamic knife cut in a pathway apparently selective for the central pressor activity of angiotensin specifically attenuates hypertension dependent upon high circulating levels of renin.

More recent data have extended these observations to other central pressor stimuli. The integrated cardiovascular responses produced by electrical stimulation of the AV3V region, consisting of muscle vasodilation and renal and mesenteric vasoconstriction, were unaffected by the knife cut [10]. We speculated that other centrally mediated pressor stimuli, such as carbachol and hypertonic sodium chloride, might use ventral descending pathways from the AV3V region not interrupted by the knife cut. However, only those knife cuts that blocked the angiotensin-induced response were capable of blocking the responses to the two other pressor stimuli. These data could be explained by several types of neuroanatomic organization. For example, cells in the AV3V region containing the receptors for angiotensin might also possess cholinergic and osmotic receptors; or axons from cells, each with different types of receptors, might project through the same region of the hypothalamus.

Although we anticipated that a midline ventral knife cut in the coronal plane along the base of the anterior hypothalamus would abolish the hemodynamic effects of electrical stimulation of the AV3V region, such cuts were ineffective. In contrast, bilateral cuts in the region of the medial forebrain bundle were effective in eliminating the response to electrical stimulation. These data indicate that a pathway completely separate from that required for pressor responses induced by angiotensin, carbachol, or hypertonic sodium chloride originates in or passes through the AV3V region. The physiological role of this projection, which descends bilaterally through ventral rostral hypothalamus, is not known. Our current working hypothesis is that this projection might participate in the development of those forms of hypertension that depend upon the AV3V region, but which are not affected by the anterior hypothalamic knife cut that severs the pathways responsible for chemically induced pressor stimuli and renin-dependent hypertension.

SUMMARY

The anterior hypothalamus contains a complex organization of pressor systems involved in mediating responses to chemical and electrical activation of the AV3V region. A midline pathway projecting from the region of the anterior commissure through the dorsal preoptic region and into the anterior hypothalamus is necessary for pressor responses produced by cerebroventricular admin-

278

istration of angiotensin, carbachol, and hypertonic sodium chloride. Integrity of this pathway is important for the development of renin-dependent forms of experimental hypertension. Other forms of experimental hypertension, such as one-kidney Grollman hypertension, neurogenic hypertension, and DOCA-salt hypertension, are not affected by this knife cut. A second pathway, activated by electrical stimulation of the AV3V region, projects bilaterally in the region of the medial forebrain bundle. The physiological role of this projection and its potential function in experimental hypertension remains to be established.

ACKNOWLEDGMENT

This work was supported in part by USPHS Grants HLB-14388, 5T-3207069, HLB-07021, and 1 R01 HL24102; Research Scientist Development award 1 K02 MH00064; and a gift from the Searle Family Trust.

REFERENCES

1. Brody MJ, Johnson AK: Role of the anteroventral third ventricle region in fluid and electrolyte balance, arterial pressure regulation and hypertension, in Martini L, Ganong WF (editors): Frontiers in Neuroendocrinology. New York, Raven Press, 1980, vol 6, pp 249-292.
2. Brody MJ, Johnson AK: Role of forebrain structures in models of experimental hypertension, in Disturbances in the Neurogenic Control of the Circulation. Clinical Physiological Series. American Physiological Society. Baltimore, Williams & Wilkins, 1980.
3. Swanson LW, Kucharczyk J, Mogenson GJ: Autoradiographic evidence for pathways from the medial preoptic area to the midbrain involved in the drinking response to angiotensin II. J Comp Neurol 178:645, 1978.
4. Fink GD, Buggy J, Haywood JR, et al.: Hemodynamic effects of electrical stimulation of forebrain angiotensin and osmosensitive sites. Am J Physiol 235:H445, 1978.
5. Knuepfer MM, Gordon FJ, Johnson AK, et al.: Identification of descending cardiovascular pathways from the anteroventral third ventricle (AV3V) region. Fed Proc 38:1446, 1979.
6. Johnson AK, Buggy J, Fink GD, et al.: Prevention of renal hypertension and central pressor effect of angiotensin by ventromedial and hypothalamic ablation. Brain Res 205:255-264, 1981.
7. Hartle DK, Lind RW, Johnson AK, et al.: Localization of the anterior hypothalamic AII pressor system. Hypertension, in press.
8. Haywood JR, Shaffer RA, Fastenow C, et al.: Regional blood flow measurement in the conscious rat with a pulsed doppler flowmeter. Am J Physiol 241:H273-H278, 1981.
9. Hartle DK, Johnson AK, Brody MJ: The angiotensin (AII) pressor pathway of the anterior hypothalamus. AHA Scientific Sessions, Dallas, TX, Nov 16-19, 1981. Circulation 64(suppl 4), 1981.
10. Hartle DK, Brody MJ: Vasoconstrictor pathways from the anteroventral third ventricle (AV3V) region. Fed Proc, in press.

DISCUSSION

Discussants: Haeusler, Brody, Denton, Sambhi, Palkovits, Sleight

Haeusler: I have difficulties in understanding that the knife cut which destroys the middle pathway does not affect the pressor response to electrical stimulation of the AV3V region, but that to local angiotensin II or carbachol. Does this mean that the neurons which mediate the effects of angiotensin II or carbachol are unresponsive to electrical stimulation (which is unlikely), or are we dealing with two distinct neuronal systems?

Brody: We share your surprise at the failure of the electrical stimulation to produce the same pattern of response as that induced chemically. We are not at all clear why that should be. One possibility is that we have a receptor mechanism which sends a projection to a neuron that ultimately carries the information. That receptor mechanism may not be easily transduced by electrical means. Thus the neurons may lie some small distance from the periventricular tissue, whereas the receptors may be on the ependymal side of the ventricle. I believe we have a current spread which must include the ependymal region which is accessible to the chemical stimulation, but I don't understand exactly why the proposed ependymal receptors might be resistant to electrical activation.

Denton: I was wondering if you might tell us a little more about the physiological condition of the animals after the AV-3 lesion and their response to other pressor stimuli. As I know you're aware, with the sheep and the ACTH hypertension, the lesion in the AV-3 region has no influence on the hypertension, but it abolishes the dypsogenic response to intercarotid NaCl.

Brody: I'm certainly aware of the recent information about species differences. Animals receiving AV3V lesions immediately lose their thirst. At the same time, they develop inappropriate diuresis and go into a period of weight loss, that we are able to attenuate by giving them sugar solutions instead of pure water to drink. We never study the animals until several weeks after an AV3V lesion, when they are fully recovered and have regained normal drinking, normal fluid and electrolyte status (save chronic hypernatremia), have normal arterial pressures, and are in every way indistinguishable from a normal rat. The pressor responsiveness to peripheral pressor stimuli except angiotensin is normal. Thus similar to what we see with the anterior hypothalamic knife cut, AV3V lesion rats lose the pressor responsiveness to intravenously and centrally administered angiotensin, but responsiveness to vasopressin, norepinephrine, phenylephrine, and so on is completely normal. Myocardial responses of AV3V lesion rats to pressure and volume loads are also normal. So we think that their cardiovascular system is in excellent condition and that their failure to develop high arterial pressure in response to the different interventions is due to interference with centrally mediated hypertensive mechanisms that are quite different for each form of hypertension.

Sambhi: I ask the question with no claim of accuracy of my recollection at all, but in his very early experiments, didn't Goldblatt show that he could produce hypertension in his spinal animals?

Brody: Yes, there are a number of studies indicating that in the absence of the nervous system it is possible to raise arterial pressure by the usual renovascular mechanism. I have never thought of those experiments as excluding a role for the nervous system when the nervous system is intact. In the absence of the nervous system, the lack of baroreflex and other compensatory mechanisms limits the ability to compensate for an increase in arterial pressure and in fact, humorally-induced pressor mechanisms are exaggerated. The data I've shown you point to the possibility that humoral and neural mechanisms interact. Our work on the central nervous system indicates that there is a coupling between a humoral system which originates with a renal enzyme and the central nervous system which contains receptors that can activate neural mechanisms. I conclude that our data and those showing development of renal hypertension in spinal or sympathetectomized animals are not mutually exclusive.

Palkovits: Could you tell me anything about the chemical nature or transmitter nature of these two pathways? And, when you used the L-shaped knife, you transected the major input from the hippocampus and probably from the amygdala to the hypothalamus. Both these regions are good candidates to modulate the hypertension. Have you ever checked these regions?

Brody: Although it is one of our long-term goals, we have no information yet about the neurotransmitters involved in projecting this information. With respect to the second question, we're very interested in other projections which may originate, for example, in the limbic system, and project into the AV3V region. We have not yet done any experiments with amygdala stimulation in rats with the anterior hypothalamic knife cut, but we intend to do that. We do have experiments, however, which indicate that lesions of the central amygdaloid nucleus attenuate the development of hypertension in spontaneously hypertensive rats.[1] We have also studied the responses to electrical activation of the amygdala, and they closely resemble those of AV-3V stimulation (unpublished observation). Finally, we have found that the exaggerated cardiovascular responses in SHR to noise stress, are normalized by a central nucleus lesion.[2]

Sleight: I wanted to ask a slightly nasty question. I am not an expert on rat's brains, but I am worried that the use of U-shaped and T-shaped knives might leave a rather less precise lesion than Derick Denton can do in a bigger brain, such as that of the sheep. Do you think that could have anything to do with the differences?

Brody: No. In fact, I'm struck by some major similarities between species with respect to some of the effects produced by the lesion. He mentioned that sheep lose the dipsogenic response to angiotensin in the same way that rats do, and they also lose some thirst behavior. Other species have behaved similarly with response to their drinking behavior. We now have evidence from the work of Greg Fink that rabbits and cats also show drinking deficits and loss of responses to central angiotensin. In preliminary studies that we have carried out in baboons with Orville Smith at the University of Washington, we found that AV3V lesions also produced the thirst deficit. So there are remarkable similarities between species with respect to the effects of AV3V lesions. It's not yet been sorted out how many of the cardiovascular similarities exist. But returning to the nasty part of your question, we do not think that the lesions are damaging the rat brain in an 'abnormal' way. We use very fine electrodes and we control for sham effects of the lesions by putting the electrodes, down to similar depths, but just above the AV3V region. These sham lesions have no effects on the cardiovascular system or responses to any pressor stimuli. Furthermore, extensive studies using overlap analysis of lesion sites show excellent site specificity.[3] Only those lesions that lie within the AV3V region produce the specific deficits and protection against hypertension that we have described. So I think that's not really a problem.

[1] Galeno TM, Van Hoesen GW, Marxier W, et al.: Contribution of the amygdala to development of spontaneous hypertension. Brain Res. In Press 1982.

[2] Galeno TM, Van Hoessen EW, Brody MJ: Bilateral lesion of central amygdaloid nucleus attenuates hemodynamic responses to noise stress in the spontaneously hypertensive rat (SHR). Society for Neuroscience Abstracts, 1982. (In Press).

[3] Hantle DK, Lind RW, Johnson AK, et al.: Localization of the anterior hypothalamic angiotensin II pressor system. Hypertension 4(Suppl II) II-159-II-165, 1982.

Sleight: In your sham animals, does the knife go in and then just come out rather than circle around?

Brody: The knife cuts are of different kinds. The one I have described here uses an 'L' shaped knife that is first inserted and then rotated through a plane of 180°. We've done many kinds of sham operations where we lower the knife, or a lesioning electrode to very similar depths, but just avoid the critical tissue, and we never get any effects. As I just described, you must invade the critical tissue.

NEUROPEPTIDES IN THE CENTRAL REGULATION OF BLOOD PRESSURE

MIKLOS PALKOVITS

INTRODUCTION

During the last few years, the possible role of neuronal peptides in the central baroreceptor regulatory mechanism has been the subject of considerable attention. Increasing evidence suggests that this mechanism could be partly mediated or controlled by neuropeptides, which are present in nerves, brain areas, and pathways that are known to be involved in cardiovascular regulation. Apart from their neurotransmitter mode of action, certain peptides - vasopressin and angiotensin - could also act as neurohormones; that is, they are released into the cerebrospinal fluid or the blood vessels. Central administration of many neuropeptides alters blood pressure and heart rate [1-8].

The central baroreceptor mechanism is constituted by multineuronal reflex arcs. To investigate and understand the role of neuropeptides in the central baroreceptor regulation, their topographical, cellular, and subcellular localizations in the baroreceptor reflex arc seem to be important.

BARORECEPTOR REFLEX ARC

This reflex arc comprises afferent and efferent fiber systems and baroreceptor centers. One short-loop and one long-loop arc can be distinguished anatomically. The afferent inputs and efferent outputs are the same in both arcs. Whereas in the short-loop reflex arc the baroreceptor inputs are switched over to the vasomoter cells directly, in the long-loop reflex arc higher centers (hypothalamus, limbic system) are inserted between the afferent and efferent fibers establishing the anatomical basis of a wide-range modulation in the baroreceptor regulatory mechanism. The reflex arc comprises:

(a) baroreceptor afferent stimuli conveyed by the aortic depressor and carotic sinus nerves carrying signals from baro- ('stretch') receptors to the medulla oblongata via vagus and glossopharyngeal nerves [9, 10];

(b) the primary baroreceptor center, which is constituted by the medial and caudal subdivisions of the nucleus of the solitary tract (NTS) where afferent inputs are integrating and forwarding;

(c) axons of NTS neurons either to the efferent (vasomotor) cells - short-loop reflex - or to the modulatory centers - ascending portion of the long-loop reflex;

(d) descending pathways from the higher centers to the vasomotor efferent cells, which are located in the medulla oblongata (dorsal vagal nucleus and nucleus ambiguus) and spinal cord (intermediolateral cell column);

(e) efferent preganglionic fibers from the above vasomotor efferent cells, which project to autonomic postganglionic neurons, which in turn project to the heart and vessels.

NEUROPEPTIDES IN THE AFFERENT BARORECEPTOR NERVES

Five neuropeptides (substance P, enkephalin, somatostatin, vasoactive intestinal polypeptide [VIP] and cholecystokinin [CCK]) have been recognized in the vagus nerve by immunocytochemistry [11-13]. Following extracranial or intracranial vagus transections (Table 1), there is a marked fall in substance P concentrations in the baroreceptor subdivisions of the NTS [15]. About 10 to 20% of the vagal fibers are immunostained with antibodies for substance P [11, 12]. A total disappearance of radioimmunoassayable CCK from the NTS one week after bilateral transection of the solitary tract (Table 1) indicates that this peptide in the NTS might be of vagus origin. A small change in VIP levels in the NTS after bilateral

Table 1. Concentrations of certain neuropeptides in the nucleus of the solitary tract after dorsal medullary deafferentation

Concetrations in sham-operated animals (ng/mg protein)		Depletions in percentage of the sham-operated rats		
		Bilateral	Transections (ipsilateral)	Unilateral (contralateral)
VIP*	2.02	− 34.2	− 15.4	− 22.8
Substance P**	4.88	− 74.2[+]	− 59.4[+]	− 18.2
Cholecystokinin†	1.25	n.d.[+]	− 40.0[+]	− 12.5

*   VIP = vasoactive intestinal polypeptide [14]
** Douglas FL, Jew JY, Williams RH et al. (unpublished data)
†   Palkovits M, Kiss JZ, Beinfeld MC et al. (unpublished data)
[+]   P < 0.01
    n.d. = not detectable

denervation (Table 1) suggests that VIP fibers among the baroreceptor afferents are less significant in number if there are any at all.

NEUROPEPTIDE-CONTAINING CELLS IN THE PRIMARY BARORECEPTOR CENTER

By immunocytochemistry, 14 neuropeptides have been visualized in the NTS (Table 2). Concentrations of many of these neuropeptides have also been measured in rats by radioimmunoassays. Data are summarized in Table 3. Neuropeptides are present either in local cells (in perikarya and dendrites) or in nerve terminals both of peripheral (vagal, glossopharyngeal) and central (descending) origins (Table 2). Substance P-, enkephalin-, somatostatin-, VIP-, neurotensin-, avian pancreatic polypeptide [APP]-, and bovine pancreatic polypeptide [BPP]-containing cell bodies have been recognized in the baroreceptor center peptide-containing [14, 17, 19, 20, 23, 26, 27]. All these cells are scattered in and around the NTS. The order of magnitude of the total number ofaning cells is not likely to exceed hundreds, less than 10% of the total, which is about 20,000 of the cells in the NTS [43]. The chemical nature of the majority of NTS cells is still unknown.

ASCENDING FIBERS FROM THE PRIMARY BARORECEPTOR CELLS TO HIGHER CENTERS

A number of brain regions have been suggested to be involved in central baroreceptor mechanisms [9]. These areas, called 'modulatory baroreceptor centers,' are present in the pons (locus ceruleus, parabrachial nuclei), diencephalon

Table 2. Immunocytochemical localization of neuropeptides in the nucleus of the solitary tract

Cell bodies (and terminals)	Only nerve terminals
Substance P [16–18]	Vasopressin [28–30]
Neurotensin [19]	Oxytocin [28–30]
Enkephalin [18, 20–22]	β-Endorphin [31]
Somaostatin [23]	ACTH [32]
VIP [14, 24, 25]	α-MSH[33]
APP [26]	Angiotensin II [34]
BPP [27]	Cholecystokinin* [35, 36]

* Paklovits MP, Kiss JZ, Beinfeld MC et al. (unpublished data)
  VIP = vasoactive intestinal polypeptide
  APP = avian pancreatic polypeptide
  BPP = bovine pancreatic polypeptide
  ACTH = adrenocorticotrophic hormone
  MSH = melanocyte-stimulating hormone

Table 3. Concentrations of certain neuropeptides in the primary baroreceptor center (nucleus of the solitary tract)

	Protein (ng/mg)	Comparison to brain average	References
Somatosatin	4.57–9.71	high	37, 38
Vasopressin	0.50–0.70	low	*
TRH	1.20	high	**
Substance P	3.20	high	39
met-Enkephalin	2.47	high	†
VIP	0.87	moderate	40
Cholecystokinin	1.25	moderate	41
α-MSH	1.07	moderate	33
Bombesin	7.62	very high	42

* Zerbe RL, Palkovits M (unpublished data)
** Eskay RL, Long RE, Palkovits M (unpublished data)
† Epelbaum J, Palkovits M (unpublished data)
  TRH = thyrotropin-releasing hormone
  VIP = vasoactive intestinal polypeptide
  MSH = melanocyte-stimulating hormone

(certain hypothalamic and preoptic nuclei), and telencephalon (amygdala, septum, hippocampus). Various neuroanatomical and electrophysiological techniques furnish evidence that all these regions are directly (monosynaptically) connected with the NTS, since neurons from this baroreceptor center project axons to these regions [9, 43, 44]. The chemical character of these ascending fibers, except those from epinephrine- and norepinephrine-containing cells in and around the NTS (so-called C2 and A2 aminergic cell groups), are unknown. As yet, no ascending peptidergic fibers from the NTS have been visualized. Whether the ascending catecholaminergic fibers are carrying any baroreceptor signals to the modulatory centers is only a matter of speculation at the present time [5, 43, 45].

FIBERS FROM THE BARORECEPTOR CENTER (NTS) TO THE VASOMOTOR CELLS

The NTS, especially its posteromedial and commissural subdivisions, project to the dorsal vagal nucleus, ambiguus nucleus, and to the spinal cord [9, 46]. In the spinal cord, fibers run lateral to the central canal. There is a rich peptidergic network in the intermediolateral cell group (Table 4), but none of the neuropeptides in these terminals has been proved to be of NTS origin. A number of neuropeptides has also been described in the dorsal vagal nucleus (Table 4). The topographical situation can lead to the speculation that the somastatin-, VIP-,

Table 4. Immunocytochemical localization of neuropeptides in the baroreceptor vasomotor centers

Medullary preganglionic cell group (dorsal vagal nucleus)		Spinal preganglionic cell group (intermediolateral cells)
Cell bodies (and terminals)	Only nerve terminals	Only nerve terminals
Substance P[17]	Vasopressin [28–30]	Vasopressin [28, 29]
APP [26]	Oxytocin [28–30]	Oxytocin [28, 29, 48]
	Enkephalin [20, 22]	Enkephalin [21]
	Somatostatin [23]	Somatostatin [49]
	VIP*	APP [26]
	Angiotensin II [34]	Angiotensin II [34]
	TRH [47]	Substance P [17]
	Neurotensin [19]	

* Palkovits M, Leranth C (unpublished data)
 APP = avian pancreatic polypeptide
 VIP = vasoactive intestinal polypeptide
 TRH = thyrotropin-releasing hormone

and neurotensin-containing nerve terminals in the dorsal vagal nucleus are projections from cells present in the neighboring NTS.

DESCENDING PEPTIDERGIC FIBERS FROM THE MODULATORY CENTERS TO THE VASOMOTOR EFFERENTS

Two descending peptidergic pathways to the medulla and spinal cord have been described: 1) oxytocin and vasopressin (with neurophysins) fibers from the hypothalmic paraventricular nucleus to the NTS, dorsal vagal nucleus, and intermediolateral cell column in the spinal cord [29, 30, 48]; 2) opiocortin (β-endorphin, adrenocorticotrophic hormone [ACTH], and melanocyte-stimulating hormone [α-MSH] fibers from the arcuate, ventral pre-mamillary nuclei to the NTS and dorsal vagal nucleus [31-33]. Angiotensin II fibers are also present in these nuclei, but the perikarya of these axons have not been localized yet. Observations are contradictory with respect to the sources of somatostatin-containing nerve, terminals in the vagal nuclei and in the spinal cord [23, 38, 49].

Baroreceptor modulatory signals from the hypothalamic regions may arrive at the medulla not only by neuronal but also by neurohumoral routes. Angiotensin may be transported by the cerebrospinal fluid down to the IVth ventricle from where it may gain access to the vagal nuclei through the area postrema. No blood-brain barrier exists in the area postrema; therefore, it may serve as an open gate to the medulla oblongata for many circulating substances, including neuropeptides.

EFFERENT BARORECEPTOR NEURONS

None of the neuropeptides have yet been recognized in vasomotor preganglionic neurons. A few substance P and APP cells in the dorsal vagal nucleus seem to be intrinsic [17, 26]. Other peptides there and in the spinal cord are present only in nerve terminals (Table 4), but not in cells or projecting axons. All these pre-ganglionic vasomotor cells are believed to be cholinergic.

CONCLUSIONS

The brain contains several vasoactive substances. An increasing number of studies indicate that the blood pressure and other cardiovascular mechanisms can be centrally influenced by neuropeptides. Their functional role, however, has not been established. Their morphological clarification in the baroreceptor reflex arc does not automatically imply the knowledge of their physiological significance there. Many neuropeptides may exert their effect through brain stem cate-cholamine cells by changing the synthesis, turnover, and firing rates. Experimen-tal manipulations (even exogenous applications of neuropeptides) in the bar-oreceptor reflex arc produce rather unspecific consequences [7]. In fact, most neuropeptides produce some influence on blood pressure [5]. Studying only one selected effect or only a single peptide may produce interesting results, but little is gained about the physiological mechanisms of the central baroreceptor regu-lation. This review has summarized the present knowledge about the distribution of neuropeptides in the baroreceptor reflex arc. It should be kept in mind that neuropeptides represent only one group of substances influencing this regulatory mechanism. A number of studies indicate that the baroreceptor reflex arc can be influenced by many others, such as biogenic amines or transmitter amino acids.

REFERENCES

1. Beale JS, White RP, Huang S-P: EEG and blood pressure effects of TRH in rabbits. Neurophar-macology 16:499-506, 1977.
2. Bolme P, Fuxe K, Agnati Lf, et al.: Cardiovascular effects of morphine and opioid peptides following intracisternal administration in chlorase-anesthetized rats. Eur J Pharmacol 48:319-324, 1978.
3. Hutchinson JS, Ganten D, Schelling P, et al.: Central pressor actions of angiotensin II. Acta Med Acad Sci Hung 33:101-109, 1976.
4. Laubie M, Schmitt H, Vincent M, et al.: Central cardiovascular effects of morphomimetic peptides in dogs. Eur J Pharmacol 46:67-71, 1977.
5. Palkovits M: Neuropeptides and biogenic amines in central cardiovascular control mechanisms, in Buckley JP, Ferrario CM (editors): Central Nervous System Mechanisms in Hypertension. New York, Raven Press, 1981, pp 73-87.
6. Schaz K, Stock G, Simon W, et al.: Enkephalin effects on blood pressure, heart rate and

baroreceptor reflex. Hypertension 2:395-407, 1980.

7. Talman WT, Reis DJ: Baroreceptor actions of substance P microinjected into the nucleus tractus solitarii in rat: A consequence of local distortion. Brain Res 220:402-407, 1981.

8. Unger T, Rockhold RW, Yukimura T, et al.: Role of kinins and substance in the central blood pressure regulation of normotensive and spontaneously hypertensive rats, in Buckley JP, Ferrario CM (editors): Central Nervous System Mechanisms in Hypertension. New York, Raven Press, 1981, pp 115-127.

9. Palkovits M, Zaborszky L: Neuroanatomy of central cardiovascular control. Nucleus tractus solitarii: Afferent and efferent neuronal connections in relation to the baroreceptor reflex arc. Prog Brain Res 47:9-34, 1977.

10. Kalia MP: Localization of aortic and carotid baroreceptor and chemoreceptor primary afferents in the brain stem, in Buckley JP, Ferrario CM (editors): Central Nervous System Mechanisms in Hypertension. New York, Raven Press, 1981, pp 9-24.

11. Gamse R, Lembeck F, Cuello AC: Substance P in the vagus nerve. Immunochemical and immunohistochemical evidence for axoplasmic transport. Naunyn Schmiedeberg Arch Pharmacol 306:37-44, 1979.

12. Lundberg JM, Hokfelt T, Nilsson G, et al.: Peptide-neurons in the vagus, splanchnic and sciatic nerves. Acta Physiol Scand 104:499-501, 1978.

13. Lundberg J, Hokfelt T, Shultzberg M, et al.: Pathways of peripheral peptide neurons to the vagus. Neurosci Lett 1(Suppl 1):S224, 1978.

14. Palkovits M, Leranth CS, Eiden LE, et al.: Intrinsic vasoactive intestinal polypeptide (VIP)-containing neurons in the baroreceptor nucleus of the solitary tract in rat. Brain Res 244:351-355, 1982.

15. Gillis RA, Helke CJ, Hamilton BL, et al.: Evidence that substance P is a neurotransmitter of baro- and chemoreceptor afferents in nucleus tractus solitarius. Brain Res 181:476-481, 1980.

16. Cuello AC, Kanazawa I: The distribution of substance P immunoreactive fibers in the rat central nervous system. J Comp Neurol 178:129-156, 1978.

17. Ljungdahl A, Hokfelt T, Nilsson G, et al.: Distribution of substance P-like immunoreactivity in the central nervous system of the rat. I. Cell bodies and nerve terminals. Neuroscience 3:861-944, 1978.

18. Pickel VM, Joh TH, Reis DJ, et al.: Electron microscopic localization of substance P and enkephalin in axon terminals related to dendrites of catecholaminergic neurons. Brain Res 160:387-400, 1979.

19. Uhl GR, Goodman RR, Snyder SH: Neurotensin-containing cell bodies, fibers and nerve terminals in the brain stem of the rat: Immunohistochemical mapping. Brain Res 167:77-91, 1979.

20. Hokfelt T, Elde R, Johansson O, et al.: The distribution of enkephalin immunoreactive cell bodies in the rat central nervous system. Neurosci Lett 5:25-31, 1977.

21. Sar M, Stumpf WE, Miller RJ: Immunohistochemical localization of enkephalin in rat brain and spinal cord. J Comp Neurol 182:17-38, 1978.

22. Simantov R, Kuhar MJ, Uhl GR, et al.: Opioid peptide enkephalin: Immunohistochemical mapping in the rat nervous system. Proc Natl Acad Sci USA 74:2167-2171, 1977.

23. Finley YWC, Maderdrnt JL, Roger LJ, et al.: The immunocytochemical localization of somatostatin-containing neurons in the rat central nervous system. Neuroscience 6:2173-2192, 1981.

24. Roberts GW, Woodhams PL, Bryant MG, et al.: VIP in the brain: Evidence for a major pathway linking the amygdala and hypothalamus via the stria terminalis. Histochemistry 65:103-119, 1980.

25. Sims KB, Hoffman DL, Said SI, et al.: Vasoactive intestinal peptide (VIP) in mouse and rat brain: An immunocytochemical study. Brain Res 186:165-184, 1980.

26. Hunt SP, Emson PC, Gilbert R, et al.: Presence of avian pancreatic polypeptide-like immunoreactivity in catecholamine and methionine-enkephalin-containing neurones within the central

nervous system. Neurosci Lett 21:125-130, 1981.

27. Olschowka JA, O'Donohue TL, Jakobowitz DM: The distribution of bovine pancreatic polypeptide-like immunoreactive neurons in rat brain. Peptides 2:309-331, 1981.

28. Buijs RM: Intra- and extrahypothalamic vasopressin and oxytocin pathways in the rat. Pathways to the limbic system, medulla oblongata and spinal cord. Cell Tissue Res 192:423-435, 1978.

29. Nilaver G, Zimmerman EA, Wilkins J, et al.: Magnocellular hypothalamic projections to the lower brain stem and spinal cord of the rat. Immunocytochemical evidence for predominance of the oxytocin-neurophysin system compared to the vasopressin-neurophysin system. Neuroendocrinology 30:150-158, 1980.

30. Sofroniew WV, Schrell U: Evidence for a direct projection from oxytocin and vasopressin neurons in the hypothalamic paraventricular nucleus to the medulla oblongata: Immunohistochemical visualization of both the horseradish peroxidase transported and the peptide produced by the same neurons. Neurosci Lett 22:211-217, 1981.

31. Finley JCW, Lindstrom P, Petrusz P: Immunocytochemical localization of β-endorphin-containing neurons in the rat brain. Neuroendocrinology 33:28-42, 1981.

32. Watson SJ, Richard CW, Barchas JD: Adrenocorticotropin in rat brain: Immunocytochemical localization in cells and axons. Science 200:I180-I182, 1978.

33. O'Donodue TL, Miller RL, Jakobowitz DM: Identification, characterization and stereotaxic mapping of intraneuronal α-melanocyte-stimulating hormone-like immunoreactive peptides in discrete regions of the brain. Brain Res 176:101-123, 1979.

34. Fuxe K, Ganten D, Bolme P: Immunohistochemical evidence for existence of angiotensin II-containing nerve terminals in the brain and spinal cord in the rat. Neurosci Lett 2:229-234, 1976.

35. Loren I, Alumets J, Hakanson R, et al.: Distribution of gastrin and CCK-like peptides in rat brain. An immunocytochemical study. Histochemistry 59:249-257, 1979.

36. Vanderhaeghen JJ, Lostra F, De Mey J, et al.: Immunohistochemical localization of cholecystokinin- and gastrin-like peptides in the brain and hypophysis of the rat. Proc Natl Acad Sci USA 77:I190-I194, 1980.

37. Douglas FL, Palkovits M: Distribution and quantitative measurements of somatostatin-like immunoreactivity in the lower brainstem of the rat. Brain Res 242:369-373, 1982.

38. Palkovits M, Epelbaum J, Tapia-Arancibia L, et al.: Somatostatin in catecholamine-rich nuclei of the brainstem. Neuropeptides, in press.

39. Douglas FL, Falkovits M, Brownstein MJ: Regional distribution of substance P-like immunoreactivity in the lower brainstem of the rat. Brain Res, submitted for publication.

40. Eiden LE, Nilaver G, Palkovits M: Distribution of vasoactive intestinal polypeptide (VIP) in the rat brainstem nuclei. Brain Res 231:472-477, 1982.

41. Beinfeld MC, Palkovits M: Distribution of cholecystokinin (CCK) in the rat lower brain stem nuclei. Brain Res 238:260-265, 1982.

42. Moody TW, O'Donohue TL, Jakobowitz DM: Biochemical localization and characterization of bombesin-like peptides in discrete regions of rat brain. Peptides 2:75-79, 1981.

43. Palkovits M: The anatomy of central cardiovascular neurons, in Fuxe K, Goldstein M, Hokfelt B, et al. (editors): Central Adrenaline Neurons: Basic Aspects and Their Role in Cardiovascular Function. New York, Pergamon Press, 1980, pp 3-17.

44. Ciriello J, Cararesu FR: Monosynaptic pathways from cardiovascular neurons in the nucleus tractus solitarii to the paraventricular nucleus in the cat. Brain Res 193:529-533, 1980.

45. Palkovits M, de Jong W, Zandberg P, et al.: Central hypertension and nucleus tractus solitarii catecholamines after surgical lesions in the medulla oblongata of the rat. Brain Res 127:307-312, 1977.

46. Norgen R: Projections from the nucleus of the solitary tract in the rat. Neuroscience 3:207-218, 1978.

47. Hokfelt T, Fuxe K, Johansson O, et al.: Distribution of thyrotropin-releasing hormone (TRH) in

the central nervous system as revealed with immunocytochemistry. Eur J Pharmacol 34:389-392, 1975.

48. Swanson LW, McKellar S: The distribution of oxytocin- and neurophysin-stained fibers in the spinal cord of the rat and monkey. J Comp Neurol 188:87-106, 1979.

49. Krisch B: Somatostatin-immunoreactive fiber projections into the brain stem and the spinal cord of the rat. Cell Tissue Res 217:531-552, 1981.

DISCUSSION

Discussants: Johnston, Palkovits, Brody, Sleight, Denton

Johnston: We've recently been attempting to see where substance P is involved in the baroreceptor pathways. After bilateral carotid denervation, we can show no change in substance P measured immunocytochemically, histochemically, or by radioimmunoassay in the nucleus of the tractus solitarius. Where else are the fibers containing substance P likely to be coming from that go into that tract or that nucleus?

Palkovits: The nodose ganglion. The ganglion nodosum has few substance P cells according to the immunocytochemistry published by Lundberg and his co-workers. So, we only know that after the intracranial transection of the vagus, we got a depletion of substance P levels in the NTS.

Brody: I would like to discuss studies which document the importance in the rat of projections from the baroreceptor regions to the hypothalamus in determining the sensitivity of the brain to angiotensin.[1] Pressor responses to peripherally administered pressor agents angiotensin, vasopressin and phenylephrine were increased in rats with chronic sinoaortic denervation. The changes in sensitivity were approximately 2-fold for phenylephrine, 4-fold for angiotensin and 8-fold for vasopressin. In contrast, the ventricular administration of angiotensin produces a pressor response which is shifted in sensitivity over 1000-fold in animals with sinoaortic denervation. This suggests that projections to hypothalamus, originating in baroreceptor regions such as NTS, modulate the central sensitivity to angiotensin. One can speculate that during hypertension, when baroreceptor sensitivity is dimished, the central pressor activity of angiotensin would be accentuated.

Sleight: I agree. In man, when we tested baroreflex sensitivity in about 60 people and examined the pressor response to a wide range of different stresses - such as intravenous phenylephrine or noradrenalin, or bicycle exercise - we found a very strong negative correlation between the pressor response and baroreflex sensitivity. When baroreflexes are poor, there are very much larger rises in pressure, which just bears out what you said.

Denton: If we inject angiotensin into the CSF and stimulate central angiotensin, we get the release of ADH and catecholamines. Fifty percent of the blood pressure response to a central angiotensin appears to be due to SADH. Now, the increase of ADH in the plasma following central angiotensin is about 10 to 50 picograms per ml which is not enough to raise blood pressure if you infuse this amount peripherally. Now, we know that ADH counteracts its own pressor effects peripherally by a central action. It appears that these data agree very well with your angiotensin data. Otherwise, we could not explain why ADH contributes so much for a central angiotensin and not for a peripheral application of ADH.

---

[1] Barron KW, Frapani AJ, Brody MJ: Sinoaortic baroreceptors produce central inhibition of the central pressor effect of angiotensin II. Fed. Proc. 41: 1094, 1982.

THE ROLE OF VARIOUS AFFERENTS IN THE REGULATION OF SYMPATHETIC TONE IN HYPERTENSION: A BRIEF REVIEW

Francois M. Abboud

INTRODUCTION

The neurons involved in cardiovascular control fall into three groups: 1) afferent neurons with cell bodies in the petrosal and nodose ganglia and projections to the nucleus tractus solitarius in the medulla (NTS); 2) neurons in the NTS that send axons to the hypothalamus and to preganglionic vagal and sympathetic efferent neurons; and 3) vagal and sympathetic efferent neurons in the medulla and spinal cord that innervate the heart and blood vessels.

The neurons in the NTS are probably the most important in the integration of sensory input from various afferent pathways and in the modulation of reflex autonomic cardiovascular functions [1].

The activity of neurons in the NTS is modulated by peripheral impulses arising from sensory receptors in the cardiovascular system, such as the arterial baroreceptors and the cardiopulmonary receptors; in skeletal muscle and skin, such as the somatic and ergoreceptors; and in the viscerae, such as the liver and kidney. These impulses regulate arterial pressure and blood flow to various organs, but the extent to which they cause or sustain hypertension is not clear.

Four aspects of these afferent impulses are reviewed here:

I. The role of arterial baroreceptors in the regulation of heart rate and vascular resistance in hypertensives.

II. The role of cardiopulmonary receptors in the early and late phases of hypertension.

III. The reflex response to stimulation of somatic afferents in hypertension.

IV. The role of afferent renal nerve activity, which may contribute a neurogenic element to renal hypertension.

ARTERIAL BARORECEPTORS IN HYPERTENSION

The role of arterial baroreceptors in the regulation of vascular resistance in hypertension has been examined for decades, but several questions remain partially answered.

Effect of baroreceptor denervation on blood pressure

The question of whether denervation of arterial baroreceptor causes hypertension has been controversial. Cowley et al. [2] reported that arterial baroreceptor denervation causes labile fluctuations in arterial pressure but not a sustained hypertension. Conversely, Ito and Scher [3] and McRitchie et al. [4] reported sustained hypertension in dogs after either aortic [3] or carotid baroreceptor [4] denervation. Krieger [5] and Fink et al. [6] described hypertension in rats after aortic baroreceptor denervation. It is possible that the failure of blood pressure to rise consistently after denervation of one or both sets of arterial baroreceptors may be caused by an exaggerated inhibitory influence on sympathetic outflow of the remaining set of arterial baroreceptors or of the cardiopulmonary receptors. In examining the influence of sequential denervation of carotid, aortic, and vagal afferents in rabbits, we observed that [7] denervation of carotid baroreceptors caused increases in arterial blood pressure averaging 27 ± 4 mm Hg (n = 8) when aortic and vagal afferents were intact and 46 ± 6 mm Hg when aortic baroreceptors were denervated. Similarly, section of cardiopulmonary afferents by bilateral vagotomy caused a rise in arterial pressure of 6 ± 3 mm Hg when arterial baroreceptors were intact and of 44 ± 5 mm Hg after sinoaortic denervation. Thus, after partial denervation of baroreceptors, a greater restraining influence of the remaining intact afferents from arterial or cardiopulmonary baroreceptors may suppress a hypertensive response [8]. This concept is supported by the observations that lesions of the NTS, where the afferents from sinoaortic and cardiopulmonary baroreceptors converge, cause severe hypertension [9, 10].

Early impairment or resetting of baroreceptors

Arterial baroreceptors are reset in hypertension; they have higher pressure threshold and reduced sensitivity to increases in pressure. This resetting is caused, at least in part, by changes in arterial distensibility secondary to the elevated arterial pressure [11]. Resetting occurs also acutely, within hours after elevation of arterial pressure, and is reversible.

An important question is whether resetting occurs *before* the onset of hypertension. Data from four separate experiments suggest that an abnormal baroreflex may precede or coincide with the onset of mild hypertension. In the early stages of hypertension, in SHR at 10 weeks of age, the strain-sensitivity of aortic baroreceptors is significantly reduced with normotensive rats [12]. The Dahl salt-sensitive rats have impaired baroreflexes on low sodium intake in the absence of hypertension [13]. Partial resetting of baroreceptors may occur in the absence of structural vascular changes, and a significant impairment of baroreflexes may occur in the very early stages of labile essential human hypertension [14].

Differential control of heart rate and resistance in hypertension

Most of the information available in the literature concerning baroreflex control of the circulation has been based on studies of reflex changes in heart rate in response to increases or decreases in arterial pressure with intravenous phenylephrine or nitroglycerin. In some studies in humans, responses to changes in transmural pressure of the neck (neck suction or neck pressure) to activate or unload the carotid sinus baroreceptors indicate that changes in cardiac output are predominant, while in others changes in total resistance are more evident [15].

In a series of recent studies, we systematically contrasted baroreflex control of heart rate and vascular resistance in normotensive and hypertensive rabbits. The data indicate that in hypertensive rabbits baroreflex control of heart rate is impaired, whereas baroreflex control of vascular resistance is preserved or augmented. These findings require reassessment of the role of arterial baroreceptors in the pathogenesis of hypertension and other pathological states where conclusions are based on changes in heart rate exclusively.

Experimental preparation and results

The reason why baroreflex control of rate is reported much more frequently than baroreflex control of resistance is the simplicity of the measurement, particularly in awake animals and humans. Phenylephrine or nitroglycerin are given intravenously, and the reflex change in rate corresponding to a change in pressure is described. Because these drugs have *direct* vascular effects, one cannot examine *reflex* changes in resistance simultaneously.

We examined reflex changes in vascular resistance in rabbits by perfusing the hindlimb with a pump, which maintains blood flow at a constant rate. We interposed along the pump a delay coil to prevent the arrival of phenylephrine or nitroglycerin to the hindlimb vessels until the peak reflex response had been noted. When a bolus of phenylephrine is given intravenously blood pressure goes up, and reflex vasodilatation can be seen before the drug reaches the hindlimb. Reflex responses were studied in renal hypertensive rabbits (unilateral nephrectomy and polyethylene wrap of remaining kidney or both kidneys wrapped). Since changes in vascular resistance in hypertensive and normotensive rabbits are difficult to compare because of the high baseline vascular resistance in the hypertensives, we also measured reflex changes in lumbar sympathetic activity.

In hypertensives, baroreflex control of heart rate was impaired both in the awake and in the anesthetized state, whereas baroreflex control of vascular resistance was not only preserved but was enhanced. After normalization of the change in resistance based on the higher baseline resistance in hypertensives, the responses were similar in both groups. Furthermore, the changes in lumbar sympathetic activity were also similar in both groups (Fig. 1).

There are many studies that show resetting of arterial baroreceptors in renal

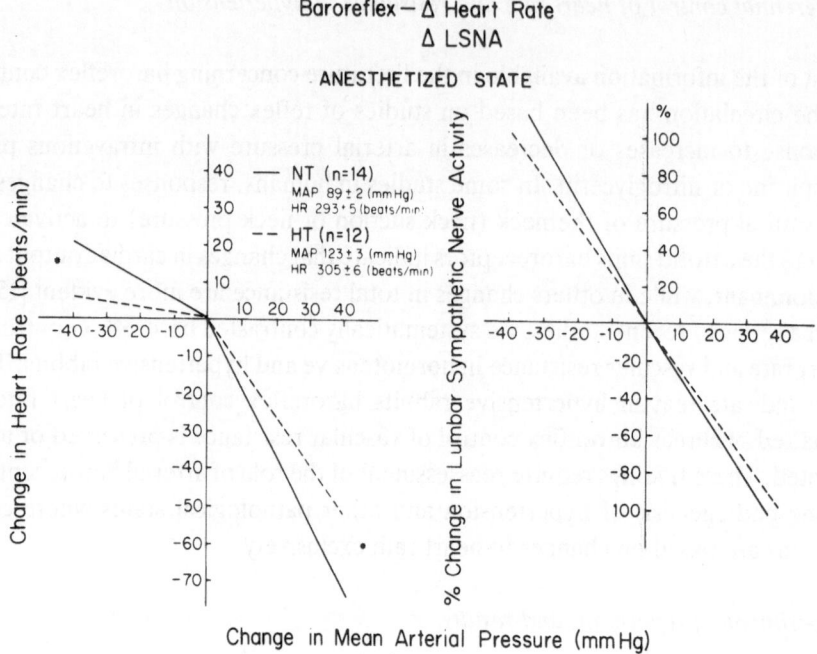

Figure 1. Impaired baroreflex control of heart rate and preserved baroreflex control of lumbar sympathetic activity in hypertensive rabbits (HT) compared to normotensive rabbits (NT). Work done in collaboration with Drs. Guo and Thames.

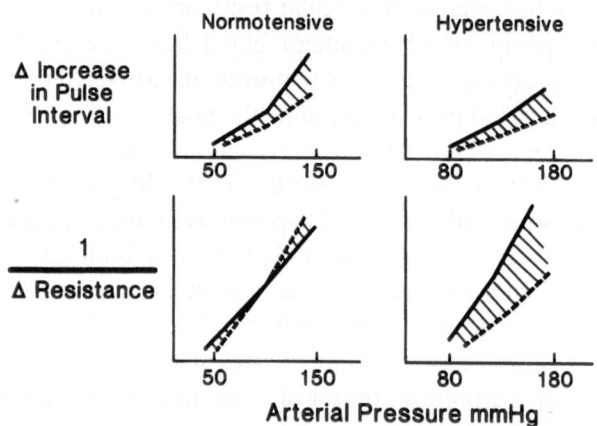

Figure 2. Diagrammatic representation of effect of denervation of aortic *or* carotid baroreceptors on baroreflex control of heart rate and vascular resistance in normotensive and hypertensive rabbits. Based on results obtained in our laboratories (Guo, Thames, and Abboud). Note that normotensive rabbits after partial denervation behave like hypertensive rabbits before denervation. Before denervation, solid line; after partial denervation, dashed line. (Reproduced from Ref. 8 by permission of authors and publisher.)

hypertension after a few weeks of elevated blood pressure. Why does this resetting affect the control of heart rate but not the control of vascular resistance or lumbar sympathetic activity?

It is interesting that in *normotensive* rabbits, a differential control of rate and resistance may be demonstrated after partial denervation of the arterial baro-receptors (either by section of the carotid sinus nerve or the aortic depressor nerves) [7, 8] (Fig. 2). The parasympathetic control of heart rate is impaired by partial denervation of baroreceptor afferents, whereas the sympathetic control of resistance is preserved. A careful analysis of these responses in normotensives after partial baroreceptor denervation and vagotomy allowed us to conclude that there is no 'redundancy' or 'overlap' in the control of vagal neurons by aortic and carotid baroreceptors, whereas there is significant 'redundancy' or 'overlap' in the control of sympathetic neurons [7, 8]. Because of these findings, the suppression of reflex control of rate but not of resistance in hypertensives may be explained on the basis of the decline in sensitivity of arterial baroreceptors. Partial denervation of arterial baroreceptors in *hypertensive* animals by sectioning one set of baroreceptors causes significant suppression of baroreflex control of both rate and resistance, suggesting that the redundancy in the control of sympathetic neurons in hypertensives is only marginal [8] (Fig. 2).

The most important finding, in these studies, is that there is preservation of reflex control of vascular resistance in hypertensive animals at a time when reflex control of heart rate is impaired. Thus, one cannot, on the basis of an evaluation of reflex control of heart rate alone, predict what is happening to the baroreceptor control of the total circulation. Furthermore, preservation of reflex control of vascular resistance minimizes the role of arterial baroreceptors in maintaining a high vascular resistance in hypertensive animals, assuming, of course, that the baroreflex control of other vascular beds besides the hindlimb is preserved in this model of hypertension as well as in others. This assumption should be tested experimentally. It is of interest, however, that in a study of the carotid barorcflex in hypertensive humans, the baroreflex control of total peripheral resistance appeared preserved or even augmented [15].

Central resetting in hypertensive rabbits

We examined the possibility of a central defect in the control of rate or lumbar sympathetic activity in hypertensives by electrically stimulating the central end of one aortic depressor nerve in rabbits that had both carotid sinuses denervated and both aortic depressor nerves cut. Preliminary results indicate that reflex responses were equivalent in the normotensive and hypertensive groups. Thus, there was no evidence of an abnormality in the central control of rate or lumbar sympathetic activity in response to stimulation of the inhibitory aortic depressor nerve in hypertensive animals. It is possible, however, that a difference between responses of normotensive and hypertensive animals might be seen if more than one inhibitory afferent input is stimulated, since the pattern of summation of afferent impulses may vary in normotensives and hypertensives. This is currently being examined.

CARDIAC SENSORY RECEPTORS IN HYPERTENSION

These endings may modulate sympathetic tone and neurohumoral drive to the circulation in important ways [16-18]. They may be activated chemically or mechanically with veratridine or nicotine, during coronary ischemia or volume expansion, and during vigorous cardiac contractions. Their activation not only suppresses sympathetic drive [19], but also changes the gain of the arterial baroreceptors such that during carotid hypotension, for example, the anticipated increase in sympathetic activity is suppressed when cardiac afferent activity is increased and vice versa [20].

Interaction between cardiac sensory receptors and arterial baroreceptors

We isolated the carotid sinuses and connected them to a pressure reservoir containing Kreb's solution. This allowed us to maintain carotid pressure at the desired level. The effect of changes in carotid sinus pressure on renal nerve activity was examined. Input from the cardiac afferents was either increased (by occluding the circumflex artery or with volume expansion) or decreased (by cooling or sectioning the vagi), and the baroreflex was studied under each

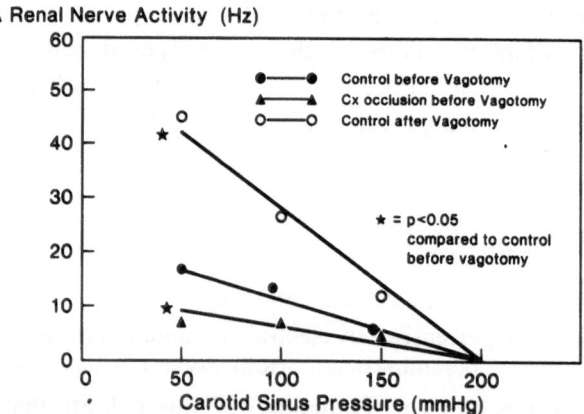

Figure 3. The carotid baroreflex control of renal nerve activity decreased during transient occlusion of the circumflex coronary artery and increased markedly following bilateral vagotomy. This established the importance of cardiac sensory input in the modulation of the arterial baroreflex (8, 20). (Reproduced from Ref. 8 by permission of authors and pusblisher.)

condition. The results indicate that the gain of the arterial baroreflex is inversely related to the vagal afferent input from cardiac or cardiopulmonary receptors [20] (Fig. 3).

Protective effect of increased cardiac afferent activity in early human hypertension

To study the role of cardiac afferents in humans, we pool blood in the lower extremities with a 'lower-body negative pressure box.' This unloads the cardiac receptors and decreases their sensory input, resulting in reflex vasoconstriction. If the *resting* cardiac sensory afferent activity is increased, one would expect that lower-body negative pressure would cause a greater vasoconstriction.

An important question is whether, in hypertensive humans, the activity of cardiac afferents is increased, thus suppressing sympathetic tone, or decreased, thus contributing to a high sympathetic drive and resistance. The results indicate that lower-body negative pressure caused greater vasoconstriction in patients with borderline hypertension than in the normotensive subjects [21, 22] (Fig. 4). This effect could not be ascribed to increased vascular reactivity [22]. Thus, in the supine position, cardiac afferent activity is increased in borderline hypertension, suppressing in part sympathetic drive and providing a 'protective' compensatory effect, which may offset the influence of impaired arterial baroreceptor activity on vascular resistance. In the upright position, on the other hand, just as during lower-body negative pressure, the sympatho-adrenal drive may be excessive. As a corollary, renin levels are reported to increase markedly in the upright position in patients with borderline hypertension, in contrast to normotensives.

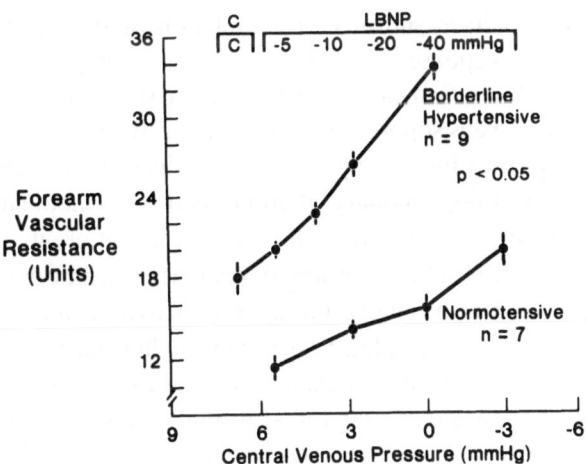

Figure 4. Withdrawal of the inhibitory influence of cardiac afferents with lower-body negative pressure (LBNP) causes a greater augmentation of forearm vascular resistance in borderline hypertensives than in normotensives (22). (Adapted from Mark and Kerber (22) by permission of authors and publisher.).

Decreased cardiac afferent activity in animal models of hypertension

What happens in late stages of hypertension after cardiac hypertrophy that may be different? The sensitivity of cardiac sensory afferents may decrease, causing a high level of sympathetic drive. Thoren et al. [16] have shown that in genetic (SHR) models of hypertension, activity of sensory cardiac C fibers is decreased during either transient aortic occlusion or volume expansion. This results in lesser inhibition of renal sympathetic activity [16] and lesser natriuresis and diuresis for equivalent increases in left atrial pressure. On the other hand, volume expansion causes a greater rise in left atrial pressure to SHR than WKY because of decreased compliance of capacitance vessels. The greater rise in left atrial pressure may cause greater activation of cardiac afferents despite their higher threshold, resulting in greater reflex inhibition of sympathetic efferents [23].

To summarize, the cardiac afferents may play an important role in inhibiting neurohumoral drive when patients with borderline hypertension are placed in the supine position. The supine position causes cardiac distension and activation of these nerve endings. During the late stages of hypertension and left ventricular hypertrophy, decreased activity of these sensory endings may contribute to the high sympathetic tone, increased vascular resistance, and greater sodium retention.

STIMULATION OF SOMATIC AFFERENTS IN HYPERTENSIVES: INFLUENCE OF INPUT FROM ARTERIAL AND CARDIOPULMONARY BARORECEPTORS

The somatic hypertensive reflex resulting from activation of group IV unmyelinated afferents may be modulated by input from arterial baroreceptors. Coote and Perez-Gonzales have shown that stimulation of the carotid sinus nerve inhibited the reflex responses [24]. We have shown in dogs that during carotid hypertension, the reflex vasoconstrictor response to stimulation of the central cut end of the sciatic nerve is suppressed [25]. Conversely, when the input from the arterial baroreceptors is impaired or suppressed, the somatic excitatory reflex is augmented [25]. Cardiopulmonary afferents may also modulate the somatic reflex. Increased activity from the cardiopulmonary afferents during volume expansion reduces the renal vasoconstrictor response to sciatic nerve stimulation, and bilateral vagotomy to remove the afferent activity from cardiopulmonary receptors augments the reflex [25]. Experiments in humans from our laboratory indicate that isometric (handgrip) exercise of one forearm causes reflex vasoconstriction in the opposite resting forearm; this reflex response is augmented during lower-body negative pressure, which decreases central blood volume and presumably reduces the activity of cardiopulmonary baroreceptors [26] (Fig. 5).

On the basis of these studies, one would expect that the response to exercise in hypertensives will be augmented if arterial baroreflexes are impaired or if there is

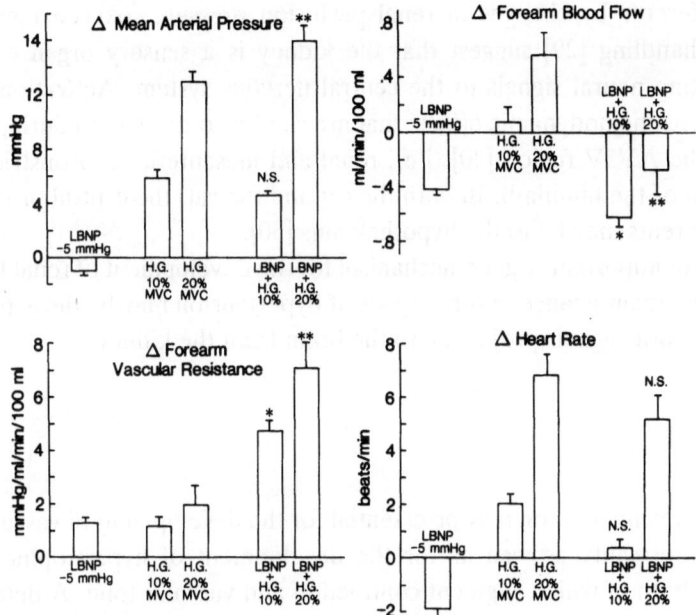

Figure 5. Changes in mean arterial pressure, forearm blood flow, forearm vascular resistance, and heart rate that resulted from LBNP at − 5 mm Hg, from isometric handgrip (H.G.) at 10 and 20% of MVC, and during concomitant LBNP and H.G. at 10 and 20% of MVC. The changes in each subject were calculated by subtracting the value obtained during the intervention from the control value. Asterisk (*) indicates that response to LBNP plus H.G. at 10% MVC is significantly greater ($P < 0.05$) than the algebraic sum of LBNP alone plus H.G. at 10% MVC alone. Double asterisk (**) indicates that response to LBNP plus H.G. at 20% MVC is significantly greater than the algebraic sum of LBNP alone plus H.G. at 20% MVC alone. Changes that are not significantly different are so indicated. Data presented as mean ± SE (26). (Reproduced from Ref. 26 by permission of authors and publisher.).

left ventricular hypertrophy with impaired cardiac sensory afferents. In support of this notion is the report of Ewing et al. [27], who showed that hypertensives with left ventricular hypertrophy respond to isometric exercise with an increase in peripheral resistance, while those without ventricular enlargement have no increase in resistance.

ROLE OF RENAL AFFERENTS IN HYPERTENSION

An increase in renal afferent activity has been implicated in the maintenance of high sympathetic tone in certain types of renal hypertension and even in SHR. The work of Katholi et al. in renal hypertension [28] suggests that renal denervation may reduce arterial blood pressure because of interruption of the afferent neural influence on sympathetic tone rather than through a direct effect on sodium and water handling by the kidney.

Responses to electrical stimulation of renal afferents and to the activation of these afferents by changes in renal perfusion pressure, oxygen tension, and sodium handling [29] suggest that the kidney is a sensory organ capable of transmitting neural signals to the central nervous system. Activation of these nerves gives hemodynamic effects that are similar to those seen during stimulation of the AV3V region [30], i.e., renal and mesenteric vasoconstriction and dilatation of the hindlimb. In both the cat and the rat, the central projection of renal afferents may be to the hypothalamus [30].

Thus, an important trigger mechanism for the development of renal hypertension or the maintenance of other types of hypertension may be the activation of sensory neural signals projecting to the brain from the kidney.

SUMMARY

Sympathetic innervation may be essential for the development of vascular membrane abnormality as well as for the development of hypertrophic vascular changes, both of which augment contraction and vascular tone. A defect at the sensory endings of arterial stretch receptors may account for impaired arterial baroreceptor reflexes seen in very early phases of hypertension or, in some genetic models, before hypertension develops. This defect may cause a decrease in baroreceptor discharge, resulting in exaggerated sympathetic drive. Further information is needed, however, on the baroreflex control of parasympathetic and various sympathetic efferents in hypertension because of the differential control of rate and resistance that we observed in renal hypertensive rabbits. Cardiac receptors may have a variable influence on sympathetic drive in the various stages of hypertension, depending on the degree of cardiac hypertrophy or cardiac size. Increased activity in the early stages of hypertension may reduce vascular resistance, but reduced activity in the late stages may increase resistance. The somatic pressor reflex may be augmented in hypertensives because of either impaired arterial baroreflexes or impaired cardiopulmonary baroreceptors, such as might occur with left ventricular hypertrophy. Finally, increased renal afferent nerve activity may provoke an increase in sympathetic activity and provide a link between humoral and neurogenic factors in renal hypertension.

ACKNOWLEDGMENT

Work referred to here from the Cardiovascular Center at Iowa was done in collaboration with Drs. G. Guo, A. Mark, M. Thames, A. Waickman, and J. Walker and was supported by Program Project Grant HL 14388 and Grant HL 21158 from the U.S. Public Health Service, Bethesda, Maryland.

Several studies referred to here have already been published in full or in part (references [18, 19, 22, 25, and 26]).

REFERENCES

1. Palkovits M: The anatomy of central cardiovascular neurons, in Fuxe K, Goldstein M, Hokfelt B, et al. (editors): Central Adrenaline Neurons: Basic Aspects and Their Role in Cardiovascular Functions. Elmsford, NY, Pergamon Press, 1980, pp 3-17.
2. Cowley AW Jr, Liard JF, Guyton AC: Role of the baroreceptor reflex in daily control of arterial blood pressure and other variables in dogs. Circ Res 32:564-576, 1973.
3. Ito CS, Scher AM: Hypertension following denervation of aortic baroreceptors in unanesthetized dogs. Circ Res 45:26-34, 1979.
4. McRitchie RJ, Vatner SF, Heyndrickx GR, et al.: The role of arterial baroreceptors in the regulation of arterial pressure in conscious dogs. Circ Res 39:666-670, 1976.
5. Krieger EM: Neurogenic hypertension in the rat. Circ Res 15:511, 1964.
6. Fink GD, Kennedy F, Bryan WJ, et al.: Pathogenesis of hypertension in rats with chronic aortic baroreceptor deafferentation. Hypertension 2:319-325, 1980.
7. Guo GD, Thames DM, Abboud FM: Differential control of heart rate and hindlimb resistance by carotid, aortic and cardiopulmonary baroreflexes in rabbits. Circ Res 50:554-565, 1982.
8. Abboud FM: The sympathetic system in hypertension. State-of-the-art review. Hypertension (suppl II) 4(3):208-225, 1982.
9. Doba N, Reis DJ: Role of central and peripheral adrenergic mechanisms in neurogenic hypertension produced by brainstem lesions in rat. Circ Res 34:293-301, 1974.
10. Carey FM, Dacey RG, Jane JA, et al.: Production of sustained hypertension by lesions of the nucleus tractus solitarii of the American foxhound. Hypertension 1:246-254, 1979.
11. Angell-James JE: Characteristics of single aortic and right subclavian baroreceptor fiber activity in rabbits with chronic renal hypertension. Circ Res 32:149-161, 1973.
12. Brown AM: Receptors under pressure; and update on baroreceptors. Circ Res 46:1-10, 1980.
13. Gordon FJ, Matsuguchi H, Mark AL: Abnormal baroreflex control of heart rate in prehypertensive and hypertensive Dahl genetically salt-sensitive rats. Hypertension 3(3):I-135-I-141, 1981.
14. Takeshita A, Tanaka S, Kuroiwa A, et al.: Reduced baroreceptor sensitivity in borderline hypertension. Circulation 51:738-742, 1975.
15. Mancia G, Ferrari A, Gregorini L, et al.: Control of blood pressure by carotid sinus baroreceptors in human beings. Am J Cardiol 44:895-902, 1979.
16. Thoren P, Ricksten S-E: Cardiac C-fiber endings in cardiovascular control under normal and pathophysiological conditions, in Abboud FA, Fozzard HA, Gilmore JP, et al. (editors): Disturbances in Neurogenic Control of the Circulation. Baltimore, Williams & Wilkins, 1981, pp 17-31.
17. Coleridge HM, Coleridge JCG, Kidd C: Cardiac receptors in the dog, with particular reference to two types of afferent endings in the ventricular wall. J Physiol (Lond) 174:323-339, 1964.
18. Abboud FM, Thames MD, Mark AL: Role of cardiac afferent nerves in regulation of circulation during coronary occlusion and heart failure, in Abboud FA, Fozzard HA, Gilmore JP, et al. (editors): Disturbances in Neurogenic Control of the Circulation. Baltimore, Williams & Wilkins, 1981, pp 65-86.
19. Thames MD, Abboud FM: Reflex inhibition of renal sympathetic nerve activity during myocardial ischemia mediated by left ventricular receptors with vagal afferents in dogs. J Clin Invest 237 (Heart Circ Physiol 6):H299-H304, 1979.
20. Waickman LA, Abboud FM: Circumflex coronary occlusion inhibits the compensatory increase in sympathetic activity during arterial hypertension. Clin Res 28(4):717A, 1980.
21. Mark AL, Abboud FM: Low-pressure baroreflex control of vascular resistance in young borderline hypertensive men. Clin Res 27(4):674A, 1979.
22. Mark AL, Kerber RE: Augmentation of cardiopulmonary baroreflex control of forearm vascular resistance in borderline hypertension. Hypertension 4(1):39-46, 1982.
23. Ricksten S-E, Noresson E, Thoren P: Inhibition of renal sympathetic nerve traffic from cardiac

receptors in normotensive and spontaneously hypertensive rats. Acta Physiol Scand 106:17-22, 1979.

24. Coote JH, Perez-Gonzalez JF: The response of some sympathetic neurons to volleys in various afferent nerves. J Physiol 208:261-279, 1970.

25. Thames MD, Abboud FM: Interaction of somatic receptors with cardiopulmonary and carotid baroreceptors in the control of the renal circulation in dogs. Am J Physiol 6:H560-H565, 1979.

26. Walker JL, Abboud FM, Mark AL, et al.: Interaction of cardiopulmonary receptors with somatic receptors in man. J Clin Invest 65:1491-1497, 1980.

27. Ewing DJ, Irving JB, Kerr F, et al.: Static exercise in untreated systemic hypertension. Br Heart J 35:413-421, 1973.

28. Katholi RE, Winternitz SR, Oparil S: Role of the renal nerves in the pathogenesis of one-kidney renal hypertension in the rat. Hypertension 3(4):404-409, 1981.

29. Recordati GM, Moss NG: Electrophysiological study of renal mechano- and chemoreceptors in the rat. Proc Int Congr Nephrol. 7th, Montreal, 1978, p 559.

30. Knuepfer MM, Mohrland JS, Shaffer RA, et al.: Effects of afferent renal nerve (ARN) stimulation and baroreceptor activation on unit activity (UA) in the anteroventral third ventricle (AV3V) region. Fed Proc 39:837, 1980.

DISCUSSION

Discussants: Folkow, Sleight, Abboud, MacGregor

Folkow: I really want to stress what you said here about the two links of the baroreceptor reflex and that both should be examined in hypertension. Peter Thorén, in our department, has looked at this in spontaneous hypertensive rats, the typical neurogenic model of hypertension. If one first explores only the heart rate upon activation of the baroreceptors, there is a very poor reflex response. It seems clear that this is due to a 'central nervous occlusion,' causing a fairly selective suppression at the bulbar level of the reflex arch to the heart, while the reflex inhibition of tonic sympathetic activity is largely normal in SHR at a given percentage increase of mean arterial pressure.

Sleight: Well, I don't disagree very much with that. All I can say is that there are other studies in humans that show some parallelism between carotid baroreceptor impairment of heart rate and peripheral resistance, as judged by arterial pressure. I'm referring really to Bevegard's work using neck suction. Some methods employ a static square-wave suction and some sine waves. It does seem that sine waves give better carotid baroreceptor stimulation in man. I was interested to see recently a paper from Wallin's group in Uppsala that showed this very elegantly with sympathetic nerve recording directly in humans. They showed that when a square-wave neck suction is applied to the carotid baroreceptors, there is very little sustained change in sympathetic nerve activity, whereas a sine wave gives sustained suppression. I don't disagree at all with what Folkow and Abboud have said. It's very obvious, but I would still say that there is some parallelism between heart rate control and peripheral resistance control in humans.

Abboud: I think that Dr. Mancia found that too.

Sleight: No, they used a square wave. I think we just have to keep an open mind on this until we have more data using sinusoidal stimulation of carotid baroreceptors with this technique in humans.

Abboud: I think it's difficult to reconcile all the findings with carotid neck suction and pressure by different groups. The point we are really trying to make with this renal hypertensive model is to try to activate the reflex like we would do in intact humans by giving phenylephrine and nitroglycerin. Under those circumstances, we see a significant differential effect on rate and resistance.

Sleight: I wondered whether you might see different effects in different vascular beds? There may be problems when we look at just one vascular bed.

Abboud: I would not necessarily presume that there is no inhibition of other sympathetic efferents, but that's precisely the point that I'm trying to make. The concept is that you cannot extrapolate from one efferent activity to the whole system, and that's the only point I'm trying to make. Maybe I should just stop there. Assessment of the baroreflex is much more complex than simply giving phenylephrine and watching the slope of a heart rate.

Unidentified discussant: As you know, Stevo Julius has managed to create some kind of hypertension by lower body compression. Now, according to what you have shown, it could be a matter of somatic afferents or cardiopulmonary or both. What would your explanation be of this high resistance type of hypertension? I think he has created it both in humans and in dogs.

Abboud: I am afraid I'm not terribly well versed on the details of his experiment. If you compress the lower extremities, you will shift volume centrally, and one would expect that you would inhibit sympathetic drive. If indeed Dr. Julius found an exaggerated sympathetic drive under those conditions, one might postulate activation of other afferents. If you compress the lower extremities severely, you could be producing ischemia of skeletal muscle that could activate somatic events. What you really have then is a complex integration of not only cardiopulmonary afferent activity but also somatic afferent activity.

MacGregor: In your experiments, you reduce central blood volume. In essential hypertension and inherited forms of hypertension in the rat, there is quite good evidence that there's an increase in central blood volume due to dimished venous compliance - in other words, the exact opposite of what you're doing when you suck.

Abboud: If you have an increase in central blood volume in hypertensive states, one would expect decreased sympathetic tone if everything else were unchanged. If the sensitivity of the cardiac nerve endings were not depressed or if there were no reduction in the contractile force of the left ventricle, which seems to activate these endings, then maybe what you say is correct. Indeed, we think from the experiment, which I just reported, that in *borderline hypertension,* there may be an increase in the cardiopulmonary afferent activity which may suppress sympathetic drive. We think, however, that in late hypertensive states, when there is left ventricular hypertrophy and possibly damaged cardiac sensory nerve endings, as was seen with the dog model of left ventricular overload by Greenberg et al., and in SHR by Peter Thorin, there is reduced firing of cardiac afferents, possibly because of damage of those endings. That damage would contribute to the rise in sympathetic drive and blood pressure.

DEFECTS IN SIGNAL GENERATION IN ARTERIAL BARORECEPTORS

PETER SLEIGHT

INTRODUCTION

The discovery of the carotid sinus nerve and the reflex effects of stimulation of carotid baroreceptors by Hering [1] and Koch [2] quickly focussed attention on the possibility that disordered function of this very powerful mechanism might be responsible for disease, particularly hypertension, in humans. Although Adrian [3] and Bronk and Stella [4] recorded from single and few-fiber baroreceptor afferent nerves, the first comparison of the discharge of the carotid sinus baroreceptors in normotensive and hypertensive animals was made by McCubbin et al. [5] in the dog. Their studies on multifiber preparations suggested that the discharge from the hypertensive sinus was the same as that of the normotensive sinus, even though the threshold and operating range of the receptors were reset to a higher level. The implication was that the receptors had adapted to the new level of pressure and were therefore similarly capable of controlling pressure at this new level.

In this paper, I will review the more recent evidence, which suggests that the former is an oversimplification, in that the reset receptors show not only a decrease in sensitivity and operating range, as is already known, but there's also a resetting of the threshold pressure at which they first discharge. I will, furthermore, review the evidence which suggests that these differences are due to mechanical changes in the arterial wall, rather than to degenerative changes in the neural elements themselves.

ANATOMICAL STUDIES

The classic papers of de Castro [6, 7] on the innervation of the carotid sinus in humans and animals showed that the receptor endings - at least those subserved by myelinated axons - were located in the border between the adventitia and the outermost layers of the media. The receptors often lay close to isolated muscle fibers in the adventitia, a finding later confirmed by Rees [8] in an electron microscopy study. Rees et al. [9] later carried out a quantitative examination of the ultrastructural changes, occurring in experimental coarctation and in experimental renal hypertension in the dog. They found no evidence of any qualitative or quantitative difference occurring in receptor endings as a result of hypertension of some months' duration. This is contrary to the evidence of Abraham [10], who suggested that there was loss of neural elements in longer standing hypertension.

It has also been reported that changes in the vessel wall may contribute to a normal baroreceptor function in hypertension. Age changes in humans have been reported by Learoyd and Taylor [11]. There is an increase in medial thickness and in overall diameter [12]. Tobian et al. [13, 14] described increased content of water and sodium in hypertensive arteries. An increase in protein synthesis can be shown in arterial wall following baroreceptor denervation [15]. However, in the larger arteries in humans, we were unable to show any increase in stiffness if measurements were made at the same transmural pressure [16].

We did careful ultrastructural examination of the wall of the carotid sinus [9]. When a quantitative count of nerve structure was carried out in both normal and hypertensive dog carotid sinuses by a 'blind' comparison, we found no significant changes, although intimal and medial changes were seen. This was in contrast to the changes seen in longer-lasting hypertension in humans [10].

PHYSIOLOGICAL STUDIES

Baroreceptor discharge under normal conditions

Landgren [17] found two types of receptors in the sinus area of the cat, and thought that these two types were probably distinguished by axons with myelinated or unmyelinated fibers. Unmyelinated fibers tended to have receptors with higher thresholds and slower firing rates, with action potentials of smaller voltage. I found no clear distinction between the action potential voltages of myelinated and unmyelinated fibers is the dog [18] (see Figs. 1 and 2). Certainly, action potential voltage seems more related to technical factors, such as the size of the filament examined, and the intraelectrode difference than by fundamental properties of the axon. In support of Landgren, we did find that the higher threshold fibers tended to have lower firing rates. A comparison of medullated and non-medullated fibers in the rat aortic arch [19] suggests that some of the differences in their discharge characteristics may be due to differences in the mechanical coupling of the receptor endings.

Baroreceptor units show very characteristic and rapid adaptation when a static pressure change is induced. This adaptation is probably largely explained by viscoelastic 'creep' in the vessel wall [20]. When a stress is applied to the wall, e.g., a sudden pressure change, the resultant deformation of the wall (or strain) has a rapid (elastic) component followed by a slower deformation, thought to be a viscous process, as different tissue and cells adapt to the new situation. This

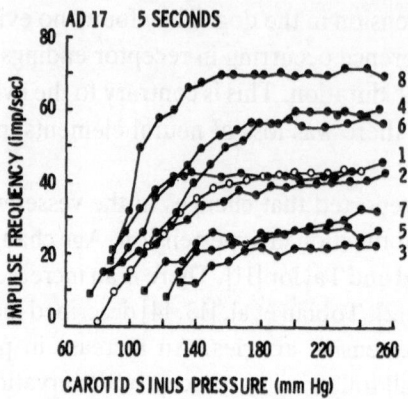

Figure 1. Pressure impulse frequency plots for eight consecutive single fibers examined in one normo-tensive dog. Note the wide range of firing characteristics. The numbers at the end of each line represent the order in which the fibers were dissected and examined. Open circles represent the mean of all eight fibers.

slower process is referred to as 'creep.' At this time, the wall tension decreases slightly, and there is less tension on receptor elements arranged in series with the tissue elements; hence, the firing rate decays or adapts. As the stress is increased, the wall becomes increasingly stiff, asymptotically reaching a plateau with no further deformation of the receptor element, so that there is no further increase in discharge. This is referred to as 'saturation.' The firing curve in response to pressure change operates from the threshold portion of the stimulus-response curve (i.e., when the discharge begins), and shows a plateau due to saturation. We have shown that if firing is related to wall strain rather than to pressure, there is no plateau phase. 'Saturation' therefore appears to be due to failure of the

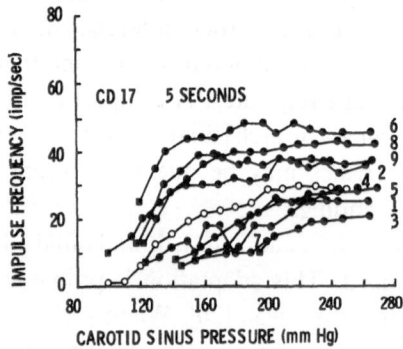

Figure 2. As in Fig. 1, nine fibers from one hypertensive dog. Note the higher threshold, loss of sensitivity, and lower maximal firing frequency.

vessel wall to stretch further in response to rise in transmural pressure.

If we correlate the changes in firing frequency with the dynamic input to the baroreceptors, we find that there is a very faithful reproduction of the mechanical changes in the sinus wall, and hence of the arterial pressure pulse. Thus, the quality of information transmitted to the central nervous system is very high (Fig. 3).

We have used a sensitive ultrasonic micrometer to relate the pressure and nerve firing changes to dimension changes in the sinus wall [21] (Fig. 3). We found that firing was linearly related to sinus dimension, and that the plateau seen when firing was related to pressure is due to the lack of wall stretch at higher pressures [22]. The carotid sinus was found to be more distensible than the adjacent carotid artery [23]. We found also that the firing frequency of the receptors could be influenced by the tone of the vascular smooth muscle, changed either by noradrenaline or by efferent sympathetic nervous stimulation [24]. We calculated sinus wall tension, and found that there was a clear relation between wall tension and firing. The data strongly argued in favor of the hypothesis that the receptor element is in series with smooth muscle, rather than in parallel. This has implications for the use of vasoactive drugs, such as phenylephrine, in the testing of the baroreflex function [25].

Changes in baroreceptor discharge induced by hypertension

The most striking characteristic of the change in baroreceptor output in hypertension is the upward resetting of the firing threshold. The speed with which this

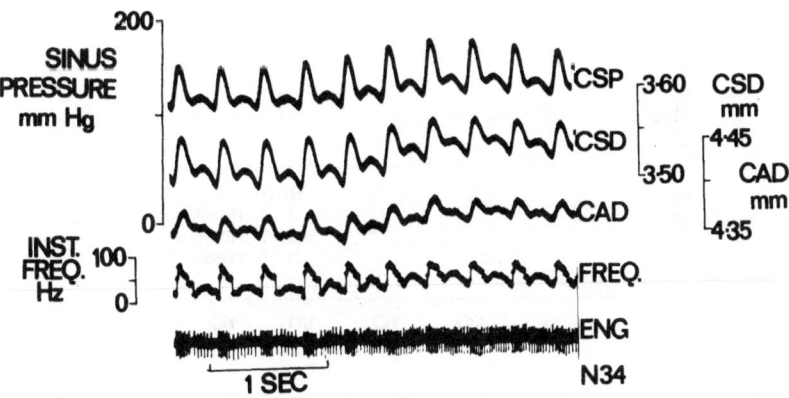

Figure 3. Records (from above down) of carotid sinus pressure (CSP mm Hg), carotid sinus diameter (CSD), and adjacent carotid artery diameter (CAD mm); instantaneous firing frequency of the single baroreceptor nerve fiber shown at ENG. Note the faithful correlation between pressure, dimension, and nerve firing frequency. (Data from Bergel et al. [21] on anesthetised dogs.)

308

occurs appears to be different in different species. In the rat, it appears to occur within 24 to 48 hours [26]. In the rabbit, it is present at 5 days of hypertension [27]. We found it became progressively more apparent after 5 days in the dog [18]. We found that the single fiber static threshold in hypertensive dogs (MAP 148 mm Hg) increased from 104 mm Hg (normotensive) to 128 mm Hg. Furthermore, the maximum firing frequency decreased from 43 to 32 impulses/second. Lowering of the animals' pressure caused a recovery towards normality in the baroreceptor characteristics (Figs. 1, 2, 4). We also compared normal and hypertensive grey-hounds, and found that the carotid sinus was stiffer in hypertensive animals, but that the relation between baroreceptor firing and wall strain was not significantly different [28].

CONCLUSION

All these data suggest that the rise in threshold and decrease in sensitivity seen in hypertension is a consequence of changes in the mechanical behavior of the sinus wall rather than in the receptors per se. Whatever the causes of the deterioration in receptor function, it is clear that this results in a deterioration in the ability to buffer changes in arterial pressure at the higher level of pressure [29].

In this review, I have not dealt with the important studies on the nonmyelinated baroreceptor afferents [30, 31]. Jones and Thoren [32] found that these fibers

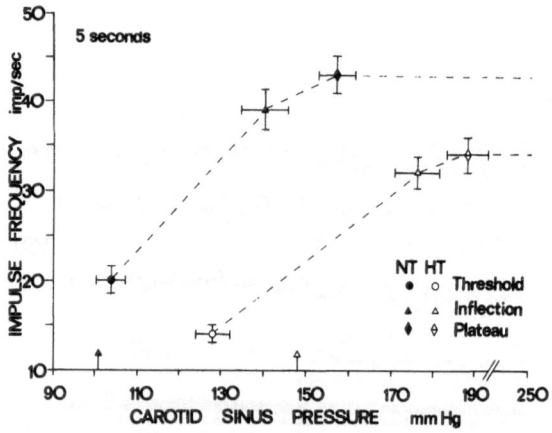

Figure 4. Impulse frequency 5 seconds after a static pressure step input to the carotid sinus, in normotensive and hypertensive dogs. The mean ± SE for the values at the threshold for firing, the end of the linear range (inflection), and plateau (maximal firing rate) are shown. The arrows on the abscissa indicate the resting conscious arterial pressure in the normotensive (filled arrow) and the hypertensive (open arrow) animals. Summary of data from Sleight et al. 1977 [18].

were reset less than myelinated fibers in hypertensive rabbits. They may therefore have a relatively greater influence in blood pressure control in hypertension.

REFERENCES

1. Hering HE: Der karotisdruckversuch. Munch Med Wochenschr 70:1287-1290, 1923.
2. Koch EH: Ueber den depressorischen gefassreflex beim karotid druck versuche am menschen. Munch Med Wochenschr 71:1924.
3. Adrian ED: The impulses produced by sensory nerve endings. Part I. J Physiol 61:49-72, 1926.
4. Bronk DW, Stella G: Afferent impulses in carotid sinus nerve. J Cell Comp Physiol 1:113-130, 1932.
5. McCubbin JW, Green JH, Page IH: Baroreceptor function in chronic renal hypertension. Circ Res 4:205-210, 1956.
6. De Castro F: Sur la structure et l'innervation de la glande intercarotidienne (glomus caroticum) de l'homme et des mammiferes et sur un nouveau systeme d'innervation autonome du nerf glossopharyngien. Trav Lab Recherch Biol Univ Madrid 24:365-432, 1926.
7. De Castro F: Sur la structure et l'innervation du sinus carotidien de l'homme et des mammiferes. Nouveaux faits sur l'innervation et la function du glonus caroticum. Trav Lab Recherch Biol Univ Madrid 25:331-380, 1928.
8. Rees PM: Observations on the fine structure and distribution of presumptive baroreceptor nerves at the carotid sinus. J Comp Neurol 131:517-548, 1967.
9. Rees PM, Sleight P, Robinson JL, et al.: Histology and ultrastructure of the carotid sinus in experimental hypertension. J Comp Neurol 181:245-252, 1978.
10. Abraham A: The structure of baroreceptors in pathological conditions in man, in Kezdi P (editor): Baroreceptors and Hypertension. London, Pergamon Press, 1967, p 273.
11. Learoyd BM, Taylor MG: Alterations with age in the viscoelastic properties of human arterial walls. Circ Res 18:278-292, 1966.
12. Bader H: Dependence of wall stress in the human thoracic aorta on age and pressure. Circ Res 20:354-361, 1967.
13. Tobian L, Redleaf PD: Ionic composition of aorta in renal and adrenal hypertension. Am J Physiol 192:325-330, 1958.
14. Tobian L, Olson R, Chesley G: Water content of arteriolar wall in renovascular hypertension. Am J Physiol 216:22-24, 1969.
15. MacLean AG, Bevan RD, Hume WR, et al.: Rapid onset of vascular wall protein synthesis with increase in lability of blood pressure in rabbits. Clin Sci 59(Suppl 6):327s-329s, Dec 1980.
16. Gribbin B, Pickering TG, Sleight P: Arterial distensibility in normal and hypertensive man. Clin Sci 56:413-417, 1979.
17. Landgren S: The baroreceptor activity in the carotid sinus nerve and the distensibility of the sinus wall. Acta Physiol Scand 26:35-56, 1952.
18. Sleight P, Robinson JL, Brooks DE, et al.: Characteristics of single carotid sinus baroreceptor fibers and whole nerve activity in the normotensive and the renal hypertensive dog. Circ Res 41(6):750-758, 1977.
19. Brown AM, Saum WR, Yasui S: Baroreceptor dynamics and their relationship to afferent fibre type and hypertension. Circ Res 42:694-702, 1978.
20. Arndt JO, Dorrenhaus A, Wiecken H: The aortic arch baroreceptor response to static and dynamic stretches in an isolated aorta-depressor nerve preparation of cats in vitro. J Physiol 252:59-78, 1975.
21. Bergel DH, Bertram CD, Brooks DE, et al.: Simultaneous recording of the carotid sinus

dimensions and the baroreceptor nerve in the anaesthetized dog. J Physiol 252:15-16, 1975.

22. Bergel DH, Brooks DE, MacDermott AJ, et al.: The relation between carotid sinus dimension, nerve activity and pressure in the anaesthetized greyhound. J Physiol 263:156-157, 1976.

23. Bergel DH, Brooks DE, MacDermott AJ, et al.: Comparison of the mechanical properties of the carotid sinus and adjacent common carotid artery, and the effects of noradrenaline. J Physiol 263:266, 1976b.

24. Bergel DH, Brooks DE, MacDermott AJ, et al.: Baroreceptor firing frequency and activation of carotid sinus vascular smooth muscle in dogs. J Physiol 275:37-38, 1977.

25. Bergel DH, Peveler RC, Robinson JL, et al.: The measurement of arterial pressure, carotid sinus radius and baroreflex sensitivity in the conscious greyhound. J Physiol 292:65-66, 1979.

26. Krieger EM: The time course of baroreceptor resetting in acute hypertension. Am J Physiol 218:486-490, 1970.

27. Angell J: Characteristics of single aortic and right subclavian baroreceptor fibre activity in rabbits with chronic renal hypertension. Circ Res 32:149-161, 1973.

28. Bergel DH, Peveler RC, Robinson JL, et al.: Resetting of arterial baroreceptors in hypertensive dogs. J Physiol 319:119-120, 1981.

29. Sleight P: Baroreceptors and Hypertension. Oxford, University Press, 1980.

30. Aars H, Myhre L, Haswell BA: The function of baroreceptor C fibers in the rabbit's aortic nerve. Acta Physiol Scand 102:84-93, 1978.

31. Thoren P, Jones JV: Characteristics of aortic baroreceptor C-fibers in the rabbit. Acta Physiol Scand 99:448-456, 1977.

32. Jones JV, Thoren PN: Characteristics of aortic baroreceptors with non-medullated afferents arising from the aortic arch of rabbits with chronic renovascular hypertension. Acta Physiol Scand 101:286-293, 1977.

DISCUSSION

Discussants: Summit, Sleight, Birkenhager, Brody, Abboud, Mark, Bohr, Williams

Summit: How long does it take for the altered setting to reset itself if you treat the hypertensive, assuming that there are no structural changes yet?

Sleight: Well, that's quite an interesting question. In some animals, like the rat, it occurs very quickly indeed. In dogs we found that it took at least four or five days before we could see any changes. John Vann Jones, who works in my department, found that the resetting of the reflex arc in the rat with renal hypertension occurred very early, indeed, much earlier than researchers in Bjorn Folkow's department had found structural changes. There were two possibilities: One seemed to be that it could be due to waterlogging or saltlogging of the wall; but another alternative, which seemed more attractive (and I believe he's got some evidence for this now), was that it had to do with the central resetting due to the rise in angiotensin. So the beginning part of the resetting might occur rather quickly on a central basis in some animals. We didn't find changes in the nerve activity in the dogs in the early stages, but I should say we didn't actually test the reflex at that stage. If we had done so with whatever test, e.g., phenylephrine, we might well have found that it was reset in that early stage because of the high levels of angiotensin at that time.

Birkenhager: You just mentioned initial hypertension, and I would like to challenge you on that a bit. Did you have a close look at those cases with extremely labile hypertension and try to find out whether the baroreflex arc in this case is abnormal?

Sleight: I find it terribly difficult to say what is labile hypertension because with our 24-hour blood pressure records, we find enormous variability in blood pressure in people. If we examine the standard deviation of the intra-arterial systolic blood pressure over 24-hours in ambulant subjects away from the hospital, there is a negative correlation with baroreflex sensitivity, the poorer the sensitivity, the more labile the blood pressure. But to partly answer your question, some others (Takeshita and Mark) have looked at borderline hypertension rather than labile hypertension and found that the reflex is reset at that stage.

Brody: I would like to amplify on the contention that there are early signs of resetting in hypertension. In the model I showed you this morning of acute hypertension produced by renal artery stenosis in the conscious rat, there is a significant resetting of the baroreflex response within two hours after elevation of the arterial pressure. Using pressor and depressor responses to trigger changes in heart rate we found a shift without any change in baroreflex slope. So, sensitivity was normal, but early resetting occurred. This mechanism could play an important role in establishing hypertension in its very early stages.

Abboud: I think the point about the change in strain sensitivity in some hypertensive models even before the onset of hypertension would be an intriguing observation. Dr. Mark, do you want to comment on the change in strain sensitivity?

Mark: Arthur Brown has some studies in young SHR which suggest that differences in strain sensitivity, which may be genetically determined, may contribute to early changes in baroreceptor properties and function. It's difficult in the SHR to separate the contribution of genetic factors and changes in pressure. I'll present some evidence when I talk on the Dahl strain.

Bohr: Your model putting the smooth muscle in series with the receptor makes the smooth muscle a candidate for altering the activity of the receptor. Is there any respect given to this tissue?

Sleight: We actually examined the influence of efferent sympathetic nerve activity upon baroreceptor sensitivity on the afferent side and we were able to show that there was quite a substantial effect of the sympathetic nervous system on tuning the afferent output. There's been a lot of controversy about this over the years. In the early days, Landgren and others showed that norepinephrine applied externally on the carotid sinus increased output from the nerve, and there was argument as to whether this was physiological or not because they used rather large concentrations. When we started to stimulate the sympathetic supply to the sinus, we started with the stellate ganglion in the dog. We got absolutely no result and were rather disappointed. Later we read of the anatomy of the supply to the carotid sinus and found that it comes from much lower down. So you have to go much lower down the sympathetics to actually show this effect on the carotid sinus. The result is rather complex and best fits a model with the receptors in series with smooth muscle blocks: low pressures, when the wall itself is not stretched very much. There is in fact a decrease in firing, but a crossover occurs fairly early on, and then there is an increase in the firing with stimulation at higher baseline transneural pressures. The decrease at low pressures is because contraction of the media of the wall decreases the carotid diameter and substantially unloads the receptors. At higher pressures, the smooth muscle is unable to reduce carotid diameter, but stimulation of muscle fibers which are in series with the receptor increases the load on the receptor with an increase in firing.

Williams: Can you show that the baroreceptor response in treated hypertensives is different after treatment, and, if so, how long a period of treatment does it take before you can detect that change in their baroreflex sensitivity?

Sleight: In man, we haven't had much success in doing that. It can be shown in animals, but in man the wall changes include fibrosis and atheroma, which are not reversible. We have studied renal hypertensive subjects who had extremely high pressure initially, which was covered by dialysis or transplantation. Baroreflex sensitivity (measured by the phenylephrine method) did not change when tested over a year or so at very different levels of pressure. So the short answer is, in man, at least in well-established and severe hypertension, there is not much chance of showing a resetting. It's possible that one might show this with early treatment of borderline hypertensives.

INFLUENCE OF SODIUM INTAKE ON THE NEUROGENIC CONTRIBUTION IN HYPERTENSION

ALLYN L. MARK

INTRODUCTION

There are multiple mechanisms by which excess dietary sodium might contribute to increased vascular resistance and hypertension. These include increases in sodium and water content of blood vessels, autoregulation of blood flow, effects on transmembrane ionic exchange in vascular muscle, and alterations in humoral mechanisms.

In addition to these mechanisms, research during the past 20 years has revealed that the autonomic nervous system is an important link between sodium and hypertension. This was initially demonstrated in deoxycorticosterone (DOC)-salt hypertension and has subsequently been confirmed in genetic models of hypertension, including the Dahl salt-sensitive rat and the Okamoto spontaneously hypertensive rat. There is also evidence implicating neural mechanisms in the effects of dietary sodium on human hypertensives. Indeed, it is now apparent that high dietary salt can unmask or aggravate underlying genetic abnormalities in central and peripheral adrenergic mechanisms. The nature of the interaction of sodium balance and neural mechanisms is not clear, but it is tempting to speculate that it may involve genetic abnormalities in humoral factors on transmembrane ionic exchange.

In this paper, I will discuss briefly some of the information implicating the autonomic nervous system in DOC-salt hypertension, Dahl salt-sensitive rats, and human hypertension.

DEOXYCORTICOSTERONE (DOC) AND SALT

The classical studies of deChamplain et al. in DOC-salt hypertensive rats were the first to clearly establish that sodium balance exerted a profound influence on the sympathetic nervous system [1, 2]. In DOC-salt hypertensive rats, the retention and storage of norepinephrine in peripheral adrenergic endings was decreased, presumably as a reflection of increased turnover of norepinephrine [1, 2]. These changes preceded the development of hypertension. The abnormalities were related to the state of sodium balance, since withdrawal of sodium lowered the blood pressure and restored a normal turnover rate of norepinephrine [1, 2]. The studies of these investigators and others thus provided convincing evidence for an effect of sodium balance on peripheral adrenergic function.

The augmentation of peripheral adrenergic function appears to relate to a defect in central adrenergic mechanisms [2, 3]. In DOC-salt rats, there was a decrease in turnover of norepinephrine in the brainstem. It was proposed that this indicated decreased activity of a central noradrenergic sympathoinhibitory system and would result in activation of the peripheral adrenergic system. Ganglionic blockade or spinal cord sectioning lowered blood pressure and normalized turnover of norepinephrine in the periphery but did not reverse the decreased turnover in the brain stem [2]. This observation excluded the possibility that the abnormalities in central adrenergic mechanisms were secondary to elevated arterial pressure and favored the view that the influence of sodium balance on central neural mechanisms plays a pivotal role in DOC-salt hypertension.

There is also evidence that neural mechanisms may be involved in the vasoconstrictor and pressor effects of vasopressin in DOC-salt hypertension. Matsuguchi and Schmid [4] found that effects of vasopressin on vascular resistance were augmented in DOC-salt hypertensive rats. This augmented effect was dependent on an intact sympathetic innervation to blood vessels. This interaction of vasopressin and neurogenic mechanisms in DOC-salt hypertension has previously been attributed to peripheral interactions or loss of a normal facilitatory influence of vasopressin on baroreflex buffering. However, recent work suggests that it may instead involve a disturbance in complex effects of vasopressin on central neural mechanisms [5].

The knowledge that the sympathetic nervous system contributes importantly in DOC-salt hypertension stimulated interest in the role of neurogenic mechanisms in human hypertension and in animal models of genetic hypertension such as the Dahl strain.

DAHL SALT-SENSITIVE RATS

The Dahl strain of sodium-sensitive, genetically hypertensive rats was developed in the early 1960s. For many years it was considered a model of renal and humoral hypertension. Based on the findings in DOC-salt rats, we began in 1975 to study the role of neurogenic mechanisms in Dahl rats. Our first study demonstrated that a substantial fraction of the salt-induced increase in hindquarters vascular resistance in Dahl-sensitive (DS) rats resulted from increased neurogenic vasoconstrictor tone [6]. It was subsequently demonstrated that 'chemical sympathectomy' with 6-hydroxydopamine prevents salt-induced hypertension in DS rats [7] and that ganglionic blockade eliminates the difference in arterial pressure between hypertensive Dahl-sensitive and resistant (DR) rats [8].

These findings in the Dahl strain indicated that the observations in DOC-salt rats on the importance of the sympathetic nervous system in the effects of sodium extend to genetic hypertension.

These observations prompted a number of studies regarding the ways in which high sodium intake and genetic factors interact to perturb neurogenic mechanisms in Dahl rats.

Takeshita and Mark [6] demonstrated that a high-sodium diet potentiates vasoconstrictor responses sympathetic nerve stimulation in DS rats but does not augment responses to norepinephrine. In DR rats, a high-sodium diet did not alter vascular responses to either sympathetic nerve stimulation or norepinephrine. The finding that high sodium potentiates responses to sympathetic nerve stimulation, but not to norepinephrine, suggests that high salt facilitates release of norepinephrine from adrenergic nerve endings. Thus, salt loading appears to unmask a genetic abnormality in peripheral adrenergic mechanisms.

As in DOC-salt hypertensive rats, the central nervous system also appears to be involved in the abnormalities of the autonomic nervous system produced by high-sodium diets. Pressor responses to cerebral ventricular administration of angiotensin II and hypertonic sodium chloride are greater in DS than DR rats on both low- and high-salt diets [9, 10]. Recent studies in our laboratory [10] suggest that these differences are exaggerated after chronic sinoaortic baroreceptor denervation. In addition, lesions of the anteroventral third ventricle attenuate salt-induced hypertension in DS rats but do not alter arterial pressure in DR rats fed high salt [11, 12]. Injection of the adrenergic neurotoxin, 6-hydroxydopamine, into the brain ventricles also prevents salt-induced hypertension in DS rats.

Gordon et al. [8, 13] have determined that baroreflex control of heart rate and vascular resistance is less in DS than in DR rats fed low-sodium diets. This difference may be of genetic origin, since it occurs before a difference in arterial pressure in DS and DR rats. It is not clear how and to what extent this difference in baroreflex control might contribute to the hypertensive effect of high salt in DS rats. It may contribute to augmented systemic pressor responses to vasoconstrictor stimuli in DS rats. In addition, it may deprive the DS rats of a compensatory mechanism that normally protects against the vasoconstrictor and hypertensive effects of high salt intake. Specifically, it is known that the gain or buffering capacity of arterial baroreflexes normally increases during high salt intake [14]; this compensatory response to high salt intake is impaired in DS rats.

Thus, studies during the last five years have demonstrated that salt-induced hypertension in Dahl rats, which was attributed to humoral and renal factors, also involves an important role for the autonomic nervous system.

HUMAN HYPERTENSION

In recent years, studies from several laboratories have extended to humans the concepts of salt-sensitivity and salt-resistance. In normotensive humans, increasing sodium intake from 10 to 400 mEq Na$^+$/24 h usually fails to increase arterial pressure [15-17] and may decrease rather than increase vascular resistance [15, 17]. This apparently occurs because of compensatory neurohumoral adjustments that prevent increases in vascular resistance and arterial pressure during a high-sodium diet [15]. For example, high sodium intake decreases renin, aldosterone, and presumably angiotensin and may thereby decrease vascular resistance. In addition, high-sodium diets appear to decrease sympathetic nervous system activity in normotensive humans. Abboud demonstrated that a high-sodium diet tends to decrease vasoconstrictor responses to tyramine and to lower body negative pressure relative to responses to the neurotransmitter norepinephrine [15]. This suggests that a high-sodium diet may decrease the storage and release of norepinephrine in normotensive subjects. In addition, a high-sodium diet decreases plasma norepinephrine concentration and urinary norepinephrine excretion in normotensive humans [18, 19]. In contrast to these observations in normotensive humans, there is evidence that many humans with hypertension may be sensitive to the deleterious effects of a high-sodium diet [17, 20, 21]. As in experimental animals, this salt-sensitivity may involve the autonomic nervous system. For example, we observed that a high-sodium diet increased forearm vascular resistance in borderline hypertensives [20], whereas it decreased forearm resistance in normotensive subjects [15]. The increase in forearm vascular resistance in the borderline hypertensives was accompanied by a selective augmentation of vasoconstrictor responses to a reflex stimulus (lower-body negative pressure) as compared with the neurotransmitter norepinephrine [20]. This suggests that high-sodium diet facilitates neurogenic vasoconstriction in many borderline hypertensives, whereas it appears to exert opposite effects in normotensive subjects [15, 20].

Fujita et al., in Bartter's laboratory, have identified contrasting behavior of sympathetic indices in salt-sensitive and salt-resistant human hypertensives [22]. With a change in sodium intake from 9 to 249 mEq/24 h, plasma norepinephrine initially decreased in both groups, but then rose significantly in salt-sensitive subjects and remained low in salt-resistant subjects. These investigators suggested that persistence of relatively normal adrenergic drive in the face of a high-sodium diet may contribute to the increase in blood pressure in salt-sensitive human hypertensives.

Thus, there is increasing evidence that the concept of salt-sensitivity and salt-resistance applies to humans as well as animal models of genetic hypertension. The phenomenon of salt-sensitivity in humans appears to involve abnormalities in adrenergic control of the circulation.

CONCLUSION

There is increasing evidence that the sympathetic nervous system participates in the vasoconstrictor and hypertensive effects of excess dietary sodium. This paper briefly reviews some of the evidence derived from models of experimental (DOC-salt) and genetic (Dahl-strain) hypertension in animals and from human hypertensives.

ACKNOWLEDGMENTS

The author's studies described in this paper were supported by Program Project Grant HL 14388, Research Grants HL 24962, and an Institutional Research Fellowship HL 07121 from the National Heart, Lung, and Blood Institute; by Research Funds from the Veterans Administration; and by Grant-in-Aid from the Iowa Affiliate, American Heart Association.

We thank Jan Ellsworth for secretarial assistance, and Jinx Tracy and Don Morgan for research assistance. Dr. Junichi Iwai kindly provided Dahl rats for the studies of the author and his colleagues.

REFERENCES

1. De Champlain J, Krakoff LR, Axelrod J: Relationship between sodium intake and norepinephrine storage during the development of experimental hypertension. Circ Res 23:479-291, 1968.
2. De Champlain J: Experimental aspects of the relationships between the autonomic nervous system and catecholamines in hypertension, in Genest J, Koiw E, Kuchel O (editors): Hypertension: Pathophysiology and Treatment. New York, McGraw-Hill, 1977, pp 76-92.
3. Nakamura K, Gerold M, Thoenen H: Experimental hypertension of the rat: Reciprocal changes of norepinephrine turnover in heart and brainstem. Naunyn Schmiedebergs Arch Pharmacol 268:125, 1971.
4. Matsuguchi H, Schmid PG: Acute interaction of vasopressin and neurogenic mechanisms in DOC-salt hypertension. Am J Physiol 242:H37-H43, 1982.
5. Sharabi F, Schmid PG: Evidence for a role of vasopressin in hypertension. Am J Nephrol, in press.
6. Takeshita A, Mark AL: Neurogenic contribution to hindquarters vasoconstriction during high sodium intake in Dahl strain of genetically hypertensive rat. Circ Res 43:186-I91, 1978.
7. Takeshita A, Mark AL, Brody MJ: Prevention of salt-induced hypertension in the Dahl strain by 6-hydroxydopamine. Am J Physiol 236:H48-H52, 1979.
8. Gordon FJ, Matsuguchi H, Mark AL: Abnormal baroreflex control of heart rate in prehypertensive and hypertensive Dahl genetically salt-sensitive rats. Hypertension 3:I135-I141, 1981.
9. Ikeda T, Tobian L, Iwai J, et al.: Central nervous system pressor responses in rats susceptible and resistant to sodium chloride hypertension. Clin Sci Mol Med 55:225s-227s, 1978.
10. Gordon FJ, Mark AL: Effect of arterial baroreceptor denervation on central nervous system pressor responses in the Dahl strain. Fed Proc 41:1518, 1982.
11. Brody MJ, Fink GD, Bugge J, et al.: Critical role of the anteroventral third ventricle (AV3V) region in development and maintenance of experimental hypertension, in Meyer P, Schmitt H (editors): Nervous System and Hypertension: Perspectives in Nephrology and Hypertension. New York, Wiley-Flammarion, 1979, pp 76-84.

318

12. Goto A, Ikeda T, Tobian L, et al.: Brain lesions in paraventricular nucleus and adrenergic neurons minimize NaCl hypertension. Circulation 64:IV-111, 1981.

13. Gordon FJ, Mark AL: Impaired baroreflex control of vascular resistance in Dahl salt-sensitive rats. Clin Res 29:722A, 1981.

14. Rocchini AP, Cant JR, Barger AC: Carotid sinus reflex in dogs with low- to high-sodium intake. Am J Physiol 233:H196-H202, 1977.

15. Abboud FM: Effects of sodium, angiotensin, and steroids on vascular reactivity in man. Fed Proc 33:143-149, 1974.

16. Murray RH, Luft FC, Bloch R, et al.: Blood pressure responses to extremes of sodium intake in normal man. Proc Soc Exp Biol Med 159:432-436, 1978.

17. Sullivan JM, Ratts TE, Taylor C, et al.: Hemodynamic effects of dietary sodium in man. A preliminary report. Hypertension 2:506-514, 1980.

18. Romoff MS, Keusch G, Campese VM, et al.: Effect of sodium intake on plasma catecholamines in normal subjects. J Clin Endocrinol Metab 48:26-31, 1979.

19. Luft FC, Rankin LI, Henry DP, et al.: Plasma and urinary norepinephrine values at extremes of sodium intake in normal man. Hypertension 1:261-266, 1979.

20. Mark AL, Lawton WJ, Abboud FM, et al.: Effects of high and low sodium intake on arterial pressure and forearm vascular resistance in borderline hypertension. Circ Res 36/37:I194-I198, 1975.

21. Kawasaki T, Dulea CS, Bartter FC, et al.: The effect of high-sodium and low-sodium intakes on blood pressure and other related variables in human subjects with idiopathic hypertension. Am J Med 64:193-198, 1978.

22. Fujita T, Henry WL, Bartter FC, et al.: Factors influencing blood pressure in salt-sensitive patients with hypertension. Am J Med 69:334-344, 1980.

DISCUSSION

Discussants: Muirhead, Mark, Langer, Williams, Birkenhager, Bohr, Abboud, Haddy, Blaustein.

Muirhead: As you know, Dahl did the cross-transplantation experiment and showed that the S rat could be made into an R rat and an R rat into an S rat. Tomorrow we'll show that the renal medullary interstitial cells of the S rat are entirely different from those of the R rat. The S rats have marked depletion in the number of these cells. They're small, they lack granules, and they lack processes. The R rats have huge cells, the largest we've seen, loaded with granules and processes. We have obtained both cells in the cell culture, and in cell culture the abnormal characteristics of each is retained. What we don't have is functional studies, which we are attempting to develop now. How do you align the neuromechanisms with the seeming abnormality in the kidney, as demonstrated by Dahl's cross-experiments and as now demonstrated by what appears to be a deficiency in the renal medullary interstitial cell system?

Mark: I think Dahl's work and your observations suggest that there may be abnormalities in renal vasodilator mechanisms. He also suggested that there was an abnormal vasoconstrictor or pressor substance which was released, he thought in the kidney. Lou Tobian has some evidence from cross-perfusion studies to support the presence of a circulating vasoconstrictor substance. I think it's tempting to speculate that abnormalities in humoral factors might play a very important role in the abnormalities in adrenergic function that I've described, perhaps facilitation of peripheral adrenergic mechanisms and perhaps even central adrenergic mechanisms in the Dahl strain. There are some observations, I believe, that suggest that the humoral factor, which Haddy and Overbeck have described in models of volume-expanded hypertension, is not the humoral factor in the Dahl strain. There is some evidence for abnormalities in vasopressin release in the Dahl strain, but not much evidence that this contributes importantly to the self-induced hypertension.

Muirhead: The presence of a pressor substance, at least hypothetically, could be due to an unmasking of that substance as a consequence of the absence of a depressor substance. So it doesn't necessarily follow that there is a pressor substance as a primary event.

Mark: It's an extremely complex series of experiments, involving not only parabiosis but nephrectomy and the like, which prompted him to suggest that there was both a deficiency of a circulating vasodilator and a pressor substance. So I think the weight of evidence suggests that both may be involved.

Langer: In your high-salt group, the S strain, you showed that the responses to sympathetic nerve stimulation are enhanced. Are these effects still observed when you inhibit norepinephrine reuptake with cocaine or desipramine, and is this increased responsiveness to nerve stimulation restricted to blood vessels, or do you see it, for instance, on accelerans nerve stimulation as well?

Mark: We have not performed experiments with cocaine or inhibition of uptake. I might note here that the selective augmentation of the responses to nerve stimulation that we observed in the hind-quarters is not seen in the renal circulation, which may provide some evidence against the hypothesis that they're related to a circulating humoral factor. We haven't performed experiments in the heart, for example.

Williams: Your results both in animals and humans are very intriguing. It would be very interesting if we could find that sort of a differentiation between individuals genetically predisposed to hypertension in a free-living population. My question is, in contrast to your laboratory methods where you can look at very extreme circumstances in terms of salt loading and have nice instrumentation with invasive instruments, do you think, in a noninvasive setting, that instruments such as cold-pressor tests or grip-pressure tests and 24-hour urinary sodiums and so forth could allow us in a free-living population to find the same kind of data that you've been finding in your laboratory studies?

Mark: You may recall the slide on the studies in humans. The differences in the effects of high sodium in the two groups were not strikingly apparent from the effects on arterial pressure. I think it obvious from studies on circulatory control that measurements of arterial pressure alone may not be a very sensitive indicator of the effects of interventions like high salt intake on the circulation. I think it's the measurements of vascular resistance that really revealed the striking difference in the vascular response of the two groups. So, I think it may not be possible simply from measurements of arterial pressure, even accurate measurements, to get a lot more information on the question of salt sensitivity and salt resistance.

Williams: What about the use of tests like the grip-pressure or cold-pressor test to sympathetically stimulate the individual? Sometimes there's a dramatic change in blood pressure in some individuals and not in others. Do you think that's related to the phenomenon?

Mark: Yes, Onesti's group at Hahnemann has some evidence that there are exaggerated responses to cold pressor tests and other stimuli in the offspring of hypertensive parents as well as mildly hypertensive young subjects.

Birkenhager: I'm going to move the ball backwards again and ask Dr. Bohr what happened to cardiac output and to the old autoregulation hypothesis that salt loading causes at first an increase in cardiac output?

Bohr: Our pigs hadn't heard of it, and they just don't act that way. Vascular smooth muscle sensitivity does increase, but DOCA or mineralocorticoids acting *in vitro* on vascular smooth muscle have no effect. They have to be in an intact animal where the nervous system can have some influence on it.

Mark: I think that in normotensive volunteers, there's no evidence to suggest that the increase in flow is a sufficient stimulus for vasoconstriction because they have very high levels of flow, presumably for prolonged periods of time. Nevertheless vascular resistance remains low. I think that the increase in cardiac output with a high-salt diet in young Dahl R rats is in fact greater than in the S rats, and yet they do not develop vasoconstriction whereas the S rats do. So it would appear that it's at least not a sufficient condition for the salt-induced vasoconstriction in either the Dahl rats or the humans.

Abboud: So, to answer the question, the total body autoregulation hypothesis is not alive and well.

Haddy: Have you looked at potassium effects? Recall that Dietz in Germany showed that in SHR, a high-salt diet reduced norepinephrine uptake by the cardiac sympathetic nerve endings in association with an accelerated rise in blood pressure, and when he also placed them on a high-potassium diet, the accelerated rise in blood pressure disappeared, as did the norepinephrine uptake defect.

Mark: Yes, we have fed rats a high-salt diet with and without high potassium, and it significantly modulates the effects of high sodium. That modulation involves, to some extent, modulation of the neurogenic vasoconstriction, but it also appears to involve direct vascular effects that may involve membrane effects, I suppose. So, it does have a significant antihypertensive effect in the Dahl strain.

Blaustein: I just wanted to clarify one point in one of your very interesting slides on the pressure-flow relationships, in which you showed the effect of denervation in the salt-sensitive strain on a high-salt diet. There was a reduction in pressure at every flow level, whereas there was no effect in the animals on the low-sodium diet. Does that mean that there's no sympathetic activity?

Mark: In those animals which were anesthetized, that does suggest that there was no resting sympathetic drive in the S rats fed normal salt or, indeed, in the R rats fed high salt. We've subsequently performed studies in conscious S and R rats with ganglionic blockage, and there the differences in the two groups and in their response to ganglionic blockage are even more pronounced. So I think that the effects of anesthesis probably masked the differences in the two groups.

Blaustein: You mean there's relatively little sympathetic control of blood pressure in low-salt Dahl S rats?

Mark: In the hind limb, resistance under urethane anesthesia. That's correct.

SOME ASPECTS OF CARDIOVASCULAR NERVOUS CONTROL IN SPONTANEOUSLY HYPERTENSIVE RATS: CENTRAL AND PERIPHERAL MECHANISMS

PETER THORÉN, GUNNAR GÖTHBERG, STEFAN LUNDIN, HOLGER NILSSON AND BJÖRN FOLKOW

INTRODUCTION

For decades, our group has been engaged in studies of central, reflex, and peripheral nervous influences on cardiovascular function, mainly because they reflect by far the most differentiated, powerful, and swift of all control systems involved [1-3]. For example, at the limbic-hypothalamic level, nervous and hormonal mechanisms are linked together to form highly specific psychoemotional response patterns, each elicited by the appropriate type of environmental stimuli and, in their actions, often overswaying the reflex control level [3].

With respect to an involvement of nervous mechanisms in primary hypertension, the polygenetic predisposition in this disorder often seems to particularly affect the limbic-hypothalamic levels of control, both in humans and in the Okamoto-Aoki spontaneously hypertensive rat (SHR) [4-7]. For example, SHR display an inherently increased sensitivity to alerting or stressful environmental stimuli, which results in exaggerated defense reactions compared with controls [8]. This type of cental hyperreactivity to environmental stimuli is evidently quite important for the development of the SHR variant of primary hypertension, because Hallback [9] could show how partial social isolation from early age, which reduces the number of 'ordinary' environmental stimuli, attenuates and delays the development of hypertension. Likewise, SHR hypertension is greatly aggravated by chronic exposure to a stressful environment [4, 10].

In this respect, at least, SHR seems to be an appropriate model for the perhaps most common variant of human primary hypertension. For example, Falkner et al. [11] have shown how normotensive, or marginally hypertensive, adolescents from families with primary hypertension commonly display accentuated and prolonged defense reactions to a standardized test of forced mental arithmetic, as compared with adolescents without such family predisposition. Further, a subsequent follow-up study [12] showed that a considerable fraction of these genetically predisposed youngsters had developed mild established hypertension some 4 years later.

This close parallel between human and SHR primary hypertension with respect to central nervous involvement seems to make SHR a particularly suitable animal model for analyzing other aspects of nervous cardiovascular control in primary hypertension. Therefore, some of our recent findings concerning altered sympathetic control in SHR will be briefly outlined below, together with some evidence suggesting that kidneys may, via hormonal mechanisms, exert a central *attenuating* influence on tonic sympathetic discharge in a way that may reflect one of the buffering mechanisms of importance in primary hypertension.

SYMPATHETIC RENAL ACTIVITY

It was mentioned above how SHR display exaggerated defense reactions to ordinary alerting or 'stressful' environmental influences, and it is well known that defense reactions normally engage the renal sympathetic supply to a considerable extent, increasing renal blood flow resistance [13]. Therefore, Thorén and Lundin [14] are presently involved in analyses of renal sympathetic fiber discharge and neurogenic effects on renal blood flow, glomerular filtration, and tubular sodium reabsorbtion in awake rats, comparing SHR and Wistar Kyoto rats (WKY) when they are exposed to standardized environmental stimulation. Both during 'rest' and during increased alertness, SHR show a clearly increased sympathetic discharge to the kidneys, as compared with WKY. Particularly during 'mental stress' (exposure to a standardized jet of air), there is increased sympathetic activity in SHR, paralleled by a more reduced renal blood flow and glomerular filtration rate and by a more extensive tubular reabsorbtion of sodium chloride than in WKY. The net effect is a markedly greater decrease of sodium chloride excretion in SHR than in WKY (Fig. 1). This is no doubt of nervous origin with respect to the increased tubular reabsorbtion, because the difference between SHR and WKY was largely abolished by renal denervation. Thus, as one important expression of the central hyperreactivity in SHR to environmental stimuli, and consequent to the accentuated sympathetic activity to the kidneys, SHR show a clear trend towards *increased* sodium chloride retention as compared with normotensive controls when alerted.

STRESS AND SALT

This means that the two major environmental influences in primary hypertension - psychosocial stimuli and habitual salt intake - are in reality closely linked at the renal level. The former type of influence in appropriately predisposed organisms neurogenically reduces the renal excretion of the latter, implying a trend towards volume increase, other things being equal. It should be remembered that findings by Axelrod and de Champlain et al. [15, 16] suggest that a salt-volume expansion can, in turn, exert a reinforcing influence on catecholamine turnover. This is also supported by findings by the groups of Mark [17] and Tobian [18]. This provides possibilities for an important positive feedback interaction between these two

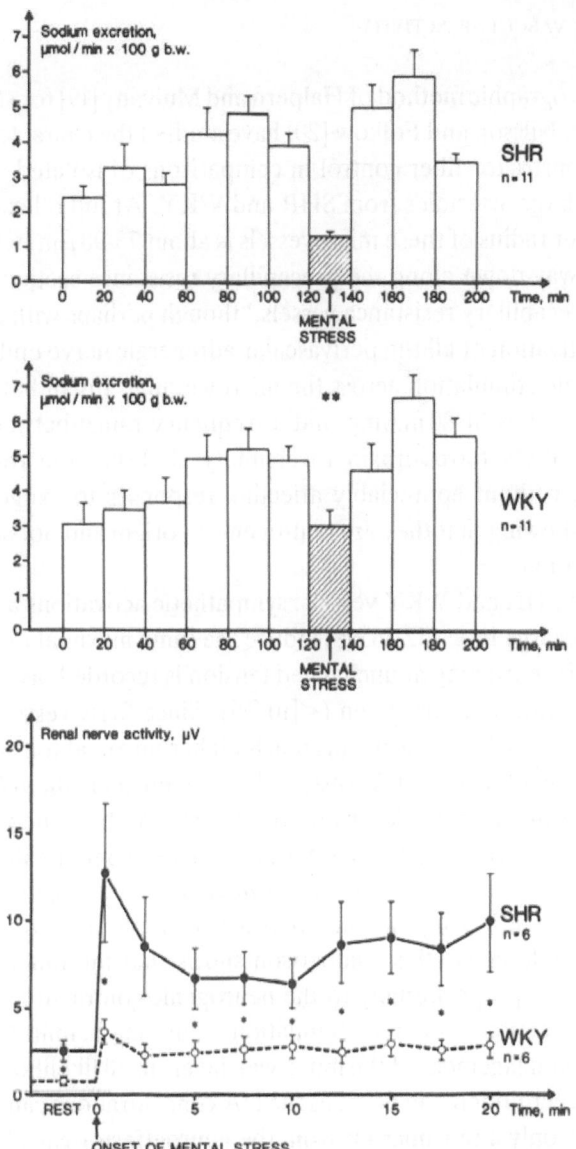

Figure 1. Upper panel shows urinary sodium excretion during awake rest and during a 20-minute period of mental stress in SHR and WKY rats. Lower panel shows renal sympathetic activity during rest and during mental stress measured in a separate group of SHR and WKY rats. Levels of statistical significance of the differences between SHR and WKY are indicated as *P <0.05 and **P <0.01.

environmental influences, once the appropriate genetic predisposition is at hand. Thus, the old 'either-or' argument concerning the importance of salt versus stress in hypertension may in reality boil down to 'both-and' because of such a close interaction between these two environmental elements.

SYMPATHETIC VASCULAR ACTIVITY

Using the myographic method of Halpern and Mulvany [19] for studies of isolated microvessels, Nilsson and Folkow [20] have studied the characteristics of sympathetic vasoconstrictor fiber control in comparisons of isolated mesenteric small arteries and large arterioles from SHR and WKY. At full relaxation and distension, the inner radius of these microvessels is about 75-90 μm, which places them roughly halfway down along the precapillary resistance section; i.e., they truly represent 'precapillary resistance vessels,' though perhaps with a fairly proximal location. Activation of all the perivascular adrenergic nerve endings was accomplished by field stimulation across the microvascular 'organ bath,' using 2-msec square wave pulses at 80 mAmp and a frequency range between 0.1 to 30 Hz. Addition of 10^{-7} M tetrodotoxin reversibility abolishes the responses to such stimulations, without appreciably affecting responses to exogenous noradrenaline (NA), showing that they are neurogenic in origin and not a matter of direct muscle excitation.

In both the SHR and WKY vessels, sympathetic activations at maximal 'physiological' discharge rates (12-16 Hz) induce the same maximal isometric response (or isotonic, if shortening at unchanged tension is recorded, as when supramaximal NA concentrations are given ($<[10^{-5M}]$). Since SHR vessels have a thicker and stronger media [21], this means much higher maximal tension levels for the SHR vessels than for the WKY vessels (Fig. 2). Further, the *relative* degrees of contraction of the microvessels were, on the whole, the same to given stimulations or NA concentrations whether they contracted isometrically or isotonically. The latter better reflects vessel behavior *in vivo*. Thus, despite the fact that the adrenergic neuro-effector junctions are restricted to the adventitial surface of the outermost muscle layer, this comparison shows that the inner, noninnervated layers contribute proportionally to the neurogenic contractions; otherwise, the isometric contractions to nerve stimulation would lag behind the isotonic contractions. This engagement of the inner-wall layers in all likelihood occurs mainly by myogenic recruitment via nexa, as the NA concentrations can be calculated to fall drastically only a few microns from the neuroeffector gaps [22].

As the wall-to-lumen ratio (w/r_i) of SHR precapillary resistance vessels at this stage of early established hypertension is increased - perhaps 40-50% as compared with WKY [21, 23] - with a correspondingly thicker smooth muscle layer, it means that neurogenic activations of SHR precapillary resistance vessels fully utilize the 'amplifying gain' inherent in the increased w/r_i. Thus, it is not only the responses to constrictor drugs which exhibit the characteristic unspecific hyperreactivity ensuing from the altered vessel design, but also the more 'physiological' ones induced by the vasoconstrictor nerves [21]. This is particularly well illustrated when the complete frequency-response curves to graded sympathetic stimulation are compared for the SHR and WKY vessels, as shown in the left part of Figure 2, which gives the absolute levels of tension increase for both vessels.

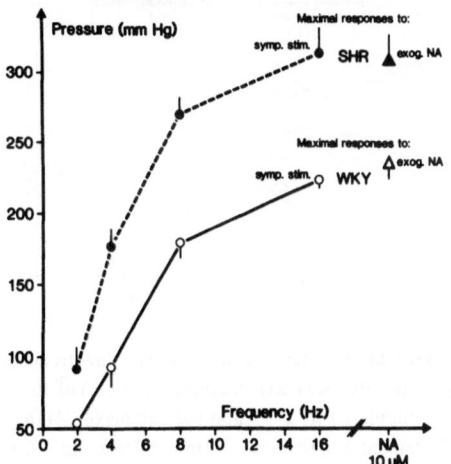
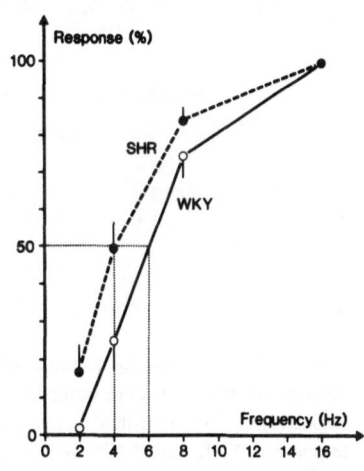

Figure 2. Frequency-response curves for seven pairs of mesenteric resistance vessels from SHR and WKY. *Left part* shows nerve responses as well as responses to a supramaximal dose of exogenous noradrenaline, in absolute values (calculated transmural pressure necessary to keep the rounded vessel isometric). *Right part* shows responses expressed as percent of maximal nerve response. Dotted lines show frequencies needed for half-maximal responses; bars indicate SEM. Note the leftward placement of the SHR curve.

Obviously, the SHR frequency-response curve is steeper and reaches a maximum that is about 30% higher than for WKY. When the SHR and WKY frequency-response curves are plotted with the maximal responses set to 100%, as shown in the right part of Figure 2, it is seen that the SHR curve is also displaced in parallel well to the left of the WKY curve, a difference present also after reuptake blockade. This displacement implies, for example, that the SHR vessels reach 50% of their maximal response at 4 Hz, when the WKY vessels have reached only some 25% of their maximal tension. As the dose-response curves for exogenous NA reveal roughly equal sensitivities in the SHR and WKY microvessels, at least before reuptake blockade [24], these results indicate that the NA release from the nerve endings per impulse may be higher in SHR than in WKY. Vanhoutte et al. [25] have arrived at similar results with respect to the SHR renal vessels, whereas the results by Brody's group [26] on SHR skeletal muscle vessels suggest a reduced NA release.

Another interesting characteristic of these precapillary microvessels is their quite rapid 'single twich' responses to individual nerve impulses, where again the SHR responses are substantially larger than the WKY responses (Fig. 3). At 2-3 Hz these 'twitches,' which even in SHR amount to only a few percent of maximal tension, fuse into a smooth 'tetanic' response. However, at least the

326

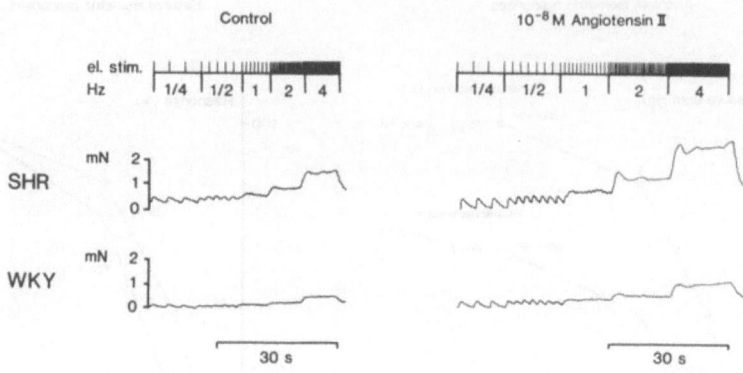

Figure 3. Records showing responses of SHR and WKY mesenteric resistance vessels to low-frequency 'field stimulation' of the sympathetic nerve endings in the absence (left) and presence (right) of 10^{-8} M angiotensin II. 'Single-twitch' responses to individual impulses were 2–3% and 1–2% of maximal (16 Hz) response in SHR and WKY, respectively. Vessel segment lengths were 1.9 mm (SHR) and 1.6 mm (WKY); normalized internal diameters were 165 μm (SHR) and 136 μm (WKY). Note the rapid 'single twitches' and their substantial potentiation by angiotensin II, which in this concentration does not directly constrict the vessels.

early phase of this 'tetanic' response reaches only some 15% of maximal tension. Obviously, only a small fraction of the contractile filaments in the media are initially brought into activation. In contrast, active tension is largely maximal in tetanic contractions of skeletal muscle. However, on continued sympathetic stimulation at the same rate, the rapid but fairly weak initial contractions markedly grow in stength within a minute or so, suggesting a gradually increasing recruitment of contractile filaments then takes place. This may reflect a gradual increase of transmitter release per impulse and/or an altered intramuscular handling of free Ca^{++} ions, so that they reach higher concentrations for each excitation but are still rapidly eliminated, because prompt vessel relaxation nevertheless occurs on interruption of stimulation. It is of interest that also *in vivo,* the more proximally placed precapillary resistance vessels show such two-phasic responses to sympathetic stimulation, in contrast to those placed closer to the capillary level, which show more prompt contraction that are soon followed by partial relaxation [21].

If angiotensin II is added in concentrations that are subthreshold to the muscle cells, it greatly reinforces the stimulation effects, clearly noted also for the 'single twitches' (Fig. 3). This is *not* mainly a consequence of, e.g., altered transmitter reuptake, because the angiotensin reinforcement is about as pronounced after cocaine blockade of NA reuptake, which per se enhances also the stimulation responses.

These results suggest that, apart from the thicker and stronger smooth muscle sheath in the SHR vessels which renders them hyperreactive because of the higher w/r_i ratio [21], the adrenergic nerve endings release larger NA amounts per stimulus than in WKY, or possibly there are more nerve endings in SHR. It is an open question whether this represents a neuronal adaptation to the relatively higher level of average sympathetic discharge in SHR, or whether it might be 'primary' in the sense that it reflects alterations directly connected to the polygenetic predisposition. If so, the interesting possibility arises that similar changes might also characterize central NA neurons, which modulate a variety of CNS mechanisms by means of their widespread arborizations. For example, a modestly increased NA release per impulse at the nerve endings of the ascending NA neurons, which seem to normally exert a facilitatory influence on limbic-hypothalamic structures, might perhaps explain the characteristic central hyper-reactivity to alerting stimuli that is often present both in human and SHR primary hypertension, as outlined above.

SYMPATHETIC TONIC ACTIVITY

Earlier studies in this department [28, 29] concerning the rapid reversal of two-kidney one-clip renal hypertension, which occurs upon renal declipping, strongly suggest that vascular smooth muscle tone then becomes considerably *sub*normal. This suggests a renal release of depressor agents, analogous with findings by Muirhead's group [30, 31], in which the interesting medullar depressor lipids isolated by Muirhead come into focus.

In a recent study [32], we showed how awake normotensive WKY rats, when extracorporally perfusing isolated, chronically clipped, renal hypertension (RHR) kidneys, became markedly hypotensive upon renal declipping. Thus, powerful depressor substances were released when the chronically hypotensive renal vascular bed was suddenly 'overperfused' at higher pressure upon declipping, again in close agreement with Muirhead's findings. Some of these data indicated that the nervous control was somehow interfered within the normotensive WKY in this situation. Therefore, these studies have now been extended, together with those of Thorén, to include also a continuous recording of efferent renal sympathetic discharge in the awake WKY rats while perfusing the clipped-declipped RHR kidneys, as well as continuous recordings of their heart rate and arterial pressure [33]. As shown in Figure 4, renal declipping induces the characteristic, often profound drop of arterial pressure, and it is associated not only with bradycardia but also with a marked *inhibition* of tonic sympathetic discharge. In sharp contrast, when equal reductions of arterial pressure were induced in these awake WKY rats by graded blood loss or by the vasodilator drug nitroprusside sodium, these pressure drops were always associated with tachycardia and a reflex *increase* of sympathetic discharge (Fig. 4).

Clearly, the blood-borne renal depressor substances, emerging from the de-

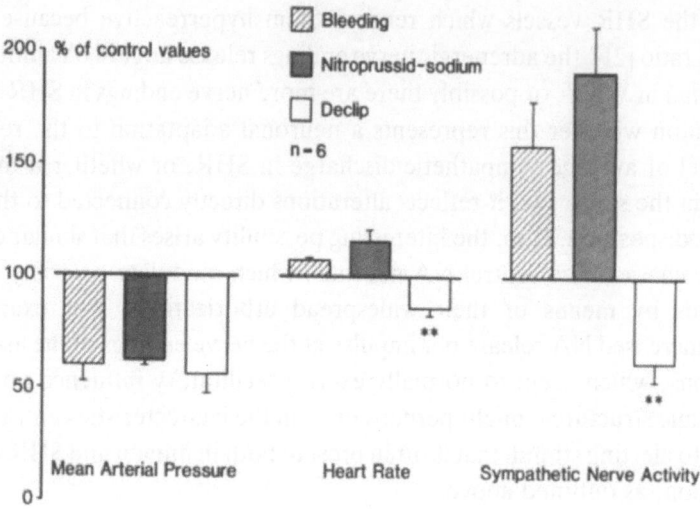

Figure 4. Relative changes (±SEM) of mean arterial pressure, heart rate, and efferent renal sympathetic nerve activity in 12 awake normotensive Wistar Kyoto rats (WKY), exposed to three different kinds of 'depressor' effects while extracorporally perfusing isolated clipped-declipped kidneys from rats with chronic two-kidney one-clip renal hypertension (RHR). Six WKY were exposed to a standardized bloodloss while perfusing *clipped* RHR kidneys (left bars in each group). The other six WKY were first exposed to a period of vasodilator drug infusion (nitroprusside sodium) while perfusing *clipped* RHR kidneys (middle bars in each group). After return to control steady state, the renal clip was removed, leading to a gradually increasing fall in arterial pressure with associated changes in heart rate and renal sympathetic activity. These changes are illustrated by the *right* bars, representing the situation 20 minutes after declipping. Note how the pressure drop caused by blood loss or nitroprusside vasodilatation leads to reflex *tachy*cardia and sympathetic *activation*, while the depressor response to renal declipping is associated with mild *brady*cardia and sympathetic *inhibition*.

clipped kidneys and presumably identical with Muirhead's medullary depressor lipids, produce an often profound, centrally conveyed inhibition of sympathetic discharge. This is, in a way, the opposite of what the hormonal renal pressor system, renin angiotensin, accomplishes. Angiotensin is known to centrally enhance sympathetic discharge, in this case acting via the bulbar area postrema and/or related hypothalamic areas [34]. Thus, the kidneys might centrally modulate tonic sympathetic discharge in *both* directions via blood-borne links.

Finally, it is not impossible that the aforementioned humorally transferred sympatho-inhibitory influence of renal origin acts as a damping influence in primary hypertension, when most other barostat mechanisms are chronically reset, with partial exception for the unmyelinated baroafferents according to Thoren's group [35].

SUMMARY

The role of the sympathetic nervous system in hypertension is discussed on the basis of three different lines of recent experimental findings:

1. The sympathetic renal activity in SHR is accentuated as compared with normotensive controls, particularly during increased alertness as a result of environmental stimuli. Thereby a *neurogenically* induced increase of sodium retention ensues in SHR, which seems to link together the two major environmental influences in primary hypertension: salt and physchosocial environment.

2. Graded sympathetic activations to isolated SHR and WKY vessels may suggest an increased NA release per impulse in SHR, which together with the structurally based vascular hyperreactivity may further potentiate sympathetic vascular influences in SHR hypertension. If generalized, such a change might also afflict the central NA neurons and thereby their psychomotor effects, perhaps explaining the central hyperreactivity to alerting stimuli that is commonly seen both in human and SHR primary hypertension.

3. The depressor substances, released from declipped kidneys when the 'chronically-hypotensive' renal vascular bed is suddenly perfused at higher pressures, can cause a powerful central inhibition of tonic sympathetic activity. It is discussed whether such blood-borne depressor agents might also exert a mild damping influence on sympathetic activity in, e.g., chronic primary hypertension and thereby represent one of the few 'barostat mechanisms' that is not fully reset.

ACKNOWLEDGMENTS

These studies were supported by grants from the Swedish Medical Research Council (14X-00016 and 14X-04764) and by AB Hassle, Molndal.

REFERENCES

1. Folkow B: Nervous control of the blood vessels. Physiol Rev 35:629-663, 1955.
2. Folkow B: Range of control of the cardiovascular system by the central nervous system. Physiol Rev 40:93-99, 1966.
3. Folkow B: Relevance of cardiovascular reflexes. Invited lecture, in Hainsworth R, Kidd C, Linden RJ (editors): Cardiac Receptors. New York, Cambridge University Press, 1979, pp 473-505.
4. Okamoto K: Spontaneous hypertension in rats. Internat Rev Exp Pathol 7:227-270, 1969.
5. Julius S, Esler M (editors): The Nervous System in Arterial Hypertension. Springfield, Ill, Charles C Thomas Publisher, 1976.
6. Folkow B: Central neuro-hormonal mechanisms in spontaneously hypertensive rats as compared with human essential hypertension. Clin Sci Mol Med 48:205s-214s, 1975.

7. Frohlich ED, Pfeffer MA: Adrenergic mechanisms in human hypertension and in spontaneously hypertensive rats. Clin Sci Mol Med 48:225s-238s, 1975.

8. Hallback M, Folkow B: Cardiovascular responses to acute mental stress in spontaneously hypertensive rats. Acta Physiol Scand 90:684-698, 1974.

9. Hallback M: Consequence of social isolation on blood pressure, cardiovascular reactivity and design in spontaneously hypertensive rats. Acta Physiol Scand 93:455-465, 1975.

10. Yamori Y: Neurogenic mechanisms of spontaneous hypertension, in Onesti C, Fernandes M, Kim KK (editors): Regulation of Blood Pressure by the Central Nervous System. New York, Grune & Stratton, 1976, p 65.

11. Falkner B, Onesti G, Angelakos ET, et al.: Cardiovascular response to mental stress in normal adolescents with hypertensive parents. Hypertension 1:23-30, 1979.

12. Falkner B: Cardiovascular responses to stress in adolescents, in Onesti G, Kim KE (editors): Phasic Pressor Mechanisms: Hypertension in the Young and the Old. Sixth Hahnemann International Symposium on Hypertensive Disease. New York, Grune & Stratton, 1981.

13. Folkow B, Neil E: Circulation. New York, Oxford University Press, 1971.

14. Lundin S, Thoren P: Renal function and sympathetic activity during 'mental stress' in normotensive and spontaneously hypertensive rats. Acta Physiol Scand 1982.

15. Axelrod J: Experimental hypertension and noradrenergic nerves, in Davies DS, Reid JR (editors): Central Action of Drugs in Blood Pressure Regulation. London, Whitefriars Press Ltd, 1975, pp 1-7.

16. Champlain J De, Krakoff LR, Axelrod J: Interrelationships of sodium intake, hypertension and norepinephrine storage in the rat. Circ Res 24(Suppl I):75-92, 1969.

17. Takeshita A, Mark AL: Neurogenic contribution to hindquarter vasoconstriction during high sodium intake in Dahl strain of genetically hypertensive rat. Circ Res 43(Suppl I):86-91, 1978.

18. Tobian L, Lange J, Iwai J, et al.: Prevention with thiazide of NaCl-induced hypertension in Dahl 'S' rats. Hypertension 1:316-323, 1979.

19. Mulvany MJ, Halpern W: Contractile properties of small arterial resistance vessels in spontaneously hypertensive and normotensive rats. Circ Res 41:19-26, 1977.

20. Nilsson H, Folkow B: Different nerve responses in elastic and muscular arteries. Acta Physiol Scand 1982.

21. Folkow B: Cardiovascular structural adaptation: Its role in the initiation and maintenance of primary hypertension. The Fourth Volhard Lecture. Clin Sci Mol Med 55:3s-22s, 1978.

22. Johsnsson B, Johansson SR, Ljung B, et al.: A receptor kinetic model of a vascular neuroeffector. J Pharmacol Exp Ther 180(3):637-646, 1972.

23. Mulvany MJ, Hansen PK, Aalkjaer C: Direct evidence that the greater contractility of resistance vessels in spontaneously hypertensive rats is associated with a narrower lumen, a thicker media and a larger number of smooth muscle cell layers. Circ Res 43:854-864, 1978.

24. Mulvany MJ, Aalkjaer C, Christensen J: Changes in noradrenaline sensitivity and morphology of arterial resistance vessels during development of high blood pressure in spontaneously hypertensive rats. Hypertension 2:664-671, 1980.

25. Collis MG, De Mey D, Vanhoutte PM: Renal vascular reactivity in the young spontaneously hypertensive rat. Hypertension 2:45-52, 1980.

26. Lais LT, Shaffer RA, Brody MJ: Neurogenic and humoral factors controlling vascular resistance in the spontaneously hypertensive rat. Circ Res 35:764-774, 1974.

27. Folkow B, Sonnenschein RR, Wright DL: Loci of neurogenic and metabolic effects on precapillary vessels of skeletal muscle. Acta Physiol Scand 81:459-471, 1971.

28. Lundgren Y, Hallback M, Weiss L, et al.: Rate and extent of adaptive cardiovascular changes in rats during experimental renal hypertension. Acta Physiol Scand 91:103-115, 1974.

29. Hallback-Nordlander M, Noresson E, Lundgren Y: Haemodynamic alterations after reversal of renal hypertension in rats. Clin Sci 57:15s-17s, 1979.

30. Muirhead EE: Antihypertensive functions of the kidney. Arthur C. Corcoran Memorial Lecture. Hypertension 2:444-464, 1980.

31. Muirhead EE, Pitcock JA: Evidence for an invovement of the renal papilla in hypertension, in Mandal AK, Bohman SO (editors): The Renal Papilla and Hypertension. New York, Plenum Press, 1980, pp 35-61.

32. Gothberg G, Lundin S, Folkow B: Acute vasodepressor effect in normotensive rats following extracorporal perfusion of the declipped kidney of two-kidney, one-clip hypertensive rats. Hypertension 1982.

33. Gothberg G, Lundin S, Folkow B, et al.: Is the antihypertensive function of the kidney elicited by renomedullary depressor substances partly acting on the central nervous system? Acta Med Scand 1982 (abstract).

34. Buckley JP, Ferrario CM: Central Actions of Angiotensin and Related Hormones. New York, Pergamon Press, 1977.

35. Thoren P: Characteristics and reflex effects of aortic baroreceptors with non-medullated afferents in rabbits and rat, in Kovach AGP, Sandor P, Kollai M (editors): Advancements in Physiological Sciences. Proceedings of the 28th International Congress of Physiological Sciences. New York, Pergamon Press, 1980, vol 9, pp 85-94.

DISCUSSION

Discussants: Folkow, Mark, Muirhead, Brody, Langer, Blaustein

Unidentified Discussant: I would like to ask a question concerning the last experiment, which is very interesting. The whole hemodynamic pattern looks like circulating beta endorphins. I know that Peter Toreg thinks along these lines, as well. A sympathetic tone and decrease of blood pressure, of course, would stimulate that. Have you tried the experiments and used naloxone or any other kind of peptide inhibitors to see if you can reverse these effects?

Folkow: Not so far, because we have only had time to complete this first series of experiments which I reported here, where we specifically wanted to see whether there were signs of inhibition of tonic sympathetic activity. We don't know what the renal blood-borne agents are, but for sure they must have come out of the declipped kidney. For good reasons, I am inclined to think that they are identical with Eric Muirhead's medullary lipids. It's probably not prostaglandins, first because these are largely inactivated in the lung circulation, second because the responses seem to be the same after, e.g., indomethacin. It is, however, an open question as to which are the factors that cause this presumably central inhibition of tonic sympathetic activity.

Mark: Dr. Folkow, have you performed the last experiment in a denervated kidney? The reason I ask is because of the possibility that renal afferent mechanisms might be involved in that response, in addition to or as opposed to humoral agents.

Folkow: No, sot so far, because this is a meeting of 'recent advances,' and we completed this first series of experiments in the last two months. So, they truly represent our own minor addition to 'recent' advances.

Muirhead: I am very grateful for these observation, obviously, but I would like to re-emphasize one of our experiments. When we use a one-kidney, one-clip hypertensive rat, in which the ureter is connected to the vena cava to slow down the recession of the blood pressure, then at some point in the slope of that drop in pressure, we can derive from the renal venous effluent a vasodepressor lipid that chromatographically is not prostaglandin. At least it is not a product of the cyclo-oxygenase pathway. (I don't know about the lipoxygenase pathway.) This lipid is in two phases - chromatographically, one phase can be changed into the other, and it is a vasodepressor lipid. I only wish we had enough of it to supply you with some at this time. But perhaps we will in the future, hopefully.

Folkow: That would be extremely interesting. I think what one must remember in our particular variant of experiment is the following: Chronically clipped but acutely declipped kidney is kept perfused at a *constant* pressure equal to that in the renal hypertensive rat, implying a considerable 'overperfusion' after declipping. It may well be loaded with depressor material, now joining the blood stream, in high concentrations. Therefore, it may well be that these depressor agents relax vascular smooth muscle at fairly low concentrations and that somewhat higher concentrations are needed for inhibition of sympathetic activity.

Muirhead: How long does that effect last after you unclip? Is that just a transient hypotension, or does it come back up?

Folkow: It lasts as long as our (and the rat's) endurance allows us to follow these animals. We cannot, however, follow them too long because they are heparinized, catheterized, etc., but they remain in good shape for perhaps six or seven hours, provided that the extracorporally perfused kidney remains unclipped. We are not able, so far, to say what may happen in the longer run with a particular technique. Then, one probably has to design another type of experiment. But here, we wanted to simply have an indicator, in an awake, largely 'intact' animal, to see whether something happens with sympathetic activity.

Brody: With your studies on the possibility that environmental factors may be important in inducing hypertension in the spontaneously hypertensive rat, we have been examining the 'defense reactions' in rats instrumented with flow probes. We can produce the classical defense reaction by an acute noise stress, which is similar to blowing on the animals like you have been doing. They exhibit an increase in blood pressure, tachycardia, renal and mesenteric vasoconstriction, and vasodilation in the muscle bed; these response are exaggerated in SHR.[1] The greatest vasoconstriction is seen in the renal bed. So, we certainly agree that there is exaggerated cardiovascular responsiveness to environmental stimuli in SHR. Unfortunately, despite our great interest in the nervous system, we have been unable to show that these animals have their arterial pressure maintained by neural mechanisms.[2]

Using the test of ganglionic blockade in conscious animals instrumented with flow probes, we can show exaggerated vasoconstrictor activity in baroreceptor denervated animals.[3] Thus we validate in a neurogenic hypertension model that ganglionic blockade unmasks increased vascular resistance of neurogenic origin. Using this test in SHR, we cannot show that the blood pressure is maintained by exaggerated neurogenic vasoconstrictor tone. So we have the paradox of exaggerated neurogenic responsiveness, but the maintenance of arterial pressure by something other than a neurogenic mechanism. I wonder about your comments.

Folkow: I agree with you here, because I look upon the autonomic nervous component, in SHR as in neurogenic variants of human primary hypertension, more as an 'intermittent triggering lash' on the cardiovascular system. That is just one cause which contributes to a gradual structural cardiovascular adaption, 'resetting' the whole system towards a higher-pressure equilibrium. Therefore, I don't think

---

[1] Galeno TM, Van Hoesen EW, Brody MJ: Bilateral lesions of central amygdaloid nucleus attenuates hemodynamic responses to stress in the spontaneously hypertensive rat. Society for Neuroscience Abstracts, 1982 (In Press).

[2] Fouw KB, Haywood JR, Shaffer RA, et al.: Contribution of the sympathetic nervous system to vasuclar resistance in the conscious young and adult spontaneously hypertensive rat. Hypertension 2: 408-418, 1980.

[3] Trapani AJ, Barron KW, Brody MJ: Regional neurogenic basis of hypertension produced by sinoaortic baroreceptor denervation (SAD). Fed. Proc 41: 1094, 1982.

one should expect the pressure equilibrium in these animals to hang on a *continuously* increased sympathetic activity. One must further remember that the so-called 'resting' awake rat in the lab is no more resting than I am just now: He or she is literally on the alert. So I think the mistake that is often made concerning the contribution of nervous mechanisms to primary hypertension is the assumption that 'it must then always be there,' especially in terms of a *continuously* increased activity, which is not at all necessary once heart and vessels become structurally reset. This happens far more rapidly than is generally considered.

Langer: In your responses to field stimulation in the microvessels, you show that angiotensin 10^{-8} potentiates responses at all the frequencies up to 4 Hz, where your frequency-response curve stops. When you subsequently show the full frequency-response curve stops, the maximal response you get is at 16 Hz. Does the potentiation by angiotensin continue at higher frequencies of stimulation than 4 Hz, and is it consistently more pronounced in the SHR when compared with the WKY as it seemed from your slide?

Folkow: We have not followed in detail the whole frequency-response curves in larger series of animals. Here we utilized the 'single twitches' to see how much they could be amplified by, e.g., angiotensin. In the limited series of animals, the whole frequency-response curve is displaced to the left for SHR, as an average, as one would expect if the quantal release per stimulus were increased.

Blaustein: Dr. Folkow, you showed this very interesting dose-response curve with no change in the sensitivity of the normotensive rats versus the SHR rats for norepinephrine. And yet we know that in human hypertension, there is some evidence for an altered sensitivity to catecholamine. Also, in relation to the angiotensin II data that you showed, there did appear to be some change in sensitivity of the muscle under those circumstances. Would you care to comment on some of those differences?

Folkow: I think one can manipulate the sensitivities of the smooth muscles over a fairly wide range. One of the things we have done is to add fairly low concentrations of ouabain to damp the membrane Na^+/K^+, ATPase 'pump,' while following the responsiveness of the true resistance vessels in SHR and WKY hindquarter vessels. If there is little or no difference in sensitivity between SHR and WKY before ouabain, its *immediate* effect is to increase the NA responsiveness, for example. Then the SHR resistance curve is slightly more displaced to the left than that of WKY so as to seemingly unmask a 'hidden' supersensitivity in SHR vascular smooth muscle. We are now looking at this in the isolated microvessel, but I cannot say what happens precisely if similar manipulations are made during nerve stimulations. The only thing I can say is that the frequency-response curve often *seems* to be dramatically shifted to the left. If this is true, it can imply striking effects concerning overall hemodynamics consequences.

Unidentified Discussant: If you clip the splanchnic circulation and then release it, would you think you elaborate the humoral factor that could suppress sympathetic drive? In other words, do you need an internal control for this experiment?

Folkow: If one produces severe regional hypotension for the gastrointestinal tract, as studied by O. Lendren's group in our department, one will disturb the oxygen delivery to the tips of the mucosal villi because of their vascular 'countercurrent' loops, so that damaged and toxic depressor agents come out in the circulation. But chronically clipped kidneys have survived in the renal hypertensive rats for many weeks and are probably not at all threatened by severe hypoxia and tissue damage. Actually, their vascular beds have been 'structurally autoregulated' downwards showing a markedly *reduced* resistance to flow. This is a very different situation, I think, from an acutely underperfused intestine.

PRE- AND POSTSYNAPTIC RECEPTORS IN HYPERTENSIVE STATES

S.Z. LANGER

INTRODUCTION

Norepinephrine released by nerve impulses acts on postsynaptic α- or β-adrenoceptors to elicit the physiological response of the effector organ. The magnitude of this response is directly related to the concentration of the transmitter in the biophase. Therefore, factors that modify the concentration of norepinephrine in the junction between the nerve-terminal varicosity and the receptor of the effector cell will influence the magnitude of the response produced.

During the last decade, evidence has accumulated in favor of the view that in addition to the classical postsynaptic receptors which mediate the response of the effector organ, there are presynaptic receptors which modulate the release of neurotransmitters from peripheral as well as central nerve terminals (for reviews, see [1-9].

In addition to the presynaptic autoreceptors involved in negative feedback mechanisms for the release of transmitters such as norepinephrine, dopamine, serotonin, and acetylcholine, there are presynaptic receptors which are sensitive to endogenous compounds other than the neuron's own transmitter. These presynaptic receptors can be acted upon by transmitters released from adjacent terminals or by various locally produced or blood-borne substances to modulate peripheral as well as central noradrenergic neurotransmission.

Several drugs currently used in therapy belong to the category of a classical receptor agonist or antagonist acting on either α- or β-adrenoceptors. These agents have different degrees of affinities for the corresponding presynaptic release-modulating receptor: α-inhibitory or β-facilitatory adrenoceptors. Therefore, the overall analysis of the pharmacological profile of these drugs should take into account both their presynaptic and postsynaptic effects.

In the noradrenergic system, the presynaptic release-modulating receptors differ pharmacologically from the corresponding postsynaptic receptors. Selective agonists or antagonists acting presynaptically can preferentially modify the release of the neurotransmitter with small or negligible effects on the corresponding postsynaptic receptor.

In the context of this article, the term presynaptic autoreceptor will be used for those receptors, probably located in axon terminals, which are involved in the regulation of the calcium-dependent release of a neurotransmitter by the transmitter itself. The term presynaptic heteroreceptors will be used for those receptors, also localized to nerve terminals, which are acted upon by other neurotransmitters or autacoids but not by the neurons' own transmitter.

NORADRENERGIC NEUROTRANSMISSION AND PRESYNAPTIC INHIBITORY AUTORECEPTORS: SUBCLASSIFICATION OF α-ADRENOCEPTORS INTO α_1- AND α_2 TYPES

Before the discovery of presynaptic release-modulating α-adrenoceptors, it was generally believed that the α-adrenoceptors represented a homogenous population. As stated in the Introduction, there is now ample evidence in support of the view that presynaptic α-adrenoceptors regulate the release of norepinephrine elicited by nerve stimulation. Both under *in vitro* and *in vivo* conditions, it has been demonstrated that α-adrenoceptor agonists inhibit norepinephrine release, while α-adrenoceptor blocking agents enhance the stimulation-evoked release of the neurotransmitter. The effects of α-adrenoceptor agonists and antagonists on norepinephrine release are observed regardless of the α- or β-type of the postsynaptic adrenoceptor that mediates the response of the effector organ.

The peripheral noradrenergic neurons offer a suitable model for these studies on the modulation of norepinephrine release because end-organ responses can be determined postsynaptically, while transmitter release elicited by sympathetic nerve stimulation can be measured at the same time.

Although both presynaptic and postsynaptic α-adrenoceptors are stimulated and blocked by α-receptor antagonists, the evidence accumulated during recent years indicates that these two receptors are not identical. Experimental evidence suggesting differences between pre- and postsynaptic α-adrenoceptors was first obtained in the perfused cat spleen [10]. Subsequently, it was shown that the α-adrenoceptor antagonist phenoxybenzamine is nearly 100 times more potent in blocking the postsynaptic α-adrenoceptors than it is in blocking the presynaptic α-adrenoceptors [11, 12]. These results with phenoxybenzamine led to the proposal that the α-adrenoceptors should be subclassified into α_1- and α_2 subtypes [1]. Originally, this proposal identified the α_1-adrenoceptor with the classical postsynaptic vascular smooth muscle receptor that mediates vasoconstriction and the α_2-adrenoceptor with the presynaptic inhibitory receptor that modulates norepinephrine release. This proposal remains essentially correct, and in recent years it was shown that α_2-adrenoceptors are also present in non-neuronal tissues.

Subsequent studies provided additional supportive evidence for the classification of α-adrenoceptors into α_1 and α_2 subtypes. Differences in the relative order of potencies of α-adrenoceptor agonists, and particularly of antagonists, represent the main pharmacological criterion for the subclassification of α-adrenoceptors [4, 5, 13, 14]. Table 1 shows the relative orders of selectivities for

Table 1. Relative orders of selectivity ratios for agonists and antogonists acting on α_1- and α_2-adrenoceptors. The data are derived from results obtained in noradrenergically innervated tissues of peripheral neuroeffector junctions of several species.

Relative order of selectivity of agonists	
M7 > guanabenz > clonidine > 6F-NE > α-CH$_3$-NE > DA $\alpha_2 > \alpha_1$	
Epinephrine = NE	$\alpha_2 = \alpha_1$
Phenylephrine < methoxamine < cirazoline	$\alpha_2 < \alpha_1$
Relative order of selectivity of antagonists	
RX 781094 > RS 21361 > rawolscine > yohimbine > piperoxan	$\alpha_2 > \alpha_1$
Phentolamine	$\alpha_2 = \alpha_1$
Penoxybenzamine < WB 4101 < prazosin	$\alpha_2 < \alpha_1$

M7 = 2-(NN-dimehylamino-5,6,dihydroxy-1,2,3,4-tetrahydronaphtalene).
RX 781094 = (2-[2-(1,4,benzodioxanyl)]-2-imidazolidine.
RS 21361 = (2-(1-ethyl-2-imidazolyl methyl)-1,4 benzodioxan).
DA = dopamine.
NE = Norepinephrine.

agonists and antagonists acting on α_1- and α_2-adrenoceptors.

Guanabenz and M7 (a tetrahydronaphtalene derivative) are among the most selective α_2-adrenoceptor agonists available at present [15, 16]. It should be noted, however, that M7, the selective α_2-adrenoceptor agonist, can also stimulate the D-2 dopamine receptor, as for example, the presynaptic dopamine autoreceptor that modulates the release of dopamine in the striatum [17].

Clonidine and α-methylnorepinephrine are preferential α_2-adrenoceptor agonists, but in higher concentrations or doses they also stimulate α_1-adrenoceptors (Table 1). Dopamine itself, which is a weak α-adrenoceptor agonist, appears to preferentially stimulate the α_2-subtype of adrenoceptor [18] (Table 1). The neurotransmitters, norepinephrine and epinephrine, activate both α_1 and α_2-adrenoceptors. The preferential α_1-adrenoceptor agonists include phenylephrine, methoxamine, and cirazoline (Table 1). It should be pointed out, however, that cirazoline, a potent α_1-adrenoceptor agonist, has α_2-adrenoceptor blocking properties in higher concentrations or doses [19]. Cirazoline, which is presently used as a nasal decongestant, associates a potent α_1-adrenoceptor agonist action with α_2-adrenoceptor antagonist activity. Until recently, rauwolscine and yohimbine were the best preferential α_2-adrenoceptor antagonists available. However, as shown in Table 1, there are at least two new compounds that have an *in vitro* selectivity ratio α_2/α_1, which is approximately 10 times superior to rauwolscine and yohimbine. Phentolamine is the classical α-adrenoceptor antagonist which blocks both α_1- and α_2-adrenoceptors under *in vitro* and *in vivo* experimental conditions [20]. On the other extreme of the spectrum, prazosin remains the most selective α_1-adrenoceptor antagonist available (Table 1).

One can therefore define the α_1-adrenoceptor as that preferentially stimulated

Table 2. Distribution and physiological effects mediated by α_1-adrenoceptors

Location	Effect
1) Postsynaptic in vascular smooth muscle	Contraction (preferentially innervated receptor subtype)
2) Postsynaptic in the heart	Positive inotropic (physiological relevance not clear)
3) Postsynaptic in the liver	Glycogen phosphorilase activation
4) Postsynaptic in the central nervous system	Stimulation

by methoxamine and cirazoline and blocked by prazosin, whereas the α_2-adrenoceptor is preferentially stimulated by M7, guanabenz, or clonidine and blocked by RX 781094 or rauwolscine. An additional advantage of compound RX 781094 over yohimbine and rauwolscine is the absence of nonspecific actions.

Table 2 shows the location as well as the physiological effects linked to α_1-adrenoceptor activation. As shown in Table 3, the presynaptic inhibitory α-adrenoceptors on noradrenergic neurons in the peripheral and central nervous systems have the pharmacological characteristics of the α_2-adrenoceptor. An interesting feature of the presynaptic α_2-adrenoceptor on noradrenergic neurons is that it modulates the calcium-dependent release of norepinephrine but not the synthesis of the neurotransmitter. On the other hand, the dopamine autoreceptor in the central nervous system is involved in the modulation of both the synthesis and the release of dopamine (for review, see [21]. As shown in Tables 3 and 4, α_2-adrenoceptors are not located exclusively on nerve terminals; they are also present postsynaptically and in non-neuronal structures such as platelets, fat cells, and pancreatic islets.

Table 3. Distribution and physiological effects mediated by neuronal α_2-adrenoceptors

Location	Effect
1) Presynaptic on peripheral and central NE nerve endings	Inhibition of NE release
2) Presynaptic on peripheral cholinergic neurons	Inhibition of Ach release
3) Presynaptic on 5HT neurons	Inhibition of 5HT release
3) Postsynaptic in the CNS	Hypotension, bradycardia
5) Somatodendritic autoreceptors	Inhibition of firing of NE neurons
6) Sympathetic ganglia	Hyperpolarization

NE = norepinephrine.
Ach = acetylcholine.
5HT = serotonin.
CNS = central nervous system.

Of particular interest are the α_2-adrenoceptors in vascular smooth muscle which (like the α_1-adrenoceptors) also mediate contractile responses. These postsynaptic α_2-adrenoceptors are easier to detect in *in vivo* studies that determine pressor effect or in studies on regional blood flow, as in the mesenteric vascular bed of the dog [16].

Differences exist between the mechanisms involved in the contractile responses of vascular smooth muscle mediated by activation of α_1- and α_2-adrenoceptors. The stimulation of α_1-adrenoceptors in vascular smooth muscle appears to induce depolarization and the release of calcium ions from intracellular stores. On the other hand, activation of postsynaptic α_2-adrenoceptors in vascular smooth muscle leads to an increase in intracellular calcium via a potential-dependent slow calcium channel which can be blocked by calcium antagonists [16].

Receptor binding studies using radiolabelled ^{3}H-WB4101 and ^{3}H-prazosin (α_1-adrenoceptors), ^{3}H-dihydroergocryptine (α_1- and α_2-adrenoceptors), ^{3}H-clonidine, ^{3}H-p-amino clonidine, ^{3}H-yohimbine, and ^{3}H-rauwolscine (α_2-adrenoceptors) have provided additional evidence for the subclassification of α-adrenoceptors into α_1 and α_2 categories. Recently, the tritiated selective α_2-adrenoceptor antagonist ^{3}H-RX 781094 became available for receptor binding studies [22, 23].

Recent autoradiographic studies using ^{3}H-WB4101 and ^{3}H-clonidine revealed that α_1- and α_2-adrenoceptors have different distributions in the rat brain [24].

PHARMACOLOGICAL IMPLICATIONS IN THE CARDIOVASCULAR SYSTEM OF THE SUBCLASSIFICATION OF α_2-ADRENOCEPTORS IN α_1 AND α_2 SUBTYPES

Clonidine is an imidazolidine which was originally designed as a nasal vasoconstrictor because of its ability to stimulate α-adrenoceptors on vascular smooth muscle [25]. Yet, the main cardiovascular effects of clonidine, which is a preferential α_2-adrenoceptor agonist (Table 1), involve hypotension, bradycardia, and a decrease in cardiac output. These cardiovascular effects of clonidine

Table 4. Distribution and physiological effects mediated by non-neuronal α_2-adrenoceptors

Location	Effect
1) Platelets	Aggregation
2) Human fat cells	Inhibition of lipolysis
3) Pancreatic islets	Inhibition of insulin secretion
4) Vascular smooth muscle	Contraction (predominantly extrasynaptic)

are predominantly due to the activation of postsynaptic α_2-adrenoceptors in the central nervous system [26, 27].

It is of interest to note that the plasma levels obtained with therapeutic doses of clonidine are in the range (nanomolar) where stimulation of peripheral presynaptic inhibitory α_2-adrenoceptors, by reducing norepinephrine release, may contribute to the hypotension and particularly the bradycardia produced by clonidine [28]. In support of this view, it was reported that in the intact dog, very small doses of clonidine injected into the artery perfusing the sinoatrial node region produce a negative chronotropic effect. This is antagonized by a low intra-arterial dose of phentolamine, which does not by itself affect blood pressure [28-30].

Similar peripheral effects of clonidine on the sympathetic tone to the vasculature are more difficult to assess because of the postsynaptic vasoconstrictor effect of clonidine related to the activation of α_2-adrenoceptors in vascular smooth muscle (Table 4). Sedation and dry mouth during the administration of clonidine involves stimulation of α_2-adrenoceptors by this drug [29, 31].

It appears that α_2-adrenoceptor agonists like clonidine are more effective in reducing noradrenergic neurotransmission in the heart than in the vasculature (Cavero, personnal communication). Therefore, peripheral acting α_2-adrenoceptor agonists are likely to reduce heart rate rather lower peripheral resistance by decreasing norepinephrine release in the blood vessels.

The sudden withdrawal of chronic clonidine administration may lead in some instances to a rebound hypertension syndrome accompanied by increased catecholamine levels in plasma and urine [32-34]. This syndrome could be related to a clonidine-induced subsensitivity of α_2-adrenoceptors both in the periphery and in the central nervous system [35]. In a recent study carried out in spontaneously hypertensive rats (SHR), it was reported that the chronic administration of antihypertensive doses of clonidine did not affect the parameters of ^{3}H-clonidine binding in the cerebral cortex [36]. It is possible that after the chronic administration of clonidine, supersensitivity of postsynaptic α_1- and β_1-adrenoceptors develops in response to the chronic reduction in noradrenergic neurotransmission produced by clonidine [37, 38].

Alpha-methyldopa is used extensively in the treatment of hypertension, and it appears that the formation of α-methyl-norepinephrine, which is an α_2-adrenoceptor agonist (Table 1), is a prerequisite for its centrally mediated antihypertensive action. It is likely that central α_2-adrenoceptor stimulation by α-methylnorepinephrine, as in the case of clonidine, is mainly responsible for the antihypertensive effects of α-methyldopa. In addition, an impairment of peripheral sympathetic neuronal function through the stimulation of presynaptic α_2-adrenoceptors by α-methyl-norepinephrine may contribute to the hypotensive action of α-methyldopa [39, 40].

Blockade by prazosin of α_1-adrenoceptors in vascular smooth muscle is most likely the mechanism of its antihypertensive action. It is possible that the effectiveness of prazosin in the chronic treatment of hypertension may be partly related to the fact that it lacks α_2-adrenoceptor-blocking properties (which would increase the neuronal release of norepinephrine). Most drugs that decrease blood pressure through a peripheral mechanism of action trigger cardiovascular reflexes which lead to tachycardia and an increase in cardiac output. Such effects are observed with vasodilators such as hydralazine and with nonselective α-adrenoceptor antagonists such as phentolamine. The absence of tachycardia when prazosin is administered to man represents a therapeutic advantage [41-43]. The lack of tachycardia in response to the blood pressure fall may be partly due to the fact that prazosin has a very low or negligible affinity for the blockade of presynaptic α_2-adrenoceptors in the heart (Table 1). Other mechanisms that may contribute to the absence of tachycardia include changes in baroreceptor sensitivity and absence of rat atrial pressure increases.

Prazosin, in low doses, preferentially blocks the responses to sympathetic nerve stimulation when compared to those elicited by exogenous norepinephrine. These results have been obtained *in vitro* in the perfused cat spleen [44, 45] as well as *in vivo* in the anesthetized dog [46]. Under these experimental conditions, prazosin effectively antagonizes responses to exogenous phenylephrine, which is a preferential α_1-adrenoceptor agonist (Table 1). Since norepinephrine is an agonist on both α_1- and α_2-adrenoceptors, these results are compatible with the view that α_1-adrenoceptors in vascular smooth muscle are preferentially innervated. In addition, these results suggest that postsynaptic α_2-adrenoceptors of predominantly extrasynaptic location are also present in vascular smooth muscle [16, 45].

The selective blockade by prazosin of vasoconstriction elicited by neuronally released norepinephrine (acting on vascular α_1-adrenoceptors) may explain the effectiveness of this drug in reducing peripheral resistance and blood pressure in hypertensive patients.

The proposed locations of postsynaptic α_1- and α_2-adrenoceptors in vascular smooth muscle may not necessarily apply to all vascular beds, and additional work is required to clarify this question. For example, in the cerebral vessels of several species, the predominant α-adrenoceptor in vascular smooth muscle is the α_2 subtype [47]. The femoral and renal vascular beds have predominantly α_1-adrenoceptors, while the mesenteric vascular bed in the dog has both α_1- and α_2-adrenoceptors postsynaptically [18].

In the vascular smooth muscle of the rat tail artery, both α_1- and α_2-adrenoceptors can be shown to be present [48]. Additionally, in spontaneously hypertensive rats, the postsynaptic α_2-adrenoceptors in the tail artery play a more important role in the vasoconstrictor responses than in the corresponding WKY normotensive control rats [49].

In blood vessels with both α_1- and α_2-adrenoceptors, the transmitter (norepinephrine) released by nerve stimulation appears to preferentially stimulate intrasynaptic α_1-adrenoceptors in the adventitial-medial border, while exogenously administered or circulating catecholamines preferentially reach post-

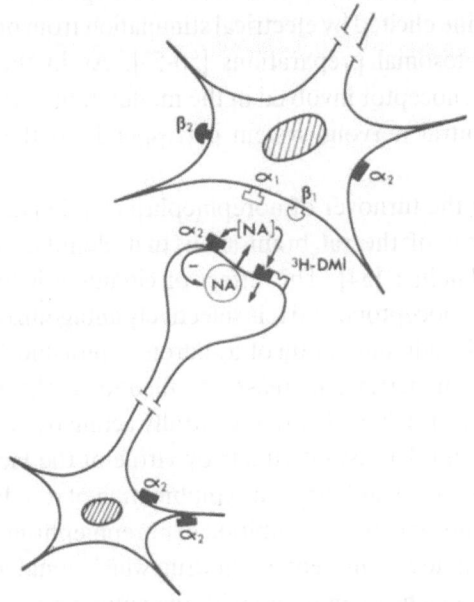

Figure 1. Schematic representation of a central noradrenergic neuron.

Note: Inhibitory α_2-adrenoceptors with somatodendritic location modulate neuronal firing. The inhibitory α_2-adrenoceptors involved in the regulation of transmitter release are probably located on the nerve terminal. Postsynaptic α_1- α_2- and β_1- β_2-adrenoceptors are shown schematically. Their presence in the same neuron and the possibility of preferential innervation of α_1- and β_1-adrenoceptors remains to be clarified. The substrate recognition site of the neuronal uptake of norepinephrine is located on nerve endings and can be labelled with high affinity with ^{3}H-desipramine.

synaptic α_2-adrenoceptors which predominate near the intima.

When neuronal uptake is inhibited by cocaine, prazosin becomes more effective in blocking the vasoconstrictor responses to exogenous norepinephrine [45]. The latter may be due to the fact that inhibition of neuronal uptake facilitates the access of exogenous norepinephrine to intrasynaptic α_1-adrenoceptors in vascular smooth muscle [45].

PRESYNAPTIC INHIBITORY α_2-ADRENOCEPTORS IN THE CENTRAL NERVOUS SYSTEM

As shown in Figure 1, central noradrenergic neurons have α_2-adrenoceptors in their cell bodies and dendrites that exert an inhibitory effect on the generation of action potentials. The presynaptic α_2-adrenoceptors, located on noradrenergic nerve terminals, modulate the calcium-dependent release of norepinephrine in a similar manner to that described in the periphery. In support of this view, it was reported that α-adrenoceptor agonists inhibit, while the antagonists increase, the release of ^{3}H-norepinephrine elicited by electrical stimulation from brain slices or by potassium from synaptosomal preparations [50-53]. As in the peripheral nervous system, the α-adrenoceptor involved in the modulation of the release of norepinephrine in the central nervous system corresponds to the α_2 subtype (Table 3).

In vivo studies in which the turnover of norepinephrine and epinephrine was determined in several areas of the rat brain show that clonidine reduces the turnover of both catecholamines [54]. This effect of clonidine is linked to the activation of central α_2-adrenoceptors, and it is selectively antagonized by yohimbine. On the other hand, the administration of α_2-adrenoceptor-blocking agents, which cross the blood-brain barrier, increase on their own the turnover of norepinephrine in the brain. It is possible that centrally acting α_2-adrenoceptor-blocking agents may have antidepressant effects by virtue of the fact that these drugs increase norepinephrine release [55]. The combination of α_2-adrenoceptor-blocking properties and neuronal uptake inhibition of norepinephrine in the same molecule may provide for a novel antidepressant drug which could act clinically with a shorter latency period when compared with the antidepressants (tricyclic and atypical) available at present. In support of this view, it has been shown recently that the administration of either tricyclic or monoamine oxidase inhibitor antidepressants in combination with α-adrenoceptor antagonists accelerates and intensifies the desensitization of β-adrenoceptors [56].

PRESYNAPTIC RECOGNITION SITES FOR THE NEURONAL UPTAKE MECHANISM FOR NOREPINEPHRINE: HIGH AFFINITY BINDING OF ^{3}H-DESIPRAMINE

Following the discovery that ^{3}H-imipramine may be used to label a specific high-affinity site associated with the neuronal uptake of serotonin [57, 58], it was recently reported that ^{3}H-desipramine labels, with high affinity, a binding site associated with the neuronal uptake of norepinephrine [59, 60].

The specific binding site of ^{3}H-desipramine is unevenly distributed in the brain, and it is present in peripheral tissues that have noradrenergic innervation [59, 60]. The high-affinity binding site of ^{3}H-desipramine is inhibited by tricyclic antidepressants and other inhibitors or neuronal uptake of norepinephrine in the low nanomolar range [60]. Nevertheless, substrates of the neuronal uptake system for norepinephrine are only active in very high concentrations to inhibit ^{3}H-desipramine binding [60]. The latter suggests that ^{3}H-desipramine does not directly label the recognition site for the substrate of neuronal uptake. It is possible that ^{3}H-desipramine binds to the recognition site of a unit that modulates neuronal uptake of norepinephrine.

The high-affinity ^{3}H-desipramine-binding sites thus appear to be localized on noradrenergic nerve endings in the peripheral and the central nervous system and to be closely associated with the neuronal uptake mechanism for norepinephrine.

PRESYNAPTIC INHIBITORY DOPAMINE RECEPTORS ON PERIPHERAL NORADRENERGIC NERVE ENDINGS

The presence of presynaptic inhibitory dopamine receptors has been reported in peripheral noradrenergic nerves of several species [10, 61-66]. Stimulation of presynaptic inhibitory dopamine receptors by agonists such as dopamine, apomorphine, N,N-di-n-propyldopamine (DPDA), and pergolide reduces the stimulation-evoked release of norepinephrine and the postsynaptic end-organ responses to nerve stimulation. These effects have been demonstrated both under *in vitro* and *in vivo* experimental conditions. Both DPDA and pergolide produce hypotensive and bradycardic effects *in vivo* in the rat and the dog [67, 68]. The reduction in noradrenergic neurotransmission elicited by dopamine receptor agonists remains unaffected after blockade of α-adrenoceptors, and it is selectively antagonized by dopamine-receptor blocking drugs, such as pimozide or sulpiride.

The presynaptic inhibitory dopamine receptors on peripheral noradrenergic nerve endings differ from the postsynaptic dopamine receptors that mediate vasodilatation in some vascular beds (renal, mesenteric, cerebral, and coronary). The S-enantiomer of sulpiride preferentially blocks presynaptic inhibitory dopamine receptors. Bulbocapnine selectively antagonizes the postsynaptic vascular dopamine receptor, and it is inactive at the presynaptic level [18]. In analogy with the subclassification already adopted for α-adrenoceptors, the postsynaptic dopamine vascular receptor corresponds to the DA_1 subtype, and the presynaptic inhibitory dopamine receptor on peripheral noradrenergic nerve endings corresponds to the DA_2 subtype [5, 69]. This nomenclature for peripheral dopamine receptors, which is based on measurable responses and on relative order of potencies of agonists and antagonists [69], may serve as a basis for the classification of dopamine receptor subtypes in the central nervous system, where a considerable controversy exists regarding multiple receptor subtypes for dopamine.

While the renal vasodilating effects of dopamine agonists are mainly due to the activation of postsynaptic vascular dopamine DA-1 receptors, the hypotensive and bradycardic effects of dopamine-receptor agonists involve the activation of presynaptic inhibitory dopamine DA-2 receptors [5].

Presynaptic inhibitory dopamine receptors could be considered as target receptors for the development of selective agonists that might be useful antihypertensive agents. These peripherally acting agonists should ideally be devoid of emetic effects. Some emetic effects might be acceptable, as it is well-known that in man, tolerance develops rapidly to the emetic effects of dopamine-receptor agonists, such as bromocriptine and pergolide.

PRESYNAPTIC FACILITATORY BETA-ADRENOCEPTORS ON PERIPHERAL NORADRENERGIC
NERVE ENDINGS

Facilitation of the stimulation-evoked release of norepinephrine through presynaptic beta-adrenoceptors was first reported by Langer et al. [70]. Additional
support for the presence of presynaptic beta-adrenoceptors was obtained in
experiments in which exposure to low concentrations of isoprenaline facilitated
the release of norepinephrine during low-frequency nerve stimulation in several
noradrenergically innervated organs [71-76]. The presence of presynaptic facilitatory beta-adrenoceptors was also reported in human vasoconstrictor nerves [77-
79] and under *in vivo* conditions [80].

As already shown for the presynaptic α-adrenoceptor, the presynaptic β-adrenoceptor appears to be stereospecific. The facilitation of noradrenergic transmission observed with (−) isoprenaline was not obtained when (+) isoprenaline was
substituted for (−) isoprenaline in the perfusion medium of the cat spleen [72].
The increase in the stimulation-evoked release of norepinephrine obtained *in
vitro* in the presence of isoprenaline is antagonized by propranolol [71] but not by
betaxolol, which is a selective β_1-adrenoceptor-blocking agent [81]. Dahlöf et al.
[82] reported that dl-, but not d-propranolol, reduced the stimulation-evoked
release of ^{3}H-norepinephrine from the isolated portal vein of spontaneously
hypertensive rats.

The experimental evidence available so far indicates that under *in vitro* conditions, the presynaptic facilitatory β-adrenoceptors might be of the β_2 type rather
than of the β_1 type. It is possible, therefore, that presynaptic β-adrenoceptors are
mainly activated by circulating epinephrine to enhance noradrenergic neurotransmission. Epinephrine taken up from the circulation and stored as a co-trans-
mitter in noradrenergic nerves could also be released by stimulation and thus
activate presynaptic facilitatory β-adrenoceptors [81].

Rats implanted with osmotic minipumps containing epinephrine develop hypertension, which can be prevented by the concomitant administration of the
β-adrenoceptor antagonist metoprolol [83]. It is possible that the increase in
blood pressure produced in rats by chronic treatment with epinephrine is partly
related to the facilitation of noradrenergic transmission to cardiovascular effector
tissues.

When peripheral noradrenergic nerve endings are labelled with epinephrine
instead of norepinephrine, blockade of β-adrenoceptors with propanolol becomes more effective in reducing transmitter release elicited by sympathetic
nerve stimulation [84, 85]. Therefore, it appears that epinephrine is part of a
positive feedback mechanism modulating the release of norepinephrine from
peripheral noradrenergic nerve endings. Beta-adrenoceptor antagonists may
thus act at this site to cause a decrease in transmitter output by blocking the
presynaptic beta-adrenoceptor-mediated positive feedback mechanism that enhances norepinephrine release. This effect at presynaptic β-adrenoceptors may

contribute to the antihypertensive effects of β-adrenoceptors antagonists, as suggested earlier [35]. The effectiveness of metoprolol in preventing the epinephrine-induced hypertension in rats [83] is compatible with the hypothesis that blockade of presynaptic facilitatory β-adrenoceptors contributes to the antihypertensive effects of β-receptor antagonists. Recently, it was reported by Kawasaki et al. [86] that the β_2-adrenoceptor-mediated facilitatory modulation of vascular neurotransmission is enhanced in spontaneously hypertensive rats.

PRESYNAPTIC FACILITATORY ANGIOTENSIN II RECEPTORS ON NORADRENERGIC NERVE ENDINGS

The facilitation by angiotensin II of peripheral noradrenergic neurotransmission has been reported by several authors [87-89].

In the rabbit heart, low concentrations of angiotensin II (1 and 10 nM) can produce up to four-fold increases of ^{3}H-norepinephrine release during nerve stimulation (Garcia-Sevilla, Dubocovich, and Langer, unpublished observations). Presynaptic facilitatory angiotensin II receptors appear to be present in central noradrenergic neurons, as recently reported in the rabbit hypothalamus [90].

Captopril, an antihypertensive drug which inhibits the angiotensin-converting enzyme, may reduce sympathetic tone through a decrease in the circulating levels of angiotensin II and by decreasing the local formation of angiotensin II, particularly in blood vessels. This effect, by reducing norepinephrine output, may contribute to the antihypertensive action of captopril and of other drugs that inhibit the angiotensin-converting enzyme.

SUMMARY

There is now a growing list of presynaptic release-modulating receptors for various neurotransmitters in the peripheral and central nervous systems. These presynaptic receptors, irrespective of whether or not they play a physiological role in neurotransmission, can be acted upon by administered agonists to modify transmitter release. On the other hand, for those presynaptic receptors that play a physiological role in regulating neurotransmission, the administration of selective receptor antagonist drugs should be expected to produce a pharmacological effect, mediated through changes in transmitter release.

Presynaptic inhibitory autoreceptors through which the neurotransmitter can regulate its own release have been reported to be present for the following neurotransmitters: norepinephrine, acetylcholine, dopamine, serotonin, and possibly epinephrine and GABA.

The antihypertensive and bradycardic effects of clonidine are linked to the activation of central, postsynaptic α_2-adrenoceptors. In addition, activation of presynaptic inhibitory α_2-adrenoceptors on noradrenergic nerves in the heart contributes to the bradycardic action of clonidine.

Prazosin, a selective α_1-adrenoceptor antagonist, is an effective antihypertensive drug which does not produce tachycardia as a side effect, possibly because it does not block presynaptic α_2-adrenoceptors on noradrenaline nerves in the heart.

Presynaptic receptors sensitive to endogenous compounds, different from the neuron's own transmitter, that modify the release of norepinephrine include: inhibitory muscarinic receptors, inhibitory dopamine receptors, inhibitory opiate receptors, inhibitory adenosine receptors, and inhibition by prostaglandins of the E series. In addition, there exist on noradrenergic nerve terminals facilitatory β_2-adrenoceptors and facilitatory angiotensin II receptors.

There is now evidence to indicate that the hypotension and bradycardia produced by dopamine-receptor agonists are linked to the activation of peripheral presynaptic dopamine receptors on noradrenergic nerves which are of the DA_2 subtype. The antihypertenive effects of beta-receptor antagonists may be related, at least partly, to the blockade of presynaptic facilitatory beta-adrenoceptors on peripheral noradrenergic nerve terminals.

Neuronal uptake of norepinephrine represents the main inactivating mechanism for the released transmitter. The substrate recognition site for neuronal uptake of norepinephrine has pharmacological characteristics different from the classical α- and β-adrenoceptors located presynaptically and postsynaptically. Drugs such as desipramine, nisoxetine, and cocaine, which inhibit neuronal uptake of norepinephrine, do not act as agonists or antagonists on the α- and β-adrenoceptor subtypes. The specific, high-affinity binding site for ^{3}H-desipramine is localized on noradrenergic nerve endings, and it is closely associated with the neuronal uptake of norepinephrine in the periphery and in the central nervous system.

REFERENCES

1. Langer SZ: Presynaptic regulation of catecholamine release. Biochem Pharmacol 23:1793-1800, 1974.
2. Langer SZ: Presynaptic receptors and their role in the regulation of transmitter release. Sixth Gaddum Memorial Lecture. Br J Pharmacol 60:481-497, 1977.
3. Langer SZ: Presynaptic receptors and the regulation of transmitter release in the peripheral and central nervous system: Physiological and pharmacological significance, in: Usdin E, Kopin IJ, Barchas J (editors), Catecholamines: Basic and Clinical Frontiers. New York, Pergamon Press, 1. 387-398, 1979.
4. Langer SZ: Presynaptic receptors and modulation of neurotransmission: Pharmacological implications and therapeutic relevance. Trends in Neurosciences 3:110-112, 1980.
5. Langer SZ: Presynaptic regulation of the release of catecholamines. Pharmacol Rev 32:337-362, 1980.

7. Starke K: Regulation of noradrenaline release by presynaptic receptor systems. Rev Physiol Biochem Pharmacol 77:1-124, 1977.

8. Vizi ES: Presynaptic modulation of neurochemical transmission. Prog Neurobiol 12:181-290, 1979.

9. Stjärne L: Basic mechanisms and local feed-back control of secretion of noradrenergic and cholinergic neurotransmitters, in Iversen LL, Iversen SD, Snyder SH (editors): Handbook of Psychopharmacology. New York, Publishing Corporation, 1975, vol 6, pp 179-233.

10. Langer SZ: The regulation of transmitter release elicited by nerve stimulation through a pre-synaptic feedback mechanism, in Usdin E, Snyder SH (editors): Frontiers in Catecholamine Research. New York, Pergamon Press, 543-549, 1973.

11. Dubocovich ML, Langer SZ: Negative feedback regulation of noradrenaline release by a nerve stimulation in the perfused cat's spleen: Differences in potency of phenoxybenzamine in blocking the pre- and postsynaptic adrenergic receptors. J Physiol Lond 237:505-519, 1974.

12. Cubeddu LX, Barnes EM, Langer SZ et al.: Release of norepinephrine and dopamine-β-hydroxylase by nerve stimulation. I. Role of neuronal and extraneuronal uptake and of alpha-presynaptic receptors. J Pharmacol Exp Ther 190:431-450, 1974.

13. Langer SZ: Presynaptic adrenoceptors and regulation of release, in Paton DM (editor): The Release of Catecholamines from Adrenergic Neurones. Oxford and New York, Pergamon Press, 1978, pp 59-85.

14. Starke K, Langer SZ: A note on terminology for presynaptic receptors, in Langer SZ, Starke K, Dubocovich ML: Presynaptic Receptors. Oxford, Pergamon Press, 1979, pp 1-3.

15. Shepperson NB, Langer SZ: The effects of the 2-aminotetrahydronaphtalene derivative M7, a selective α_2-adrenoceptor agonist in vitro. Naunyn Schmiedebergs Arch Pharmacol 318:10-13, 1981.

16. Langer SZ, Shepperson NB: Recent developments in vascular smooth muscle pharmacology - the postsynaptic α_2-adrenoceptor. Trends in Pharmacological Sciences 3:440-444, 1982.

17. Lehmann J, Briley MS, Langer SZ: Characterization of classical and novel dopamine receptor agonists at dopamine autoreceptor and at ^{3}H-spiperone binding sites in vitro. Eur J Pharmacol (in press).

18. Shepperson NB, Duval N, Massingham R, et al.: Differential blocking effects of several dopamine receptor antagonists for peripheral pre- and postsynaptic dopamine receptors in the anaesthetized dog. J Pharmacol Exp Ther 221:753-761, 1982.

19. Cavero I, Langer SZ: Lefevre-Borg F, et al.: Cirazoline possesses α_2-adrenoceptor blocking properties in addition to its α_1-adrenoceptor agonist activity. Br J Pharmacol 75:153P, 1982.

20. Massingham R, Dubocovich ML, Shepperson NB, et al.: In vivo selectivity of prazosin but not of WB 4101 for postsynaptic α_1-adrenoceptors. J Pharmacol Exp Ther 217:467-474, 1981.

22. Langer SZ, Pimoule C: Pharmacology and biochemistry of noradrenergic receptors. Br J Dermatol 107:145-151, 1982.

23. Langer SZ, Pimoule C, Scatton B: [^{3}H]-RX781094, a preferential α_2-adrenoceptor antagonist radio-ligand, labels α_2-adrenoceptors in the rat brain cortex. Br J Pharmacol 78:109P, 1983.

24. Young WS, Kuhar MJ: Noradrenergic α_1 and α_2 receptors: Autoradiographic visualization. Eur J Pharmacol 59:317-319, 1979.

25. Graubner W, Wolf M: Kritische Betrachtungen zum Wirkungsmechanisms des 2-(2,6-Dichlorophenylamino)-imidazolinhydrochlorids. Arzneimittelforsch 16:1055-1058, 1966.

26. Schmitt H: The pharmacology of clonidine and related products, in Gross F (editor): Antihypertensive Agents. Berlin, Springer-Verlag, 1977, pp 229-378.

27. Kobinger W: Central alpha-adrenergic systems as targets for hypotensive drugs. Rev Physiol Biochem Pharmacol 81:40-100, 1978.

28. Langer SZ, Cavero I, Massingham R: Recent developments in noradrenergic neurotransmission and its relevance to the mechanism of action of certain antihypertensive agents. Hypertension 2:372-382, 1980.

348

29. Cavero I, Roach AG: The effects of prazosin on the clonidineinduced hypotension and bradycardia in rats and sedation in chicks. Br J Pharmacol 62:468P, 1980.

30. Cavero I, Roach AG: Effects of clonide on canine cardiac neuroeffector structures controlling heart rate. Br J Pharmacol 70:269-276, 1980.

31. Green GJ, Wilson M, Yates MS: The mechanism of the clonidine-induced reduction in peripheral parasympathetic submaxillary salivation. Eur J Pharmacol 56:331-345, 1979.

32. Hansson L, Hunyor SN, Julius S, et al.: Blood pressure crisis following withdrawal of clonidine (Catapres, Catapresan) with special reference to arterial and urinary catecholamine levels, and suggestions for acute management. Am Heart J 85:605-610, 1973.

33. Reid JL, Dargi HJ, Davis DS, et al.: Clonidine withdrawal in hypertension: Changes in blood pressure and urinary noradrenaline. Lancet 1:1171-1174, 1977.

34. Whitsett TL, Chrysant SG, Dillard BL, et al.: Abrupt cessation of clonidine administration: A prospective study. Am J Cardiol 41:1285-1290, 1978.

35. Langer SZ: The role of α- and β-presynaptic receptors in the regulation of noradrenaline release elicited by nerve stimulation. Clin Sci Mol Med 51:423s-426s, 1976.

36. Amstrong JM, Atkinson J, Langer SZ, et al.: Prolonged supramaximal antihypertensive doses of clonidine are needed to change α_2-adrenoceptors in SHR. Br J Pharmacol 78:26P, 1983.

37. Langer SZ: Denervation supersensitivity, in Iversen LL, Iversen SD, Snyder SH (editors): Handbook of Psychopharmacology. New York, Plenum Publishing Corporation, 1975, pp 245-280.

38. Langer SZ, Massingham R: α-adrenoceptors and the clinical pharmacology of clonidine, in Turner P (editor): Clinical Pharmacology and Therapy, 1980, pp 158-164.

39. Lokhandwala MF, Buckley JP, Jandhyala BS: Effect of methyldopa treatment on peripheral sympathetic nerve function in the dog. Eur J Pharmacol 32:170-176, 1975.

40. Lokhandwala MF, Buckley JP, Jandhyala BS: Studies on the mechanism of the cardiovascular effects of methyldopa. Eur J Pharmacol 37:78-89, 1976.

41. Constantine JW, McShane WK, Scriabine A, et al.: Analysis of the hypotensive action of prazosin, in Onesti J, Kim KE, Myoer JH (editors): Hypertension: Mechanisms and Management. New York, Grune and Stratton, 1973, pp 429-443.

42. Massingham R, Hayden ML: A comparison of the effects of prazosin and hydralazine on blood pressure, heart rate and plasma renin activity in conscious renal hypertensive dogs. Eur J Pharmacol 30:121-124, 1975.

43. Brogden RN, Hell RG, Speight TM, et al.: Prazosin: A review of its pharmacological properties and therapeutic efficacy in hypertension. Drugs 14:163-197, 1977.

44. Langer SZ, Massingham R, Shepperson NB: Preferential, long-lasting blockade of neuronally released but not exogenously administered noradrenaline in vitro: Further evidence that the α_1-adrenoceptor subtype predominates intrasynaptically. Br J Pharmacol 73:281P-282P, 1981.

45. Langer SZ, Shepperson NB: Post-junctional α_1 and α_2-adrenoceptors: Preferential innervation of α_1-adrenoceptors and the role of neuronal uptake. J Cardiovasc Pharmacol 4:S8-S13, 1982.

46. Langer SZ, Massingham R, Shepperson NB: Differential sensitivity to prazosin blockade of endogenously released and exogenously administered noradrenaline: Possible relationship to the synaptic location of α_1 and the extrasynaptic location of α_2-adrenoceptors in dog vascular smooth muscle. Br J Pharmacol 72:123P, 1981.

47. Medgett IC, Langer SZ: Characterization of smooth muscle adrenoceptors and of responses to electrical stimulation in the cat isolated perfused middle cerebral artery. Naunyn Schmiedebergs Arch Pharmacol (in press).

48. Langer SZ, Medgett IC: Subclassification of smooth muscle α-adrenoceptors of the rat tail artery. Br J Pharmacol 78:44P, 1983.

49. Hicks P, Langer SZ, Medgett IC: Greater contribution of smooth muscle α_2-adrenoceptors to vasoconstrictor responses in SHR than in WKY rat tail arteries. Br J Pharmacol (in press).

50. Taube HD, Starke K, Borowski E: Presynaptic receptor systems on the noradrenergic neurones

of rat brain. Naunyn Schmiedebergs Arch Pharmacol 299:123-141, 1977.

51. Mulder AH, Wemer J, de Langen CDJ: Presynaptic receptor-mediated inhibition of noradrenaline release from brain slices and synaptosomes by noradrenaline and adrenaline, in Langer SZ, Starke K, Dubocovich ML: Presynaptic Receptors. Oxford, Pergamon Press, 1979, pp 219-224.

52. Pelayo F, Dubocovich ML, Langer SZ: Inhibition of neuronal uptake reduces the presynaptic effects of clonidine but not of α-methylnoradrenaline on the stimulation-evoked release of ^{3}H-noradrenaline from rat occipital cortex slices. Eur J Pharmacol 64:143-155, 1980.

53. Galzin AM, Dubocovich ML, Langer SZ: Presynaptic inhibition by dopamine receptor agonists of noradrenergic neurotransmission in the rabbit hypothalamus. J Pharmacol Exp Ther 221:461-471, 1982.

54. Scatton B, Pelayo F, Dubocovich ML, et al.: Effect of clonidine on utilization and potassium-evoked release of adrenaline in rat brain areas. Brain Res 176:197-201, 1979.

55. Langer SZ: Presynaptic receptors. Nature 275:479, 1978.

56. Crews FT, Paul SM, Goodwin FK: Acceleration of β-receptor desensitization in combined administration of antidepressants and phenoxybenzamine. Nature 290:787-789, 1981.

57. Langer SZ, Zarifian E, Briley M, et al.: High-affinity binding of ^{3}H-imipramine in brain and platelets and its relevance to the biochemistry of affective disorders. Life Sciences 29:211-220, 1981.

58. Langer SZ, Briley MS: High-affinity ^{3}H-imipramine binding: A new biological tool for studies in depression. Trends in Neurosciences 4:28-31, 1981.

59. Langer SZ, Raisman R, Briley M: High-affinity ^{3}H-DMI binding is associated with neuronal noradrenaline uptake in the periphery and the central nervous system. Eur J Pharmacol 72:423-424, 1981.

60. Raisman R, Sette M, Pimoule C, et al.: High-affinity ^{3}H-desipramine binding in the peripheral and central nervous system: A specific site associated with the neuronal uptake of noradrenaline. Eur J Pharmacol 78:345-351, 1982.

61. Enero MA, Langer SZ: Inhibition by dopamine of ^{3}H-noradrenaline release elicited by nerve stimulation in the isolated cat's nictitating membrane. Naunyn Schmiedebergs Arch Pharmacol 289:179-203, 1975.

62. Long JP, Heintz S, Cannon JG, et al.: Inhibition of the sympathetic nervous system by 5,6-dihydroxy-2-dimethyl-amino tetralin (M-7), apomorphine and dopamine. J Pharmacol Exp Ther 192:336-342, 1975.

63. Hope W, McCulloch MW, Story DF, et al.: Effects of pimozide on noradrenergic transmission in rabbit isolated ear arteries. Eur Pharmacol 46:101-111, 1977.

64. Fuder H, Muscholl E: The effect of dopamine on the overflow of endogenous noradrenaline from the perfused rabbit heart evoked by sympathetic nerve stimulation. Naunyn Schmiedebergs Arch Pharmacol 305:109-115, 1978.

65. Langer SZ, Dubocovich ML: Physiological and pharmacological role of the regulation of noradrenaline release by presynaptic dopamine receptors, in Imbs JL, Schwartz J (editors): Peripheral Dopaminergic Receptors. New York, Pergamon Press, 1979, pp 233-245.

66. Dubocovich ML, Langer SZ: Dopamine and α-adrenoceptor agonists inhibit neurotransmission in the cat spleen through different presynaptic receptors. J Pharmacol Exp Ther 212:144-152, 1980.

67. Massingham R, Dubocovich ML, Langer SZ: The role of presynaptic receptors in the cardiovascular action of N,N-di-n-propyldopamine in the cat and dog. Naunyn Schmiedebergs Arch Pharmacol 314:17-28, 1980.

68. Cavero I, Lefevre-Borg F: Functional and pharmacological role of cardiovascular dopamine receptors, in Worcel M, et al (editor): New Trends in Arterial Hypertension. New York, Elsevier/North-Holland, Biomedical Press B.V., 1981, pp 87-99.

69. Langer SZ, Arbilla S: Pharmacological significance of pre- and postsynaptic dopamine receptors.

Proceedings of Smith Kline & French Laboratories Research Symposia I. Dopamine Receptor Agonists. (in press).

70. Langer SZ, Adler-Graschinsky E, Enero MA: Positive feed-back mechanism for the regulation of noradrenaline released by nerve stimulation, abstract. Jerusalem Satellite Symposia. XXVIth International Congress of Physiological Sciences, 1974, p 81.

71. Adler-Graschinsky E, Langer SZ: Possible role of a β-adrenoceptor in the regulation of noradrenaline release by nerve stimulation through a positive feedback mechanism. Br J Pharmacol 53:43-50, 1975.

72. Celuch SM, Dubocovich ML, Langer SZ: Stimulation of presynaptic β-adrenoceptors enhances ³H-noradrenaline release during nerve stimulation in the perfused cat spleen. Br J Pharmacol 63:97-108, 1978.

73. Dahlöf C: Studies on β-adrenoceptor mediated facilitation of sympathetic neurotransmission. Acta Physiol Scand 500 (suppl.):1-147, 1981.

74. Dahlöf C, Ablad B, Borg KO, et al.: Prejunctional inhibition of adrenergic nervous vasomotor control due to β-receptor blockade, in Almgren O, Carlsson A, Engel J (editors): Proceeding of a Symposium on Chemical Tools in Catecholamine Research. Amsterdam, North-Holland Publishing Company, 1975, vol 2, pp 201-210.

75. Dalhöf C, Ljung B, Ablad B: Increased noradrenaline release in the rat portal vein during sympathetic nerve stimulation due to activity of presynaptic β-adrenoceptors by noradrenaline and adrenaline. Eur J Pharmacol 50:75-78, 1978.

76. Westfall TC, Peach MJ, Titermary V: Enhancement of the electrically induced release of norepinephrine from the rat portal vein: Mediation by β₂-adrenoceptors. Eur J Pharmacol 58:67-74, 1979.

77. Stjärne L, Brundin J: Dual adrenoceptor-mediated control of noradrenaline secretion from human vasoconstrictor nerves: Facilitation by β-receptors and inhibition by α-receptors. Acta Physiol Scand 94:139-141, 1975.

78. Stjärne L, Brundin J: β₂-adrenoceptors facilitating noradrenaline release from human vasoconstrictor nerves. Acta Physiol Scand 97:88-93, 1976.

79. Stjärne L, Brundin J: Additive stimulating effects of inhibitor of prostaglandin synthesis and of β-adrenoceptor agonist on sympathetic neuroeffector function in human omental blood vessels. Acta Physiol Scand 97:267-269, 1976.

80. Yamaguchi N, De Champlain J, Nadau PA: Regulation of norepinephrine release from cardiac sympathetic fibers in the dog by presynaptic alpha and beta receptors. Circ Res 41:108-117, 1977.

81. Langer SZ, Galzin AM: Importance physiologique et pharmacologique des récepteurs β-présynaptiques dans la modulation de la libération de la noradrénaline. Thérapie 37:523-532, 1982.

83. Majewski H, Tung LH, Rand J: Adrenaline activation of prejunctional β-adrenoceptors and hypertension. J Cardiovasc Pharmacol 4:99-106, 1982.

84. Guimaraes S, Brandao F, Paiva MO: A study of the adrenoceptor-mediated feed-back mechanisms by using adrenaline as a false transmitter. Naunyn Schmiedebergs Arch Pharmacol 305:185-188, 1978.

85. Rand MJ, Majewski H, McCulloch MW, et al.: An adrenaline-mediated positive feedback loop in sympathetic transmission and its possible role in hypertension, in Langer SZ, Starke K, Dubocovich ML (editors): Presynaptic Receptors. Oxford, Pergamon Press, 1979, pp 263-269.

86. Kawasaki H, Cline WH, Su C: Enhanced presynaptic beta-adrenoceptor-mediated modulation of vascular adrenergic neurotransmission in spontaneously hypertensive rats. J Pharmacol Exp Ther 223:721-728, 1982.

87. Zimmerman BG, Whitmore L: Effect of angiotensin and phenoxybenzamine on release of norepinephrine in vessels during sympathetic nerve stimulation. Int J Neuropharm 6:27-38, 1967.

88. Starke K, Werner U, Hellerforth R, et al.: Influences of peptides on the output of noradrenaline

from isolated rabbit hearts. Eur J Pharmacol 9:136-140, 1970.

89. Campbell WB, Jackson EK: Modulation of adrenergic transmission by angiotensin in the perfused rat mesentery. Am J Physiol 236:211-217, 1979.

90. Garcia-Sevilla AJ, Dubocovich ML, Langer SZ: Angiotensin II facilitates the potassium-evoked release of ³H-noradrenaline from the rabbit hypothalamus. Eur J Pharmacol 56:173-176, 1979.

DISCUSSION

Discussants: Starke, Langer, Hauesler, Birkenhager

Starks: When you compare the pharmacological properties of the dopamine receptors at peripheral noradrenaline neurons with the autoreceptors in the striatum, do you find any difference, or do they seem to be identical? What about the effects of the so-called selective autoreceptor agonist 3PPP [3-(3-hydroxyphenyl)-N-n-propylpiperidine] either centrally or peripherally?

Langer: So far we have no indication that the dopamine receptor that inhibits norepinephrine release in the periphery differs pharmacologically from the dopamine autoreceptor that modulates the release of dopamine in the central nervous system. Both would seem to belong to the D_2 subtype of dopamine receptor. The only difference that we find, and we have no explanation for that, is that when one inhibits reuptake of norepinephrine, the presynaptic effects of dopamine-receptor agonists in the periphery in reducing noradrenergic neurotransmission remains unaffected. However, in the CNS, when one inhibits the reuptake of dopamine with nomifensine, the presynaptic inhibitory effect of some of these dopamine agonists is decreased.

Starke: Might that be due to the rise in the concentration of dopamine at the autoreceptors in the CNS, which would not happen in the periphery?

Langer: This is likely to be one possible explanation.

Starks: What about 3PPP - did you study it?

Langer: Yes, we looked at 3PPP, and in our hands it is not a dopamine-receptor agonist *in vitro* on the model of dopamine release from the striatum by electrical stimulation or on adrenergic neurotransmission peripherally. The effects of 3PPP *in vivo* are likely, therefore, to be due to a metabolite that may be active. We cannot pick it up *in vitro*. They may be due to an effect that does not involve the dopamine receptors which modulate transmitter release.

Hauesler: We have studied apomorphine as a stimulant of presynaptic dopamine receptors in the isolated nictitating membrane of the cat and found inhibition of contraction in response to low frequency (0.5 to 2 Hz) sympathetic nerve stimulation, but no inhibition at higher frequencies. This makes me doubt the therapeutic impact of a stimulant of presynaptic dopamine receptors in, for example, a hypertensive individual. One would expect that an imminent fall in blood pressure (as a result of inhibition of norepinephrine release through activation of presynaptic dopamine receptors) leads to a reflex activation of the sympathetic nervous system. Thereby, the discharge rate in sympathetic nerves may well increase above 2 Hz and move out of the discharge range that is affected by presynaptically-acting drugs.

Langer: We have found that the dopamine-receptor agonists inhibits noradrenergic neurotransmission and that this effect is clearly frequency dependent. Yet, it is less frequency dependent than the effects mediated by alpha-2 agonists. In other words, the intermediate and the high frequencies of stimulation are decreased by dopamine agonists slightly more than by α-2 adrenoceptor agonists. This may be considered in fact a therapeutic advantage provided you have efficacy - namely, you produce a hypotensive effect. Because of the frequency dependency, you are not likely to produce postural hypotension to the extent that this mechanism is less operational in the intermediate and high frequencies of stimulation. I'm in favor of the view that stimulation of presynaptic dopamine receptors is an effective mechanism to lower blood pressure because you produce both hypotension and bradycardia in models of hypertensive animals under *in vivo* conditions - namely, the baroreceptor reflexes are unable to cope with this frequency-dependent decrease in sympathetic output. This is reflected both at the level of peripheral resistance and at the level of heart rate, and this bradycardia may be undoubtedly a desirable effect.

Birkenhager: A simple clinical question referring to your final slide: If we assume that indeed the release of noradrenalin during beta blockade is decreased, what would your prediction be as to systemic noradrenalin levels? In our hands, the response of circulating noradrenalin has been very erratic. It can rise, and it can decrease. What would your prediction and your ideal timing of sampling be?

Langer: It is well known that, in contrast to clonidine, a decrease in plasma norepinephrine levels has not been demonstrated with β-adrenoceptor blockade. This is, I think, well accepted except for the fact that groups like Dr. Champlain in Canada would claim that if you separate your hypertensive patients in what he calls hyperadrenergic and normoadrenergic groups, then you can demonstrate that β-adrenoceptor antagonists will decrease plasma catecholamine levels in the hyperadrenergic group and fail to decrease those levels in the normoadrenergic group. Whether this is an artificial sort of separation that favors a given hypothesis or whether this is a reasonable approach remains an open question. The second factor that should be taken into account is the effect of acute administration against the effect of chronic administration, and perhaps it is a question of time for this effect on noradrenergic neurotransmission to be clear and to become detectable. On the other hand, epinephrine may play a more important role than norepinephrine, and one should measure carefully and separately epinephrine and norepinephrine levels in plasma.

ELECTRICAL EVENTS OF VASCULAR SMOOTH MUSCLE IN RESPONSE TO α_1-ADRENOCEPTOR STIMULATION

GUENTHER HAEUSLER

INTRODUCTION

The biochemical processes triggered by β-adrenoceptor stimulation and initiated by an increase in intracellular cyclic AMP are rather well understood for a variety of organs [1]. Much less is known about the events occurring subsequent to α-adrenoceptor stimulation of vascular smooth muscle. In particular, it is a matter of debate whether the elevation of free intracellular Ca^{++}, required for the induction of contraction, is brought about by electrical changes of the surface membrane or is equally possible in their absence.

In the present study, strips of rabbit main pulmonary artery have been used to measure contractile and electrical events over the entire concentration-response curve of agonists at α-adrenoceptors. Previous studies have shown that the rabbit main pulmonary artery responds to α-adrenoceptor stimulation with maintained contraction and its individual smooth muscle cells with graded depolarization, but not with generation of action potentials [2-8].

Since vascular smooth muscle cells may possess both α_1- and α_2-adrenoceptors [9-11] and since the physiological transmitter noradrenaline activates both subtypes of α-adrenoceptor, methoxamine [12] and prazosin [13] as rather selective α_1-adrenoceptor agonist and antagonist, respectively, have been used in addition. The results suggest that the rabbit main pulmonary artery contains predominantly, or even exclusively, α_1-adrenoceptors. The membrane events described in this study are therefore considered to be typical for α_1-adrenoceptor stimulation.

METHODS

Rabbits (Burgunder) of either sex supplied by the breeding unit Füllinsdorf and weighing 2.3-3 kg were stunned and bled. The main pulmonary artery was excised, transferred immediately to an oxygenated physiological salt solution, cleaned from adhering tissue under a dissecting microscope, and opened along its length axis. Strips 2-mm wide from the middle part of the vessel were then cut parallel to the circular muscle coat. For isometric recording of mechanical responses, the vascular strips were mounted in a 10-ml organ bath and connected to a Statham force transducer under a resting tension of 2 g. Noradrenaline or methoxamine were injected into the organ bath in volumes of 0.05 ml for each concentration. Only one cumulative concentration-response curve was obtained in a single strip.

Intracellular recordings of the membrane potential were obtained from the endothelial side of the vessel with glass capillary microelectrodes filled with 3 M potassium chloride. The resistance of the electrodes varied between 25 and 60 Ω and the tip potentials between 5 and 10 mV. The electrodes were tested at regular intervals for tip potentials in order to avoid systematic errors. The criterion for a successful cell impalement was the occurrence of an instantaneous change in voltage. Only those penetrations were included into the calculations in which the membrane potential had stabilized after impalement for at least 1 minute. In many cases, much longer recordings were obtained. Upon withdrawal of the electrode, the initial zero line was regained and the electrode resistance was unchanged. Changes in membrane potential and in contractile state were both displayed on the screen of an oscilloscope and on the recording paper of a polygraph. All data were stored on magnetic tape.

Changes in membrane resistance were assessed by changes in the space constant λ. For the measurement of the space constant, the vascular strips were introduced in a partition chamber apparatus which was previously described in detail [7].

The standard solution was a physiological salt solution of the following composition (mM concentrations): NaCl 135, KCl 5.4, $CaCl_2$ 2.25, $MgSO_4$ 0.8, NaH_2PO_4 0.4, $NaHCO_3$ 12, glucose 5.5. The solution was gassed with 95% O_2 and 5% CO_2, its pH was 7.3-7.4, and its temperature 37° C.

The following drugs were used: (±)-methoxamine hydrochloride (Burroughs Wellcome), (−)-noradrenaline base (Fluka), prazosin hydrochloride (Pfizer), (±)-propranolol hydrochloride (ICI), reserpine (CIBA-Geigy), 6-hydroxydopamine hydrobromide (Hoffman-La Roche).

RESULTS

The effects of noradrenaline on mechanical tone and on membrane potential were studied over a wide concentration range from 10^{-8} M to 10^{-4} M (Fig. 1). In virtually all experiments, the intracellular microelectrode was dislodged from the contracting smooth muscle cells when noradrenaline was added to the bath solution. Therefore, values for membrane potentials, sampled under control conditions and after contraction in response to a given concentration of noradrenaline, had become stable. In three cases, it was possible to keep the microelectrode within a vascular smooth muscle cell throughout an entire contraction-relaxation cycle. This occurred at low concentrations of noradrenaline

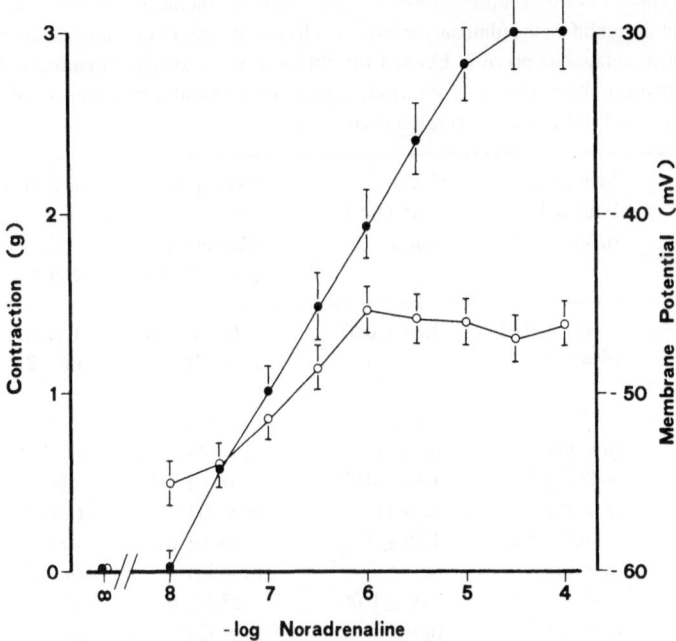

Figure 1. Strips of rabbit main pulmonary artery. Cumulative concentration-response curves for the effects of noradrenaline on tension development (left ordinate, closed symbols) of the vascular strips and on membrane potential (right ordinate, open symbols) of the smooth muscle cells. Shown are the mean values ± S.E.M. (as vertical bars) of 10 strips (contraction) and of 100–150 measurements of membrane potential with intracellular microelectrodes.

(3×10^{-8} M in two cells, 10^{-7} M in one cell) and consequently with rather feeble contractions of the vascular strips. In all three cells, a slight depolarization, corresponding in magnitude to that shown in Figure 1, preceded the noradrenaline-induced contraction. After rinsing the bath, both membrane potential and tension returned to the resting values.

The most conspicuous finding, however, was the different response to noradrenaline of tension and membrane potential. While contraction increased in a concentration-dependent manner from 10^{-8} to 3×10^{-5} M noradrenaline, depolarization was observed only up to 10^{-6} M noradrenaline (Fig. 1); i.e., over the upper segment of the concentration-response curve, contraction to noradrenaline occurred in the absence of changes in membrane potential.

The resting membrane potential of the vascular smooth muscle cells of the rabbit main pulmonary varied within rather narrow limits (-56 to -62 mV) with a mean value of -60.1 mV (Table 1). Depolarization in response to noradrenaline was concentration-dependent up to 10^{-6} M, where membrane potential decreased to 45.3 ± 1.4 mV (n = 112). Above this noradrenaline concentration, no further depolarization was observed (Fig. 1).

Table 1. The effects of various concentrations of methoxamine on the membrane potential of the smooth muscle cells of the rabbit main pulmonary artery, as well as on the space constant λ of this arterial vessel. The α_1-selective antagonist prazosin blocked the effects of methoxamine. Membrane potential was measured with intracellular glass microelectrodes, space constant with a partition chamber apparatus. The mean values $\pm$ S.E.M. of n measurements are given.

	Membrane Potential (mV)	Space Constant λ (mm)	In the presence of prazosin 10^{-6} M	
			Membrane potential (mV)	Space constant λ (mm)
Controls	60.1 $\pm$ 0.04 (n = 110)	1.89 $\pm$ 0.03 (n = 25)	61.5 $\pm$ 1.02 (n = 34)	1.91 (n = 2)
Methoxamine				
3×10^{-7} M	$-$55.1 $\pm$ 1.3 (n = 61)	1.68 $\pm$ 0.1 (n = 7)	$-$59.8 $\pm$ 0.4 (n = 36)	1.91 (n = 2)
10^{-6} M	$-$48.3 $\pm$ 1.5 (n = 75)	1.45 $\pm$ 0.07 (n = 7)	$-$59.3 $\pm$ 1.2 (n = 31)	2.00 (n = 2)
10^{-5} M	$-$46.2 $\pm$ 1.6 (n = 50)	1.25 $\pm$ 0.09 (n = 6)	$-$60.0 $\pm$ 0.9 (n = 24)	1.89 (n = 2)
3×10^{-5} M	$-$47.1 $\pm$ 1.5 (n = 57)	1.08 $\pm$ 0.06 (n = 5)	$-$58.3 $\pm$ 0.4 (n = 13)	1.95 (n = 2)

Methoxamine, which is thought to be a rather selective agonist at α_1-adreno-ceptors, induced contractions of the pulmonary artery strips with a maximum similar to that produced by noradrenaline (Fig. 2). Maximal contractions in response to noradrenaline and methoxamine were 3.01 $\pm$ 0.21 (n = 10) and 2.9 $\pm$ 0.23 g (n = 6), respectively, and did not differ significantly from each other. The potency of methoxamine was approximately one third that of noradrenaline (Figs. 1 and 2).

The maximal depolarization in response to methoxamine was reached at a concentration of 10^{-6} M or somewhat higher. Similar to noradrenaline, the contractions in the upper segment of the methoxamine concentration-response curve occurred in the absence of changes in membrane potential (Fig. 2). This finding, however, does not necessarily indicate that high concentrations of methoxamine (or noradrenaline) are without any influence on the electrical properties of the membrane of the vascular smooth muscle cells. Therefore, it was necessary to obtain further information from measurements of membrane resistance.

The cable properties of the rabbit main pulmonary artery [4, 7] allow the determination of the space constant λ. Changes of λ reflect in first-line changes in membrane resistance. However, it has to be noted that the possible occurrence of alterations in low-resistance pathways between cells and the rather unlikely event of a change in cytoplasmatic resistance will, to some extent, also affect λ.

For the determination of λ, the pulmonary vascular strips were stimulated

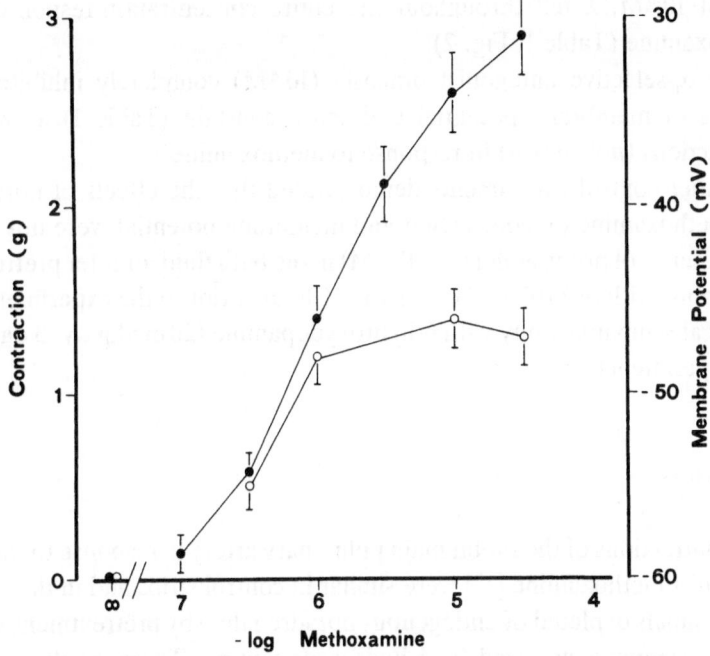

Figure 2. Strips of rabbit main pulmonary artery. Cumulative concentration-response curves for the effects of the selective agonist at α_1-adrenoceptors methoxamine on tension development (left ordinate, closed symbols) of the vascular strips and on membrane potential (right ordinate, open symbols) of the smooth muscle cells. Shown are the mean values $\pm$ S.E.M. (as vertical bars) of six strips (contraction) and of 50–75 measurements of membrane potential with intracellular microelectrodes.

though agar bridges with constant-current pulses of 3-second duration and a strength of 30, 50, 70, and 90 μA. The resulting electrotonic potentials were recorded with intracellular microelectrodes at distances of 0.8, 1.2, 1.6, and 2 mm from the stimulating electrode. The amplitude of the electrotonic potentials decreased with increasing distance from the stimulating electrode. A plot of this distance against log mV amplitude of the electrotonic potential yielded a straight line; its intercept with the ordinate indicates the (extrapolated) amplitude of the electrotonic potentials under the stimulating electrode. The space constant λ is defined as the distance from the stimulating electrode at which the amplitudes of the electrotonic potentials decline to a relative size of 1/e or to 37% of the extrapolated amplitude at 0 distance. In the present study, the average value for λ measured in the rabbit main pulmonary artery was 1.89 ± 0.03 mm (Table 1). Methoxamine reduced λ in a concentration-dependent manner, indicating a decrease in membrane resistance. A minimal value of 1.08 ± 0.06 mm for λ was found for the highest concentration of methoxamine (Table 1). In contrast to the methoxamine-induced depolarizations, which were found only up to a concentration of 10^{-6} M, λ fell throughout the entire concentration-response curve of methoxamine (Table 1, Fig. 2).

The α_1-selective antagonist prazosin (10^{-6} M) completely inhibited the decreases of membrane potential and space constant (Table 1) as well as the contractions (not shown) in response to methoxamine.

Further control experiments demonstrated that the effects of noradrenaline and methoxamine on contraction and membrane potential were not altered by the presence of propranolol (3×10^{-7} M) in the bath fluid, or after pretreatment of the rabbits with reserpine (3 mg/kg i.p. 16 hours prior to the experiment), or after chemical sympathectomy with 6-hydroxydopamine (20 mg/kg i.v. 3 days prior to the experiment).

DISCUSSION

The contractions of the rabbit main pulmonary artery in response to the selective α_1-agonist methoxamine [12] were similar in control strips and in those obtained from animals depleted of endogenous noradrenaline by pretreatment with reserpine or sympathectomized by 6-hydroxydopamine. These results characterize methoxamine as a directly-acting sympathominetic agent. Furthermore, methoxamine is a full agonist at α-adrenoceptors of the pulmonary artery, since maximal contractions to noradrenaline and methoxamine were indentical. However, noradrenaline is three times more potent than methoxamine.

Docherty and Starke [14] obtained no evidence for the presence of α_2-adrenoceptors in the rabbit main pulmonary artery. Thus, both the present results as well as those of Docherty and Starke [14] strongly suggest the existence of only one α-adrenoceptor subtype in the rabbit main pulmonary artery. It is therefore justified to conclude that the electrical and contractile events elicited by noradrenaline in this arterial vessel result from stimulation of α_1-adrenoceptors. The concomitant activation of β-adrenoceptors by noradrenaline does not seem to contribute to the recorded effects, since blockade of β-adrenoceptors by propranolol had no influence on noradrenaline-induced depolarization and contraction.

Methoxamine decreased space constant λ, and hence membrane resistance, over the entire range of the concentration-response curve, while depolarization occurred only over the lower segment. Obviously, alterations of membrane potential do not fully reflect the membrane changes produced by activation of α_1-adrenoceptors. It is suggested that low concentrations of α_1-agonists depolarize the vascular smooth muscle cells and decrease membrane resistance mainly by an increase in sodium and calcium permeability. The resultant progressive rise in free internal calcium concentration, which is reflected by increasing contraction, raises the potassium permeability of the cell membrane. This process, secondary to α-adrenoceptor stimulation, tends to hyperpolarize the cell membrane and in this way prevents further α_1-adrenoceptor-mediated depolarization. A direct positive relationship between increasing internal calcium and an elevation of potassium permeability has been demonstrated for various tissues (see [15] for cardiac muscle as an example). Thus, the stable membrane potential at high α-agonist concentrations may be explained by the simultaneous operation of two opposing processes. According to this explanation, one would expect blockade of potassium channels to eliminate the mechanism opposing α_1-adrenoceptor-mediated depolarization. This was in fact borne out in our recent experiments, where the potassium channel blocker tetraethylammonium allowed for a noradrenaline-induced depolarization over the entire concentration range of the agonist [6, 7].

Although the present study shows that contraction in response to α_1-adrenoceptor stimulation occurs with concomitant electrical events at the cell membrane, two observations question whether the latter can fully account for contraction. First, the threshold concentration of potassium to induce contractions in the rabbit main pulmonary artery is 15 mM. At this potassium concentration, the membrane potential is reduced from -60 mV to approximately -45 mV [17], i.e., to a value at which contraction in response to noradrenaline is already maximal. The corresponding threshold concentrations of noradrenaline or methoxamine are 3×10^{-8} M and 3×10^{-7} M, respectively, which depolarize the membrane from -60 mV to only -55 mV (present experiments). Second, small rabbit mesenteric arteries, chemically skinned with saponin, and thus being devoid of membrane potential, responded to α-adrenoceptor stimulation with contractions which reached approximately 50% of the maximum of unskinned preparations [16]. These observations indicate that at least part of the contraction induced by activation of α-adrenoceptors in vascular smooth muscle occurs independently of electrical processes at the cell membrane.

SUMMARY

The mechanical and electrical events occuring in smooth muscle of the rabbit main pulmonary artery in response to α-adrenoceptor stimulation were studied *in vitro* over the whole concentration-response curve of noradrenaline and the α_1-selective methoxamine. Contraction of the vascular strips was measured isometrically. Membrane potential with intracellular glass microelectrodes and changes in membrane resistance were determined as changes in space constant λ. Mechanical and membrane responses characterized methoxamine as a full agonist with approximately one third of the potency of noradrenaline. Both agonists depolarized the vascular smooth muscle cells over the lower segment of the concentration-contraction curve without further depolarization over the upper segment, indicating that part of the contraction occurred in the absence of changes in membrane potential. By contrast, λ was decreased by methoxamine over the entire range of the concentration-response curve. The similarity between methoxamine and noradrenaline with regard to induction of electrical and mechanical events as well as blockade of the two types of response by the α_1-antagonist prazosin suggest that the effects of both agonists are mediated in the rabbit main pulmonary artery mainly, if not exclusively, by α_1-adrenoceptors. Stimulation of this subtype of α-adrenoceptor in vascular smooth muscle causes concentration-dependent decreases in membrane resistance and increases in mechanical tension over an identical range of agonist concentrations and with a similar concentration-response relationship.

REFERENCES

1. Williamson JR: Effects of epinephrine on glycogenolysis and myocardial contractility, in Blaschko H, Sayers G, Smith AD (editors): Handbook of Physiology. Washington, D.C., American Physiological Society, 1975, vol 6, Sect 7, pp 605-636.
2. Somlyo AV, Somlyo AP: Electromechanical and pharmacomechanical coupling in vascular smooth muscle. J Pharmacol Exp Ther 159:129-145, 1968.
3. Somlyo AV, Vinall P, Somlyo AP: Excitation-contraction coupling and electrical events in two types of vascular smooth muscle. Microvasc Res 1:354-373, 1969.
4. Casteels R, Kitamura K, Kuriyama H, et al.: The membrane properties of the smooth muscle cells of the rabbit main pulmonary artery. J Physiol (Lond) 271:41-61, 1977.
5. Casteels R, Kitamura K, Kuriyama H, et al.: Excitation-contraction coupling in the smooth muscle cells of the rabbit main pulmonary artery. J Physiol (Lond) 271:63-79, 1977.
6. Haeusler G: Relationship between noradrenaline-induced depolarization and contraction in vascular smooth muscle. Blood Vessels 15:46-54, 1978.
7. Haeusler G, Thorens S: Effects of tetraethylammonium chloride on contractile, membrane and cable properties of rabbit artery muscle. J Physiol (Lond) 303:203-224, 1980.
8. Haeusler G, Kuhn H, Thorens S: The effect of tetraethylammonium chloride on calcium fluxes in smooth muscle from rabbit main pulmonary artery. J Physiol (Lond) 303:225-241, 1980.
9. Drew GM, Whiting SB: Evidence for two distinct types of postsynaptic α-adrenoceptor in vascular smooth muscle in vivo. Br J Pharmacol 67:207-215, 1979.
10. Timmermans PBMWM, Kwa HY, Van Zwieten PA: Possible subdivision of postsynaptic α-adrenoceptors mediating pressor responses in the pithed rat. Naunyn-Schmiedeberg's Arch Pharmacol 310:189-193, 1979.
11. Kobinger W, Pichler L: Investigation into different types of post- and presynaptic α-adrenoceptors at cardiovascular sites in rats. Eur J Pharmacol 65, 393-402, 1980.
12. Starke K, Endo T, Taube HD: Relative pre- and postsynaptic potencies of α-adrenoceptor agonists in the rabbit pulmonary artery. Naunyn Schmiedebergs Arch Pharmacol 291:55-78, 1975.
13. Cambridge D, Davey MJ, Massingham R: Prazosin, a selective antagonist of post-synaptic α-adrenoceptors. Br J Pharmacol 59:514P-515P, 1977.
14. Docherty JR, Starke K: Postsynaptic α-adrenoceptor subtypes in rabbit blood vessels and rat anococcygeus muscle studied in vitro. J Cardiovasc Pharmacol 3:854-866, 1981.
15. Bassingthwaighte JB, Fry CH, McGuigan JAS: Relationship between internal calcium and outward current in mammalian ventricular muscle; a mechanism for the control of action potential duration. J Physiol (Lond) 262:15-37, 1976.
16. Haeusler G, Richards JG, Thorens S: Noradrenaline contractions in rabbit mesenteric arteries skinned with saponin. J Physiol (Lond) 321:537-556, 1981.

DISCUSSION

Discussants: Folkov, Haeusler, Mulvani, Langes

Folkow: You have here a system in which you can follow in detail both the electrical membrane events and the contractile response. Have you performed studies along these lines comparing arteries from SHR with normotensive ones? After all, there is presently much to indicate that there are modest but perhaps functionally important membrane changes in SHR.

Haeusler: I have presented the effects of adrenergic agonists on mechanical-tension development, membrane potential, and membrane resistance over a wide concentration range covering full concentration-response curves. The electrophysiologic part of such experiments is extremely laborious and possible only in blood vessels which, like the rabbit main pulmonary artery, allow intracellular measurements with relative ease. In my experience, rat arteries are more difficult to handle in this respect, and I don't have results from normotensive or hypertensive rats.

Folkow: I fully understand the great difficulties, but such studies could perhaps provide interesting information.

Mulvani: I was very interested in your results. We've been examining electrical properties in these very small rat arteries and have been getting rather similar results. I wonder if you could answer a question which we've been asked. How do the results you obtain with exogenous noradrenaline relate to what happens with endogenous noradrenaline.

Haeusler: I don't think that this is of particular relevance for the rabbit main pulmonary artery. The neuromuscular distance in this blood vessel is very large (10,000-20,000 Å) and the adrenergic innervation rather sparse. I doubt that sympathetic nerve stimulation would induce maximal contractions in this preparation.

Mulvani: Did I understand correctly that your saponin-treated small vessels were in calcium-free solution?

Haeusler: Yes.

Mulvani: And in calcium-free solution, norepinephrine causes contraction?

Haeusler: Yes. The maximal contractile response of the skinned preparation to norepinephrine in calcium-free solution is 50% of the maximal contraction obtained with norepinephrine in the presence of calcium in unskinned preparations.

Malvuni: The other thing I remember you saying is that in discussion you might tell us how they do this.

Haeusler: I don't have a precise explanation. Electrical events in response to α-adrenoceptor stimulation are barely conceivable in skinned cells. The signal from the α-adrenoceptor to the contractile apparatus must, therefore, be of non-electric nature. It might be α-adrenoceptor mediated release of calcium from the surface membrane. This calcium could either be in itself sufficient to activate the contractile proteins or induce release of a greater amount of calcium from the sarcoplasmic reticulum. Of course, both mechanisms could operate in parallel.

Langer: In cerebral arteries, it has been reported that there is a high density of postsynaptic

α_2-adrenoceptors and that they contribute significantly to the contractile responses to norepinephrine. Is it technically possible to carry out similar experiments to the ones you did in the main pulmonary artery with dog vascular arteries, where it has been shown that there are a significant number of α_2-adrenoceptors, and to see whether norepinephrine would be acting on the so-called voltage-dependent channels that induce a contractile response?

Haeusler: That's what we are trying to do. Suitable vessels could be veins or cerebral arteries.

III. RECENT ADVANCES IN RESEARCH ON RENIN SYSTEM

INTRODUCTION

Edgar Haber

Renin is a venerable concept, dating back to the perceptive, but soon forgotten, work of Tiegerstadt and Bergman at the end of the nineteenth century, and to its revival by the elegant physiological experiments of Goldblatt and his colleagues in the 1930s. There have been other milestones that have affected the transition of renin from a debated hypothesis to the solid underpinning of human cardiovascular regulation: the determination of the sequence of angiotensin and of part of its substrate; the measurement of renin activity; the discovery of inhibitors of the renin-angiotensin system that helped uncover its contribution to the genesis of hypertension. Yet, there has seldom been a time analogous to the present moment when so many initiatives have come to fruition and when all of these were being discussed at a single session.

Today we witness the uncovering of the complete amino acid sequence of renin and the sequence of the DNA copied from the RNA that is responsible for its synthesis. Now the structure of preprorenin is known, and objective questions may be asked concerning both the transition of the precursor to the enzyme and the relationship of the prohormone to the inactive species that circulates and has provided such a puzzle to clinical investigators.

The structure of human renin substrate has been revealed, and the very substantial differences that exist between its sequence and that of other mammalian substrates will give insight into the unique specificities of human renin.

Until relatively recently renin was perceived as a kidney enzyme acting on an intravascular substrate to yield a circulating hormone. This concept has now been broadened. There appear to be many sites for renin synthesis outside the kidney, and there are interesting clues that the entire system may be somewhat different when examined in detail outside the kidney. A renin-angiotensin system is clearly present in the brain, though its precise regulatory role needs to be clarified.

While highly significant discoveries have been presented today to an excited audience, none marks the end of a line of investigation. Rather, each is likely to be a stimulus to further inquiry. Although renin has been with us as a concept for 83 years, research in the field is but at a vigorous adolescent state: activity is great, potential is apparent, some important knowledge has been gained, but the end is not in sight.

STUDIES OF RENIN BIOSYNTHESIS AND RELEASE

Victor J. Dzau and Richard E. Pratt

INTRODUCTION

Most secretory proteins are synthesized as a large molecular weight (MW) precursor. The translational product of messenger RNA is the preproform, which contains a nascent fragment of 15 to 30 amino acid extensions at the N-terminus. This prefragment is cleaved shortly after attachment and penetration of the forming protein into the endoplasmic reticulum (ER). The resultant proform, located intracisternally, is transported through the ER, Golgi apparatus, condensing vacuoles, and finally packaged into secretory granules [1, 2]. During this sojourn, glycosylation of glycoproteins occurs. The proform is usually converted into the mature protein intracellularly and stored as such in the granules. However, many enzymes remain as the inactive precursor (zymogen) and are only activated extracellularly after release. The process by which the inactive precursor is converted to the active product is limited proteolysis [3]. Secretion usually occurs by the fusion of secretory granules with plasma membrane (exocytosis). In many systems, several intracellular pools of secretory granules exist. The usual pathway of secretion in response to a stimulus is first the release of the contents of the old stored secretory granules followed by the later release of newly synthesized proteins. However, the early release of new proteins, 'bypassing' the usual secretory pathway, have also been described in several systems [4-6]. The entire process from synthesis to storage in mature granule usually takes several hours [1, 7].

RENIN: LARGE MOLECULAR WEIGHT FORMS

Studies of renin biosynthesis have been limited by several factors. Renin is present in very small quantities in the kidney, and it is extremely unstable after tissue extraction. Therefore, the purification of this enzyme in significant quantities is difficult [8-11]. Little is known about the structure of the renal enzyme or its large MW precursor. Large MW forms of renin ranging from 50,000 to 140,000 daltons have been reported [12, 13]. The difficult task is to identify which of these forms are renin precursor, renin-inhibitor complex, or artefact of extraction.

Indeed, most of these forms have not been purified, and demonstration of their existence and MW have been previously dependent on fractionation by gel filtration chromatography and enzymatic activity. One approach to this analysis is to divide the large MW renins into two general categories based on the presence or absence of intrinsic enzymatic activity.

The first category consists of all the large MW renins that possess intrinsic activities. The specific activities of these forms may be the same or lower than the small MW renin. Treatment with trypsin, pepsin, or acidification may increase, decrease, or have no effect on the renin activity, depending on the particular form studied. This category includes the 60,000-dalton form [12, 13]. The conversion of 60,000 daltons to 40,000 daltons appears to be reversible and dependent on the conditions of extraction and the protease inhibitors employed in the buffers. These forms are most likely renin-inhibitor complex or *in vitro* artefacts due to protein-protein interaction during extraction. Indeed, Yamamoto and his colleagues [14, 15] demonstrated that a 60,000-dalton form of high molecular weight renin (HMWR) was the product of the binding of small molecular weight renin (SMWR) with a renin-binding protein (RBP) present in the cytosol of the renal cortex. This HMWR is active and is the dominant from in dog, rat, and hog kidney when extracted in the presence of sulfhydryl oxidizing agents such as N-ethylmaleimide or sodium tetrathionate. Extraction in the absence of thiol oxidizing agents prevented this interaction, yielding the SMWR as the dominant form. The significance of the interaction between renin and RBP is unclear, since these proteins are usually sequestered from each other *in vivo*. Ueno et al. [16] demonstrated that RBP in the appropriate concentration inhibited renin activity and suggested that RBP may provide protection against sudden rupture of renin granules and massive intrarenal release of renin under abnormal conditions. An alternative explanation is that HMWR is an artefact of extraction resulting from the exposure of two otherwise sequestered proteins.

The second category includes large MW form(s) with no enzymatic activity. Completely inactive renin(s) has been demonstrated in plasma and in kidneys of hog, human, and possibly dog and rats [12, 13]. Treatment with trypsin, pepsin, acid, or prolonged cold exposure can result in activation of enzymatic activity. Evidence suggests that plasma inactive renin originated primarily from the kidney [17-19]. Since this form of renin is completely inactive and can be activated by limited proteolysis at the moment, it appears to be the best candidate for the biologic precursor (zymogen) of the active SMWR. However, definitive proof is still lacking. No structural or biosynthetic studies on purified inactive renin has been performed. The remarkable accomplishment of the complete purification of the inactive renin in hog kidneys will enable such definitive studies to be performed [20].

Molecular biological studies have enhanced our understanding of the bio-synthesis of renin. Most of these studies have been performed on the mouse submaxillary gland. This gland is particularly suitable for these studies, since the renin isoenzyme constitute up to 5% of total glandular protein. This isoenzyme is identical to the renal enzyme in physiochemical and immunochemical properties [21]. To first examine if renin is synthesized as a large MW precursor, we studied the translational product of renin mRNA [22, 23]. Total poly A$^+$ mRNA from male mouse glands were isolated using guanidine and phenyl-chloroform extrac-tion followed by oligo dT chromatography. The mRNAs were translated in the presence of ^{35}S-methionine using a cell-free rabbit reticulocyte lysate system. The translational products were subjected to immunoprecipitation using specific anti-serum raised against pure glandular SMWR (37,000) and *Staphylococcus aureus* (Cowen's Strain I). Analysis by 6-11% SDS polyacrylamide (PAGE) and fluo-rography revealed a single protein band of MW 48,000 daltons. This protein is the renin precursor, since it was not precipitated by preimmune serum and pure SMWR blocked its binding to antirenin antibody (Fig. 1). Similar observations were made by other investigators [24, 25]. Further evidence that this 48,000-dalton protein is preprorenin was obtained from *in vitro* translation of mRNA in the presence of pancreatic microsomes (rough ER). This procedure resulted in the conversion of the 48,000-dalton protein to a 46,000-dalton protein (prorenin), presumably by the cleavage of the prefragment by the signal peptidase [26]. To examine if this 46,000-dalton protein is converted to SMWR, we performed pulse chase labelling experiments of submaxillary gland tissue [27]. In this experiment, submaxillary glands were removed from female mice injected with testosterone in order to stimulate renin synthesis. The glands were minced, and separate portions were incubated in Delbecco's modified Eagle's medium (DMEM) with 250 μCi of ^{35}S-methionine at 37° C for 30 minutes, 3 hours, 6 hours or 6 hours followed by 12 hours in the presence of excess unlabelled methionine. Samples of tissue homoge-nates and media, removed at the different times, were subjected to immu-noprecipitation and SDS PAGE analysis (Fig. 2). The data revealed that within minutes, the 46,000-dalton prorenin was synthesized. By 30 minutes, a 41,000-dalton form of renin appeared, constituting approximately 40% of total newly synthesized renin. At 3 hours, the 41,000-dalton renin formed 75% of total radiolabelled renin and was the sole form secreted into the medium. By 6 hours, a small quantity of the SMWR (37,000 daltons) appeared in the tissue. The ratio of 46,000:41,000:37,000-dalton proteins was approximately 15:70:15. After another 12 hours of incubation in the presence of unlabelled methionine, renin existed primarily (90%) as the 37,000-dalton species, which was also the major secretory form. However, small amounts of the 46,000 and 41,000-dalton renins were still present. In a separate study, we analyzed the MW of pure submaxillary gland renin isolated by the method of Cohen et al. [28]. Ninety five percent of pure

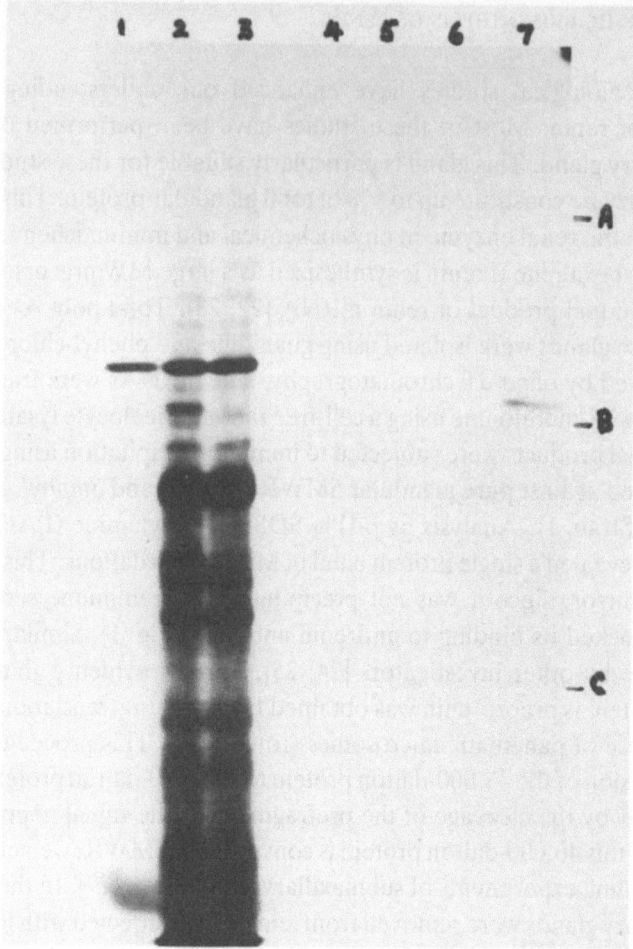

Figure 1. **SDS/polyacylamide geld electrophoresis and fluorographic analysis of translation products of poly (A)+ mRNA from mouse submaxillary glands. Lane 1: control, lysate without mRNA addition. Lanes 2 and 3 show total translation products from control male mouse SWR/J and renin-deficient mouse C57 BL/10J mRNA respectively. Lanes 4 and 5 represent immunoprecipitate of mouse C57 BL/10J total products with preimmune and antirenin sera, respectively. Lanes 6 and 7 represent immunoprecipitate of mouse SWR/J total translation products with pre-immune and antirenin sera, respectively. Arrow at right indicates the location of the 48,000-dalton renin precursor. Bars at the left indicate the position of molecular weight standards: A, phosphorylase 'a' (92,500); B, ovalbumin (45,000); C, trypsinogen (24,500).**

renin exists as the 37,000-dalton form, while only 5% are of the 41,000-dalton form [26]. Taken together, the above data suggest that renin is synthesized as a 48,000-dalton preproform, which is rapidly processed to the 46,000-dalton pro-form. The 46,000-dalton prorenin is converted intracellularly to an intermediate 41,000-dalton form for immediate secretion. A slow intracellular process converts

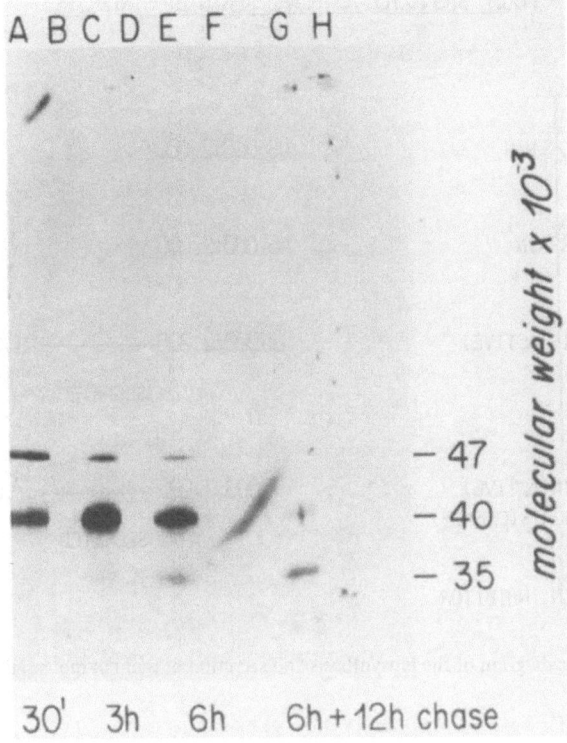

Figure 2. **Autoradiographs of mouse submaxillary gland samples** after 30 min, 3 hr, and 6 hr in [35S] methionine; and 6 hr in [35S] methionine followed by 12 hr in excess unlabelled methionine. The samples had been treated with immune serum and precipitated with staphylococcus aureus before separation by SDS polyacrylamide gel electrophoresis.

the intermediate 41,000-dalton form to the smaller 37,000 renin, which is the predominant storage and secretory form (Fig. 3).

Attempts at studying cell-free translation of total kidney poly A+ mRNA have been less sucessful. This is because renin mRNA constitutes only a minor percentage of total kidney mRNA. Despite this drawback, Poulsen et al. [29] and Dykes et al. [30] detected, by immunoprecipitation of renal mRNA translation products, a renin precursor of molecular weight similar to the submandibular gland preprorenin. These studies, which suggest that renal renin is synthesized as preprorenin, are impractical because of the long fluorographic exposure times (up to 14 weeks). We have performed pulse chase labelling experiments on isolated dog glomeruli in suspension [31]. Indeed, a proform of 55,000 daltons was first synthesized, which was converted intracellularly to a 48,000-dalton form and finally to the SMWR (38,000 daltons). The complete conversion of precursor to the 38,000-dalton product in the unstimulated state was observed to be slow; i.e.,

MOUSE SUBMAXILLARY GLAND RENIN BIOSYNTHESIS

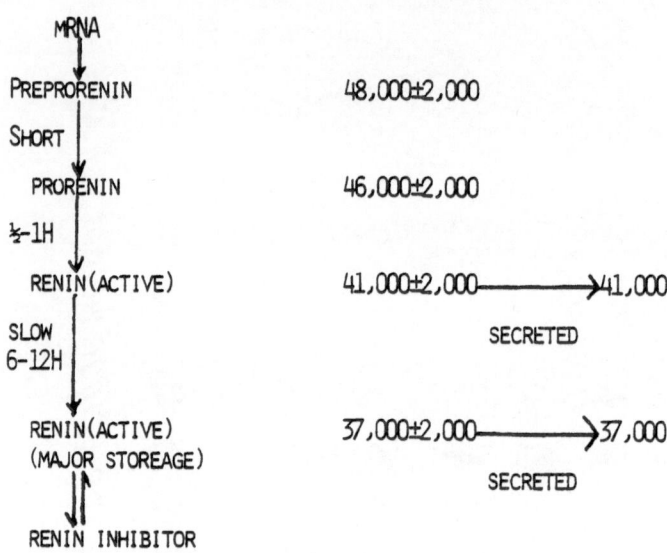

Figure 3. Schematic diagram of the biosynthesis and secretion of renin in mouse submaxillary gland.

small amounts of precursor forms were still present at 26 hours after initial pulse. The ratio of 55,000:48,000:38,000 daltons was 1:2:3. The generally lower MWs of submaxillary gland prorenin and renin as compared to their counterparts in the dog kidney can be explained by the fact that submaxillary gland renin is not a glycoprotein.

Since most of the physiologic and biochemical studies on large MW inactive renin have been performed on human plasma and kidneys, parallel studies of biosynthesis are of obvious significance. The major limitation here is the availability of fresh tissue sample. Recently, we had the opportunity of obtaining a chronically ischemic kidney from a hypertensive patient with severe renal artery stenosis and thrombosed aortorenal bypass undergoing nephrectomy. Immediately after nephrectomy, the kidney was sliced and incubated in DMEM containing 1 mCi of ^{35}S-methionine. Pulse-labelling experiments were performed as described for the submaxillary gland. Immunoprecipitation was accomplished using antihuman renin antibody. We observed that within 45 minutes of pulse, the newly synthesized renin was already predominantly in the 43,000-dalton form and was readily secreted into the medium (Fig. 4). This is the active form, since biochemical analysis of the ischemic kidney tissue and the media, as well as renal vein plasma samples, revealed very high active renin levels with little to no inactive renin [26]. This is in contrast to the findings in the normal human kidney and plasma in which inactive renin accounts for 30 to 60% of total renin concen-

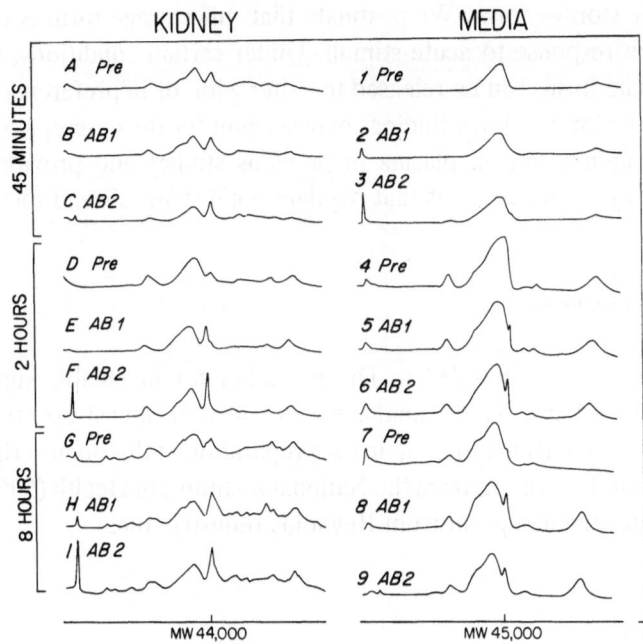

Figure 4. Densitometer tracings of autoradiographs of SDS PAGE of ischemic human kidney and media samples after 45 min, 2 hr, and 8 hr of incubation in [^{35}S]-methionine. The samples had been treated with preimmune serum (pre) or antihuman renin antisera (Ab 1, generous gift of Drs. P. Corvol and J. Menard; Ab 2 raised to pure human renin in our laboratory). Note the peak of radioactivity corresponding to MW 44,000 daltons in kidney and 45,000 daltons in media in the antisera treated samples but not in the preimmune treated samples.

tration [13, 26]. Human renal active renin from normal subjects exists predominantly as a 40,000-dalton species (by G-100 and SDS PAGE analysis) when extracted in the presence of a mixture of protease inhibitors and avoiding harsh acidification steps [26]. Under these circumstances, inactive renin has a MW of 56,000 daltons. Thus, it appears that during renal ischemia in man, the inactive renin precursor is short-lived and is rapidly converted to active renin, ready for secretion and 'bypassing' storage.

SUMMARY

In summary, renin is synthesized as a preprorenin and rapidly converted to prorenin. Prorenin is cleaved intracellularly to an intermediate form ready for immediate secretion under certain circumstances. The time required for synthesis, processing, and release of this secretory form can be as early as 30 minutes. Usually, a slower intracellular process converts this intermediate form into the small MW storage form. We postulate that this storage form is the first to be released in response to acute stimuli. Under certain conditions, however, the intermediate forms can be released together with, or in preference to, the small MW storage form. Above findings may account for the descrepancies in MW of renins in kidney and in plasma in previous studies and provide insight into possible control mechanisms that regulate renin synthesis and release.

ACKNOWLEDGMENTS

The authors are indebteded to Dr. E. Haber for invaluable suggestions and support. We thank Atau Tanaka for excellent technical assistance. We are grateful to Diane Rioux for help in the preparation of this manuscript. This work was supported by a grant from the National Institutes of Health (5 KO8 HL00750 and HL 19259) and a grant from Reynolds Industry, Inc.

REFERENCES

1. Steiner DF, Kemmler W, Tager HS, et al.: Proteolytic processing in the biosynthesis of insulin and other proteins. Fed Proc 33:2105, 1974.
2. Cohn DV, MacGregor RR: The biosynthesis, intracellular processing and secretion of parathormone. Endocr Rev 2:1, 1981.
3. Neurath H, Walsh K: Role of proteolytic enzymes in biologic regulation (a review). Proc Natl Acad Sci USA 73:3825, 1976.
4. MacGregor RR, Hamilton JW, Cohn DV: The bypass of tissue hormone stores during the secretion of newly synthesized parathyroid hormones. Endocrinology 97:178, 1975.
5. Morrisey JJ, Cohn DV: Regulation of secretion of parathormone and secretory proteins from separate intracellular pools by calcium, dibutyl cyclic AMP and (1)-isoproterenol. J Cell Biol 82:93, 1979.
6. Sharoni U, Eimerl S, Schramir M: Secretion of old versus new exportable protein in rat parotid slices. J Cell Biol 71:107, 1976.
7. Tartakoff AM, Greene LJ, Jamieson JD, et al.: Parallelism in the processing of pancreatic proteins, in Ceccarelli D, Clementi F, Meldoles J (editors): Advances in Cytopharmacology. New York, Raven Press. 1974, vol 2, p 177.
8. Inagami T, Murakami K: Isolation of pure and stable renin from hog kidney. J Biol Chem 252:2978, 1977.
9. Dzau VJ, Slater EE, Haber E: Complete purification of dog renal renin. Biochemistry 18:5224, 1979.
10. Galen FX, Devaux C, Guyenne T, et al.: Multiple forms of human renin. J Biol Chem 254:4848, 1979.
11. Yokosawa H, Holladay LA, Inagami T, et al.: Human renal renin. Complete purification and characterization. J Biol Chem 255:3498, 1980.
12. Inagami T, Murakami K: Prorenin (review). Biomed Res 1:456, 1980.
13. Sealey JE, Atlas SA, Laragh JH: Prorenin and other large molecular weight forms of renin (review). Endocr Rev 1:365, 1980.
14. Kawamura M, Ikemoto F, Funakawa S, et al.: Characteristics of a renin-binding substance for the conversion of renin into a higher molecular weight form in the dog. Clin Sci 57:345, 1979.

15. Yamomoto K, Ikemoto F, Takaori K, et al.: Nature of renin-binding substance in dog renal cortex, in Sambhi M (editor): Heterogeneity of Renin and Renin-Substrate. New York, Elsevier North-Holland, 1981, p 113.

16. Ueno N, Miyazaki H, Hirose S, et al.: A 56,000 dalton renin-binding protein in hog kidney is an endogenous renin inhibitor. J Biol Chem.

17. Atlas SA, Sealey JE, Dharmgrongartama B, et al.: Detection and isolation of inactive, large molecular weight renin in human kidney and plasma. Hypertension 3(suppl I):I-30-40, 1981.

18. Chang JJ, Kirsoragi M, Okamoto H, et al.: Isolation and activation of inactive renin from human kidney and plasma. Hypertension 3:509, 1981.

19. Hseuh WA, Carlson EJ, Dzau VJ: Characterization of inactive renin from human kidney and plasma: Evidence for a renal source of circulating inactive renin, to be published.

20. Inagami T, Takii Y, Yokosawa N, et al.: Purification of prorenin (in this volume).

21. Inagami T, Murakami K, Yokosawa H, et al.: Purification of renin and precursors, in Gross, Vogel (editors): Enzymatic Release of Vasoactive Peptides. New York, Raven Press, 1980, p 7.

22. Dzau VJ, Ouellete A, Pratt R: Studies of biosynthesis of renin with a cell-free translation system. Clin Sci 61:241s, 1981.

23. Pratt RE, Dzau VJ, Ouellete A: Abundant androgen regulated mRNA's in mouse submandibular gland: Cell-free translation of renin precursors mRNA. Nucleic Acids Res 9:3433, 1981.

24. Poulsen K, Vunst J, Lykkegaard S, et al.: Renin is synthesized as a 50,000 dalton single chain polypeptide in cell-free translation systems. FEBS Lett 98:135, 1979.

25. Morris BJ, Catanzaro DF, Richards RI, et al.: Kallikrein and renin: Molecular biology and biosynthesis. Clin Sci 61:351s, 1981.

26. Pratt RE, Dzau VJ: Unpublished data.

27. Pratt RE, Ouellete AJ, Dzau VJ: Biosynthetic processing of renin precursors. Fed Proc 41: ??, 1982. (in press)

28. Cohen S, Taylor JM, Murakami K, et al.: Isolation and characterization of renin-like enzymes from mouse submaxillary glands. Biochemistry 11:4286, 1972.

29. Poulsen K, Vuust J, Lund T: Renin precursor from mouse kidney identified by cell-free translation of messenger RNA. Clin Sci 59:297, 1980.

30. Dykes CW, Bhat K, Taylor JM, et al.: Mouse kidney renin is synthesized in precursor form in the wheat germ cell-free protein synthesis systems. Biomed Res 1:565, 1980.

31. Carlson W, Quay S, Dzau VJ, et al.: Biosynthesis of renin in dog kidney: Evidence for the existence of prorenin, in Sambhi M (editor): Heterogeneity of Renin and Renin-Substrate. New York, Elsevier North-Holland, 1981, p 33.

DISCUSSION

Discussants: Sambhi, Dzau, Haber, Corvol, Eggena, Inagami, Bumpus

Sambhi: Did you mean to say that plasma prorenin is the best candidate for being a precursor zymogen?

Dzau: I think, at this moment, that the plasma prorenin appears to be the best candidate for being a zymogen because we also see an inactive renin in the kidney, and this inactive form in the kidney, for all intents and purposes, looks very much like a precursor. Definitive evidence is clearly lacking, and one has to remember that we are dealing with impure substances and that there are a lot of speculations and extrapolations involved with this kind of analysis.

Sambhi: I am not sure that plasma prorenin qualifies as the best candidate at this time.

Haber: What do you think the relative difference in function is between the very small form of renin that you postulate being secreted after prolonged storage and the somewhat larger form that is secreted immediately? Do they have different kinetic properties? Do you have any evidence to believe that they are different functionally, or is this just an accident of long residence in the cell?

Dzau: My answer would be clearly speculative since we have little data in this area. I think that the active form, 37,000, in the mouse submaxillary gland is the storage form and is released in response to acute stimulus. I don't have any kinetic data comparing the two forms of renin to show this, but I suspect that the 41,000 may be less efficient than the 37,000.

Corvol: If I remember well, in your experiments on biosynthesis of renin in cell culture, you found small molecular weight renins. Did you find such species in human experiments or in submaxillary gland experiments?

Dzau: Not with our antibody but with yours. In fact, using your antibody we not only isolated the 44,000 precursor but also a 25,000 fragment. Using the antibody we raised, we only isolated the 44,000 dalton form.

Eggena: We did a study with human plasma and looked at inactive forms with isoelectric focusing. I just want to show with a few slides that the heterogeneity of the inactive forms is tremendous. You see five forms of inactive renin of plasma in nephrectomized patients which you can activate. When you treat normal plasma with trypsin, you get the same pattern as seen on nephrectomy. So, there isn't a great deal of difference in prorenin or inactive renin from renal and nonrenal sources that is trypsin activatable. It's in numerous forms. You might say that this heterogeneity merely reflects different glycosylation, but I don't think that's true.

Haber: I'd like Dr. Dzau to speculate some more. Dr. Eggena raised a very embarrassing question for a major candidate as a precursor of renin. Once the kidney is removed in man, apparently some humans carry a very high concentration of so-called inactive renin. Where does it come from? What's its function?

Dzau: As I've demonstrated in extrarenal renin biosynthesis experiments, renin is certainly present in the mouse submaxillary gland and in the canine aortic smooth muscle. Also, Dr. Inagami has shown the presence of inactive renin in the brain. So it is possible that we have release of renin from extrarenal sites. I think that would be one possible explanation.

Haber: And yet, as Dr. Eggena suggested, the concentration was very high even in the absence of a kidney. Would you be willing to accept the fact that a large part of the circulating inactive renin is indeed from another source than the kidney?

Dzau: I still think so, yes.

Inagami: You raised the question concerning the disposal of renin. Some time ago, we, Dr. Taugner, and Dr. Corvol saw renin in the proximal tubules of the kidney. Since then Dr. Taugner and we were able to show that labeled renin, administered intravenously, is filtered and then taken up in the proximal tubules. If that is the case, this is a physiological process. We wonder why nature elaborated this low-molecular-weight renin which can pass through the glomeruli and then just goes into the urine. Can you speculate on this? It's sort of puzzling - why does it form in that area and then it's immediately exposed to the danger of being filtered through?

Dzau: Anything I say would be speculative. Many proteins or small polypeptides that are filtered are degraded and the amino acids taken up into an amino acid pool, particularly in the proximal tubule. I presume that's nature's way of conserving its products. I also have an alternate hypothesis: We have recently studied active and inactive renin in the renal interstitium by examining the contents of the renal lymph. We were able to demonstrate high concentrations of inactive and active renin in the renal lymph. So another possible function would be reabsorption by proximal tubule, transport into the renal intertitium for intrarenal actions, i.e., the intrarenal renin angiotensin system.

Bumpus: Along similar lines, why would we need to secrete a prorenin or an inactive renin? What purpose does it have in circulation?

Dzau: First, I would say that it could be an accident of nature, as in the case of proinsulin, that, depending on the maturity of the granules and on the length of the storage of the granules, some of the inactive form may not be totally converted. Secondly, inactive renin may be activated in the periphery for immediate local action. I don't really want to go into any more speculation, except to say that we have some experimental data suggesting that peripheral activation of prorenin is possible. If so, a high concentration of active renin can be produced in a local vascular bed for immediate regulation of local blood flow.

MOLECULAR CLONING OF SUBMAXILLARY RENIN cDNA

P. Corvol, B. Chambraud, S. Foote, J.J. Panthier and F. Rougeon

INTRODUCTION

Renin is synthesized in the juxtaglomerular cell apparatus, but because it represents a very small percentage of the total proteins (1/100,000-1/400,000), separation from contaminating proteases has been very difficult. However, it has been shown that there is a high renin concentration in the submaxillary gland of the mouse and that this enzyme is indistinguishable from the kidney enzyme by immunological and physiochemical criteria [1, 2]. Acellular biosynthesis of renin by Poulsen [3, 4] showed that renin was synthesized as a 50,000-dalton precursor, whereas the enzyme extracted and purified from the gland had a molecular weight of 38,000 [5]. It was therefore the aim of this study to clone submaxillary renin cDNA in order to determine the structure of the renin gene.

As submaxillary renin is under androgenic control, acellular biosynthesis of renin was compared in males and females. A comparison was made between inbred stains known not to contain renin in submaxillary gland but in the kidney only (Balb/c [6]. Taking advantage of the sexual dimorphism and of the selective expression of an RNA encoding renin in the submaxillary gland and in the kidney of different mouse strains, a mouse cDNA encoding submaxillary renin was cloned.

IN VITRO TRANSLATION OF MESSENGER RNA ISOLATED FROM SUBMAXILLARY GLANDS OF MALE AND FEMALE MICE

Total RNA was extracted from seven-week-old mouse submaxillary glands and mouse kidneys. Poly (A)-containing RNA was selected by oligo (dT)-cellulose chromatography and translated in a mRNA-dependent rabbit reticulocyte lysate [7].

Translation products were immunoprecipitated by a renin antibody prepared in the laboratory. The results show that Poly (A)-containing RNAs from male submaxillary gland and from kidney codes for a renin-like material. The submaxillary gland renin and the kidney enzyme appear to be synthesized as a preprorenin of 45,000 daltons, a molecular weight which is slightly lower than that

Table 1. Renin activity and renin synthesis by mRNAs from submaxillary gland and kidney in various mice species

Organ	Sex	Species	Renin	
			Activity (from 6)	Synthesis (45,000 daltons)
submaxillary gland	male	AKR	+	+
submaxillary gland	male	Swiss	+	+
submaxillary gland	male	BALB/c	–	–
submaxillary gland	female	AKR, Swiss, BALB/c	–	–
kidney	Male + female	AKR, Swiss, Balb/c	+	+

reported by Poulsen et al. [3]. This renin precursor was not synthesized in the cell-free system in response to poly (A)-containing RNA prepared from either Balb/c submaxillary gland or female submaxillary gland (Table 1).

CLONING OF A MOUSE SUBMAXILLARY RENIN CDNA FRAGMENT

The strategy used for cloning a mouse submaxillary gland renin cDNA fragment has been described elsewhere [8]. Briefly, the following steps were carried out:

• Partial purification of the mRNA encoding mouse submaxillary gland renin. Total poly (A)-containing RNA was purified from Swiss male submaxillary glands on sucrose gradient. The mRNA encoding for renin (16S) was detected by its ability to translate renin in the rabbit reticulocyte lysate system.

• Molecular cloning of the cDNA of renin submaxillary gland RNA. Partially purified renin on RNA as transcribed into mRNA converted into double-stranded DNA, and the nuclear S 1-resistant cDNA was inserted into the Pst I site of pBR 322 by dC/dG tailing procedure. Recombinant containing renin sequence was selected by differential screening (Table 2). Furthermore, the renin recombinant was identified by hybrid-arrest translation: recombinant containing a 1,200 base pair-insert and poly (A)-containing RNA were hybridized. The hybrids were translated into the rabbit reticulocyte lysate, and *in vitro* translation of the precursor was selectively abolished when total Poly (A)-containing RNA from male submaxillary gland was hybridized with its recombinant DNA.

Table 2. Differential screening and characterization of a renin cDNA clone

---

(1) Hybridization + cDNA complementary to:
 – Swiss male submaxillary gland mRNA: Yes
 – Swiss female submaxillary gland mRNA: No
 – BALB/c male submaxillary gland mRNA: No
(2) Hybridization to mRNA (1,600 nucleotides) from:
 – Swiss male submaxillary gland,
 Kidney of male and female mice.
(3) Hybrid arrest translation.

CHARACTERISTICS OF SUBMAXILLARY GLAND AND KIDNEY RENIN mRNAs

Kidney and submaxillary gland renin mRNAs have the same length, 1,600 nuclotides. They also have sequence homology, according to the stability of the hybrids in solution at 50° C. The level of renin mRNAs is higher in the female kidney than in the male kidney, showing a balance of the renin mRNAs amount between the two main organs of renin biosynthesis, the kidney, and the submaxillary gland.

This study has then been completed by the obtention of the entire renin cDNA clone. Such a clone allowed the determination of the gene structure of renin which has been compared to the primary amino-acid sequence of pure renin from the submaxillary gland [9]. The structure of the prorenin and the prerenin fragments have then been deduced. Comparison of the primary structure of renin to that of other acid proteases (pepsins, prochymosin) showed a high homology.

REFERENCES

1. Michelakis AM, Yoshida H, Menzie J, et al.: A radioimmunoassay for the direct measurement of renin in mice and its application to submaxillary gland and kidney studies. Endocrinology 25:1101-1105, 1974.
2. Malling C, Poulsen K: Direct measurement of high molecular weight forms of renin in plasma. Biochim Biophys Acta 491(2):542-550, 1977.
3. Poulsen K, Vuust J, Lykkegaard S, et al.: Renin is synthesized as a 50,000 dalton single-chain polypeptide in cell-free translation systems. FEBS Lett 98(1):135-138, 1979.
4. Poulsen K, Vuust T, Lund T: Renin precursor from mouse kidney identified by cell-free translation of messenger RNA. Clin Sci 59(4):297-299, 1980.
5. Cohen S, Taylor JM, Murakami K, et al.: Isolation and characterization of renin-like enzymes from mouse submaxillary glands. Biochemistry 11:4286-4293, 1972.
6. Wilson CM, Erdos EG, Wilson JD, et al.: Location on chromosome 1 of Rnr, a gene that regulates renin in the submaxillary gland of the mouse. Proc Natl Acad Sci USA 75(11):5623-5626, 1978.
7. Pelham HR, Jackson RJ: An efficient mRNA-dependent translation system from reticulocyte lysates. Eur J Biochem 67(1):247-256, 1976.

8. Rougeon F, Chambraud B, Foote S, et al.: Molecular cloning of a mouse submaxillary gland renin cDNA fragment. Proc Natl Acad Sci USA 78(10):6367-6371, 1981.
9. Panthier JJ, Foote S, Chambrand B, et al.: (submitted for publication).

DISCUSSION

Discussants: Haber, Corvol, Dzau, Inagami, Tosteson, Sambhi, Genest

Haber: Is it possible to remove the second chain of submaxillary renin by mild reduction and demonstrate whether the remaining fragment is still active as an enzyme?

Corvol: We don't have the answer yet. It's difficult in our experience to separate both fragments, because if you don't alkylate the protein after reduction, you have a reassociation of both chains. I guess it will be difficult to obtain chain A separately and to show that it is active per se.

Inagami: You had the B chain attached at the carboxyl terminal. Are you assuming that this is a continuation of the main chain which is connected by a disulfide bridge?

Corvol: In the mature enzyme, we have not determined the C-terminus of renin. So we are obliged at the present time to speculate which are the C-terminae of A and B chains.

Inagami: So that's why the tail beyond the residue no. 354 is still attached.

Corvol: Yes.

Haber: But is not the DNA sequence continuous?

Corvol: Oh, yes.

Haber: So 353 goes directly to 354 and so forth.

Corvol: Exactly.

Dzau: Have you done hybridization of the DNA from mouse submaxillary gland with human kidney?

Corvol: Yes.

Dzau: Is there much cross homology?

Corvol: There seems to be a very good homology. There is a very good hybridization.

Tosteson: Is the mouse submaxillary gland renin-secreted? Is that known?

Corvol: I don't know.

Haber: Dr. Dzau says it works as an exocrine organ and secretes renin into the salivary duct.

Tosteson: But not into the plasma.

Haber: Dr. Dzau says that only under unusual circumstances when mice are aggressive to one another, as shown by Dr. Paulson, does renin come out into plasma.

Sambhi: When you start with the purified messenger RNA, are there any chances that you may miss a particular kind of messenger because you have excluded it during the process of purification?

Corvol: One has to be very careful because you can degrade a little bit of messenger RNA. I think that everybody agrees that in *in vitro* systems, renin is coded by a single messenger RNA because there is a single renin product with, say, a molecular size between 45 and 50 kilodaltons. I doubt that there are several renin genes with several messenger RNAs coding for several different renins in the submaxillary gland.

Haber: You have indicated that there is rather perfect hybridization between the DNA of the submaxillary renin and the RNA from kidney. Now, we know that the submaxillary renin is not glycosylated and the kidney renin is. That difference may be due to the absence of glycosylating machinery in the submaxillary gland, although it may also be due to the absence or a difference in a few amino acid residues that are necessary as a signal for glycosylation. Did you examine several conditions of hybridization to be sure that the degree of binding was absolutely equivalent between the submaxillary and the kidney RNA?

Corvol: No, we have not done these studies. I think you are certainly right - one should question hybridization techniques because you can also get false positive if you are not very strict in the hybridization conditions. The conditions which were used here were very strict, so we feel comfortable about this hybridization. But let's say a molecular homology sequence of 80% would be sufficient to produce hybridization, and yet you would have a difference in the final product.

Haber: Have you gone back into genomic DNA to see how many games there are?

Corvol: Not yet.

Genest: There is a great deal of homology between tonin, a serine protease from submaxillary gland of rat, and other serine proteases. Now that tonin has been almost completely sequenced and its tertiary structure nearly elucidated with the help of the MRC protein group in Edmonton, it poses the question that in submaxillary glands of mouse, as well as of rats, we have proof that there are two enzymes, one renin and the other tonin, which are excreted in saliva. Both enzymes are present respectively in high amounts. Tonin is about 7% of the total protein content of rat submaxillary gland. We have to ask ourselves, what is the relationship between these two hormones which yield one angiotensin I and the other directly angiotensin II, and what do they do in saliva? They must play a role in digestion. This is a fallout from the work on the renin angiotensin system in hypertension. Tonin has been shown to be excreted in the saliva as well as being secreted in the venous effluent.

PRIMARY STRUCTURE OF MOUSE SUBMAXILLARY GLAND RENIN

TADASHI INAGAMI, KUNIO MISONO, JIN-JYI CHANG AND WILLIAM A. BURKHART

INTRODUCTION

Although the active site of renin shares properties common to acid proteases [1, 2], renin is unique in that it has little, if any, general protease activity and does not function in an acidic pH range. The structural basis for these unique properties is unclear. Extremely limited quantity of renin in the kidney and lengthy purification procedures prevented the determination of its complete structure. Mouse submaxillary gland contains a relatively large amount of a renin, which may be considered a model of renin in other tissues. We have devised a rapid and large-scale purification method for renin from this gland; which made it possible to determine its complete amino acid sequence. The result will be compared with the structure of the acid protease porcine pepsin.

MATERIALS AND METHODS

Renin A [3] was purified from 600 submaxillary glands of adult male mice by ion-exchange chromatography on DEAE-cellulose at a pH of 6.5 and then on CM-cellulose at a pH of 5.38, both eluted with NaCl concentration gradients [4].

CLEAVAGE AND SEPARATION OF PEPTIDE CHAINS

Since active mouse submaxillary gland renin has been found to consist of two polypeptide chains linked by a disulfide bridge [5], lyophilized renin was reduced with 0.1 M dithiothreitol and 6 M guanidine HCl; sulfhydryl groups were carboxymethylated with [14C]iodoacetic acid. Two polypeptide chains were separated by gel filtration on a column of Sephacryl S-200 (2.5 × 100 cm) in 3 M guanidine HCl. The light (L) chain had a molecular weight of 5,500 as determined by SDS gel electrophoresis and by gel filtration on a calibrated Sephadex G-75 column. The heavy (H) chain had a molecular weight of 30,000 as determined by SDS gel electrophoresis and sedimentation equilibrium studies in 6 M guanidine HCl.

The L chain (800 nmol) was fragmented by cyanogen bromide (BrCN) cleavage and digestion with *Staphylococcus aureus* protease V-8. The H chain was fragmented by BrCN cleavage, by the *S. aureus* protease, and by tryptic cleavage after citraconylation.

Peptide fragments of the L chain were separated by gel filtration on a column of Sephadex G-25 superfine (1.8 × 200 cm) in 20 mM HCl. BrCn peptides from the H chain were purified on Sephadex G-50 and then on G-75 in 50% acetic acid. This was followed by ion-exchange chromatography on OAE-Sephadex A-25 in 6 M urea (freshly deionized), 0.05 M ammonium bicarbonate buffer at a pH of 9.3, and with an NaC concentration gradient. Peptides were further purified by high-pressure liquid chromatography on a Syn Chropak RP-P column (Syn-Chrom) in 0.1% trifluoroacetic acid, eluted with a linear concentration gradient of acetonitrile (0 to 70% in 40 min). The tryptic peptides were purified by the same chromatography sequence, maintaining the pH at 9.3 with 50 mM ammonium bicarbonate buffer during gel filtration. The purity of separated peptides were determined by alkaline-urea gel electrophoresis, amino-terminal analysis by the dansyl method and automated Edman degradation.

Peptide amino acid sequences were determined by automated Edman degradation in a Beckman 890B sequencer, using a 0.55 M Quadrol buffer, combined with benzene-ethyl acetate wash. Polybrene (Aldrich), 3 mg, was used to minimize extractive loss of sample peptides. Phenylthiohydantoin amino acids were identified by high-pressure liquid chromatography on a Zorbax CN column (0.46 × 15 cm, Du Pont) by isocratic elution with a mixture of 0.01 M sodium acetate buffer, a pH of 4.2, tetrahydrofuran, acetonitrile, and methanol at a volume ratio of 66:23 × 8:6 × 8:3 × 4. Phenylthiohydantoins of aspartic acid and carboxymethylcysteine were distinguished by chromatography on an Ultrasphere ODS column (0.46 × 25 cm, Altex) using a linear methanol gradient (0 to 40% in 20 min) in 5 mM sodium acretate buffer and a pH of 4.8. Carboxyl-terminal sequence was determined using carboxypeptidase A and B (Worthington).

RESULTS

L-chain

Three overlapping sequences (Fig. 1) obtained by automated Edman degradations of the intact L-chain, the BrCN peptide LCB-2, and the *S. aureus* protease peptide LSP-2 gave a complete amino acid sequence of the L-chain as shown in Figure 2. Its carboxyl-terminal residues were confirmed as Ala-Arg by sequential degradation by carboxypeptidase B followed by carboxpeptidase A. Aligned with the carboxy-terminal sequence of porcine pepsin [6], 22 residues, out of a total of 48, were identical. Identical residues are indicated by underlines. The single 1/2 Cys residue was also homologous. Thus, the L-chain sequence is shown in Figure 2 using residue numbers of corresponding amino acids in the carboxyl-terminal sequence of porcine pepsin [6].

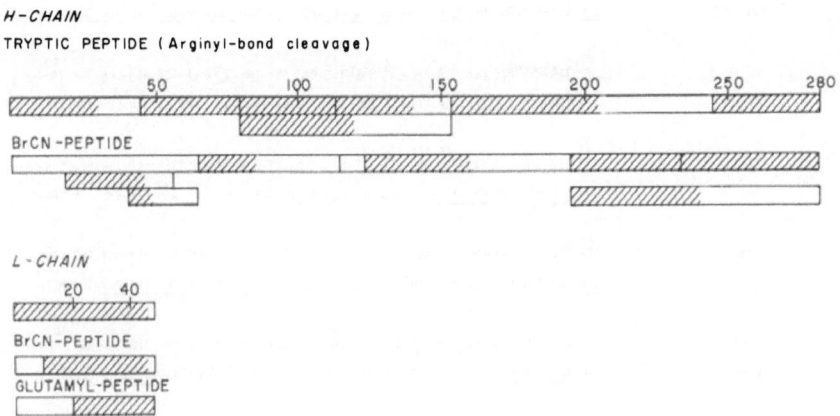

Figure 1. Overlaps of peptides obtained by BrCN and tryptic digestion of citraconylated H-chain. Shadowed areas indicate regions whose amino acid sequences have been determined. Complete overlaps of all peptides provide continuous amino acid sequence.

H-chain

As shown in Figure 1, overlapping amino acid sequences covering the entire length of the H-chain were obtained by Edman degradations of six tryptic peptides obtained from citraconylated H-chain, six BrCn peptides, and two subfragments of the amino-terminal BrCN peptide produced by cleavage with *L. enzymogenes* endoproteinase Lys-C and with *S. aureus* protease.

The renin structure was found to contain two sequences Val-Ile-Phe-Asp-Thr-Gly (residues No. 29 through 35 in Fig. 2) and Val-Asp-Thr-Gly (residues No. 214-217), which are homologous to the sequences containing the catalytically essential aspartyl residues in pepsin, Asp_{32}, which had been shown to be reactive by 1,2 epoxy-3-(p-nitrophenoxyl) propane [7], and Asp_{215}, which had been esterified with diazoacetyl-norleucine methyl ester [8] with a concomitant loss of peptic activity. Furthermore, Ser_{35}, which has been shown hydrogen-bonded to Asp_{32} [9] in penicillopepsin, and Tyr_{75}, which has been implicated in the catalytic mechanism of pepsin [9], were conserved in renin. The amino acid sequence shown in Figure 2 is aligned to obtain maximal homologous sequences, including the active site regions, and residues are numbered by the pepsin system(s). Of the 284 amino acid residues in the H-chain, 117 residues are homologous to those of porcine pepsin [6]. This represents a 41% homology. Residues 50, 206, 210, 250, and 284 of 1/2 Cys are also conserved in comparison with pepsin, in which residues 206 and 210, and 250 and 284 form disulfide bridges. It is likely that the intrachain disulfide bridge linking the L- and H-chains is the one between residues 250 and 284. On the other hand, two additional residues are inserted between cysteinyl residues 45B and 50 compared with the corresponding sequence of pepsin. The

384

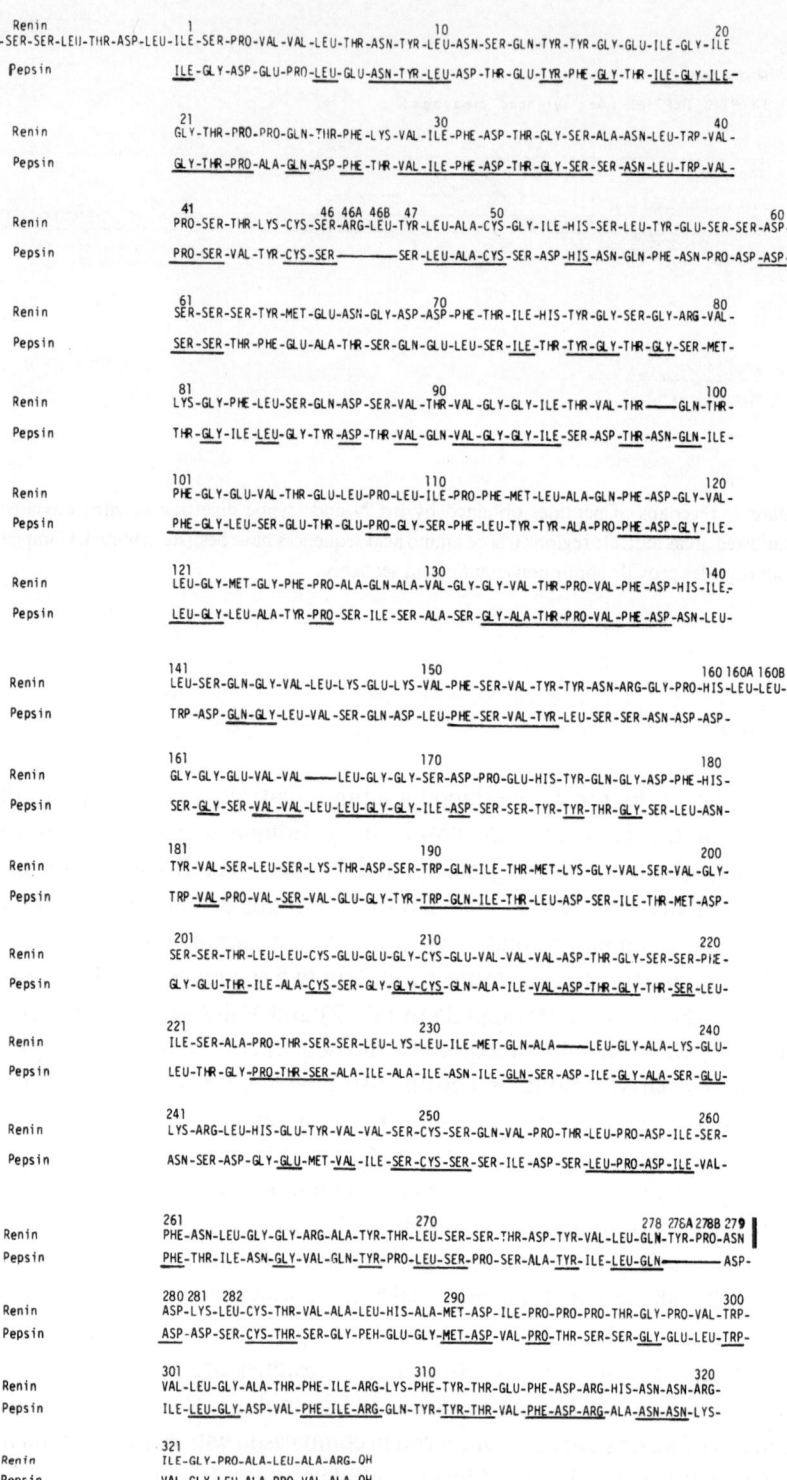

Figure 2. Amino acid sequence of mouse submaxillary gland renin, and comparison with the amino acid sequence of porcine pepsin. Residues are numbered to obtain maximum homology between renin and pepsin. Amino acid residues identical between pepsin and renin sequences are underlined.

presence of free sulfhydryl groups has been reported as a unique structural feature of renin [2]. Cys_{45B} and Cys_{50} may represent these free sulfhydryl groups [2]. In contrast to renal renin, the mouse submaxillary gland renin is not a glycoprotein [4]. The fact that the renin structure does not contain a typical glycoprotein site Asn-X-Thr or Asn-X-Ser is compatible with the absence of carbohydrate. Heterogeneity was observed in the sequence involving the first two to five amino-terminal residues. This was due to minor components whose amino terminal sequences were truncated by one, three or four amino acid residues.

The two-chain structure may arise from a precursor consisting of a single polypeptide by a proteolytic cleavage. It is quite possible that a few intervening amino acid residues have been lost during the proteolytic processing of the parent molecule. The proteolytic cleavage to form the two-chain structure may not be essential for the activation of prorenin.

SUMMARY

To determine the structural basis for the highly specific action of renin, the amino acid sequence of mouse submaxillary gland renin was determined. The active renin was found to consist of one heavy chain ($M_r = 30,000$) and one light chain ($M_r = 5,500$). Amino acid sequences of these chains were determined using overlapping peptides generated by cleavage with cyanogen bromide, trypsin, *Staphylococcus aureus* protease, and *Lysobacter enzymogenes* endoproteinase Lys-C. Sequences involving two catalytically essential aspartyl residues 32 and 215, characteristic to acid proteases, were found identical with pepsin, penicillopepsin, and chymosin. The sequence of L-chain was homologous with the carboxyl terminal region of porcine pepsin in 46% of amino acid residues. The H-chain showed 41% homology with 284 residues on the amino-terminal side of the porcine pepsin molecule.

ACKNOWLEDGMENT

This work was supported by research grants from the National Heart, Lung and Blood Institute HL-22288 and HL-14192, a Grant-in-Aid and an Investigatorship (K.S.M.) from the Tennessee Chapter of The American Heart Association, and a postdoctoral research fellowship (J.-J.C.) from the Middle Tennessee Affiliate of The American Heart Association.

REFERENCES

1. Inagami T, Misono K, Michelakis AM: Definitive evidence for similarity in the active site of renin

and acid protease. Biochem Biophys Res Commun 56:503-509, 1974.

2. Misono K, Inagami T: Characterization of the active site of mouse submaxillary gland renin. Biochemistry 19:2616-2622, 1980.

3. Cohen S, Taylor J, Murakami K, et al.: Isolation and characterization of a renin-like enzyme from mouse submaxillary glands, 1972.

4. Misono K, Holladay LA, Cohen S, et al.: Large scale purification and physicochemical characterization of mouse submaxillary renin, abstracted. Fed Proc 37:1436, 1978.

5. Misono K, Inagami T: Unpublished observations.

6. Sepulveda P, Marciniszyn J Jr, Liu D, et al.: Primary structure of porcine pepsin III. Amino acid sequence of a cyanogen bromide fragment, CB2A, and the complete structure of porcine pepsin. J Biol Chem 250:5082-5088, 1975.

7. Cheng KCS, Tang J: Amino acid sequence around the epoxide-reactive residues in pepsin. J Biol Chem 247:2566-2574, 1972.

8. Bayliss RS, Knowles JR, Wybrandt GB: An aspartic acid residue at the active site of pepsin. Biochem J 113:377-386, 1969.

9. James MNG, Hsu IN, Delbaere TJ: Mechanism of acid protease catalysis based on the crystal structure of penicillopepsin. Nature 267:808-813, 1977.

DISCUSSION

Discussants: Haber, Inagami, Corvol, Eggena, MacGregor, Dzau, Bumpus

Haber: I'd like to initiate the questions by asking you about the difference in the isoelectric point of the several species that occur on enzymatic activation of the inactive form of renin. Now, to my way of thinking, the only way that one can change an isolectric point by enzymatic treatment is to cleave a peptide bond and to expose new amino or carboxy terminae. Doesn't that pretty well prove that you are nicking the enzyme and thereby activating it, even though a polypeptide chain may still be held there either by covalent forces, such as disulfides, or by noncovalent forces?

Inagami: Yes. I think that's the most likely explanation available at this point. For example, the mouse submaxillary gland renin we have sequenced was one of the five isoenzymes and, as you have seen in the carboxyl terminal region of the light chain, there are several arginine residues which were good candidates for cleavage by the abundant arginine-specific esterases in the tissue. Thus, it is likely that partial nicking or partial cleavage may have taken place, and it may account for the multiplicity.

Haber: Dr. Corvol, looking at the length of the proenzymes - say, looking all the way down towards the stop codon in your DNA sequence - what would you predict the molecular weight to be of the mouse submaxillary proenzyme?

Corvol: It was over 44,000, which fits very well with the 45 kilodaltons of the preproenzyme that we identified in cell-free systems. We found very good hybridization between the submaxillary C-DNA renin and the human renin in RNA with the same nucleotide length, which is 1600 nucleotide sequence, corresponding to a 45,000 molecular weight human renin in the kidney. So, I wonder if glycosylation in the case of human renin would explain the slight discrepancy between this 45 and the 51 kilodaltons that you are speculating for the prorenin?

Inagami: That is much too large a difference to be accounted for by glycosylation if the carbohydrate accounts for the very small portion of the molecular weight. Of course, this is speculative. Our knowledge is limited to the carbohydrate content in the active enzyme, while we are talking about inactive protein. In the active enzyme, carbohydrate is but just a few percent of the total molecular weight, and I don't think it would affect the molecular weight readings either by Sephadex gel filtration or SDS electrophoresis. But I wonder if there is any possibility that more carbohydrates are attached during precursor processing.

Eggena: I have a comment regarding the shift in isoelectric points. We find, like you did, that when you treat with trypsin you get a downward shift in pH. This shift is into a pH range where you normally don't see active renin in normal plasma. When we activate by cold storage, there doesn't appear to be a shift in the isoelectric points. I don't want to say that cold storage is more physiologic than trypsin but, at least as far as isolectric points are concerned, they remain in the normal range. I was wondering if you have any indication at all or would like to speculate on what may activate renin *in vivo*.

Inagami: Are you asking about the plasma prorenin?

Eggena: In plasma system, yes.

Inagami: I just can't speculate.

MacGregor: Is there any evidence that prorenin in the plasma is converted to active renin? The reason I ask is that we've recently developed a highly sensitive cytochemical bioassay for angiotensin II. In anephric subjects there are around 200 fmoles/liter of angiotension II, which compares in normal subjects to a range of 10 to 20 pmoles/liter, i.e., there are two orders of magnitude less in anephric subjects. Yet according to results presented today, anephric subjects have the same amount of prorenin in the plasma as normal subjects.

Inagami: Are you asking about the source of the prorenin?

MacGregor: No, I'm asking in an inverted way, whether you think prorenin in the plasma plays any physiological role whatsoever.

Inagami: A very wild speculation is that the prorenin may find its way to the vascular bed and may be bound. As Dr. Hsueh said, it is a peculiarity of prorenin that it can be activated by a conformational change. This is one wild speculation which we are very anxious to examine, but that's one of the reasons for preparing protenin.

Corvol: I cannot accept that all the work we have done has nothing to do with blood pressure. It will be possible to crystallize renin within a few years, and then we'll get some ideas about the active site of renin compared to other proteases. And hopefully when you get a high blood pressure, you might very well receive a renin inhibitor, rather than captopril or anything like that.

Dzau: I'd like to emphasize that one has to be very cautions about interpreting molecular size, especially when using different techniques, and in using plasma. Steve Atlas has shown clearly that if you subject plasma to gel filtration chromatography, you will elute a peak of angiotensinogen followed by a peak of trypsin inhibitor. However, both these peaks overlap with the inactive and active renin peaks. So, if you try to determine the size of inactive renin, you have to add different quantities of trypsin to overcome variable trypsin inhibitor concentrations in different fractions to get an accurate size. This, of course, can easily result in experimental artifacts. We also know that acidification can create inaccuracies in that the process is readily reversible and that it can also lead to a spurious change in size if you don't pursue the conditions correctly. Therefore, I just wanted to make this specific point and suggest that people not spend too much time arguing on molecular weights.

Inagami: I appreciate your mentioning this point. It is one of the reasons why we wanted to purify it, though not completely, but free from the plasma components which Dr. Atlas has shown inhibit or shift the molecular weight estimation.

Bumpus: I'm surprised Dr. Sambhi didn't make this comment. We often ignore the possibility that the kidney may secrete something other than renin. As Dr. Sambhi has suggested, there may be a renin activator, another enzyme that could convert prorenin to renin. So, I don't think that this work is all in vain.

PURIFICATION OF PRORENIN

Tadashi Inagami, Yukio Takii, Ji-Jiy Chang and Masatsugu Kisaragi

INTRODUCTION

In the first report of activatable renin in 1971, Lumbers raised a question concerning the nature of the substance in human amniotic fluid, which showed marked increase in renin-like activity upon prolonged dialysis at pH 3.3 [1]. Since untreated amniotic fluid already showed a finite level of renin-like activity, at least three possible mechanisms were advanced to explain the activation: [1] further activation of already active renin by a conformational change, [2] dissociation of an enzyme-inhibitor complex, or [3] activation of a zymogen.

Activation of activatable renin in human amniotic fluid [2] and human plasma [3] by proteases suggested the possibility of a zymogen-type precursor. The discovery of 'big renin (molecular weight = 63,000)' as the activatable form in human plasma [4] also seemed to support the zymogen-type precursor. Puzzling was the fact, however, that proteolytic activation did not change the molecular weight of big renin as determined by gel filtration [3]. Furthermore, big renin with clearly demonstrable renin activity was not compatible with the definition of zymogen, which should be totally inactive. The property of big renin was compatible with a partially active renin with a potential for further activation by conformational change.

Activatable renins were also found in the kidney. Renin activity in crude extracts of rabbit [5] and hog [6] kidneys was found to undergo varying degrees of activation by nonproteolytic agents such as urea, high concentration of salt, detergent, ion-exchange chromatography, etc. [6, 7], suggesting the possibility of a renin-inhibitor complex. Reversible dissociation and reassociation of an inhibitor peptide have been reported [7]. On the other hand, completely inactive 'big renin' with a molecular weight of 63,000 was found in some but not all of Wilms' tumors in human kidney [8]. No single model seemed to explain all of these observed properties associated with various forms of activatable renin in various tissues.

Thus, studies on activatable renin was mired by unclear views on its molecular nature and activation mechanisms. This was because the studies were performed with crude preparations, which were mixtures of at least two forms of renin, none of which had been purified or characterized individually for studies on their molecular peoperties. The term 'prorenin' was coined without knowledge of the molecular properties of the activatable renin. 'Inactive renin' was also used while it was not known whether it was inactive or partially active. Obviously, clarification of these multifold problems had to be sought in studies based on purified or partially purified material. Reviews on the early stage of studies on activatable renin were published [9-11].

METHODOLOGICAL DEVELOPMENT

The development of prorenin studies and clarification of the problems heavily depended on development of new methods in three key areas: [1] isolation and purification, [2] stabilization, and [3] detection and assay of inactive renin.

Isolation methods

Although the method of isolation of inactive renin turned out to play a decisive role in clarifying the nature of prorenin and its relationship with active renin, the early approach was merely to fractionate human plasma by gel filtration according to molecular size of activatable renin. This method failed to separate active renin from inactive renin. Ion-exchange chromatography on DEAE-cellulose was also applied [12, 13]. However, complete separate active renin of inactive from active renin was not obtained. Much of the development had to await introduction of affinity chromatographic methods to deal wenin, which were present in tissues or plasma in very limited quantities.

Affi-Gel Blue

Cibacron Blue F3GA-agarose (Bio-Rad) was found to bind inactive renin in preference to active renin at a neutral pH and to release it in 0.5-1.4 M NaCl or by NaCl concentration gradient. This discovery was made by Norio Takahashi in our laboratory in 1977, and its application for the purification of human plasma prorenin was presented in 1978 in the International Kinin Symposium in Tokyo [14]. Independently, Carlson et al. found the utility of Affi-Gel Blue in their studies on prorenin [15]. It was used for partial purification of prorenin in human plasma [16-18], amniotic fluid [19], human kidney [18], and hog kidney [20].

Octyl-Sepharose

Octyl-Sepharose was also found to bind prorenin in 1M ammonium sulfate or NaCl solution, while active renin was more loosely bound or not bound at all [21]. Prorenin was released from the column by decreasing salt concentration or by 50% ethylene glycol [20, 22] as shown in Figure 1.

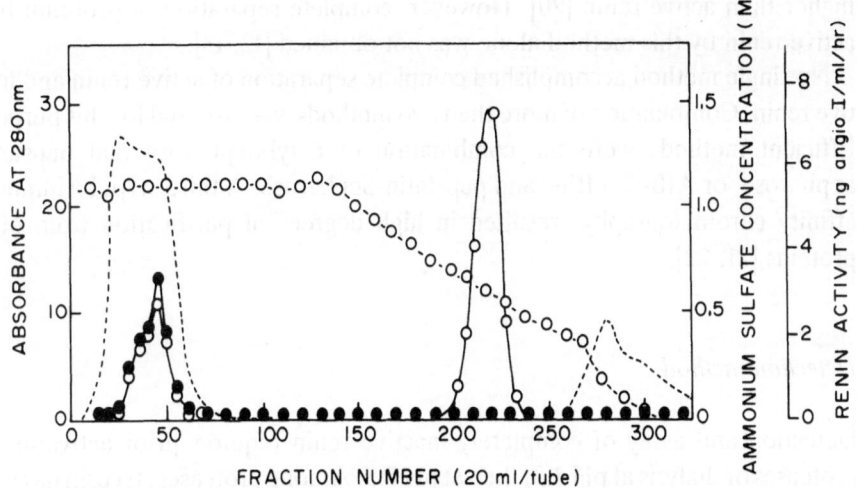

Figure 1. Separation of active renin and prorenin by an octyl-Sepharose column. Samples were applied in
1 M ammonium sulfate, washed thoroughly with the same solution, then eluted with a decreasing
concentration gradient (-- O--). (---) absorbance at 280 nm, (●) renin activity before trypsin activation.
(O) renin activity after trypsin activation. (From ref. [22] with permission of *J Clin Endocrinol Metab*)

Pepstatin Sepharose

Pepstatin Sepharose binds active renin but not inactive renin (prorenin). Thus, it
was very useful to eliminate active renin from an inactive renin preparation [15].

Concanavalin A-Sepharose

Concanavalin A-Sepharose is useful in isolating renin and prorenin, since both of
them have affinity to the gel and are eluted with 0-methyl-glucose or mannose in
1M NaCl.

Immuno-affinity chromatography

Immuno-affinity chromatography with antirenin IgG-Sepharose is useful for
highly specific isolation of renin and prorenin. Elution of renin and prorenin is
obtained by glycine buffer below pH 3.0 or by 4M $MgCl_2$. Neither of these
methods distinguish prorenin from renin.

DEAE-cellulose and DEAE-Sephacel

DEAE-cellulose and DEAE-Sephacel particularly the latter, are useful in separating active renin and inactive renin, since the isoelectric point of prorenin is

higher than active renin [20]. However, complete separation of prorenin from active renin by this method alone was not obtained [12, 13].

No single method accomplished complete separation of active renin and inactive renin. Combination of more than two methods was essential for this purpose. Efficient methods were the combination of octyl-Sepharose and pepstatin-Sepharose, or Affi-Gel Blue and pepstatin-Sepharose. A third step, by immuno-affinity chromatography, resulted in high degrees of purification from other proteins [21, 22].

Detection method

Detection and assay of completely inactive renin requires prior activation by proteases or dialysis at pH 3.3, then at pH 7.5. Among proteases, trypsin has been used most frequently. Its concentration and duration of reaction require optimization, since excessive trypsin treatment destroys both renin and prorenin, while the danger of less than maximal activation exists due to trypsin inhibitors in tissues and plasma. This problem was studied by Sealey and Atlas et al [10, 18]. One of the objectives of the purification of prorenin is to eliminate such a problem. Activation of highly purified prorenin by trypsin requires protection by serum albumin. Thus, for raw plasma, 1 mg/ml of trypsin is usually optimal at 25° C for a reaction of 5-10 minutes, whereas extensively purified prorenin needed protection by added serum albumin (0.5 to 1%), and 50 μg of trypsin per ml of solution was sufficient for the activation [16, 17, 21, 22]. Pepsin used on a relatively crude prorenin preparation does not destroy renin [23, 24]. However, pure renin is not stable at acidic pH required by pepsin action. Pure plasmin seems to be a safer activator [21, 25, 26].

Electrophoresis of prorenin on polyacrylamide gel with the detergent sodium dodecyl sulfate (SDS) and subsequent detection of migration distance by immuno-staining or direct radioimmunoassay of prorenin containing slices cut out of the gel also provide another dimension for the determination of the molecular weight of renin and/or prorenin.

Protection of prorenin from proteases

Numerous studies reported in recent years indicate that prorenin is activated by many proteases [9-11]. The kidney is known to be particularly rich in proteases of all types. Blood plasma also contains zymogens of various proteases in large quantities. Lysosomal and other proteases are present in practically all types of tissues. To prevent activation of prorenin during homogenization and purification, EDTA (10 mM), diisopropylfluorophosphate (2-5 mM), or phenylmethanesulfonylfluoride (1 mM), N-ethylmaleimide (5 mm), and soybean trypsin inhibitor, or aprotinin, were added in our laboratory. Dimercaprol and 8-hydroxy quinoine were also used [27]. Without these inhibitors, the yield of prorenin was considerably lower, as it was readily converted to active renin.

RECOGNITION OF ACTIVATABLE RENIN AS COMPLETELY INACTIVE ZYMOGEN

Isolation of human plasma inactive renin

We have focused our studies to find out if the activatable renin was a partially active enzyme or completely inactive one. If it is completely inactive, then we wanted to find out if it is an enzyme-inhibitor complex or a zymogen.

We were able to isolate inactive renin from human plasma by two steps of affinity chromatography using Affi-Gel Blue followed by pepstatin-Sepharose [14]. Inactive renin, bound to Affi-Gel Blue, was eluted with 1.4 M NaCl and was freed from small amounts of active renin by passing through a pepstatin-Sepharose column. This method separated inactive renin from active renin completely. Inactive renin was found to be totally devoid of renin activity but expressed the activity by acid dialysis or limited proteolysis by trypsin, pepsin, or kallikrein.

Active renin, which passed through Affi-Gel Blue, was found to have no potential for activation. Thus, this was the first demonstration that activatable renin was a totally inactive form of renin, which, as will be shown later, was not activated by dissociative processes such as urea, high salt concentration, or detergent. Since the total lack of enzyme activity and activation by proteases were the properties characteristic to and criteria for the zymogen of a protease, these results indicated that the inactive renin is a renin zymogen or prorenin. No findings contradicted this postulate.

Octyl-Sepharose was equally useful for separating active renin and inactive renin (Fig. 1). Totally inactive prorenin and fully activated renin were separated from human plasma [21, 22], and results obtained above were confirmed. This method depends on the hydrophobic interaction of proteins to the octyl group. The fact that the prorenin is preferentially bound to octyl-Sepharose, whereas active renin is not bound or bound only very weakly, indicates that prorenin has a hydrophobic space accessible to the octyl group.

Prorenin in human kidney

The octyl-Sepharose was found particularly useful in isolating inactive renin from the kidney where quick work-up was required, since prorenin in the crude renal extract tended to be activated by endogenous proteases. Human kidney extract in a mixture of protease inhibitors was fractionated by ammonium sulfate, dissolved

394

in a small amount of water, then applied to octyl-Sepharose without time-consuming dialysis, desalting or concentration steps. Active and inactive renin were separated by elution with negative salt gradient [21] (Fig. 1). The immunoaffinity column using Sepharose coupled with antibody to renin [22, 28] greatly increased the extent of purification. The antibodies to active renal renin had been shown to cross-react with inactive plasma prorenin [24]. Thus, this column does not discriminate between prorenin and renin. However, subsequent passage of the sample through a pepstatin-Sepharose produced a prorenin sample without active renin (Fig. 2). Both renal and plasma prorenin were activated by various proteases such as trypsin, pepsin [16, 17], plasmin, plasma kallikrein, catheps in B_1, etc. [22]. Again, dissociative reagents were not effective in inducing the activation except for the acid treatment. Thus, the zymogen nature of human renal inactive renin was demonstrated.

Complete purification of prorenin from hog kidney

Isolation of completely pure prorenin will clarify many problems related to

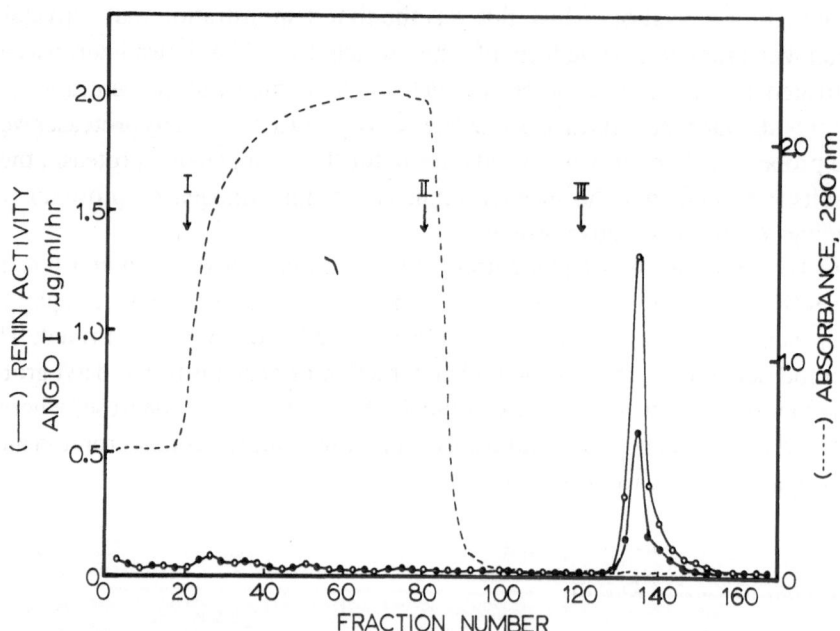

Figure 2. Separation of prorenin from active renin by pepstatin-aminohyxyl-Sepharose. The first peak contains inactive renin but no active renin. The second peak, eluted with 0.1 M acetic acid or 0.5 M Tris buffer, pH 7.5, contains active renin. (●) renin activity before trypsin activation, (○) renin activity after trypsin activation. (From ref. [21] with permission of *Hypertension*)

molecular characteristics of prorenin and its activation mechanism. Since prorenin concentration in human plasma is extremely limited and supply of human kidney is not sufficient for this purpose, a large quantity of hog kidney was used as the source for the purification of inactive prorenin.

A method consisting of a combination of various affinity chromatographic steps was developed, using pepstatin-Sepharose, ocytl-Sepharose, Affi-Gel Blue, and concanavalin A-Sepharose. With additional steps of gel filtration and ion-exchange chromatography on DEAE Sephacel, it became possible for us to obtain an electrophoretically homogeneous prorenin [29]. As shown in Table 1, approximately 3-million-fold purification was necessary to produce the pure hog renin zymogen (prorenin). Partially purified prorenin had been isolated prior to the complete purification [20, 30]. Hog renal prorenin is activated by various proteases but not by dissociative processes, as discussed later.

The partially or completely purified prorenin preparations were shown to be free from protease inhibitors. The removal of the protease inhibitors was one of the major objectives of purification required for evaluating various proteases for their ability to activate prorenin without acidifying the prorenin preparation, a procedure necessitated for the removal of plasma protease inhibitors. The absence of the inhibitors also removes the complication in molecular weight determination, as discussed by Sealey and Atlas et al. [10, 18].

Table 1. Purification of inactive renin from hog kidney

Step	Total protein (mg)	Specific[b] activity	purification	Yield (%)
Crude extract[a]	1,600,000	0.0015[c]	1	100
DEAE batch	125,000	0.016[c]	10	82
Pepstatin-Sepharose	60,000	0.03	20	75
DEAE-Sephacel	18,000	0.08	53	63
Octyl-Sepharose	1,000	1.43	950	59
Sephadex G-100	208	5.29	3,530	46
Affi-Gel Blue	16.0	62,9	41,900	42
Con A-Sepharose	0.750	1,000	666,700	31
Sephadex G-100	0.170	2,400	1,600,000	17
DEAE-Sephacel	0.030	5,000	3,333,000	6.3

[a] Prepared from 20 kg of fresh hog kidney.

[b] Activity of inactive renin as defined by, inactive renin = total renin activity after activation − renin activity before activation; expressed as μg angiotensin I/mg of protein/hr.

[c] Determined after removal of contaminating renin by using affinity chromatography; see details in 'MATERIAL AND METHODS.'

This table was taken from ref. [28] by permission of *Biochem Biophys Res Commun.*

Molecular weight of prorenin

Lack of pure prorenin severely limited methods available for molecular weight determination. Until very recently, gel filtration and identifying prorenin-containing fractions by potential activity after activation with proteases, such as trypsin or acid treatment, was the only method available to this study. Pure preparation can be studied by electrophoretic methods. Antibodies permitting detection of renin even in an impure preparation were developed by this method. Accuracy of molecular weight determination was greatly improved by inclusion of radiolabeled internal molecular weight standards [14, 16, 18, 21, 22] and consideration of uneven localization of protease inhibitors in fractionated plasma [10, 18]. These problems were resolved when pure prorenin was used. Until these problems were resolved, there had been quite a variation in apparent molecular weights of human plasma prorenin determined by gel filtration under a variety of conditions in different laboratories, as summarized in Table 2.

As extensively purified materials were introduced, the value obtained by Yokosawa et al. [16], Takii et al. [17], Atlas et al. [18], Hsueh et al. [31], and Chang et al. [21] began to converge to 55,000 to 56,000. This preparation seems to be a complex of 50,000-dalton inactive renin and a small protein. Activation by various means caused only very limited or no change in molecular weight [16-18, 21, 31].

The reason for the discrepancy between the higher molecular weight (56,000) of activated prorenin compared with the lower value (50,000 to 45,000) of active plasma renin is not immediately clear. However, the molecular weights of activation products obtained by a variety of plasma or other proteases were all in the range of 54,000 to 56,000. These proteases include plasmin, trypsin, plasma kallikrein, cathepsin B_1, arginine-specific esteropeptidases from mouse submaxillary gland, and urinary kallikrein. These findings indicate that activation by plasma proteases of plasma prorenin in blood does not produce the active renin found in blood. This result can be interpreted to indicate that activation of prorenin does not take place in the plasma.

The fact that *in vitro* activation of plasma prorenin with an apparent molecular weight of 56,000 does not result in reduction of its molecular weight may offer an explanation for an earlier report by Day and Luetscher [3] that activation of 'big renin' does not result in drastic reduction of molecular weight to 40,000.

Plasma of nonhuman mammals also seems to contain activatable renin as summarized in Table 2. Barrett et al. [38] have reported two types of trypsin-activatable renins in rat plasma with molecular weights of 58,000 and 44,000 as determined by gel-filtration on ACA44 gel. Potter et al. report their observation of activatable renin with molecular weights of 43,000 [39] and 65,000 [40] in dog plasma. We have separated 50,000-dalton prorenin from hog plasma. Gallagher et al., however, report that the trypsin activation of renin activity in dog plasma is due to an artifact of modification of angiotensinogen [41].

Table 2. Molecular weight of inactive activatable and active renin in plasma

Source and conditions	Inactive or activatable	Activated	Active renin	References
Human plasma				
Wilms' tumor and diabetic				
nephropathy	63000 partially active	63000	43000	[3]
Pregnancy	55000 partially active	38000	43000	[32]
Normal	43000 partially active	46000	41000	[12]
Normal	46000 partially active		46000	[13]
Diabetic nephropathy	60000 & partially active		60000 &	[33]
or pregnancy	40000		40000	
Normal	60000 partially active		60000	[34]
	40000 partially active		40000	
Normal	56000 completely inactive			[16]
Normal	50000 partially inactive			[35]
Normal	62000 partially inactive	59000	43000	[36]
	46000 partially inactive			
Normal	58000 partially inactive	58000	41000	[37]
Diabetic nephropathy	58000 partially inactive	58000	40000	[23]
Normal	56000 completely inactive	56000	54000	[17]
Normal	56000 completely inactive	53000[a]	48000	[18]
		49500[b]		
Normal	55000 completely inactive		48000	[31]
Normal	56000 completely inactive	56000[a]	51000	[21]
		56000[b]		
Rat normal	43000 & 65000		43000	[38]
Dog normal	43000 & 65000			[39, 40]
Pig normal	50000	39000	38000	This study

[a] Trypsin activation

[b] Acid activation

As shown in Table 3, the molecular weight of inactive renin isolated from human kidney was found to be approximately 51,000, significantly smaller than that of plasma prorenin [21]. Atlas et al. also obtained a similar value of 49,500 to 50,000 [18]. Activation of renal inactive prorenin by plasmin produced active renin with little change in molecular weight (51,000), whereas trypsin produced a smaller active enzyme 47,000 [21]. However, when the kidney extract is processed very rapidly, we found that the majority is in the 56,000-dalton form (Table 4), suggesting that 56,000-dalton prorenin may be an ultimate form of prorenin.

Active human renal renin purified from normal kidney in the past were reported to have several different forms. Multiple molecular weights of 50,000, 40,000, and 20,000 were reported by Slater et al. [51]. Thoroughly acid-treated kidney extract produced a renin of molecular weight 40,000 [52]. However, it is the natural form of active renin in human kidney that seems to be of higher

Table 3. Molecular weight of inactive, activatable, and active renin in the kidney

Species	Inactive or activatable	After activation	Active renin	References
Human kidney				
	150000 active			[42]
	63000 inactive	63000		[8]
	58000 partially active	40000		[43]
	49500 inactive	46500ª	39500	[18]
	50000 inactive, prefusate		41000	[18]
	51000 inactive	47000ª 51000ᵇ	45000	[21]
Hog kidney				
	60000 partially active 58000-	400 0		[6]
	60000 active 140000 partially	40000		[44, 45]
	& 60000 active	37000		[46]
	62000 partially active			[47]
	53000 inactive	41000		[29]
	50000 inactive	40000		[20]
	50000 inactive	40000		[29]
Hog brain				
	49000 inactive	40000	40000	[48]
Rabbit kidney				
	57000 inhibitor complex	37000	37000	[7]
Dog				
	60000 binding protein complex			[49]
	60000 active	40000		[50]

ª Trypsin Activation.
ᵇ Acid Activation.

molecular weight. The extract of human kidney subjected to octyl-Sepharose and immunoaffinity chromatography produced an active enzyme with a molecular weight of 45,000 to 50,000 (depending on the method of determination). A similar but somewhat smaller value was obtained by Atlas et al. [18]. The smaller sizes of renal prorenin, as compared with the plasma counterpart, is also puzzling. However, our recent studies of prorenins by SDS-gel electrophoresis followed by immunostaining indicates 56,000-dalton plasma prorenin contains 50,000-dalton prorenin, whereas rapid treatment of human kidney produces a 54,000-dalton substance that strongly reacts with antirenin antibodies. These results suggest that a 54,000 to 56,000-dalton molecule may be the ultimate form of prorenin attainable by state of the art technique. It is likely that 51,000-dalton prorenin in renal cortical extract, as shown in Table 4, may be a breakdown product or

Table 4. Molecular weights of human renin

Renin	Kidney	Plasma
Inactive	51,000 and 54,000**	50,000** and 56,000
Acid-treated*	51,000	56,000
Activated		
Trypsin-treated	47,000	56,000
Plasmin-treated	51,000	56,000
Active	50,000 and 45,000	51,000

* Acid-treated first by dialyzing against pH 3.2 buffer overnight and then against pH 7.5 buffer overnight. Values are mean ± standard deviation (SD).
** Determined by SDS-gel electrophoresis of crude extract followed by immunostaining. Other values were determined by gel filtration and determination of renin activity after trypsin activation.

intermediate of transition from 54,000-dalton prorenin to 50,000-dalton active renin or even to smaller molecules.

The molecular weight relationship between plasma prorenin and renal pro-renin, and between plasma active renin and renal active renin, deserves further attention. This problem is summarized in Table 4. The molecular weight of purified hog renal prorenin was determined both by gel filtration and SDS-gel electrophoresis as 50,000, which is very close to that of the intermediate form of human renal prorenin. The SDS-electrophoresis indicates that the prorenin molecule consists of a single continuous polypeptide chain of molecular weight 50,000. Activation takes place only by proteases [20, 30] (Table 5). Also, the 54,000-dalton prorenin exists in hog kidney.

No activation was observed by dissociative procedures such as treatment with 3 M urea, 3 M guanidine, 0.05% Triton X-100, or 4 M NaCl or thiocyanate, which had been shown to dissociate renin-inhibitor complex [7]. The fact that 'inactive renin' or 'prorenin' is a completely inactive form of renin consisting of a single polypeptide chain, which is activated by proteolysis with a concomitant reduction

Table 5. Molecular weights of hog renin

	Kidney	Plasma
Inactive	50,000	50,000
Activated	38,000	39,000
Active (native)	38,000	38,000

in molecular weight, is consistent with the definition of zymogen quite analogous to pepsinogen. Although the activation peptide(s) is yet to be isolated, it is likely that it may be fragmented to more than one piece due to nonspecific catalysis by trypsin, a situation analogous to those encountered in the activation of some other protease zymogens. Thus, these studies favor the zymogen nature of prorenin rather than an enzyme inhibitor complex.

The relationship of the completely inactive renin zymogen (prorenin) and high-molecular-weight renin isolated from kidneys may deserve a comment. The reversibly activatable complexes with molecular weight approximately 60,000 may have been either a complex of active renin and high-molecular-weight renin inhibitor [6, 7] or a complex with renin-binding protein [49]. It is also possible that the activation peptide was loosely bound to renin. Since rapid activation of prorenin takes place in a crude extract of kidney due to abundance of protease, it is likely that most of big renin in crude renal extracts in earlier studies may represent intermediates of degradation or activation of prorenin. However, it is noteworthy that in some but not all of Wilms' tumors, a completely inactive renin with a high molecular weight was observed by Day et al. [8].

Isoelectric points

Isoelectric focusing of human plasma inactive renin isolated by affinity chromatography on octyl-Sepharose and antirenin antibody-Sepharose revealed that it consists of three major components with pI values of 6.4, 6.1, and 5.8 plus two minor components with pI values of 5.2 and 5.4 (Fig. 3). Activation by trypsin or plasmin shifted pI values to very low values of 5.0, 5.3, 5.36, and 5.5 as illustrated in Figure 3. As shown in Figure 4, activation of renal prorenin is also accompanied by similar downward shifts in pI. Interesting is the fact that pI valves of renal prorenin are practically identical with those of plasma prorenin. The isoelectric point is a very sensitive index of a molecular change. Thus, the agreement in molecular weight (56,000) and isoelectric points between renal prorenin and plasma prorenin supports the concept that renal prorenin is the source of plasma prorenin. The isoelectric focusing is another method for separating active renin from inactive renin. Interestingly, the reversible activation method of Hsueh et al. [31] did not cause any shifts in the pI values of prorenin while full enzymatic activity was expressed.

The downward shift in pI upon proteolytic activation indicates loss of portions of the prorenin molecule containing basic amino acids by peptide-bond cleavage, whereas activation without a shift in pI indicates reversible conformational change, as demonstrated by Hsueh et al. [31]. This finding also provides further evidence for the zymogen nature of prorenin.

The partial purification methods have been applied to tissues other than the kidney, plasma, and amniotic fluid. Prorenin was demonstrated in the brain [48],

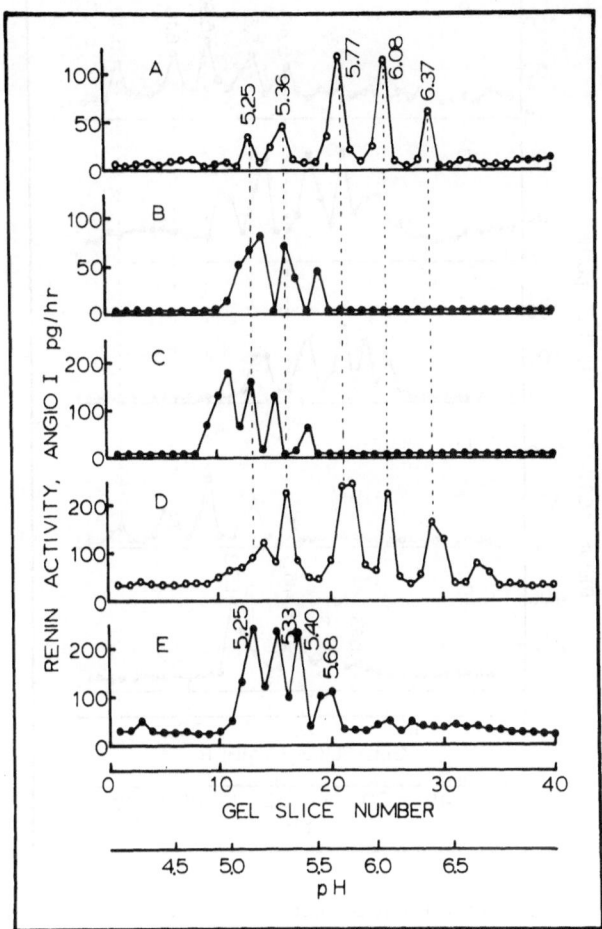

Figure 3. Isoelectric focusing of human plasma inactive renin and active renin. A. Inactive renin. B. After plasma activation. C. After trypsin activation. D. After acid activation. E. Active renin directly isolated from plasma. Closed circles indicate activity measured without activation; open circles represent activity determined after trypsin activation of inactive renin solutions eluted from 2.5-mm wide electrofocusing gel slices. (From ref. [21] with permission of *Hypertension*).

neuroblastoma cells, and adrenal glands detection of prorenin was not possible without the purification technique.

From studies summarized above, the following conclusions will be extracted: Several affinity chromatographic methods, useful for complete or partial purification of prorenin to a state free from protease inhibitors, have been developed. Molecular and functional properties of inactive renin purified and stabilized by these methods agree well with the expected properties of a zymogen rather than an enzyme-inhibitor complex. These properties include complete lack of activity, single polypeptide structure of prorenin, activation by proteolysis but not by

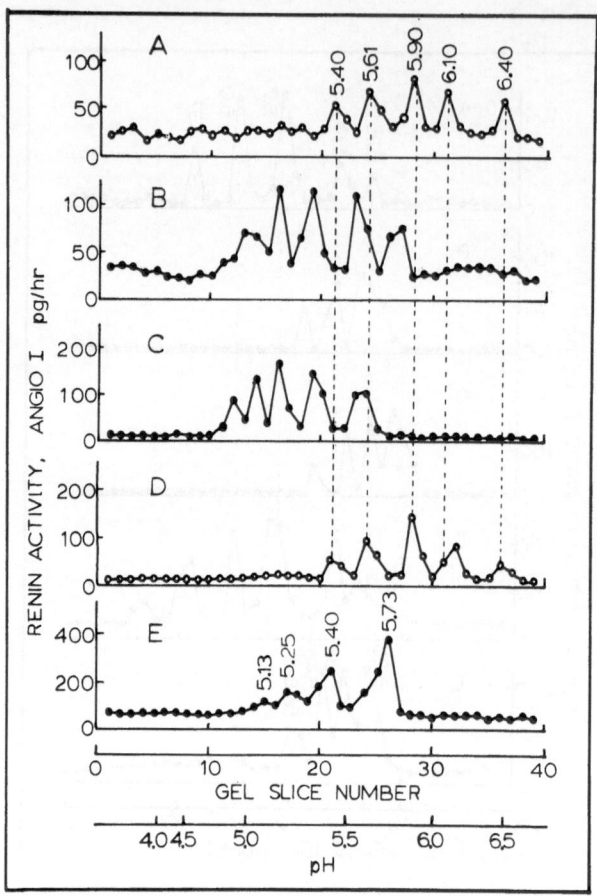

Figure 4. Isoelectric focusing of human renal inactive and active renin. A. Inactive renin. B. After plasmin activation. C. After trypsin activation. D. After acid activation. E. Active renin directly isolated from the kidney. Closed circles indicate activity measured without activation; open circles represent activity determined after trypsin activation of inactive renin solutions eluted from gel slices 2.5 mm wide. (From ref. [21] with permission of *Hypertension*)

dissociative processes, drastic change in isoelectric points, and close agreement between molecular weights of preprorenin (50,000) synthesized *in vitro* [53-56] and prorenin isolated from the kidney. These, observations provide persuasive proof that inactive renin is the renin zymogen or prorenin. It is now clear that activatable renin or 'big renin' in human plasma is a mixture of completely inactive prorenin and active renin without potential for further activation, rather than a partially active and activatable enzyme. Human renal prorenin isolated by slow processes has a molecular weight considerably lower than the ultimate prorenin, yet it is inactive. The activation of prorenin may not be a one-step mechanism.

In vitro activation of plasma prorenin produces an active renin whose molecular weight is considerably greater than that of active renin of plasma. It indicates that plasma prorenin is not the source of plasma active renin. It is more likely that the activation takes place in the kidney. The molecular weight of human active plasma renin (50,000) is considerably higher than that of hog renal or plasma active renin (38,000). Structure of human renin may be considerably different from that of hog renin. The molecular weight of hog prorenin (50,000) is compatible with that of preprorenin observed with the products of *in vitro* synthesis using renin mRNA from mouse submaxillary gland [53-56] or mouse kidney [54-56]. The messenger for human prorenin (54,000) should be much larger than that of nonprimate mammalian species.

SUMMARY

1. Affinity chromatography methods have been developed to separate active renin from prorenin. Cibacron Blue-Sepharose and octyl-Sepharose adsorbed prorenin in exclusion of active renin. Pepstatin-Sepharose adsorbed active renin in exclusion of prorenin.

2. These selective affinity gels were used to demonstrate completely inactive prorenin and active renin without potential for further activation.

3. Combinations of several affinity gels and conventional ion-exchange chromatography permitted complete purification of inactive prorenin from hog kidney by 3-million-fold purification.

4. The molecular weight of hog renal prorenin (50,000) is reduced to 38,000 upon activation by proteases. Dissociative processes such as brief treatment with 3 M urea, guanidine, detergent, or salt did not produce active renin, indicating that prorenin is a zymogen rather than an enzyme inhibitor complex.

5. Activatable 'big renin' in human plasma is a mixture of inactive renins (apparent molecular weight: 56,000) and 50,000-dalton active renin.

6. Inactive prorenin was isolated from human kidney. It has a molecular weight of 54,000. A lower value of 50,000 was obtained after further purification.

7. Activation of prorenin in human plasma and kidney by trypsin, plasmin, plasma kallikrein, cathepsin B, etc. caused little change in molecular weight.

8. Molecular weight of active renin in human plasma is 51,000 to 45,000, whereas that of active renin in human kidney extract was 50,000.

9. Isoelectric points of prorenin are considerably higher than those of active renin. The isoelectric point is a good index for the characterization of prorenin-renin conversion.

404

ACKNOWLEDGMENT

This work was supported by research grants from NIH HL-14192, HL-22288, and HL-24112 and a fellowship from the American Heart Association Middle Tennessee Chapter to JJC.

REFERENCES

1. Lumbers ER: Activation of renin in human amniotic fluid by low pH. Enzymologia 40, 329-336, 1971.
2. Morris BJ, Lumbers ER: The activation of renin in human amniotic fluid by proteolytic enzymes. Biochim Biophys Acata 289:385-391, 1972.
3. Day RP, Luetscher JA: Biochemical properties of big renin extracted from human plasma. J Clin Enocrinol Metab 40:1085-1093, 1975.
4. Day RP, Luetscher JA: Big renin: A possible prohormone in kidney and plasma of a patient with Wilms' tumor. J Clin Endocrinol metab 38:923- 926, 1974.
5. Leckie B: The activation of a possible zymogen of renin in rabbit kidney. Clin Sci 44:301-304, 1973.
6. Boyd GW: A protein-bound form of porcine renal renin. Circ Res 35:426-438, 1974.
7. Leckie BJ, McConnell A: A renin inhibitor from rabbit kidney. Conversion of a larger inactive renin to a smaller active enzyme. Circ Res 36:513-519, 1975.
8. Day RP, Luetscher JA, Gonzales CM: Occurrence of big renin in human plasma, amniotic fluid and kidney extract. J Clin Endocrinol Metab 40:1078-1084, 1975.
9. Inagami T, Murakami K: Prorenin. Biomed Res 1:456-457, 1980.
10. Sealey JE, Atlas S, Laragh JH: Prorenin and other large molecular weight forms of renin. Endocr Rev 1:365-391, 1980.
11. Leckie B: Inactive renin: An attempt at a perspective. Clin Sci 60:119-130, 1981.
12. Boyd GW: An inactive high-molecular weight renin in normal subjects and hypertensive patients. Lancet 1:215-218, 1977.
13. Shulkes AA, Gibson RR, Skinner SL: The nature of inactive renin in human plasma and amniotic fluid. Clin Sci Mol Med 55:41-50, 1978.
14. Inagami T, Takahashi N, Yokosawa N, et al.: Partial purification of prorenin and activation by kallikreins: A possible new link between renin and kallikrein systems. Abstracts of the International Symposium on Kinin, Tokyo, November 1978, p 79.
15. Carlson EJ, Hsueh WA, Luetscher JA: Separation of active and inactive renins in human plasma, abstracted. Circulation 57/58(suppl 2):250, 1978.
16. Yokosawa N, Takahashi N, Inagami T, et al.: Isolation of completely inactive plasma prorenin and its activation by kallikrein. Biochim Biophys Acta 569:211-219, 1979.
17. Takii Y, Takahashi N, Inagami T, et al.: A new form of renin in normal human plasma: 'Big renin' is a mixture of inactive prorenin and the new active high molecular weight renin. Life Sci 26:347-353, 1980.
18. Atlas SA, Sealey JE, Dharmgrongartama B, et al.: Detection and isolation of inactive, large molecular weight renin in human kidney and plasma. Hypertension 3(suppl I):I30-I40, 1981.
19. Johnson RL, Poisner AH, Crist RD: Partial purification and chromatographic properties of inactive renin from human amniotic fluid. Biochem Pharmacol 28:1791-1799, 1979.
20. Murakami K, Takahashi S, Hirose S, et al.: Renin precursor and its activation mechanism in hog kidney. Clin Sci 000:000, 1980.
21. Chang JJ, Kisaragi M, Okamoto H, et al.: Isolation and activation of inactive renin from human

kidney and plasma: Plasma and renal inactive renin have different molecular weights. Hypertension 3: 509-515, 1981.

22. Inagami T, Okamoto H, Ohtsuki K, et al.: Human plasma inactive renin: Purification and activation by proteases. J Clin Endocrinol metab, in press.

23. Hsueh WA, Carlson EJ, Luetscher JA, et al.: Activation and characterization of inactive big renin in plasma of patients with diabetic nephropathy and unusual active renin. J Clin Endocrinol Metab 51:535-543, 1980.

24. Morris BJ: Activation of human inactive ('pro') renin by cathepsin D and pepsin. J Clin Endocrinol Metab 46:153-157, 1978.

25. Sealey JE, Atlas SA, Laragh JH, et al.: Plasmin can activate plasma prorenin but is not required for alkaline phase of acid activation. Clin Sci 57:97s-99s, 1979.

26. Morris BJ, Day RP: Activation of inactive renin by fibrinolysin. IRCS Med Sci 7:188, 1979.

27. Slater EE, Haber E: A large form of renin from normal human kidney. J Clin Endocrinol Metab 47:105-109, 1978.

28. Yokosawa H, Yokosawa N, Inagami T: Specific antibody to human renal renin and its cross-reactivity with inactive human plasma prorenin. Proc Soc Exp Biol Med 164:466-470, 1980.

29. Takii Y, Inagami T: Purification of a completely inactive renin from hog kidney and identification as renin zymogen. Biochem Biophys Res Commun 104:133-140, 1982.

30. Takii Y, Inagami T: Evidence for a completely inactive renin zymogen in the kidney by affinity chromatographic isolation. Biochem Biophys Res Commun 94:182-188, 1980.

31. Hsueh WA, Carlson EJ, Israel-Hagman M: Mechanism of acid activation of renin: Role of kallikrein in renin activation. Hypertension 3(suppl I):I22-I30, 1981.

32. Leckie BJ, McConnell A, Grant J, et al.: An inactive renin in human plasma. Circ Res 40 (suppl I):46-51, 1977.

33. Hsueh WA, Luetscher JA, Carlson E, et al.: A comparison of cold and acid activation of big renin and of inactive renin in normal plasma. J Clin Endocrinol Metab 47:792-799, 1978.

34. Hsueh WA, Luetscher JA, Carlson EJ, et al.: Big renin in plasma of healthy subjects on high sodium intake. Lancet 1:1281-1284, 1978.

35. Eggena P, Barrett JD, Wiedman GE, et al.: Modification of the enzymatic activity of renin by acidification of plasma and by exposure of plasma to cold temperatures. Hypertension 1:190-196, 1979.

36. Day RP, Morris B: Properties of inactive renin in human plasma. Clin Exp Pharmacol Physiol 6:611-624, 1979.

37. Hsueh WA, Luetscher JA, Carlson EJ, et al.: Inactive renin of high molecular weight (big renin) in normal human plasma. Hypertension 2:750-756, 1980.

38. Barrett JD, Eggena P, Sambhi MP: Trypsin activatable renin in rat plasma, in Sambhi MP (editor): Heterogeneity of Renin and Renin-Substrate. New York, Elsevier-North Holland, 1981, pp 73-81.

39. Potter DM, McDonnald WJ, Dunn PM, et al.: Chemical characterization of a high molecular weight renin from the renal cortex of the dog. Circ Res 43:832-839, 1981.

40. Potter DM, Bagby SP, McDonald WJ, et al.: Circulating trypsin-activatable inactive renin in the dog, in Sambhi MP (editor): Heterogeneity of Renin and Renin-Substrate. New York, Elsevier-North Holland, 1981, pp 83-88.

41. Gallagher JF, Laragh JH, Atlas SA, et al.: Effect of trypsin or acid treatment on dog plasma renin activity measurements. Endocrinology 107:147-154, 1980.

42. Barrett JE, Eggena P, Sambhi MP: 'Big renin' enzymatic and partial physical characterization of a new high molecular weight renin from normal human kidney. Circ Res 41(suppl II):7-11, 1977.

43. Slater EE, Haber E: A large form of renin from normal human kidney. J Clin Endocrinol Metab 47:105-109, 1978.

44. Levine M, Lentz KE, Kahn JR, et al.: Partial purification of a high molecular weight renin from hog kidney. Circ Res 38(suppl II):90-94, 1976.

406

45. Levine M, Lentz KE, Kahn JR, et al.: Studies on high molecular weight renin from hog kidney. Circ Res 42:368-375, 1978.
46. Inagami T, Hirose S, Murakami K, et al.: Native form of renin in the kidney. J Biol Chem 252:7733-7737, 1977.
47. Overturf M, Druilhet RE, Fitz A: The effect of kallikrein, plasmin and thrombin on hog kidney renin. J Biol Chem 254:12078-12083, 1979.
48. Hirose S, Naruse H, Ohtsuki O, et al.: Totally inactive renin zymogen and different forms of active renin in hog brain tissues. J Biol Chem 256:5572-5576, 1981.
49. Funakawa S, Funae Y, Yamamoto K: Conversion between renin and high-molecular-weight renin in the dog. Biochem J 176:977-981, 1978.
50. Potter DM, McDonald WJ, Dunn PM, et al.: Chemical characterization of a high-molecular weight renin from renal cortex of the dog. Circ Res 43:832-839, 1978.
51. Slater EE, Strout HV: Pure human renin: Identification and characterization of two molecular weight forms. J Biol Chem 266:9164-9171, 1981.
52. Yokosawa H, Holladay LA, Inagami T, et al.: Human renal renin: Complete purification and characterization. J Biol Chem 255:3498-3502, 1980.
53. Poulsen K, Vuust J, Lykkegaard S, et al.: Renin is synthesized as a 50,000 dalton single-chain polypeptide in cell-free translation systems. FEBS Lett 98:135-138, 1979.
54. Dykes C, Kohar C, Taylor JM, et al.: In vitro synthesis of the precursor of mouse renal renin from kidney mRNA. Biomed Res 1:565-568, 1980.
55. Poulson K, Vuust J, Lund T: Renin precursor from mouse kidney identified by cell-free translation of mRNA. Clin Sci 59:297-299, 1980.
56. Pratt RE, Dzau VJ, Ouellette AJ: Abundant androgen-regulated mRNA's in mouse submaxillary gland: Cell-free translation of renin precursor mRNA. Nucleic Acids Res 9:3433-3449, 1981.

EXTRARENAL RENIN-ANGIOTENSIN SYSTEM: COMMENTS ON ITS OCCURRENCE AND CARDIOVASCULAR ROLE

F. Merlin Bumpus and Carlos M. Ferrario

INTRODUCTION

The discovery of renin in the arterial wall by Jimenez-Diaz et al. [1], salivary gland renin by Werle et al. [2], and brain renin by Ganten et al. [3] has given rise to speculation that angiotensin formed locally, and not of plasma origin, must have a significant physiological role. Sufficient proof is available for its occurrence in these areas, but its exact role is yet to be determined.

To prove that arterial renin is synthesized in the vascular wall is difficult, but its elevated levels have been demonstrated [4-6] in chronic two-kidney, one-clip renal hypertensive animals and in spontaneously hypertensive rats. This observation has been used as an explanation for the reduction of blood pressure in these experimental hypertensive models, even though plasma renin activity may be important in the maintenance of normal or low plasma renin hypertension. This evidence is not conclusive by any means. Evidence must be given in support of the hypothesis that arterial renin does not arise from the kidney. Even though arterial levels may not parallel plasma levels, the former could concentrate in the vessel. Such phenomena are known. For example, the concentration of fibrinogen is known to be high intravascularly.

Converting enzyme activity has been shown to occur in vessels. Ryan et al. [7] and Caldwell et al. [8] have shown that the enzyme is localized in the vascular endothelial cells. Johnson and Erdos [9] demonstrated that endothelial cells grown in culture produce this same enzyme. More recently, Miyauchi et al. [10] have shown a variation in concentration of converting enzyme in various vessels, with the pulmonary and renal arteries containing the highest levels.

However, crucial experiments are needed to prove that cells of vascular wall can synthesize components of renin and its substrate, and to determine the physiological control mechanism that regulates this system.

Considerable progress has been made in recent years in characterizing the presence of a renin-angiotensin system in the brain. Since the existence of angiotensin-like bioactivity and immunoreactivity was first reported in cerebrospinal fluid (CSF) by Finkielman et al. [11] and in brain by Fischer-Ferraro et al. [12], much research has been carried out to determine the origin and identity of this angiotensin. In 1977, Hutchinson et al. [13] reported that the immunoreactive angiotensin in canine cerebrospinal fluid was des-Asp[1] Ang II. Their proof was based on comparison of angiotensin-like activity of CSF to that of authentic heptapeptide by polyacrylamide-slab gel electrophoresis using Tris/borate buffers at pH 8.87.

A surprising report was made by Semple and Macrae [14] suggesting that the detection of angiotensin II in CSF arises from an immunoassay artifact. Employing a paper-chromatographic method, they observed that CSF angiotensin migrated differently from plasma angiotensin. They, of course, did not take into acount the previous report of Hutchinson nor the possibility that there may be a sequence difference between plasma and brain angiotensin.

The occurrence of angiotensinogen in brain tissue and CSF is well established. The question has remained as to the source of its biosynthesis. Printz et al. [15] injected ^{125}I-rabbit plasma angiotensinogen intravenously into rabbits and measured its uptake in brain and CSF. Although they detected radioactivity crossing into these areas, they were unable to show that the labeled protein crossed the blood-brain barrier. Printz et al. [16] demonstrated by isoelectric focussing that the microheterogeneity of CSF angiotensinogen and that of plasma substrate of sheep are different. However, most of this microheterogeneity disappeared after removal of sialic acid by neuraminidase.

With regard to the source of angiotensin I prohormone, Printz and colleagues [16] have shown by a variety of techniques that plasma angiotensinogen does not flux readily into the central nervous system. Experiments entailing either adrenalectomy, nephrectomy, or chronic treatment with reserpine revealed a clear dissociation between changes in plasma and brain renin substrates with these maneuvers. Ito et al. [17] determined that in man, CSF angiotensinogen was immunogenically different from plasma angiotensinogen, and that removal of the sialic acid residue by treatment with neuraminidase did not abolish this immunological difference. Consideration of the present data should conclude that an angiotensin is synthesized in the brain and may be different structurally from that of plasma angiotensin. Leakage of some plasma renin substrate into CSF has not been completely ruled as one considers similarity of the electrophoretic protein patterns of CSF and plasma.

Recently, Ganten et al. [18] reported that brain angiotensin has the same mobility on HPLC as that of plasma angiotensin. However, Phillips (personal communication) has found that angiotensin activity, as assayed by rat assay and radioimmunoassay, moves on a molecular sieve column as an entity of mol wt 5 000. Obviously, until brain angiotensin is isolated and characterized, we cannot speculate as to its structure.

In 1971, Ganten et al. [3] reported renin-like activity in brain extracts. In 1977, Ian Reid [19] wrote an editorial entitled 'Is there a brain renin-angiotensin system?' He correctly pointed out that Ganten's group and those who reported brain renin afterward were more than likely measuring cathepsin D. This subject has been reviewed by Phillips et al. [20], presenting evidence both for and against the existence of brain renin, and they conclude that there is an isorenin in brain different from cathepsin D. This has been sufficiently established now by Hirose et al. [21] and by Osman et al. [22], who have separated cathepsin D from isorenin. In 1980, a widespread distribution of renin in human brain was demonstrated by use of indirect peroxidase-antiperoxidase complex immunocytochemical technique. The first suggestion that angiotensin acts on brain came from Bickerton & Buckley [23], using a cross-circulation experiment in two dogs. In one dog, whose brain was perfused by the dog receiving Ang II injections, body circulation was disestablished with brain circulation. In this experiment, the action of angiotensin on the brain was clearly shown to produce a pressor response in the entire animal. Later, Severs et al. [24], showed that a direct injection of Ang II in the brain had a great pressor effect. Booth [25] first observed that angiotensin induced rats to drink, and Epstein [26] more carefully studied the drinking phenomenon related to angiotensins.

In addition to the above effects, angiotensin also releases adrenocorticotrophic hormone (ACTA) and antidiuretic hormone (ADH). Greg and Malvin [27] demonstrated that Ang II releases ADH by an action on the hypothalamus and not by direct action on the neurohypophysis.

This widespread distribution of angiotensin action sites in brain correlates with a wide distribution of angiotensin-binding sites. Bennett and Snyder [28] studied high-affinity angiotensin-binding sites in bovine and rat brain membranes. In calf brain, ^{125}I-angiotensin II binding was observed almost exclusively in the cerebellum, while in rat brain the binding was highest in thalamus-hypothalamus, midbrain, and brain stem. This original paper and later ones add to the body of evidence that angiotensin II probably plays a physiological role in the central nervous system. It is interesting that des-Asp^1-angiotensin II binds more strongly than angiotensin II in brain. Furthermore, if it is true that this heptapeptide is so prevalent in CSF, then is it a significant hormone?

FUNCTIONAL ROLE OF ANGIOTENSIN IN THE BRAIN

Angiotensin has a variety of actions on the autonomic nervous system, most of which were discovered two decades after the demonstration of its well-known vasconstrictor effects. Aside from the lucid and convincing demonstration by Braun-Menendez et al. [29] that angiotensin can stimulate discharge of catecholamine by the adrenal medulla, other effects of the parent hormone upon the autonomic nervous system were to remain unrecognized for another 20 years. At this time, an interrelationship between the peripheral autonomic nervous system and angiotensin was found by the contemporary work of Zimmerman [30] and McCubbin and Page [31], who showed that the vasoconstrictor action of angiotensin II was reduced by sympathectomy. Later experiments indicated that the most probable explanation of this phenomenon was that angiotensin acted on the peripheral sympathetic nervous system to intensify cardiovascular responsiveness to efferent sympathetic disharges [31]. Prevention of norepinephrine uptake by sympathetic nerve terminals may also play a role. (For review see reference [32].)

In 1961, Bickerton and Buckley [23] noticed that injections of angiotensin into the isolated circulation of a dog's brain caused increased central sympathetic vasomotor discharge. The technique they employed was a laborious one, and the amounts of angiotensin used were very high; both factors prevented a more timely recognition of the neurogenic effects of the peptide in the central nervous system. The subject remained dormant until recent years, when the actions of angiotensin on the central nervous system again attracted the interest of many investigators. Research carried out in the last 10 years has provided convincing proof that the actions of angiotensin II upon the central nervous system (CNS) comprise an important facet of the neuroendocrine mechanisms involved in the regulation of cardiovascular function and body fluid volumes. From what has been learned thus far, we cannot safely say whether the main biological effects of the hormone angiotensin are due to either the local generation of the peptide in brain parenchyma or the passage of the circulating hormone into the extracellular spaces of the brain via 'gaps' on the blood-brain barrier. Convincing arguments for and against each of these two possibilities are complied elsewhere [33]. In this review, we will summarize the present evidence and outline some ideas for future research.

CENTRAL ACTIONS OF ANGIOTENSIN II

Putative brain receptors involved in the expression of the cardiovascular action of angiotensin II may be stimulated in theory by the arrival of the peptide into the brain parenchyma from either the cerebrospinal fluid or the bloodstream. In the first case, the hormone enters the intercellular spaces of the brain through the CSF-brain barrier; in the other case, the molecule comes into contact with receptors via functional 'gaps' in the blood-brain barrier. While there is evidence for both routes of approach, the second possibility is more likely.

Infusion or injection of Ang II into either a cerebrolateral ventricle or the vertebral artery circulation causes in mammals, including humans, a number of physiological responses, such as increased blood pressure, thirst, sodium appetite, and enhanced secretion of hypophysial hormones. In both rats and dogs, IVT infusion of angiotensin II appears to elicit effects that are related more to body fluid regulation than blood pressure control. By this route, prominent responses entail stimulation of drinking behavior, natriuresis, and secretion of ACTH and vasopressin (AVP). These changes are accompanied by a rise in arterial blood pressure; we suspect, however, that the elevation in arterial pressure may be either a consequence of the behavioral effects associated with the introduction of the peptide in the ventricular spaces of conscious animals or secondary to an effect of AVP upon vascular resistance.

Via Vertebral Arteries

The demonstration many years ago by Yu and Dickinson [34] that angiotensin given into the vertebral arteries of the unanesthetized rabbit produced rises in blood pressure that were considerably larger than those due to the systemic infusion of the peptide led Dickinson [35] to believe that angiotensin could have important effects on the CNS. Because they were not successful in reproducing these effects in other species, these observations were relegated until the contemporaneous work of Scroop and Lowe [36] and Ferrario et al. [37].

Both groups of investigators showed that infusion of angiotensin into the vertebral arteries produced a rapid rise in arterial pressure which, in the mongrel dog, could be prevented by the administration of an adrenergic neuron-blocking agent [38]. Lowe and his colleagues [39, 40] were inclined instead to attribute most of the pressor effects of angiotensin to inhibition of vagal inhibitory activity. In their animals, the rises in arterial pressure were due to increased cardiac rate and cardiac output; peripheral resistance did not change. Ferrario et al. [37] observed that the pressor response in mongrel dogs was accompanied consistently by increases in peripheral resistance without significant changes in heart rate or cardiac output. This latter hemodynamic pattern suggested activation by angiotensin of vasoconstrictor sympathetic pathways, a fact later confirmed by prevention of the pressor response to intravertebral administration of angiotensin by either section of the spinal cord at about C2 or administration of the adrenergic blocking agent, bretylium tosylate. To prove the case further, Ferrario et al. [38] measured efferent activity from cardiac, renal, and splanchnic sympathetic nerve twigs; in the majority of cases, administration of angiotensin into a vertebral artery did not change cardiac nerve activity but increased preganglionic splanchnic vasomotor discharge.

The previous experiments provided the basis for elucidating the site at which angiotensin exerts pressor effects at concentrations that are ineffective when given intravenously. Gildenberg et al. [41] observed that the pressor responses persisted after sectioning of the dog's brain stem; hence, the hypothalamus and the midbrain were ruled out as the site of angiotensin activity. They then conducted a series of experiments in which the distribution of the circulation of the vertebral arteries was altered to reveal the site at which the hindbrain of the dog received blood from either the vertebral or carotid artery territories [42]. This permitted narrowing the possible site of action to the lower medulla where the area postrema, the nucleus of the solitary tract, and the dorsal motor nucleus of the vagus are within close anatomical proximity. Since angiotensin would not be expected to penetrate the blood-brain barrier, the area postrema having a deficient blood-brain barrier appeared the most likely site. Joy [43] discovered that bilateral ablation of the area postrema abolished the specific pressor response to infusion of angiotensin into the vertebral arteries. Shortly thereafter, Gildenberg et al. [44] were able to block the response reversibly by local cooling of this structure. With regard to the mechanism by which angiotensin II acts, Ferrario and McCubbin [45] have proposed that the area postrema may serve as a gate through which angiotensin reaches neurons in the solitary tract involved with the control of baroreceptor afferent traffic to the vasomotor center. In this manner, angiotensin may modulate (inhibit?) baroreceptor impulses by permitting an increase in the traffic of sympathetic discharges from medullary vasomotor neurons. During following years, Ferrario and colleagues showed that this area of the dog brain stem contains an angiotensin-sensitive pressor pathway that acts to increase the activity of either bulbar vasomotor or spinal preganglionic sympathetic neurons. The hemodynamic effects of intravertebral angiotensin II are mimicked by the delivery of electrical impulses into the area postrema [46]. The pressor response appears to be due to the activation of a polysynaptic pathway which might originate in the area postrema itself [47]. Additional proof for an important role of the area postrema in the control of autonomic function is the demonstration that in conscious trained dogs, surgical inactivation of this structure causes mild hypotension and reduced blood pressure lability [48]. These hemodynamic features were sustained for a 30-day period of study and were accompanied by a remarkable change in peripheral vascular reactivity to systemic pressor doses of angiotensin II. The effect entailed a downward shift of the dose-response curve to angiotensin II given intravenously. Norepinephrine responses were not modified by ablation of the area postrema.

There exists the possibility of an important participation of the area postrema to the cardiovascular response due to renal hypertension in the dog. Preliminary data obtained by Ferrario (unpublished observations) indicate that ablation of the area postrema causes a significant attenuation of the rises in blood pressure following clipping of one renal artery and associated removal of the contralateral kidney. Confirmation of these initial findings may provide strong support to the hypothesis of increased neurogenic drive as the major factor accounting for the hemodynamic onset transients of renal hypertension [45].

Via Cerebrolateral Ventricles

There is in the midbrain of both cats and dogs another area which responds to angiotensin by causing a rise in blood pressure [24, 41]. Unlike the effect obtainable in the area postrema, the phenomenon can be elicited by direct application of the peptide into either the lateral cerebral ventricle or, more specifically, by bathing the third ventricle with angiotensin. Credit is due to Buckley and his co-workers [24] for first demonstrating that angiotensin could produce a pressor response after intraventricular injection and later localizing the site in cats to the nucleus mesencephalicus in the midbrain [49]. In contrast with the pressor response elicited via the vertebral arteries, stimulation by angiotensin of this suprapontine structure requires that relatively large doses of the peptide be given into the cerebrospinal fluid. In the dog [41, 50], 100 to 200 ng of angiotensin were required to produce rises in arterial pressure comparable to those elicted following intravertebral infusion of the peptide (average dose: 3.0 ng/kg/min). Gildenberg et al. [41] showed that heat coagulation of the area postrema did not alter the pressor response elicited by the administration of angiotensin into a cerebral lateral ventricle. The response could be abolished by transection of the midbrain. It is known, therefore, that both areas can respond to angiotensin and that the route of administration determines which is affected. It is not known, however, whether or not there is a functional interrelationship between these two areas.

Angiotensin appears to evoke different hemodynamic responses according to whether the nervous structure stimulated by angiotensin is either above (midbrain) or below (area postrema) the tentorium. In the anesthetized cat, intraventricular infusions of angiotensin II at doses between 50 and 200 ng/kg produced rises in blood pressure that mediated chiefly by increased peripheral resistance. Heart rate and cardiac output did not change [51] Brosnihan et al. [50] have now recorded in the anesthetized dog the hemodynamic effects of angiotensin given into a lateral cerebral ventricle at doses similar to those reported previously [41]. The pressor response is slow in onset, its peak is sustained for only a short time, and the rises in arterial pressure disappear gradually over several minutes. The increase in blood pressure is due to increased peripheral resistance but, in contrast with the pressor response following intravertebral infusion, cardiac rate is reduced. These hemodynamic changes suggest that a different mechanism is involved.

While the mechanism of the pressor action of angiotensin above the tentorium remains largely unknown, it is pertinent to note that delivery of angiotensin into the midbrain region appears to evoke a far more complex cardiovascular response than that produced by administration of the peptide into the vertebral arteries. Injection of angiotensin II into the cerebral ventricle produces drinking, increased secretion of vasopressin and ACTH, and, of course, increased blood pressure [33]. Similar responses are produced by intraventricular administration of renin. It is not clear at present whether or not the site at which angiotensin acts to cause a rise in blood pressure involves the same neural structure responsible for increased thirst and/or release of AVP. The latter effects have been attributed to the subfornical organ, another area outside the blood-brain barrier (for review, seen Buckley and Ferrario [33]). The functional pathways, the anatomical and physiological links of these various actions of angiotensin above the midbrain, have yet to be elucidated; but significant progress is being made now due to the demonstration of Brody and colleagues [35] that a region close to the anterior portion of the third ventricle (AV3V) in the rat plays a crucial role in the development of several forms of experimental hypertension. A number of important nuclei are contained within the boundaries of the AV3V region, namely the organum vasculosum of the lamina terminalis, the nucleus medianus, projection to and from the subfornical organ, and even the most rostral part of the anterior hypothalamus. Many of these nuclei appear to be involved in the regulation of water and salt metabolism as well as having a modulatory influence on central vasopressinergic pathways. Considering that these periventricular nuclei subserve key functions as regulators of neuroendocrine hormones, it is not surprising that angiotensin could have a multiplicity of effects at this level.

INTERPLAY BETWEEN THE KIDNEY AND BRAIN RENIN-ANGIOTENSIN SYSTEMS

The evidence presented thus far indicates that blood-borne angiotensin II does affect central nervous system autonomic and endocrine functions. Most, but not necessarily all, of the known central effects of this peptide can be explained by the penetration of angiotensin II into the fluid matrix of the brain via specialized conduits in either the blood-brain or the blood-CSF barrier. It is, however, possible that some of the effects that are observed by acute introduction of angiotensin II into the cerebrospinal fluid only mimic the intrinsic action of locally synthesized angiotensin II in the brain. These data suggest that brain stem autonomic reflexes and hypothalamic neuroendocrine factors could be under the dual influence of both blood- and brain-generated angiotensin II. A comprehensive hypothesis that takes into consideration the direct interaction of the kidney renin-angiotensin system with brain stem cardiovascular nucleus and the endogenous brain angiotensin system has been proposed by Ferrario et al. [53]. While a variety of experiments do provide support for this hypothesis [54, 55], further work will be necessary to establish the site(s), mechanism(s), and neuronal structures subserving these effects.

REFERENCES

1. Jimenez-Diaz C, De la Barreda P, Molina AF: La regulación química de la presión arterial. Rev Clin Esp 24:417, 1947.
2. Werle E, Vogel R, Goldel LF: Uber ein blutdrucksteigerndes Prinzip in Extrakten aus der Glandula Submaxillaris der weissen Maus. Arch Exp Pathol Pharmacol 230:236, 1957.
3. Ganten D, Marques-Julio A, Granger P, et al.: Renin in dog brain. Am J Physiol 221:1733-1737, 1971.
4. Thurston H, Swales JD, Bind RF, et al.: Vascular renin-like activity and blood pressure maintenance in the rat. Hypertension 1:643-649, 1979.
5. Garst JB, Koletsky S, Wissenbaugh PE, et al.: Arterial wall renin in the hypertensive rat. Clin Sci 56:41-46, 1979.
6. Asaad MM, Antonaccio MJ: The effects of captopril (SQ 14,225) on vascular tissue renin in spontaneously hypertensive (SHR) and WKY-normotensive (NTR) rats: Relationship to systolic

blood pressure (SBP) and plasma renin activity (PRA). Pharmacologist 21:212, 1979.

7. Ryan JW, Ryan US, Schultz DR, et al.: Subcellular localization of pulmonary angiotensin-converting enzyme (Kininease II). Biochem J 146:497, in 7-499, 1975.

8. Caldwell PRB, Seegal BC, Hsu KC, et al.: Angiotensin-converting enzyme: Vascular endothelial localization. Science 191:1050-1051, 1976.

9. Johnson AR, Erdos EG: Metabolism of vasoactive peptides by human endothelial cells in culture: Angiotensin I-converting enzyme (Kininease II) and angiotensinase. J Clin Invest 59:684-695, 1977.

10. Miyauchi Y, Nishimura K, Ueda E, et al.: Angiotensin-converting enzyme activity in the vascular tissue from rabbits. Biomed Res 2:364-366, 1981.

11. Finkielman S, Fischer-Ferraro C, Diaz A, et al.: A pressor substance in the cerebrospinal fluid of normotensive and hypertensive patients. Proc Natl Acad Sci USA 69:3341-3344, 1972.

12. Fischer-Ferraro C, Nahmod VE, Goldstein DJ, et al.: Angiotensin and renin in rat and dog brain. J Exp Med 133:353-361, 1971.

13. Hutchinson JS, Csicsmann J, Korner PI, et al.: Characterization of immunoreactive angiotensin in canine cerebrospinal fluid as des-Asp[1] Ang II. Clin Sci Mol Med 54:147-151, 1978.

14. Semple PF, MacRae WA: VIIth Scientific Meeting of the International Society of Hypertension, New Orleans, 1980.

15. Printz MP, Lewicki JA, Wallis CJ: in Gross F, Vogel HG (editors): Enzymatic Release of Vasoactive Peptide. New York, Raven Press, 1980, pp 193-207.

16. Printz MP, Printz JM, Gregory TJ: Identification of angiotensinogen in animal brain homogenates. Circ Res 43(Suppl I):21-27, 1978.

17. Ito T, Eggena P, Barrett JD, et al.: Studies on angiotensin of plasma and cerebrospinal fluid in normal and hypertensive human subjects. Hypertension 2:432-436, 1980.

18. Ganten D, Printz M, Philips MI, et al. (editors): The Renin Angiotensin System in the Brain. Heidelberg, Springer-Verlag, 1982.

19. Reid IA: Is there a brain renin-angiotensin system? Circ Res 41:147-153, 1977.

20. Phillips MI, Weyhenmeyer J, Felix D, et al.: Evidence for an andogenous brain renin-angiotensin system. Fed Proc 38:2260-2266, 1979.

21. Hirose S, Yokosawa H, Inagami T: Immunochemical identification of renin in rat brain and distinction from acid proteases. Nature 274:392-393, 1978.

22. Osman MY, Sen S, Smeby RR: Separation of renin activity from acid protease activity in brain extracts. Fed Proc 37:354, 1978.

23. Bickerton RK, Buckley JP: Evidence for a central mechanism in angiotensin-induced hypertension. Proc Soc Exp Biol Med 106:834-836, 1961.

24. Severs WB, Daniels AE, Smoobler HH, et al.: Interrelationship between angiotensin II and the sympathetic nervous system. J Pharmacol Exp Ther 155:530-537, 1966.

25. Booth D: Mechanism of action of norepinephrine in eliciting an eating response on injection into rat hypothalamus. J Pharmacol Exp Ther 160:336-348, 1968.

26. Epstein AN, Fitzsimmons JT, Ralls BJ: Drinking caused by the intracranial injection of angiotensin into the rat. J Physiol (Lond) 200:98-100, 1969.

27. Greg CM, Malvin RL: Localization of central sites of action of angiotensin II on ADH release in vitro. Am J Physiol 234:F135-F140, 1978.

28. Bennet JP Jr, Snyder SH: Angiotensin II binding to mammalian brain membranes. J Biol Chem 251:7423-7430, 1976.

29. Braun-Menendez E, Fasciolo JC, Leloir LF, et al.: Farmacología de la hipertensina. Rev Soc Argent Biol 16:398-410, 1940.

30. Zimmerman BG: Effect of acute sympathectomy on responses to angiotensin and norepinephrine. Circ Res 11:780-787, 1962.

31. McCubbin JW, Page IH: Neurogenic component of chronic renal hypertension. Science 139:210-215, 1963.

32. McCubbin JW: Peripheral effects of angiotensin on the autonomic nervous system, in Page IH, Bumpus FM (editors): Angiotensin. New York, Springer-Verlag, 1974, pp 417-423.

33. Buckley JP, Ferrario CM (editors): Central Nervous System Mechanisms in Hypertension. New York, Raven Press, 1981.

34. Yu R, Dickinson CJ: Neurogenic effects of angiotensin. Lancet 2:1276-1277, 1965.

35. Dickinson CJ: Neurogenic Hypertension. Oxford, Blackwell Scientific Publications, 1965, p 7.

36. Scroop GC, Lowe RD: Central pressor effect of angiotensin mediated by the parasympathetic nervous system. Nature (Lond) 220:1331-1332, 1968.

37. Ferrario CM, Dickinson CJ, McCubbin JW: Central vasomotor stimulation by angiotensin. Clin Sci 39:239-245, 1970.

38. Ferrario CM, Gildenberg PL, McCubbin JW: Cardiovascular effects of angiotensin mediated by the central nervous system. Circ Res 30:257-262, 1972.

39. Lowe RD, Scroop GC: Cardiovascular response to vertebral artery infusions of angiotensin in the dog. Clin Sci 37:593-603, 1969.

40. Scroop, GC, Lowe RD: Efferent pathways of the cardiovascular response to vertebral artery infusions of angiotensin in the dog. Clin Sci 37:605-619, 1969.

41. Gildenberg PL, Ferrario GM, McCubbin JW: Two sites of cardiovascular action of angiotensin II in the brain of the dog. Clin Sci 44:417-420, 1973.

42. Gildenberg PL, Ferrario CM: A technique for determining the site of action of angiotensin and other hormones in the brainstem, in Buckley JP, Ferrario (editors): Central Actions of Angiotensin and Related Hormones. New York, Pergamon Press, 1977, pp 157-164.

43. Joy MD: Intramedullary connections of the area postrema involved in the central cardiovascular response to angiotensin II. Clin Sci 41:89-100, 1971.

44. Gildenberg PL, Ferrario CM, Alfidi RJ, et al.: Localization of central nervous system vasopressor activity of angiotensin. Proceedings of the 25th International Congres of Physiological Science, 1971, p 203.

45. Ferrario CM, McCubbin JW: Neurogenic factors in hypertension. Hosp Pract 9:71-81, 1974.

46. Barnes KL, Ferrario CM, Conomy JP: Comparison of the hemodynamic changes produced by electrical stimulation of the area postrema and nucleus tractus solitarii in the dog. Circ Res 45:136-143, 1979.

47. Barnes KL, Ferrario CM: Anatomical and physiological characterization of the sympatho-facilitative area postrema pathways in the dog, in Buckley JP, Ferrario CM (editors): Central Nervous System Mechanisms in Hypertension. New York, Raven Press, 1981, pp 25-36.

48. Ferrario CM, Barnes KL, Szilagyi JE, et al.: Physiological and pharmacological characterization of the area postrema pressor pathways in the normal dog. Hypertension 1:235-245, 1979.

49. Deuben RR, Buckley JP: Identification of a central site of action of angiotensin II. J Pharmacol Exp Ther 175:139-146, 1970.

50. Brosnihan KB, Berti GA, Ferrario CM: Hemodynamics of central infusion of angiotensin II in normal and sodium-depleted dogs. Am J Physiol 6:H139-H145, 1979.

51. Buckely JP, Lokhandwala MF, Jandhyala BS, et al.: Circulatory effects of chronic intraventricular administration of angiotensin II in dogs, in Buckley JP, Ferrario CM (editors): Central Nervous System Mechanisms in Hypertension. New York, Raven Press, 1981, pp 363-376.

52. Brody MJ, Johnson AK: Role of the anteroventral third ventricle region in fluid and electrolyte balance, arterial pressure regulation, and hypertension. Front Neuroendocrinol 6:249-292, 1980.

53. Ferrario CM, Barnes KL, Brosnihan KB, et al.: An analytical description of the role of neurogenic factors in the control of arterial pressure, in Villarreal H (editor): Hypertension. New York, John Wiley & Sons Inc., 1981, pp 185-194.

54. Brosnihan KB, Szilagyi JE, Ferrario CM: Effect of chronic sodium depletion on cerebrospinal fluid and plasma catecholamines. Hypertension 3:233-239, 1981.

55. Brosnihan KB, Smeby RR, Ferrario CM: Effects of chronic sodium depletion on canine brain renin and cathepsin D activities. Hypertension (in press).

DISCUSSION

Discussants: Haber, Bumpus, Ganten, Eggena, Laragh

Haber: Are you convinced that there is a different form of angiotensin in the central nervous system?

Bumpus: I didn't want to leave in your mind that we definitely know the brain angiotensin structure - these are very preliminary experiments. It could be that that is an active peptide, des-Asp[1] angiotensin I which has the properties we've described. If true, this is surprising since the substrate preparation used had all angiotensinase as well as converting enzyme inhibited. Does that mean that des-Asp substrate occurs in the CSF? It does certainly appear that there's something present other than human type angiotensin I.

Haber: One of the major questions you're posing is whether the central actions of angiotensin are related to angiotensin transported there from plasma pools or whether it's an intrinsic system. In your extensive review of this question, have you found any experiments in which anephric subjects, anephric animals perhaps, were studied in such a way that inhibitors of the angiotensin system, either of renin of angiotensin itself, had significant effects when introduced at the central nervous system?

Bumpus: No, I'm not aware of specific studies of this sort using anephric patients or animals. Injections of angiotensin centrally produce effects as I've reported, and I'm sure you're aware of the blood pressure lowering effects of angiotensin II antagonists given centrally. It is more difficult to prove that angiotensin II produced locally in brain is involved in blood pressure control.

Ganten: Did you say that there is no angiotensin II and no angiotensin I in the brain and that there is only this peptide which you just described?

Bumpus: It's CSF that I've referred to in the presentation. We have a fraction from HPLC that moves as does human angiotensin I. There's also a fraction that is very hydrophobic which does not correspond to nonapeptide. It might possibly be the corresponding octapeptide, which would be des-[Asp[1], Arg[2]]-Ang I.

Ganten: But this is upon incubation of renin with CSF angiotensinogen; this is not endogenous brain or CSF angiotensin.

Bumpus: That's right.

Eggena: I'm not exactly sure if this is an answer to Dr. Haber's question, but we have looked at CSF of anephric humans. These samples were sent to us by Dr. Villarreal. We find a certain amount of circulating angiotensin II in CSF, whereas we don't find any angiotensin II in the plasma. In other words, angiotensin II does seem to be locally synthesized. Angiotensin II was identified by RIA not HPLC.

Laragh: I guess I feel the same way Dr. Haber does. I don't know whether the question has been answered. You have to study anephric animals that have been nephrectomized for 48 hours or more, at which point you can be sure that the renin activity might have come from the kidneys. Only then can you determine that there might be sui generis brain renin in that animal. That's really what I think is the relevant issue.

Ganten: There is renin and there is angiotensin in the brain of nephrectomized rats and other species. Actually, if you give converting-enzyme inhibitor in nephrectomized rats, you increase angiotensin I, generation. So, there is an active turnover of angiotensin peptides in the nephrectomized brain, 24-hours after nephrectomy. These endogenous brain peptides have been clearly identified as angiotensins on several different HPLC systems.

Eggena: Again, on the CSF samples from Dr. Villarreal - some of these patients have been anephric for ten years and they still show 40 picograms angiotensin II per ml.

STUDIES ON THE PURIFICATION AND CHARACTERIZATION OF HUMAN ANGIOTENSINOGEN

Duane A. Tewksbury

INTRODUCTION

Angiotensinogen is a plasma protein which serves as the substrate for renin. Renin cleaves one peptide bond to release angiotensin I (AI). Procedures for the purification of human angiotensinogen have been previously reported [1-4], but the physical and chemical parameters reported for the final product have varied considerably. This paper describes an improved procedure for the isolation of human angiotensinogen and some of the physical and chemical properties of the isolated protein.

METHODS

Purification procedure

All of the following steps were carried out at 4°C.

Step 1: Ammonium sulfate precipitation
Outdated blood bank plasma (1 L) was diluted with 1 L 0.85% NaCl and filtered through glass wool. This solution was brought to 1.5 M $(NH_4)_2SO_4$ by the slow addition of 3.8 M $(NH_4)_2SO_4$ with stirring. The solution was stirred for at least 4 hours, centrifuged, and the precipitate discarded. The supernatant was brought to 2.4 M $(NH_4)_2SO_4$ by the addition of 3.8 M $(NH_4)_2SO_4$ and the precipitate recovered as above. The precipitate was dissolved in 350 ml H_2O and dialyzed against H_2O. The dialyzate was centrifuged to remove precipitated protein and the supernatant used in the next step.

Step 2: Blue Dextran-Sepharose
The supernatant from the previous step was applied to a Blue Dextran-Sepharose column (5 × 70 cm) which had been equilibrated with 0.05 M tris-HCl-0.1 M NaCl, ph 8. The column was eluted with the equilibrating buffer at a flow rate of 1.5 ml/min with 10 min fractions being collected. An aliquot of each fraction was subjected to immunodouble diffusion against sheep antihuman angiotensinogen

serum. Those fractions showing a precipitin line were pooled and concentrated on an Amicon ultrafilter with a PM 10 membrane.

Step 3: Phenyl-Sepharose

The material from the previous step was equilibrated with $0.8\,M$ $(NH_4)_2SO_4$-$0.05\,M$ sodium phosphate, pH 7.0, and applied to a phenyl-Sepharose column equilibrated with $0.2\,M$ $(NH_4)_2SO_4$-$0.05\,M$ sodium phosphate, pH 7.0. The volume of the packed column was determined by the amount of protein applied, $4.3\,mg$ protein per $1\,cm^3$ phenyl-Sepharose. After the sample was applied, the column was eluted with $0.025\,M$ $(NH_4)_2SO_4$-$0.01\,M$ sodium phosphate, pH 7.0, until the $A_{280\,nm}^{1\,cm}$ of the effluent was <0.05. The column was then eluted with H_{20} until $A_{280\,nm}^{1\,cm}$ was <0.05. This latter effluent was pooled and concentrated on an Amicon ultrafilter with a PM 10 membrane.

Step 4: Hydroxylapatite

The material from the previous step and a hydroxylapatite column were equilibrated with $1\,mM$ sodium phosphate, pH 6.8. The ratio of protein to packed volume was $2\,mg$ protein/$1\,cm^3$ hydroxylapatite. After application of the sample, the column was eluted with $30\,mM$ sodium phosphate, pH 6.8, at a flow rate of $0.3\,ml/min$ with 12 min fractions being collected. Those fractions with $A_{280\,nm}^{1\,cm}$ >0.05 were pooled and concentrated as above.

Step 5: Sephadex G-200

The concentrated sample (5 ml) from the previous step was applied to a Sephadex G-200 column ($3 \times 85\,cm$) equilibrated with $0.05\,M$ tris-HCl-$0.1\,M$ NaCl, pH 8.0, at a flow rate of $0.2\,ml/min$ with 12 min fractions being collected. The $A_{280\,nm}^{1\,cm}$ of each fraction was determined and those fractions under the major peak pooled and stored at $-20°\,C$ until used.

Electrophoresis

Sodium dodecyl sulfate polyacrylamide gel electrophoresis (SDS-PAGE) and polyacrylamide gel electrophoresis (PAGE) were performed according to the procedure of Laemmli [5] using a Bio-Rad protein electrophoresis cell. The gels were stained with 0.2% Coomassie Blue R-250. The following proteins were used as standards in the determination of molecular weights: phosphorylase B (M_r 92,500), bovine serum albumin (M_r 66,200), ovalbumin (M_r 45,000); carbonic anhydrase (M_r 31,000), soybean trypsin inhibitor (M_r 21,500), and lysozyme (M_r 14,400).

Protein determination

The protein concentration of all samples except the final product was determined by the method of Bradford [6]. The protein concentration of the final product was determined by dry-weight measurement. An aliquot was extensively dialyzed against H_2O and 1 ml placed in an aluminum boat. The boat was dried in a desiccator over P_2O_5. The boat was then heated at 110° C in a vacuum oven until a constant weight was achieved. A control containing only buffer was also carried through this procedure. Amino acid analysis and $A_{280\ nm}^{1\ cm}$ was determined for the solution placed in the boat. Thus a relationship between these two parameters and dry weight was established.

Angiotensinogen assay

The incubation buffer, 0.6 M sodium phosphate, 36 mM EDTA, pH 6.0, containing gelatin (4 mg/ml) was brought to a boil and cooled to room temperature. A mixture containing 0.25 ml buffer, angiotensinogen (0.8 to 10 ng AI), 20 μl of human renin, and H_2O to bring volume to 1.0 ml was incubated at 37° C for 3 hours. Aliquots were assayed for AI by the radioimmunoassay (RIA) procedure of Haber et al. [7], except that lysozyme (Sigma grade 1) (mg/ml was used as carrier protein. The buffer, 1 L, containing the lysozyme was treated with 1 ml phenylmethylsulfonyl fluoride (PMSF), 50 mg/ml ethanol, and then filtered through a 0.45 μm membrane. An aliquot of an incubation blank containing renin but no angiotensinogen was added to each RIA tube comprising the standard curve. A control plasma was assayed in each run. Human renin was prepared by procedure A of Haas et al. [8]. The renin, 2 ml, was treated with 10 μl PMSF, 50 mg/ml ethanol. It was ascertained that each batch of renin would release all of the AI in 5 μl of normal human plasma within 1.5 hours under the above assay conditions.

Immunoaffinity chromatography

Sheep were immunized with purified angiotensinogen according to the method of Vaitukaitis et al. [9]. The IgG fraction was isolated by the procedure of Livingston [10]. The IgG fraction was coupled to Affi-Gel 10 (Bio-Rad). The gel, 6.5 ml, was washed with five volumes isopropranol and then with five volumes H_2O. The gel was added to 61 mg IgG in 10 ml 0.1 M HEPES, pH 7.5, and stirred overnight at 4° C. One ml 1 M ethanolamine · HCl, pH 8.0, was added and stirred for 1 hour. The gel was washed in order with 7 M urea, 1 M NaCl, and 0.1 M Na acetate-0.1 M NaCl, pH 5.5. Plasma, 5 ml, was diluted with 5 ml 0.1 M Na acetate-0.1 M NaCl, pH 5.5, and applied to an IgG-Affi-Gel column (1 × 20 cm) equilibrated with the same buffer. The column was eluted with equilibrating buffer until $A_{280\,nm}$ of effluent returned to baseline value. The effluent was assayed for angiotensinogen. Purified angiotensinogen was chromatographed in a similar manner.

Other analytical procedures

Other procedures including amino acid analysis and carbohydrate analysis were performed as previously described [11-13].

RESULTS

A summary of the purification of human angiotensinogen is given in Table 1. The previously reported procedure of Tewksbury et al. [4] has been modified by elimination of a DEAE-Sephadex chromatography step and optimization of the phenyl-Sepharose and hydroxylapatite step. These modifications have increased the overall yield to 22% and yields the same product as the previous procedure. The mean specific AI content of the product is equivalent to the theoretical value of 21 μg AI/mg protein (based on $M_r = 61,000$).

The typical protein pattern exhibited by purified angiotensinogen on PAGE is shown in Figure 1. One heavy band with a faint trace of a second slower moving band is seen. The protein pattern exhibited by angiotensinogen on SDS-PAGE is shown in Figure 2. These preparations of purified angiotensinogen have consistently exhibited two closely spaced bands. The molecular weights of these two bands as determined by SDS-PAGE in 11 different preparations of angioten-

Table 1. Summary of the purification of human angiotensinogen

Step	Protein (mg)	Angiotensinogen μg AI	μgAI/mg	Fold purification	Percent recovery
Plasma	48312[a]	1,850	0.0383	–	–
1	5616[a]	1,150	0.205	5.3	62
2	2716[a]	1,024	0.377	9.8	55
3	189[a]	910	4.81	126	49
4	20.0[a]	439	21.9	572	24
5	19.1[b]	399	20.9	546	22

[a] Protein determined by method of Bradford.
[b] Protein determined by relating $A_{280\,nm}$ to dry weight.
The above values are means of at least six values.
AI = angiotensin I.

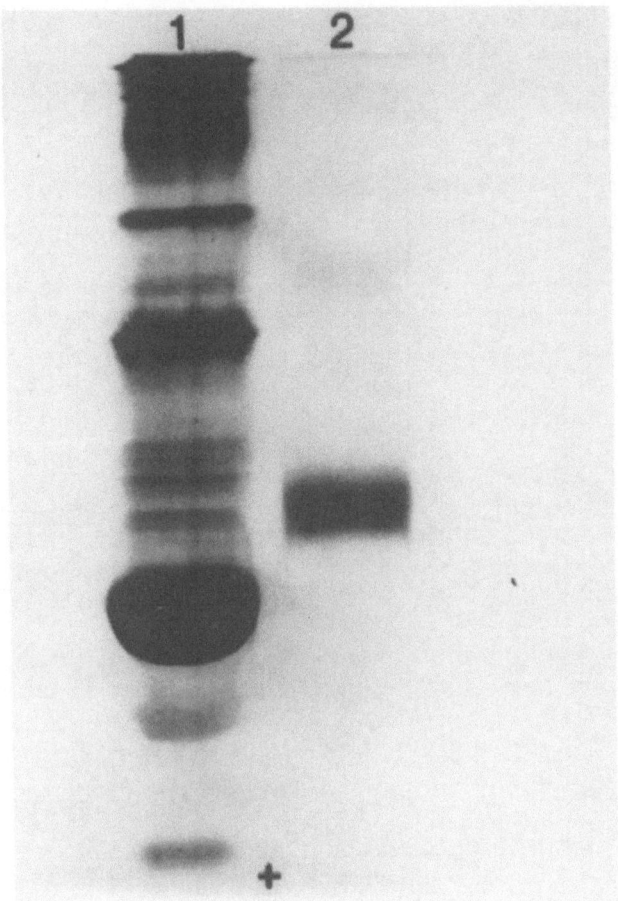

Figure 1. PAGE of human plasma (#1) and purified human angiotensinogen (#2) on a 9% gel. The albumin content of the plasma had been reduced by approximately 40% by passage through a Blue Dextran-Sepharose column.

sinogen are $61,400 \pm 330$ and $65,400 \pm 360$ (mean $\pm$ SEM). Thus, the apparent difference in the molecular weight of these two components is 4,000.

The amino acid and carbohydrate composition of purified human angiotensinogen is given in Table 2. On a weight basis, 14% of human angiotensinogen is carbohydrate. The amino acid composition of two other preparations of human angiotensinogen which have been reported to be homogeneous and that of a partially purified preparation are also presented. Since different molecular weights have been used for the derivation of these numbers, the ratios of amino acids, and not the absolute numbers, should be noted when comparing the amino acid composition of these preparations.

The results of immunoaffinity chromatography of plasma and purified an-

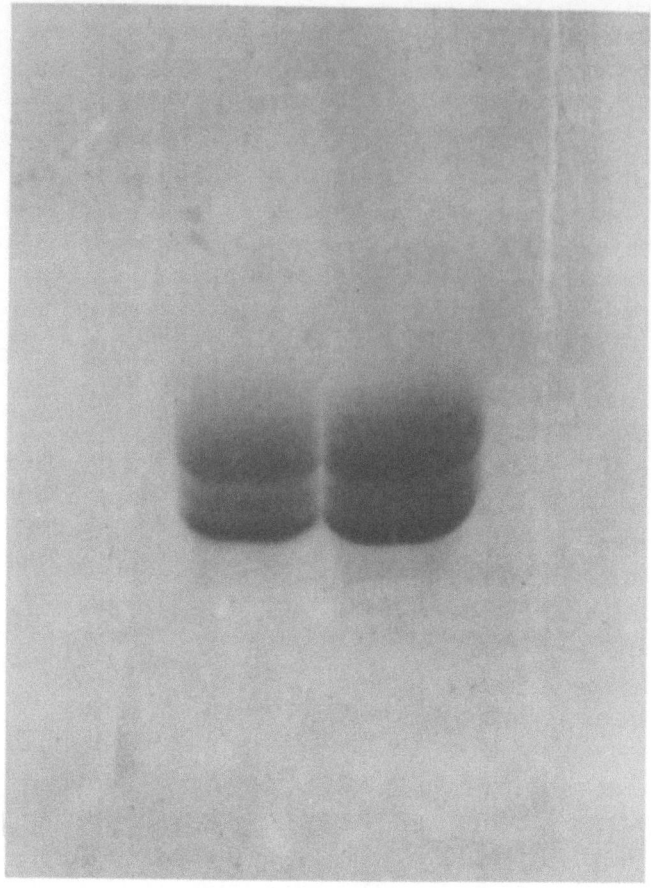

Figure 2. SDS-PAGE of two different preparations of purified human angiotensinogen on a 9% gel.

giotensinogen is given in Table 3. The IgG fraction of sheep antihuman angiotensinogen serum and nonimmune sheep serum were conjugated to agarose. The immune IgG-agarose column removed angiotensinogen from human male plasma and from purified angiotensinogen equally well. Since the nonimmune IgG-agarose did not bind angiotensinogen in either sample, this removal is due to specific binding by the antibody. Thus, almost all of the angiotensinogen in male plasma shares common antigenic determinants with the purified human angiotensinogen.

Table 2. Composition of human angiotensinogen

Residue	Residue/Molecule Human Angiotensinogen			
	Tewsbury[a]	Eggena et al.[b]	Kokubu et al.[c]	Tewksbury et al.[d]
Aspartic acid	44	92	26	33
Threonine	31	64	28	28
Serine	32	80	30	33
Glutamic acid	53	138	66	54
Proline	28	NR	32	42
Glycine	29	96	37	37
Alanine	44	96	34	40
Half-cystine	8	NR	0	8
Valine	42	54	28	34
Methionine	11	10	1	4
Isoleucine	17	13	7	10
Leucine	68	138	58	60
Tyrosine	10	24	6	7
Phenylalanine	21	39	14	19
Tryptophan	4	NR	NR	6
Lysine	25	34	9	14
Histidine	14	31	12	15
Arginine	15	62	32	31
Hexose	21	NR	NR	26
Hexosamine	19	NR	NR	12
Sialic acid	7	NR	NR	4

[a] Present study based on a molecular weight of 61, 400.

[b] Reference (1).

[c] Reference (3).

[d] Reference (11).

NR = not reported.

DISCUSSION

Previously Tewksbury et al. [12] reported a procedure for the purification of human plasma angiotensinogen. This preparation had a mean specific AI content of only 7 µg AI/mg protein but appeared to be homogeneous by electrophoretic, immunochemical, and analytical ultracentrifuge techniques. However, when amino terminal amino acid analysis was done, the presence of two amino acids, aspartic acid and alanine, could be demonstrated [11]. This indicated that these preparations of angiotensinogen consisted of a mixture of two proteins with similar physical properties. The amino acid composition of this preparation of angiotensinogen is given in Table 2. Subsequently it was demonstrated that these two proteins could be separated by chromatography on a zinc chelate-Sepharose

Table 3. Immunoaffinity chromatography of human angiotensinogen and human male plasma

Sample	Column (igG-agarose)	Angiotensinogen (μg angiotensin I)		
		Applied	Recovered in effluent	Percent bound
Purified angiotensinogen	Immune[a]	6.87	<0.46	>93
Purified angiotensinogen	Nonimmune[b]	6.87	7.37	0
Plasma	Immune[a]	9.32	<0.50	>95
Plasma	Nonimmune[b]	9.32	9.38	0

[a] IgG prepared from sheep antihuman angiotensinogen sera.
[b] IgG prepared from nonimmune sheep sera.

[14] or by chromatography on phenyl-Sepharose [4]. The protein with amino terminal alanine has tentatively been designated alanine-protein. This protein has been isolated and characterized [14].

Eggena et al. [1] and Kokubu et al. [3] have reported the amino acid composition of preparations of human angiotensinogen which were claimed to be homogeneous. The specific AI content of these preparations were 12 and 11 μg AI/mg protein, respectively. As will be noted from Table 2, there are very significant differences in the ratio of glycine to alanine and in the ratio of lysine to arginine between the present preparation of angiotensinogen and those of Eggena et al. or Kokubu et al. It should also be noted that the amino acid composition of these latter two preparations closely resemble the amino acid composition found for the preparation of angiotensinogen, which contained significant quantities of the alanine-protein and had a specific angiotensin content of 7 μg AI/mg protein. Amino terminal amino acid analysis was not reported by Eggena et al. [1], while the preparation of Kokubu et al. [3] has been reported to contain amino terminal alanine, valine, and leucine in addition to the expected aspartic acid [15]. Thus, it is suggested that the differences in the properties of the different preparations of human angiotensinogen may be due in large part to differences in purity of the preparations. Since previous experience has shown that mixtures of alanine-protein and angiotensinogen may appear to be homogeneous, it is believed that before any claim of homogeneity for preparations of human angiotensinogen can be accepted, it should be demonstrated that the preparation contains only one amino terminal amino acid and also contains, within experimental error, the theoretical amount of AI.

The current study of human angiotensinogen reveals some interesting properties. Angiotensinogen binds strongly to phenyl-Sepharose. This would indicate the presence of a hydrophobic region on the surface of the molecule. It has become apparent during the course of these studies that angiotensinogen will from aggregates. The last step in the purification procedure is a gel filtration step which separates proteins on the basis of size. It has been observed that if purified angiotensinogen from this last step is concentrated to 1 to 2 mg/ml and stored at −20° C, the presence of high molecular components will be detected upon gel filtration, thus indicating the formation of aggregates. Heating solutions of angiotensinogen at 60° C will also cause the rapid conversion of angiotensinogen to high molecular components. Preparations which contain aggregates exhibit multiple bands on PAGE which migrate more slowly than native angiotensinogen. The very light slow-moving band seen in Figure 2 is most likely an aggregate of angiotensinogen. The tendency of angiotensinogen to aggregate could be due to the presence of the hydrophobic region in angiotensinogen. This behavior increases the likelihood that the presence of some of the high molecular forms of angiotensinogen that have been observed [16] may be the result of aggregation of angiotensinogen.

The other interesting observation is that the purified angiotensinogen contains two components which exhibit a difference in molecular weight of 4,000. These two components most assuredly represent two forms of angiotensinogen. The purified angiotensinogen has the theoretical specific AI content. A mixture of angiotensinogen and an unrelated protein cannot meet this criteria unless angiotensinogen contains more than 1 mol AI/mol angiotensinogen. There is no evidence to support this suggestion. Only one amino terminal amino acid was detected by either the dansyl technique or by the Edman degradation, and only one amino terminal amino acid sequence was obtained during sequence studies [4]. The yield of the first amino acid, aspartic acid, was 65%, which is in the range expected for glycoproteins under the conditions employed [4]. It should also be noted that Printz et al. [17] prepared a partially purified preparation of human angiotensinogen containing two forms of angiotensinogen in which isoelectric points differed by 0.15 units. Bouhnik et al. [18] have purified rat angiotensinogen and have documented the presence of two forms of angiotensinogen with a difference in M_r of 2,000 and a difference in isoelectric points of 0.2 pH units. Thus, it appears that purified angiotensinogen not only exhibits a type of microheterogeneity with respect to isoelectric points but also exhibits a type of microheterogeneity with respect to molecular weight. It has been established that angiotensinogen in native plasma exhibits microheterogeneity in isoelectric points, but is has not been established that the microheterogeneity in molecular weights exists in native plasma.

Angiotensinogen has now been isolated from human, hog [19], and rat plasma [18]. All three angiotensinogens share the common traits of being glycoproteins with molecular weights between 56,000 and 64,000, with AI constituting the sequence of the first 10 amino terminal amino acids. In all of these studies, multiple forms of angiotensinogen have been detected. Whether these different forms of angiotensinogen are significant in the function of the renin-angiotensin-aldosterone system or whether they represent the variation normally seen in plasma glycoproteins remains to be established.

SUMMARY

A purification procedure for human plasma angiotensinogen is presented which produces a product with 19 µg angiotensin I/mg protein in a 22% yield. The purified angiotensinogen exhibits two components on sodium dodecyl sulfate polyacrylamide gel electrophoresis (SDS-PAGE) with molecular weights of 61,400 and 65,400. Since this preparation of human angiotensinogen contains the theoretical amount of angiotensin I (AI) and contains only one amino terminal amino acid, aspartic acid, it is suggested that this preparation of purified angiotensinogen contains two forms of angiotensinogen which differ by a molecular weight of 4,000. Human angiotensinogen is a glycoprotein which contains 14% carbohydrate.

ACKNOWLEDGMENTS

The author wishes to acknowledge the excellent technical assistance of Michael Premeau, Wayne Frome, and Michael Dumas and the secretarial and editorial assistance of Alice Stargardt.

REFERENCES

1. Eggena P, Chu CL, Barrett JD, et al.: Purification and partial characterization of human angiotensinogen. Biochim Biophys Acta 427:208, 1976.
2. Dorer F, Lentz KE, Kahn JR, et al.: Purification of human renin substrate. Anal Biochem 87:11, 1978.
3. Kokubu T, Hiwada K, Sogo Y: Isolation and characterization of human renin substrate. Jpn Circ J 44:274, 1980.
4. Tewskbury DA, Dart RA, Travis J: The amino terminal amino acid sequence of human angiotensinogen. Biochem Biophys Res Commun 99:1311, 1981.
5. Laemmli UK: Cleavage of structural proteins during the assembly of the head of bacterial phage T4. Nature 227:680, 1970.
6. Bradford M: A rapid and sensitive method for the quantitation of microgram quantities of protein utilizing the principle of protein-dye binding. Anal Biochem 72:248, 1976.
7. Haber E, Koerner T, Page LB, et al.: Application of a radioimmunoassay for angiotensin I to the physiologic measurements of plasma renin activity in normal human subjects. J Clin Endocrinol Metab 29:1349, 1969.
8. Hass E, Goldblatt H, Gipson EC, et al.: Extraction, purification and assay of human renin free of angiotensinase. Circ Res 19:739, 1966.
9. Vaitukaitis J, Robbins JB, Nieschlag E, et al.: A method for producing specific antisera with small doses of immunogen. J Clin Endocrinol Metab 33:988, 1971.
10. Livingston DM: Immunoaffinity chromatography of proteins. Methods Enzymol 34:723, 1974.
11. Tewksbury DA, Frome WL, Dumas ML: Characterization of human angiotensinogen. J Biol Chem 253:3817, 1978.
12. Tewksbury DA, Premeau MR, Dumas ML, et al.: Purification of human angiotensinogen. Circ Res 41:II-29, 1977.

13. Tewksbury DA, Premeau MR, Dumas ML: Isolation of human angiotensinogen. Biochim Biophys Acta 446:87, 1976.
14. Tewksbury DA, Dart RA: Human plasma angiotensinogen: A review of purification procedures. Mol Cell Biochem 27:47, 1979.
15. Hiwada K, Sogo Y, Takada Y, et al.: Lack of inhibition of human renin by human des-angiotensin I renin substrate. Biochem Pharmacol 30:2630, 1981.
16. Gordon DB, Sachin IN: Chromatographic separation of multiple renin substrates in women: Effect of pregnancy and oral contraceptives. Proc Soc Exp Biol Med 156:461, 1977.
17. Printz MP, Printz JM, Dworschack RT: Human angiotensinogen. J Biol Chem 252:1654, 1977.
18. Bouhnik J, Clauser E, Strosberg D, et al.: Rat angiotensinogen and des (angiotensin I) angiotensinogen: Purification, characterization and partial sequencing. Biochemistry 20:7010, 1981.
19. Skeggs LT, Lentz KE, Hochstrasser H, et al.: The purification and partial characterization of several forms of hog renin substrate. J Exp Med 118:73, 1963.

DISCUSSION

Discussants: Eggena, Tewksbury, Laragh, Denton

Eggena: We find that high-molecular-weight renin substrate can be generated in two ways. One that I'll discuss in a little while, doesn't cross-react with an antibody. The other one was obtained when we freeze dried normal-molecular-weight renin substrate and stored it in the freezer at −40° for several months. This latter high-molecular-weight form does cross-react with the antibody, suggesting that this form probably represents an aggregate. Does this agree with your findings?

Tewksbury: Right. I would like to point out that within the plasma sample that is being stored, the relative proportions do stay constant. You can store either normal plasma or plasma from a pregnant women for as long as a year at −20° without seeing any change in the relative amounts of the two forms of angiotensinogen.

Laragh: Do you have any data on the relative affinity of the high-molecular-weight form of angiotensinogen for renin as compared to the low-molecular-weight renin substrate? Also, I'd like to point out that it looks like your high-molecular-weight substance is almost a test for pregnancy. It goes up very early in pregnancy, just as prorenin seems to do. There have been other situations where people have noted a correlation between prorenin levels and substrate levels, so maybe there is another possible biological relevance here.

Tewksbury: To answer your first question, we do not have any kinetic data that would indicate what the relative affinity of these various types of substrate is for renin. Obviously, prorenin and the angiotensinogen, at least in this form, are both estrogen-sensitive proteins. This reminds one a little bit of the kallikrein-kininogen system in which there is a low-molecular-weight kininogen and a high-molecular-weight kininogen. I call your attention to the fact that the high-molecular-weight kininogen does possess a unique function in that it serves not only as a substrate for kallikrein but it also binds Hagemann factor and prekallikrein and participates in the activation of the prekallikrein. I don't think there would be duplication of substrate unless there was some unique function for the high-molecular-weight form.

Denton: What was the dose of premarin you used in these studies?

Tewksbury: I believe it was 1.25 milligrams per day. I'm not a physician but that's the number I recall.

ENZYMATIC STUDIES WITH RENIN SUBSTRATE

PETER EGGENA, JACK D. BARRETT, HIROSHI SHIONOIRI AND MOHINDER P. SAMBHI

INTRODUCTION

The contribution of renin substrate to the *in vivo* rate of angiotensin I production has recently gained further significance with the determination of the kinetic parameters of the renin reaction [1, 2]. Under normal physiological conditions, the concentration of renin substrate has been shown to represent a rate-limiting step for the renin reaction *in vivo* [2, 3]. The postulate that altered forms of renin substrate may also contribute to elevated blood pressure has led to a closer examination of the physical and chemical nature of these proteins.

In this study, we have compared the kinetic rate constants of the renin reaction in plasma from normal subjects, patients with several forms of hypertension, and subjects with elevated levels of plasma renin substrate induced by elevated plasma estrogens, and we have attempted to assess the role of various forms of renin substrate.

MATERIALS AND METHODS

Clinical Material

Several groups of subjects were studied: 1) normotensive healthy men and women between the ages of 25 and 50, not taking any medication (n = 31); 2) male subjects with essential hypertension (n = 12), renovascular hypertension (n = 6), or hypertension associated with uremia (n = 4); 3) normotensive women (n = 20) receiving estrogens either as oral contraceptives or ethinyl estradiol (50 μg); 4) five women (three on various oral contraceptive preparations, two on ethinyl estradiol, 50 μg) who became hypertensive on estrogen therapy (diastolic blood pressure >90 mm Hg); discontinuation of medication led to normalization of blood pressure (<90 mm Hg) in all cases. In addition to these groups, blood was collected from pregnant normotensive women at term and the plasma pooled. This plasma was also used as a source of high-molecular-weight renin substrate. All blood samples were collected in 15 mM EDTA, centrifuged at 4°, and plasma samples were stored at −20°.

Methods

Renin substrate was measured by radioimmunoassay of generated angiotensin I, following an incubation at 37% in the presence of semipurified human kidney renin [4] and angiotensinase inhibitors [5].

Polyacrylamide gel (7% monomer) electrophoresis was performed as previously described [6] at pH 8.6 using the albumin front to determine R_f values.

Gel exclusion chromatography was performed with Ultrogel AcA 44 (LKB) as the support medium equilibrated in 0.05 M Tris-HCl, pH 7.4, in a 1.6×100 cm glass column [2]. Molecular weights were estimated by the method of Ackers [7]. High-molecular-weight renin substrate (HMS) was defined as the substrate fraction which eluted in the void volume; normal-molecular-weight substrate (NMS) eluted with an apparent molecular weight of 60,000 daltons [8]. Renin-substrate fractions isolated by gel exclusion chromatography were concentrated by ultrafiltration using a PM 30 membrane (Amicon). Isoelectric focusing (pH range 4-6) was performed on an LKB 8101 (110 ml) column according to the method of Vesterberg and Svensson [9].

Michaelis-Menten constants (K_m and V_{max}) were determined in plasma buffered at pH 7.4 with 1/10 volume 1M sodium phosphate, as previously described [10]. K_m and V_{max} were determined by the statistical method of Wilkinson [11]. All data is given with standard deviation of the mean [12]; for comparison of different groups the unpaired t method was employed [12].

RESULTS

A comparison of the Michaelis-Menten constants of the renin reaction in the plasma of normotensive subjects and several hypertensive states are summarized in Table 1. No statistically significant differences in either the M_m or V_{max} of the renin reaction were observed between normotensive subjects (male or female) and subjects with essential hypertension, renal hypertension, or hypertension associated with uremia. In contrast, a significant elevation in both K_m and V_{max} was apparent in normotensive women receiving estrogen therapy, women with estrogenic hypertension, and of normotensive pregnant women at term. In these latter groups, a significant elevation in renin substrate was also evident (Table 1).

To determine whether qualitative differences in renin substrate could contribute to the altered kinetic parameters of the renin reaction in states of elevated plasma estrogens, several physical chemical parameters of renin substrate were investigated. Plasma renin substrate from subjects in Groups 1-5 of Table 1 indicated a single molecular weight species (MW 60,000) on gel exclusion chromatography (Fig. 1A). In subjects with elevated plasma estrogen levels (Groups 6, 7, 8 of Table 1), varying concentrations of an additional high-molecular-weight

Table 1. Kinetic parameters of the renin rection in plasma

		K_m ng AI/ml	V_{max} ng AI/ml · hr	Renin substrate ng AI eq/ml	Percent HMS	S/K_m	Initial velocity* ng AI/ml · hr
1. Normal M	n = 13	1573 ± 436	138.6 ± 34.5	1957 ± 222	0	1.2	76.8
2. Normal F	n = 18	1560 ± 410	158 ± 64	2160 ± 490	<2	1.4	91.7
3. Essential hypertensive M	n = 12	1551 ± 575	109.5 ± 21.9	1459 ± 235	0	1.0	53.1
4. Renovascular hypertension	n = 6	1523 ± 661	111 ± 30.3	1822 ± 440	0	1.2	60.5
5. Hypertension associated with uremia	n = 4	1354 ± 360	124 ± 35.1	2595 ± 610	0	1.9	81.5
6. Normotensive F on estrogens	n = 20	2610 ± 190†	162 ± 52‡	5150 ± 1530†	3.4	2.0	114.1
7. Estrogenic hypertension	n = 5	3320 ± 720†	360 ± 144†	6800 ± 2450†	7.3	2.0	241.9
8. Term pregnancy plasma pool	n = 2	4150	434	10,170	12.0	2.5	308.2

* $V = \dfrac{S \cdot V_{max}}{K_m + S}$.

† Significantly elevated from 1–5.

‡ Significantly elevated from 3.

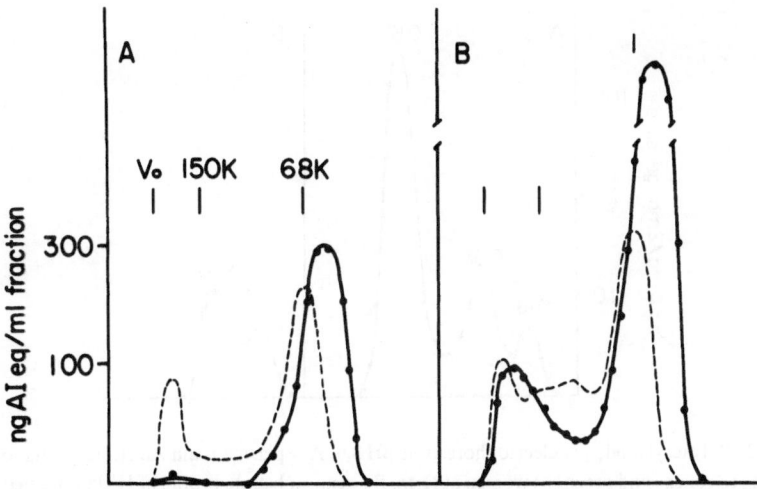

Figure 1. Separation of plasma renin substrate by gel exclusion chroma tography (--- optical density at 280. A – renin substrate molecular weight prefile of normal plasma and normotensive women taking estrogen. B – profile of normotensive pregnant women at term or women with estrogenic hypertension.

form of renin substrate (HMS) were observed (Fig. 1B). Molecular weight of this speecies was estimated to be in excess of 150,000 daltons, since it was present in the void volume of the Ultrogel AcA44 column. HMS was present in all subjects with elevated plasma estrogen levels; however, this increase was significantly higher in women with estrogenic hypertension and in normotensive term pregnancy plasma when compared to nonpregnant normotensive women receiving estrogens. This increase in HMS cannot be attributed to the general increase in renin-substrate synthesis induced by estrogens, since no statistically significant difference in total renin substrate was apparent when comparing groups 6 and 7 of Table 1. HMS was also found to be immunologically distinct from the 60,000 MW form of renin substrate (NMS); HMS did not cross-react with an antiserum specific for NMS. HMS could be quantitated solely by its ability to generate angiotensin I in the presence of renin.

On polyacrylamide gel electrophoresis at pH 8.6, we have previously shown normal renin substrate to migrate as a single band with $R_f = 0.65$. In plasmas of patients with elevated estrogen levels, two additional forms of renin substrate with Rf values of 0.16 and 0.35 were evident (Fig. 2A). Polyacrylamide gel electrophoresis of the HMS isolated from a pool of term pregnancy plasma revealed two components with Rf valves of 0.16 and 0.35 (Fig. 2B). Heterogeneity was also evident following isoelectric focusing (Fig. 3). Isolated NMS or normotensive control plasma demonstrated a single species of renin substrate with an isoelectric point at pH 4.41. Isolated HMS, on the other hand, separated into two forms of renin substrate with isoelectric points at pH 3.78 and 4.23. HMS

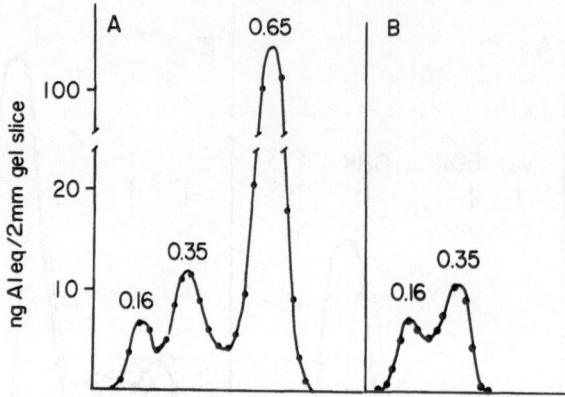

Figure 2. Polyacrylamide gel electrophoresis at pH 8.6. A – plasma renin substrate profile of women receiving estrogens and pregnant women at term. B – renin substrate profile of HMS obtained from gel exclusion chromatography.

and NMS partially purified by gel exclusion chromatography of term pregnancy plasma were employed for a comparison of K_m values. In an isolated system (0.1 M Tris-HCl, pH 7.4), HMS was found to have a significantly higher affinity for isolated homologous kidney renin than the normal form of renin substrate ($K_m = 1800 \pm 290$ for HMS vs 3520 ± 260 for NMS, $p < 0.05$).

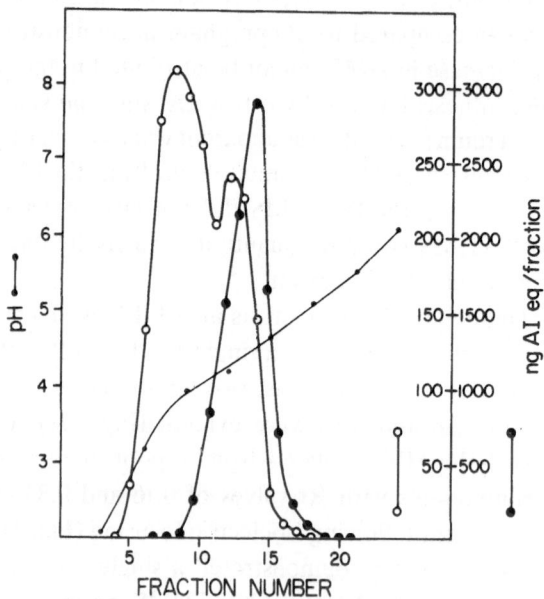

Figure 3. Isoelectric focusing pattern of renin substrate. HMS O–O–O; normal plasma ●–●–●.

DISCUSSION

The kinetic data presented in Table 1 indicate that the plasma renin substrate concentration/K_m ratio ranges from 1.0 to 2.5. These results clearly confirm the results of others [2, 3] indicating that under normal physiological conditions, renin substrate concentrations represents a rate-limiting step of the renin reaction. Even in term-pregnancy plasma, where renin substrate attains concentrations in excess of 10 μg angiotensin I equivalents/ml (S/K_m = 2.5), only 71% of the maximum velocity is reached (Table 1). To obtain zero-order kinetics with respect to renin substrate, concentrations of more than 10 times the K_m value are required. These results reemphasize the importance of the renin substrate concentration to plasma renin activity measurements.

We have previously reported an increased rate of angiotensin I production in certain subjects with renovascular and essential hypertension [1, 13], and have postulated the presence of modifiers of the renin reaction in these plasmas. We also reported that in renovascular hypertension, des-angiotensin I renin substrate is present in sufficient concentrations to act as a competitive inhibitor of plasma renin [14]. In the present study, using different methodology, no statistically significant differences in the K_m and V_{max} values of normal, essential, and renovascular hypertensive patients were apparent. The relationship of these findings to our previous results on modifiers of the renin reaction deserves comment. In those studies, an accelerated rate of angiotensin production was apparent (a) when fresh whole plasma from hypertensive subjects was incubated with an excess of exogenous homologous renin or (b) when small aliquots of plasma from hypertensive patients were added to an isolated system consisting of partially purified renin and renin substrate [1]. The latter methods, using the purified renin and renin substrate, were designed to demonstrate the existence of renin activators and, although nonphysiological, possessed the required sensitivity to demonstrate small but significant changes in K_m and V_{max}. The former experiments on whole plasma did not allow for the determination of kinetic parameters of the renin reaction due to the large excess of added renin. The present study was focused not on the presence of modifiers, but rather, on the kinetic parameters of the renin reaction in whole plasma, with particular emphasis on the influence of the composition and the concentration of renin substrate. Our failure to observe the contribution of modifiers of the renin reaction in the present study is unexplained, but may be attributable to the large and subject-dependent variation in the kinetic parameters of the renin reaction resulting from both the composition and the concentration of renin and renin substrate in plasma in addition to methodological differences. Our data on uremic subjects indicates no significant change in K_m and V_{max}. On the basis of reactivity data, Kotchen et al. [15] have postulated that the lack of a neutral lipid renin inhibitor in uremic plasma may be responsible for the hypertension associated with uremia. Our results do not support the concept of a renin inhibitor in these patients, but support our previous finding that when lipids are removed from normal plasma by centrifugation, the kinetic parameters of normal plasma are not altered [10].

When plasma renin substrate synthesis was stimulated by elevated plasma estrogen levels, induced either therapeutically or by pregnancy (Groups 6, 7, 8 of Table 1), a sharp rise in both K_m and V_{max} of the renin reaction was apparent. These data are in agreement with those of McDonald et al. [16], indicating an increase in K_m and V_{max} following administration of estrogenic compounds. Although one might expect the increased K_m value to reduce the rate of angiotensin production for a constant renin concentration, the simultaneous increase in V_{max} results in a significant increase in the relative velocity of angiotensin generation, as shown in Table 1.

An investigation was performed to determine whether alterations in renin substrate were responsible for the observed shifts in K_m and V_{max} of the renin reaction of plasmas from subjects with elevated plasma estrogen levels. Renin substrate from the plasma of normal, essential hypertensive, and renovascular hypertensive patients could not be distinguished on the basis of molecular weight, isoelectric point, mobility on polyacrylamide gel electrophoresis, or antigenic cross-reactivity with an antibody specific for NMS [6]. When plasma renin substrate was stimulated by estrogen administration however, several additional forms of renin substrate could be distinguished in plasma on the basis of immunological cross-reactivity and electrophoretic mobility [17]. In the present study, we have shown that estrogens can also induce a high molecular weight form of renin substrate, which can be separated by isoelectric focusing into two components. Printz et al. [18] have reported differences in the kinetics of isoelectrically distinct forms of renin substrate, but these forms do not appear to be related to HMS, since HMS was found to have lower isoelectric points (3.78, 4.23 vs 4.65, 4.8).

We have previously shown [8] that the induction of HMS is very dependent on the estrogen composition; e.g., at equally stimulated renin substrate levels, ethinyl estradiol is significantly more potent than premarin in HMS stimulation. The differences in the literature regarding estrogens and kinetic rate constants of the renin reaction may possibly be accounted for by the degree of HMS stimulation of the estrogen preparations employed, since HMS was found to have a significantly higher affinity for renin in an isolated system.

Although estrogens significantly elevate renin substrate levels, no statistically significant difference was observed in total renin substrate concentration of normotensive women receiving estrogens and women with estrogenic hypertension. These two groups did differ, however, with respect to their plasma concentration of HMW renin substrate, which was twofold higher in the hypertensive group. These data therefore suggest that the estrogen-mediated elevation of total renin substrate does not result in a corresponding increase in HMW. However, in term-pregnancy plasma pools, total renin substrate was 1.5-fold higher than in plasma of women receiving estrogens, and a corresponding 1.6-fold increase in

HMW was evident. It is therefore possible that at very high plasma levels of total renin substrate, a correlation may exist between these two forms of renin substrate. When estrogen therapy was discontinued in three subjects with estrogen-associated hypertension, both blood pressure and HMS levels returned to normal. It is not known, at present, whether reduction of blood pressure by other pharmacological agents while simultaneously maintaining estrogen therapy would also have reduced HMS levels. HMS, however, does not appear to be a general marker for hypertension, since this protein is not elevated in essential hypertension. The high levels of HMS in normotensive term pregnancy plasma do not refute a possible relationship between HMS and estrogen-induced hypertension, since during pregnancy many other hormonal and physiological changes may compensate for elevated HMS levels, e.g., decreased sensitivity to the vasopressor action of angiotensin II [19].

To clearly assess the influence of HMS on the renin reaction will require its purification and the determination of kinetic parameters, not only with partially purified homologous kidney renin but the also with the recently discovered multiple forms of plasma and tissue renins.

ACKNOWLEDGMENTS

This study was supported by research funds from the Veterans Administration, PHS grant HL22773 and a fellowship from the Los Angeles Chapter of the American Heart Association.

REFERENCES

1. Sambhi MP, Eggena P, Barrett JD, et al.: A circulating renin activator in essential hypertension. Circ Res 36 & 37:128-137, 1975.
2. Eggena P, Chu CL, Barrett JD, et al.: Purification and partial characterization of human angiotensinogen. Biochim Biophys Acta 427:208-217, 1976.
3. Krakhoff LR: Measurement of plasma renin substrate by radioimmunoassay of angiotensin I. Concentrations in syndromes associated with steroid excess. J Clin Endocrinol Metab 37:110-117, 1973.
4. Eggena P, Barrett JD, Wiedeman CE, et al.: The validity of comparing the measurements of angiotensin I generated in human plasma by radioimmunoassay and bioassay. J Clin Endocrinol Metab 39:865-870, 1974.
5. Barrett JD, Eggena P, Sambhi MP: Influence of angiotensinase inhibitors on the enzymatic activity of renin. Biochem Med 16:157-168, 1976.
6. Eggena P, Hidaka H, Barrett JD, et al.: Multiple forms of human plasma renin substrate. J Clin Invest 62:367-378, 1978.
7. Ackers GK: Molecular sieve studies of interacting protein systems. I. Equations for transport of associated systems. J Biol Chem 242:3026-3034, 1967.
8. Eggena P, Barrett JD, Shionoiri H, et al.: The influence of estrogens on plasma renin substrate, in Sambhi MP (editor): Heterogeneity of Renin and Renin Substrate. New York, Elsevier-North Holland, 1981, pp 255-260.

438

9. Vesterberg O, Svensson H: Isoelectric fractionation analysis and characterization of ampholytes in a natural pH gradient. IV. Further studies on the resolving power in connection with separation of myoglobins. Acta Chem Scand 20:820-834, 1966.

10. Eggena P, Barrett JD, Sambhi MP: The influence of plasma lipoproteins on the renin reaction in normal human plasma. Biochem Med 21:247-351, 1979.

11. Wilkinson GN: Statistical estimations in enzyme kinetics. Biochem J 80:324-332, 1961.

12. Snedecor GW: Statistical Methods. Ames, LA, Iowa University Press, 1962.

13. Sambhi MP, Wiedeman CE: Renin activation in the venous plasma from the involved kidney in the patient with renal hypertension. J Clin Invest 51:22-30, 1972.

14. Barrett JD, Eggena P, Hidaka H, et al.: In vitro inhibition of renin by human des-angiotensin I renin substrate. J Clin Endocrinol metab 48:96-100, 1979.

15. Kotchen TA, Talwalker RT, Miller MC, et al.: Modification of renin reactivity by lipids extracted from normal, hypertensive, and uremic plasma. J Clin Endocrinol Metab 43:971-981, 1976.

16. McDonald WJ, Cohen EL, Lucas CP, et al.: Renin-renin substrate kinetic constants in the plasma of normal and estrogen-treated humans. J Clin Endocrinol Metab 45:1297-1304, 1977.

17. Eggena P, Barrett JD, Hidaka H, et al.: A direct radioimmunoassay for human renin substrate and identification of multiple substrate types in plasma. Circ Res 41(Suppl II):34-37, 1977.

18. Printz MP, Printz JM, Dworschack RT: Human angiotensinogen. Purification, partial characterization, and a comparison with animal prohormones. J Biol Chem 252:1654-1662, 1977.

19. Everett RB, Worley RJ, McDonald PC, et al.: Modification of the vascular responsiveness to angiotensin II in pregnant women by intravenously infused 5 alpha-dihydroprogesterone. Am J Obstet Gynecol 131:352-357, 1978.

DISCUSSION

Discussants: Corvol, Eggena, Tewksbury, Johnston, Luetscher, MacGregor

Corvol: We treated rats with estrogen, glucocorticoids and thyroid hormones and were unable to find any difference between direct angiotensinogen assay and angiotensinogen determined by angiotensin I RIA. Did you check in rats to see whether or not you got this high molecular weight?

Eggena: Our antibody is made to the normal form of human substrate, and it doesn't cross-react with the rat substrate. With regard to looking at animal models, we've tried to develop an animal model to see if we could generate high-molecular-weight substrate. We have looked in pigs treated with estrogens and we found very little. We have also looked in rat plasma and could not detect any high-molecular-weight substrate. In rhesus monkeys we found very small amounts, but they don't seem to be stimulated by estrogens.

Tewksbury: We've looked for high-molecular angiotensinogen in a number of animals, including rats, in the late stages of pregnancy. Some animals show it and some do not. The horse and the cow show 7 to 10 percent of the total being high molecular weight, and the rat did not show a high-molecular-weight component that was discretely resolved. However, there was an unusual shoulder on the leading edge of the low-molecular-weight component, which indicated there was some other component there, but it wasn't well separated in the systems that we use. Do you have any evidence that your antibody will detect an aggregate of low-molecular-weight angiotensinogen?

Eggena: All I can say is that the antibody does recognize what appears to be an aggregate generated on storage. It is a well-known fact that a lot of proteins, such as albumin, do aggregate on storage – especially in the freeze-dried form. This is the only evidence I have at present.

Tewksbury: It may be that certain antibodies will not recognize the aggregate form.

Eggena: Certainly.

Johnston: I wonder if you could give us some idea of how important you think the rate-limiting step of substrate is *in vivo*? How quickly is substrate regenerated or replaced *in vivo* in plasma? One of the reasons I ask is that most of the people who measure plasma angiotensin actually find a very good correlation between the active renin and the level of angiotensin in the plasma, suggesting that the substrate is continuously being replenished and doesn't actually become rate limiting as it does in the test tube.

Eggena: No, renin substrate is always rate limiting. If you take a normal plasma and you add substrate to it, which is renin-free, you will find that the amount of angiotensin I you generate goes up. In other words, the available renin has the capacity to increase angiotensin I production if the substrate concentration is increased. This is what the KM data indicates.

Johnston: Yes, I'm not questioning your data, I was wondering how important you thought it was *in vivo* where there was a continuous supply of substrate. How good is the continuous supply of substrate?

Luetscher: Your're looking at two ends of the relationship. If substrate is depleted severely, that will certainly reduce the rate of reaction. This depletion must be very rare. But then there's also the question of whether increasing the concentration of substrate above normal will drive the reaction faster. This occurs quite regularly in the circumferences which Dr. Eggena has pointed out to us.

MacGregor: We should be looking at plasma renin activity as an index of circulating angiotensin II rather than plasma renin concentration.

Eggena: Yes, in general I agree with you.

THE BRAIN RENIN-ANGIOTENSIN SYSTEM: PROBLEMS AND ANSWERS

D. Ganten, M. Printz, Th. Unger and R.E. Lang

INTRODUCTION

The existence of a brain renin-angiotensin system (RAS)[1] was originally proposed in 1971 [1-4] on the basis of the discovery of the components required for the formation of angiotensin II (ANG II) in the brain. At that time, none of the individual components of this complex enzyme peptide system had been obtained in pure form, and their physiochemical properties were still unclear.

In the last ten years progress has been made, especially with respect to the characterization of the enzymes and peptide precursors of the RAS and with respect to the methodology of their measurement. The RAS can now be considered an unusually well-defined peptide hormone-generating system [5]. The enzyme, high-molecular-weight precursor proteins, the effector peptides, as well as the receptors are well known, and pharmacological agents are available which interfere specifically with the system at the various levels of peptide generation and ANG II action.

Several questions, however, remain to be answered concerning the *in vivo* activity and the biological and pathophysiological role of the brain RAS. It is the purpose of this paper to address some of these questions and discuss recent data which solve some of the problems, or may lead to answers.

PROBLEMS

Brain renin was measured in most of the early experiments using methods which were originally devised for plasma renin measurement and which did not distinguish between nonspecific cathepsin D-like activity and true renin. In fact, it has been argued that most if not all of the brain renin activity was due to cathepsin D-like enzymes [6-8]; the distribution of immunoreactive renin appeared to be

---

[1] *Abbreviations used:* ANG I - angiotensin I; ANG II - angiotensin II; HPLC - high pressure liquid chromatography; RS - renin substrate; SHRSP - spontaneously hypertensive rats stroke-prone strain; RAS - renin-angiotensin system; CSF - cerebrospinal fluid.

quite similar to the distribution of immunocytochemically localized cathepsin D [9]. The distribution of renin as studied by immunocytochemistry did not completely agree with the data obtained by biochemical methods [10-20]. It has also been suggested that renin in the brain could partly be explained by contamination with plasma renin [8]. Finally, even if renin or renin-like enzymes were present in the brain, it remained to be demonstrated that the enzyme functions as an angiotensin-forming enzyme *in vivo* by reacting with brain angiotensinogen.

Brain angiotensinogen is less problematic than renin [5, 21-23], but the immunocytochemical localization has not been achieved. From ultracentrifugation and biochemical studies it has been concluded by some authors that most of the peptide precursor was in the extracellular space [24, 25]. This distribution could pose difficulties with respect to the interactions of renin with angiotensinogen and might point to a peripheral origin of the protein. Also, the regulation of brain angiotensinogen seemed to be only partly independent of plasma angiotensinogen [7, 23, 26, 27].

Converting enzyme (CE) is a ubiquitous enzyme with apparently limited specificity [28-34]. In most studies on CE, artificial peptides have been used to measure enzyme activity [32], and different results may be obtained when the natural substrates are utilized. Again, a discrepancy was noted between the immunocytochemical localization as studied with antibodies raised against lung CE and its distribution assayed biochemically [35].

Angiotensin had been extracted from brain and characterized by conventional methods [1, 3], but several authors failed to confirm the results [8, 36]. Definite evidence for the presence and local synthesis of ANG II was lacking. The partial discrepancy between the localization of ANG II-like material and renin-like immunofluorescence [12, 13, 17, 20] was used as an argument against the peptide being synthesized endogenously in the brain by an interaction of brain renin with brain angiotensinogen *in vivo*.

Renin

Many of the initial observations on brain renin activity probably reflected the activities of both, a ubiquitous cathepsin D-like enzyme and true brain renin. The relative contributions of these two enzymic pathways depend on the assay conditions. Recent results indicate a close structural similarity of renin with other acid proteases. Submandibular renin, for example, has a catalytic site almost identical with that of pepsin and exhibits approximately 30% sequence homology with porcine pepsin. Hence, it should be closely homologous to cathepsin D [11].

A specific assay method for true renin and the elimination of the nonspecific activity has therefore become essential for the identification of brain renin and the future evaluation of its pathophysiological role. On the other hand, it is possible that enzymes different from kidney renin can generate ANG I from angiotensinogen *in vivo,* and these should also be investigated. In this respect, the mainly negative discussion of cathepsin-D-like enzymes in the brain was misleading.

The separation of renin from cathepsin activity is largely a result of advances in the application of affinity chromatographic procedures. True renin in human, rat, hog, beef, dog, and mouse brain have been separated from renin-like activity by affinity chromatography [13, 15, 19, 37-40]. True renin, defined by its similarity to purified kidney or submandibular gland renin, does not bind to casein-Sepharose. Evidence of renin activity was confirmed by direct inhibition with specific antisera to renin. Another separation method, Blue-Sepharose, with known affinity for inactive prorenin but not for active renin in the plasma and kidney, was found to preferentially bind active renin of mouse brain but not cathepsin [40]. Thus, these affinity techniques provide a reliable methodology for the identification and specific measurement of brain renin. The use of such chromatographic separation methods is, however, cumbersome and requires large amounts of tissues. Specific renin activity has been estimated in a more simple procedure by inhibition of ANG I-generating activity with antibodies directed against kidney renin and by the use of unfractionated plasma from nephrectomized rats as a source of renin substrate at an incubation pH over 7. An acid protease inhibitor in unfractionated plasma reduces the nonspecific renin-like activity considerably [11, 37].

Complete purification of bovine pituitary renin and an 850,000-fold enrichment of the enzyme has recently been achieved by Hirose et al. [19]. The pure renin had a specific activity of 146 μmol ANG I/mg/h and a K_m of 1 μMol with rat angiotensinogen. The molecular weight was 36,000, the pI 5.25; the pH optimum was between 6.5 and 7.5. The amino acid composition was similar but not identical to kidney renin with a high content of Leu, Gly, and Glu, and relatively low content of Cys, Met, and His. A lower Val and Ser content was found in brain renin than in kidney renin. The pituitary enzyme did not bind to agarose-bound lectins; antibodies raised against pituitary renin cross-reacted with bovine and hog kidney renin.

The concentration of renin in the brain is relatively low. There are marked species differences, however, with respect to brain renin content. Bovine and hog anterior pituitary, for example, have high-renin content (45.3 and 42.7 ng ANG I/mg/protein/h), while rabbit, sheep, and rat pituitary exhibit low-renin activity (5.2, 1.3, 0.7, respectively) [11, 19]. A contamination with plasma renin is unlikely, because nephrectomy has repeatedly been shown to cause no change or even an increase in brain renin concentration [11]. The amino acid composition, pH optimum, pI values, and other physiochemical characteristics of purified brain renin are different from kidney renin [15-17, 38, 40]. In addition, brain renin has been localized intracellularly by immunocytochemical techniques [12, 20, 41], and the existence of prorenin in the brain [17, 18] is indicative of its local synthesis.

Haulica et al. [42] suggested the *de novo* endogenous formation of brain renin in monolayer cultures of pineal glands, which produced increasing amounts of the enzyme when kept over 30 days in culture. Recent reports on the presence of renin and other components of the RAS in neuroblastoma cells also support the local synthesis or renin in nervous tissue [5, 11]. Finally, the data on angiotensin in the brain as discussed below and the stimulation of ANG I in the brain of nephrectomized rats and after converting enzyme blockade are clearly in favor not only of the presence but also the *in vivo* activity of brain renin.

Converting enzyme

Converting enzyme is a dipeptidyl-carboxy-peptidase which cleaves the COOH-terminal dipeptides from various substrates and splits the carboxy-terminal histidyl-leucine from the decapeptide ANG I, thus generating ANG II, the effector peptide of the RAS. CE has been demonstrated to be ubiquitously distributed in the organism of various species, including man, with particularly high concentrations in lung, plasma, kidney, and testis [32, 33]. Besides these peripheral tissues, CE is also present in the brain. In the rat, enzyme activities were found in the striatum, posterior lobe of the hypophysis, and cerebellum; lower activities were found in the midbrain, medulla oblongata, and hypothalamus [28, 35, 43, 44].

A particularly rich source of CE in the brain is the chorioid plexus [29, 35], but high CE activity has also been reported in cortical microvessels of calf and rabbit brain [45, 46]. CE has been shown to be bound to vascular endothelial cells (e.g., lung) and to epithelial cells from the brush border of proximal tubules (kidney) or of epithelial plexus cells facing the ventricular space (plexus, chorioideus); it also exists in soluble form in plasma, seminal fluid, cerebrospinal fluid (CSF), and lymph [30, 33, 35, 44].

When brain tissue was subjected to subcellular fractionation, the highest CE activities were associated with the microsomal fractions containing the synaptosomes while there was little activity in the supernatant [30, 44]. Converting enzyme isolated and purified from brain tissue exhibited similar characteristics as CE from different peripheral sources with respect to molecular weight, pH optimum, chloride dependency, and inhibition by chelating agents such as EDTA and o-phenantroline or by inhibitors like SQ20881 and SQ14225 [29, 30, 44]. Converting enzyme may act on a variety of substrates in the brain as it does in the periphery, but its activity on ANG I in the brain is undisputed and has been shown by various authors under different experimental *in vitro* and *in vivo* conditions [29, 34, 44, 47].

Angiotensinogen

The primary method currently in use to identify and quantify renin substrate (RS) is to incubate the preparation with sufficient homologous kidney renin to release all the ANG I and to quantitate the latter by specific radioimmunoassay [5]. If the resulting peptide is then identified by additional methods (e.g., HPLC, amino acid analysis) as ANG I, there is little doubt that angiotensinogen is indeed being measured. As a matter of fact, one of the strongest pieces of evidence in favor of a brain RAS has for some time been the evidence that RS (angiotensinogen) is present in the central nervous system [2, 3, 21-23, 48, 49]. The contamination with plasma can introduce artificially high results. This is a severe problem with brain RS, since the concentration of RS in plasma, although quite low in terms of specific concentration (e.g., per mg protein), is still appreciable. Depending upon the endocrine state of the animal and prior surgical procedures (e.g., nephrectomy or adrenalectomy), the plasma RS can vary from 50 to 1000 ng ANG I/ml.

There are several approaches to this problem. Traditionally, most laboratories working on such plasma/brain located substances either ignore plasma contamination or perform a perfusion of the cerebral vascular bed. This perfusion, while esthetically satisfying by the greatly diminished color of the tissue, still leaves much of the contaminating plasma present. In fact, in a recent study, Gregory et al. [50] and Wallis et al. [51, 52] found that such perfusions, even when done carefully and with maximal attention to all details, still left much of the contaminating plasma in the brain tissue as monitored either by radioiodinated albumin or tritiated inulin. An alternative approach is to quantify the actual amount of plasma present in brain tissue and, with the knowledge of the plasma RS concentration, subtract the latter to obtain net brain RS [23, 30]. Such an approach is essential for regional and for whole-brain RS analyses. Renin substrate constitutes 1.5 to 3% of the total cerebrospinal fluid (CSF) protein in several mammalian species [27, 43]. This selective enrichment over plasma is of primary interest. There is a possibility that CSF RS contains some plasma RS which may enter either via the choroid plexus or directly from brain parenchyma at sites devoid of a blood-brain barrier. Studies of the latter phenomena are continuing, and caution must be exercised on the use of CSF as a source of brain RS. But data described below show that brain and CSF angiotensinogen can be dissociated from the plasma angiotensinogen concentration and are therefore probably regulated independently.

The first regional distribution analysis of brain RS was reported by Lewicki et al. [49] and indicated both that many areas of rat brain contain the protein and that some areas have an 8- to 15-fold higher concentration than other regions. These studies were extended and replicated by Gregory et al. [50], and recently by Chen et al. [48] following the development of methods to obtain a net brain substrate concentration. Further, the work of Gregory et al. [50] indicated that brain RS was extravascular. In fact, calculations indicated that the protein must be intracellular, most likely in a cytosolic compartment. Utilizing the release rate analysis, Sernia and Reid [53] found that highest RS concentrations were in the pons, midbrain, diencephalon region, medulla, and cerebellum, while less was released from the cerebral hemispheres and olfactory lobes; lowest concentrations were released from the cerebrospinal cord. This distribution is very similar to that found by Printz and collaborators using direct brain RS analysis [22, 48, 50].

We may conclude from these studies that the concentration of the brain RS exhibits a unique topographical distribution in the rat and rabbit and that release occurs from an extravascular and most likely cytosolic compartment of the brain. The concentrations of the protein in CSF and in some brain areas are appreciable. In CSF, it can comprise 3% of the total protein, while in some brain regions the concentration is approximately 0.04 to 0.1% of total soluble protein.

The first indications were that the RS from plasma and brain are very similar as judged by chromatography using gel filtration, apparent molecular weight, and binding to concanavalin A-Sepharose [5, 21, 54]. However, differences were noted in the distribution of isoelectric pH of the brain, CSF, and plasma RS [5, 21]. Since both plasma and brain RS exhibit properties of a glycoprotein (concanavalin A-binding and sensitivity to neuraminidase digestion), it was anticipated that they would show heterogeneity in isoelectric point distributions. Indeed, in the human, rabbit, sheep, and hog, the plasma and brain renin substrates are quite different by isoelectric focusing analysis [5, 21]. Along these same lines, there is evidence that human CSF renin substrate does not cross-react with antibodies directed against human plasma renin substrate [55, 56]. This finding is supported by an independent study using antisera directed against human plasma angiotensinogen and employing partially purified human CSF angiotensinogen (unpublished results). At this time, we must conclude that brain and plasma renin substrates exhibit many similarities but important differences. The differences in antigenic cross-reactivity and isoelectric point microheterogeneity are what might be expected for similar proteins which arise from different cellular origins. These findings support a brain origin for brain RS.

Studies of the endogenous regulation of brain renin substrate are important for several reasons, one being that such investigations may provide a further differentiation between plasma and brain RS. Wallis and Printz [51] and Printz et al. [22] reported that selected rat brain areas exhibit marked decreases in apparent brain RS following adrenalectomy. Replacement of glucocorticoids restored the levels and in some regions led to elevated brain RS concentrations over control values. In these experiments, plasma RS levels decreased by 50%. Since many brain regions exhibited no change following adrenalectomy, this provides an additional argument that brain RS does not simply reflect plasma RS contamination of brain tissue. Schelling et al. [26, 27, 43] recently replicated these studies and quantified rat CSF RS levels. They demonstrated that the combined effects of adrenalectomy and nephrectomy dissociated the plasma and brain RS changes: Nephrectomy alone increased both plasma RS and CSF RS; however, the combined effects of nephrectomy and adrenalectomy resulted in a dissociation of brain and plasma RS, i.e., in a decrease in CSF RS, while plasma RS was still increased over control values [27].

It is thus clear that a pool of RS is present in the central nervous system of man, sheep, dog, rats, and rabbits. All evidence to date indicates that the protein is of central origin, although caution must be exercised until direct intracellular bio-synthesis is established. Brain RS probably fluxes into the CSF and constitutes a significant percentage of CSF protein. What is of special interest is the evidence indicating that regional brain CSF is regulated in a highly specific manner by steroids. CSF RS may reflect short time variatons in local synthesis and/or release of brain RS.

Brain angiotensin

Angiotensin and its fragments, as well as a number of other neuropeptides, can be separated from each other in a reproducible way on high-pressure liquid chro-matography (HPLC). This technique was used to clarify the controversy as to whether angiotensin was indeed present in the brain or not [8, 14, 36, 57]. For all angiotensin peptides, baseline separation was achieved on the chromatographic systems used by Hermann et al. [58]. It is noteworthy that [Ile⁵]-ANG II was separated from [Val⁵]-ANG II and from [Ile⁵]-ANG III, the latter having a longer retention time than [Ile⁵]-ANG II on a methanol gradient and a shorter retention time on an isopropanol gradient system. This provided confidence that peptides extracted from the brain and CSF, and eluted with retention times identical to synthetic [Ile⁵]-ANG I, [Ile⁵]-ANG II, and [Ile⁵]-ANG III on at least these two HPLC systems, corresponded to the standard peptides and probably have the same amino acid sequence.

The levels of angiotensin in CSF in rats have been reported to vary between undetectable levels to 200 fmol/ml or higher [26]. The variability of angiotensin concentration in native CSF has been confirmed in the study by Hermann et al. [58], and frequently undetectable levels of angiotensin have been observed in some but not all samples of native CSF of rats and human. In those cases where angiotensin-like immunoreactivity was detected, this could be identified as true angiotensin on HPLC. In a series of CSF angiotensin measurements, mean values of 17.6 ± 1.5 fmol/ml (Ile⁵]-ANG I and 29.5 ± 5.9 fmol/ml [Ile⁵]-ANG II were reported [58]. There was no relationship between the CSF levels and plasma angiotensin concentration or blood pressure [26].

If renin was injected into the brain ventricles and CSF was collected 15 min later, significant amounts of [Ile⁵]-ANG I and [Ile⁵]-ANG II were detected in CSF, and the peptides eluted identically with the synthetic standard peptides previously added to the CSF. Small amounts of [Ile⁵]-ANG III were also formed under these conditions. When CSF was incubated under *in vitro* conditions with the addition of inhibitors of CE and angiotensinase, only [Ile^5]-ANG I was generated from CSF angiotensinogen. [Ile^5]-ANG I and [Ile^5]-ANG II extracted from both rat plasma and CSF had identical retention times. It can therefore be concluded that their physicochemical properties, i.e., their amino acid sequence, are similar or identical.

The identification of [Ile^5]-ANG I as the cleavage product of renin from CSF angiotensinogen and from plasma angiotensinogen could indicate that the high-molecular-weight precursors of angiotensin in plasma and in brain are identical and that they originate from the plasma. This is unlikely, however, as has been discussed elsewhere in detail [5] and as will be shown below.

Similar to the rat, human CSF also contains variable amounts of angiotensin. In those samples where angiotensin levels were sufficiently high, the CSF peptide could be shown to be identical with synthetic [Ile^5]-ANG I and [Ile^5]-ANG II standards. This is in contrast to other reports in which it was claimed that the peptides cross-reacting with the angiotensin antibody in the radioimmunoassay were neither ANG I, ANG II, nor ANG III [36].

Rat brain tissue itself contained significant amounts of angiotensin which was identified as being [Ile^5]-ANG I, [Ile^5]-ANG II, and to a lesser extent [Ile^5]-ANG III upon rechromatography on two different HPLC systems [58]. Concentrations per gram brain tissue vary between 50 and 500 fmol and are thus in a similar order of magnitude as in the plasma. The recovery of ANG was carefully monitored using ^{125}J-labelled peptide and was found stable at $62.4 \pm 1.5\%$. The relatively constant ratio between [Ile^5]-ANG I and [Ile^5]-ANG II of less than 1 in the hypothalamus confirms that the extraction rate is similar for both peptides. This also supports previously reported data, namely that brain angiotensin does not originate from the plasma since the ratio of [Ile^5]-ANG I [Ile^5]-ANG II in the plasma is above 1.

The dissimilarity of the [Ile^5]-ANG I over [Ile^5]-ANG II ratio in plasma and in brain, apart from the intracellular localization of the peptide and its increase after nephrectomy, is an additional argument speaking against the uptake of angiotensin from plasma into the brain and in favor of local synthesis of the peptide. The immunohistochemical data reported previously [13, 57] are thus strengthened by these biochemical results. When the converting-enzyme inhibitor Captopril was given intracerebroventricularly to nephrectomized rats, an increase of ANG I has been measured in the brain. This confirms that ANG I is being generated endogenously in the brain and shows that the peptide acumulates if its conversion to ANG II is blocked.

In summary, [Ile^5]-ANG I, [Ile^5]-ANG II, and [Ile^5]-ANG III have been identified in the brain and CSF of rats and in human CSF. This solves the controversy as to whether angiotensin is present in the brain and supports the idea that the brain renin-angiotensin system is active *in vivo*.

In vivo function of the brain ras

To answer the question of the functional significance of the brain renin-angiotensin system, two questions needed to be answered: 1) Do the components of this enzyme-peptide system interact *in vivo,* and is angiotensin being formed under physiologic conditions through hydrolysis of angiotensinogen by renin? 2) Is the pharmacologic interference with the biosynthesis or with the action of endogenous brain angiotensin followed by a biologic effect on, for example, blood pressure? Part of these questions have been discussed in previous sections of this review. Additional evidence will be described below.

Brain renin from various species, purified by different procedures and tested under varying *in vitro* assay conditions, differ in their pH optimum of enzyme activity. To answer the first question, and to test whether these enzymes can cleave ANG I from endogenous brain angiotensinogen under physiologic conditions, we have elaborated an '*in vivo* test' of enzyme activity [40]. For this, a permanent cannula was implanted into the lateral brain ventricle of rats, and purified renin from various sources was injected into the CSF. Due to the high angiotensinogen concentrations, ANG I will be locally formed if the enzyme is active. ANG I will then be converted into ANG II by brain CE. The *in vivo* activity of an enzyme preparation can thus be tested by its bochemical activity, that is, by the increase of CSF ANG I and ANG II and by the decrease of angiotensinogen concentration, all of which can be measured precisely after withdrawal of CSF at different time intervals following injection of the enzyme. The biologic effects of the newly generated brain angiotensin on drinking and on blood pressure can also be measured.

It was found that renin from human, rat, and mouse brain, from mouse submaxillary gland, and from hog and mouse kidney clearly exhibited biologic and biochemical activity in this '*in vivo* enzyme-activity test' paradigm [5, 38, 40, 54]. All enzymes tested led to increases of angiotensin I formation and simultaneous decrease of CSF angiotensin concentrations, and they induced drinking and pituitary hormone release, increase of sympathetic tone, and pressor responses. These biologic effects could be inhibited by central angiotensin receptor blockade with saralasin and by blockade of the brain CE. It was thus concluded that brain renin is active *in vivo* like kidney renin and produces biologic effects specific for ANG II [40].

Cathepsin-like enzymes were also tested in this *in vivo* enzyme assay. They were not active at the concentrations used. This does not exclude the possibility, however, that they could generate ANG I *in vivo* in the brain. It has, indeed, been hypothesized that two different types of enzymes may be active intracellularly and extracellularly. Like kidney renin, so-called 'true' brain renin might be segregated in certain conditions (e.g., hypertension) and initiate a neurohormonal action of the brain RAS. This would be analogous to renin secretion from the kidney into the blood following, e.g., renal artery stenosis.

In addition to this hormonal action, kidney renin is believed to have a local role in the kidney. In the brain, most of the evidence available points in fact to a local intracellular role of the RAS. Here, an enzyme could be active in intracellular compartments with lower pH, and these enzymes may well have similarity to the cathepsins. The fact that several renin-like enzymes have been identified in the brain and that these may even vary from brain region to brain region certainly supports the conclusion that more than one enzyme has to be considered as ANG I-generating enzyme in the brain as well as in other tissues.

Pharmacologic interference with the brain RAS was chosen as an approach to answer the second question as to whether or not this system was involved in blood pressure regulation. When the angiotensin II-receptor blocker saralasin was injected into the brain ventricles of spontaneously hypertensive rats of the stroke-prone strain (SHRSP), a significant and dose-dependent decrease of blood pressure was observed [59-61]. This effect was not due to inhibition of plasma angiotensin, because the central blood pressure-lowering action of saralasin persisted after nephrectomy, and because intravenous administration of even higher doses of saralasin did not cause a decrease but, in contrast, an increase of blood pressure [61]. The latter can be explained by the low plasma renin levels in SHRSP when tested at the age of 4 to 8 months [13, 59].

In separate experiments, saralasin was not injected but, instead, was continuously infused into the brain ventricles during 6 days, using osmotic mini-infusion pumps. Blood pressure decreased to nearly normotensive levels in SHRSP [59, 60]. In view of the increased renin activity in certain brain areas [43], but not in the plasma of SHRSP, these results are in harmony with the concept that the brain participates in the maintenance of high blood pressure in these rats, and that the observed decrease of blood pressure was due to blockade of a stimulated brain RAS in SHRSP [59].

Recent results with the CE inhibitor Captopril corroborate this conclusion [34, 62]. When low doses of Captopril were injected into the brain ventricles of SHRSP, a significant fall of blood pressure was observed. The brain CE activity was blocked by 70% at this dose centrally, while under the same conditions plasma CE activity remained unchanged. It can therefore be concluded that the lowering of blood pressure in SHRSP by central Captopril was brought about by the inhibition of brain ANG II biosynthesis. Several other authors have reached the same conclusions, and similar blood pressure-lowering effects, as described with centrally applied angiotensin receptor blockers and converting enzyme inhibitors, have also been observed with the renin inhibitor pepstatin [5, 60, 63].

Pharmacologic inhibition of the brain RAS appears also to affect other biologic functions such as thirst, memory, and pain, the possible significance of which is discussed elsewhere [42, 47, 64-68].

450

The first publications on the presence of renin, angiotensinogen, and angiotensin-like material in brain tissue appeared about ten years ago [1-4]. This coincided with the discovery of new biological actions of angiotensin on the brain [64]. The possibility that angiotensin could be generated within the brain itself had, therefore, exciting implications. The hypothesis of the existence of a complete endogenous RAS in the brain did not remain unchallenged, and for several years there was ardent discussion on whether such a RAS existed in the brain or not [6, 8, 14].

Several components of the RAS have not been dealt with in this paper at all, but the data briefly discussed above show that many of the questions have been answered positively by experimental results.

More detailed reviews have recently been published [5, 11, 43, 61, 69, 70]. Major advances have been made with respect to the characterization of the brain RAS and definition of its ANG II-generating pathway. In fact, our knowledge of the brain RAS appears to be more advanced in several aspects than other brain peptides, where in general, little is known on the biosynthetic pathways or on methods of specific pharmacologic intervention. The enzymes, high-molecular-weight precursor proteins, and the effector peptides, as well as the receptors, are well characterized now for the brain RAS. Pharmacological agents that interfere specifically with the system *in vivo* are known. In this respect, the RAS may be considered a model for enzyme-peptide systems in the brain. This is not to say that all problems are solved and all questions are answered, but the present state of the art makes us confident that the past research efforts in this field were worthwile and that there are many years of fruitful research ahead of us.

ACKNOWLEDGMENT

This work was supported by the Deutsche Forschungsgemeinschaft, Sonderforschungsbereich 90, Cardiovasculäres System.

The secretarial help of Mrs. I. Rüchler is gratefully acknowledged.

REFERENCES

1. Fischer-Ferraro C, Nahmod VE, Goldstein DJ, et al.: Angiotensin and renin in rat and dog brain. J Exp Med 133:353-361, 1971.
2. Ganten D: Studies on the Existence of an Independent Brain Renin-Angiotensin System: A Model for Extrarenal Tissue Renin, thesis. McGill University, Montreal, Canada, 1972.
3. Ganten D, Marquez-Julia A, Granger P, et al.: Renin in dog brain. Am J Physiol 221:1733-1737, 1971.
4. Ganten D, Minnich JL, Granger P, et al.: Angiotensin-forming enzyme in brain tissue. Science 173:64-65, 1971.

5. Printz MP, Ganten D, Unger TH, et al.: Minireview: The brain renin angiotensin system 1982, in Ganten D, Printz MP, Phillips MI, et al. (editors): Experimental Brain Research, Suppl 4: The Renin Angiotensin System in the Brain. Heidelberg, Springer Verlag, 1981, pp 3-52.

6. Hackenthal E, Hackenthal R, Hilgenfeld U: Purification and partial characterization of rat brain protease (isorenin). Biochem Biophys Acta 522:561-573, 1978.

7. Reid IA, Day RP: Interactions and properties of some components of the renin-angiotensin system in brain, in Buckley JP, Ferrario CM (editors): Central Actions of Angiotensin and Related Hormones. New York, Pergamon Press, 1977, pp 267-282.

8. Reid IA, Brownfield MS: The brain renin angiotensin system: Some unresolved problems, in Ganten D, Printz MP, Phillips MI, et al. (editors): Experimental Brain Research, Suppl 4: The Renin Angiotensin System in the Brain. Heidelberg, Springer Verlag, 1981, pp 284-293.

9. Slater EE, Defendini R, Zimmermann EA: Wide distribution of immunoreactive renin in nerve cells of human brain. Proc Natl Acad Sci USA 77:5458-5460, 1980.

10. Celio MR, Clemens DL, Inagami T: Renin in anterior pituitary, pineal and neuronal cells of mouse brain. Biomed Res 1:427-431, 1980.

11. Deboben A, Inagami T, Ganten D: Tissue renin, in Genest J, Kuchel O, Hamet P, et al. (editors): Hypertension, Physiopathology and Treatment. New York, McGraw-Hill Book Co., 1977, pp 240-256.

12. Fuxe K, Ganten D, Hokfelt T, et al.: Renin-like immunocytochemical activity in rat and mouse brain. Neurosci Lett 18:245-250, 1980.

13. Ganten D, Fuxe K, Phillips MI, et al.: The brain isorenin angiotensin system: Biochemistry, localization, and possible role in drinking and blood pressure regulation, in Ganong WF, Martini L (editors): Frontiers in Neuroendocrinology. New York, Raven Press, 1978, vol 5, pp 61-99.

14. Ganten D: Is there a brain iso-renin angiotensin system? Circ Res 42(5):732-733, 1978.

15. Hirose S, Yokosawa H, Inagami T: Immunochemical identification of renin in rat brain and distinction from acid proteases. Nature 274:392-393, 1978.

16. Hirose S, Workman RJ, Inagami T: Specific antibody to hog renal renin and its application to the direct radioimmunoassay of renin in various organs. Circ Res 45:275-279, 1979.

17. Hirose S, Yokosawa H, Inagami T, et al.: Renin and prorenin in hog brain: Ubiquitous distribution and high concentration in the pituitary and pineal. Brain Res 191:489-499, 1980.

18. Hirose S, Naruse M, Ohtsuki K, et al.: Totally inactive renin zymogen and different forms of active renin in hog brain tissues. J Biol Chem 256:5572-5576, 1981.

19. Hirose S, Ohsawa T, Murakami K, et al.: Pituitary renin: Purification and characterization, in Ganten D, Printz MP, Phillips MI, et al. (editors): Experimental Brain Research, Suppl 4: The Renin Angiotensin System in the Brain. Heidelberg, Springer Verlag, 1982, pp 53-63.

20. Inagami T, Clemens DL, Celio MR, et al.: Immunohistochemical localization of renin in mouse brain. Neurosci Lett 18:91-98, 1980.

21. Printz MP, Printz JM, Gregory TJ: Identification of angiotensinogen in animal brain homogenates. Circ Res 42(Suppl I):21-27, 1978.

22. Printz MP, Lewicki JA, Wallis CJ: Brain angiotensinogen: Origin and evidence for an influence by adrenal corticosteroids, in Gross F, Vogel G (editors): Enzymatic Release of Vasoactive Peptides. New York, Raven Press, 1980, pp 193-207.

23. Printz MP, Gregory TJ: Brain angiotensinogen: Evidence for an independent and functional central angiotensin system, in Buckley JP, Ferrario CM (editors): Central Nervous System Mechanisms in Hypertension. New York, Raven Press, 1981, pp 311-326.

24. Morris BJ, Reid IA: The distribution of angiotensinogen in dog brain studied by cell fractionation. Endocrinology 103:492-500, 1978.

25. Smeby RR, Husain A, Speth RC: Properties and subcellular localization of brain renin and its substrate, in Ganten D, Printz MP, Phillips MI, et al. (editors): Experimental Brain Research. The Renin-Angiotensin System: A Model for the Synthesis of Peptides in the Brain. Heidelberg, Springer-Verlag, 1982.

26. Schelling P, Ganten U, Sponer G, et al.: Components of the reninangiotensin system in the cerebrospinal fluid of rats and dogs with special consideration of the origin and the fate of angiotensin II. Neuroendocrinology 31:297-308, 1980.

27. Schelling P, Felix D, Liard JF: Regulation of angiotensinogen in cerebrospinal fluid and plasma: Some regulatory aspects, in Ganten D, Printz MP, Phillips MI, et al. (editors): Experimental Brain Research, Suppl 4: The Renin Angiotensin System in the Brain. Heidelberg, Springer Verlag, 1982, pp 178-191.

28. Arregui A, Barer GR: Chronic hypoxia in rats: Alterations in striato-nigral angiotensin converting enzyme, GABA, and glutamic acid decarboxylase. J Neurochem 34:740-743, 1980.

29. Arregui A, Iversen LL; Angiotensin converting enzyme: Presence of high activity in chorioid plexus of mammalian brain. Eur J Pharmacol 52:147-150, 1978.

30. Benuck M, Berg MJ, Marks N: A distinct peptidyl dipeptidase that degrades enkephalins: Exceptionally high activity in rabbit kidney. Life Sci 28:2643-2650, 1981.

31. Couture R, Regoli D: Inactivation of substance P and its C-terminal fragments in rat plasma and its inhibition by Captopril. Can J Physiol Pharmacol 59:621-625, 1981.

32. Depierre D, Roth U: Fluorometric determination of dipeptidylcarboxypeptidase (angiotensin I converting enzyme). Enzyme 19:65-70, 1975.

33. Erdos EG: Angiotensin I converting enzyme. Circ Res 36(2):247-254, 1975.

34. Unger T, Kaufmann-Buhler I, Scholkens B, et al.: Brain converting enzyme inhibition: A possible mechanism for the antihypertensive action of captopril in spontaneously hypertensive rats. Eur J Pharmacol 70:467-478, 1981.

35. Rix E, Ganten D, Schull B, et al.: Converting enzyme in the chorioid plexus, brain and kidney. Immunocytochemical and biochemical studies in rats. Neurosci Lett 22:125-130, 1981.

36. Semple PF, Macrae WA, Morton JJ: Angiotensin II in human cerebrospinal fluid may be an immunoassay artifact. Clin Sci 59:61s-64s, 1980.

37. Dzau VJ: Isolation and regulation of brain renin, in Ganten D, Printz MP, Phillips MI, et al. (editors): Experimental Brain Research, Suppl 4: The Renin Angiotensin System in the Brain. Heidelberg, Springer Verlag, 1981, pp 92-108.

38. Ganten D, Speck G: The brain renin-angiotensin system: A model for the synthesis of peptides in the brain. Biochem Pharmacol 27:2379-2389, 1978.

39. Osman MY, Smeby RR, Sen S: Separation of dog brain renin-like activity from acid protease activity. Hypertension 1:53-60, 1979.

40. Speck G, Poulsen K, Unger T, et al.: In vivo activity of purified mouse brain renin. Brain Res 219:371-384, 1981.

41. Naruse K, Takii Y, Inagami T: Immunohistochemical localization of renin in luteinizing-hormone containing cells of rat pituitary. Proc Natl Acad Sci USA (in press).

42. Haulica I, Petresu G, Stratone A, et al.: Possible functions of brain renin, in Ganten D, Printz MP, Phillips MI, et al. (editors): Experimental Brain Research, Suppl 4: The Renin Angiotensin System in the Brain. Heidelberg, Springer Verlag, 1981, pp 335-352.

43. Schelling P, Speck G, Unger T, et al.: The brain angiotensin system: Biochemistry, localization and functional aspects, in Parvez H, Parvez S (editors): Advances in Experimental Medicine: A Centenary Tribute to Claude Bernard. Amsterdam, Elsevier/North Holland, 1980, pp 243-288.

44. Yang H-Y, Neff NH: Distribution and properties of angiotensin converting enzyme of rat brain. J Neurochem 19:243-250, 1972.

45. Brecher P, Tercyak A, Chobanian A: Properties of angiotensin converting enzyme in intact cerebral microvessels. Hypertension 3:198-204, 1981.

46. Gimbrone MA, Majeau GR, Atkinson WJ, et al.: Angiotensin converting enzyme activity in isolated brain microvessels. Life Sci 25:1075-1084, 1979.

47. Barney CC, Katovich MJ, Fregly MJ: The effect of acute administration of an angiotensin converting enzyme inhibitor, Captopril (SQ14225) on experimentally induced thirst in rats. J Pharmacol Exp Ther 212:53-57, 1980.

48. Chen FM, Hawkins R, Printz MP: Evidence for a functional independent brain angiotensin system. Correlation between brain angiotensin receptors, angiotensin and drinking in the estrous cycle of rats, in Ganten D, Printz MP, Phillips MI, et al. (editors): Experimental Brain Research, Suppl 4: The Renin Angiotensin System in the Brain. Heidelberg, Springer Verlag, 1982, pp 157-168.

49. Lewicki JA, Fallon JH, Printz MP: Regional distribution of angiotensinogen in rat brain. Brain Res 158:359-371, 1978.

50. Gregory TJ, Wallis CJ, Printz MP: Regional changes in rat brain angiotensin following bilateral nephrectomy. Hypertension (submitted for publication).

51. Wallis CJ, Printz MP: Adrenal regulation of regional brain angiotensinogen content. Endocrinology 106:337-342, 1980.

52. Wallis CJ, Gregory TJ, Printz MP: (submitted for publication).

53. Sernia C, Reid IA: Release of angiotensinogen by rat brain in vitro. Brain Res 192:217-225, 1980.

54. Reid IA, Ramsay DJ: The effects of intracerebroventricular administration of renin on drinking and blood pressure. Endocrinology 97:536-542, 1975.

55. Eggena P, Ito T, Barrett ID, et al.: A comparison of human renin substrate in plasma and cerebrospinal fluid, in Ganten D, Printz MP, Phillips MI, et al. (editors): Experimental Brain Research, Suppl 4: The Renin Angiotensin System in the Brain. Heidelberg, Springer Verlag, 1982, pp 169-172.

56. Ito T, Eggena P, Barrett JP, et al.: Studies on angiotensinogen of plasma and cerebrospinal fluid in normal and hypertensive human subjects. Hypertension 2:432-436, 1980.

57. Phillips MI, Quinlan JT, Weyhenmeyer J; An angiotensin-like peptide in the brain. Life Sci 27:2589-2594, 1980.

58. Hermann K, Ganten D, Bayer C, et al.: Definitive evidence for the presence of Ile[5]-angiotensin I and Ile[5]-angiotensin II in the brain of rats, in Ganten D, Printz MP, Phillips MI, et al. (editors): Experimental Brain Research, Suppl 4: The Renin Angiotensin System in the Brain. Heidelberg, Springer Verlag, 1982, pp 112-207.

59. Ganten D, Unger T, Rockhold R, et al.: Central peptidergic stimulation: Its possible contribution to blood pressure regulation, in Albertini A, Daprada M, Peskar BA (editors): Radioimmunoassay of Drugs and Hormones in Cardiovascular Medicine. Amsterdam, Elsevier/North Holland, 1979, pp 33-43.

60. McDonald WJ, Aumann SK: Centrally administered angiotensin antagonists in hypertensive rats, in Ganten D, Printz MP, Phillips MI, et al. (editors): Experimental Brain Research, Suppl 4: The Renin Angiotensin System in the Brain. Heidelberg, Springer Verlag, 1981, pp 311-323.

61. Phillips MI, Weyhenmeyer J, Felix D, et al.: Evidence for an endogenous brain renin-angiotensin system. Fed Proc 38:2260-2266, 1979.

62. Stamler JF, Brody MJ, Phillips MI: The central and peripheral effects of captopril (SQ 14, 225) on the arterial pressure of the spontaneously hypertensive rat. Brain Res 186:499-503, 1980.

63. Tonnaer JADM, Wiegant VM, De Jong W: Angiotensin generation in the brain and drinking: Indications for the involvement of endopeptidase activity distinct from cathepsin D. Brain Res 226: (in press).

64. Buckely JP, Smookler HH, Severs WB, et al.: A central site of action of angiotensin II and its possible role in the central regulation of the cardiovascular system, in Buckley JP, Ferrario CM (editors): Central Actions of Angiotensin and Related Hormones. New York, Pergamon Press, 1978, pp 149-155.

65. Camacho A, Phillips MI: Separation of drinking and pressor responses to central angiotensin by monoamines. Am J Physiol 240:R106-R113, 1981.

66. Fitzsimons JT: Angiotensin stimulation of the central nervous system. Rev Physiol Biochem Pharmacol 87:117-167, 1980.

67. Koller M, Krause HP, Hoffmeister F, et al.: Endogenous brain angiotensin II disrupts passive avoidance behaviour in rats. Neurosci Lett 14:71-75, 1979.

68. Severs WB, Summy-Long J, Taylor JS, et al.: A central effect of angiotensin: Release of pituitary pressor material. J Pharmacol Exp Ther 174:27-34, 1970.
69. Phillips MI: Angiotensin in the brain. Neuroendocrinology 25:354-377, 1978.
70. Sirett NE, McLean AS, Bray JJ, et al.: Distribution of angiotensin II receptors in rat brain. Brain Res 122:299-312, 1977.

DISCUSSION

Discussants: Haber, Ganten, Inagami, Laragh, Corvol, Denton, Palkovits

Haber: There's an interesting issue which should be emphasized in the difference between the renin system as elaborated by the kidney and utilized in the plasma and in the brain, as you demonstrated today. The brain system seems to generate all of its angiotensin intracellularly. At least - you've demonstrated the presence of angiotensin intracellularly. Presumably, the enzyme renin and its substrate are also there, and angiotensin is then released from dendrites in order to stimulate other cells. None of the components exist extracellularly except perhaps converting enzyme, which I think I've seen you demonstrate on the outside of cells, whereas in the more classical renal system everything happens in free solution in the plasma. Do you think that there's any action at all in the central nervous system that occurs extracellularly?

Ganten: Yes, I do believe so. I believe that the brain renin system may function in a similar dual way as the renal renin system i.e., as a local system and as a true hormonal system. There is now good evidence to show that in the kidney there is a local renin system, but in emergency situations such as hemorrhage or sodium depletion, you have a stimulated release of the local kidney renin into the blood. In analogy to the kidney, the brain renin angiotensin system may be mainly a local enzyme-peptide system, but under certain conditions its components, especially the effector peptide angiotensin II, may get into the extracellular space and exert neurohormonal effects. In the New Zealand strain of hypertensive rats and in some human essential hypertensive patients, for example, elevated CSF angiotensin levels have been reported. So, in certain situations the local brain system may also be active extracellularly.

Inagami: I would like to respond to Dr. Haber's question. Studies on neuroblastoma show that true cells contain all the components of the renin-angiotensin system within the neuroblastoma, except that the substrate seems to be leaking out rather easily compared with the other components. We are not completely sure about the substrate, but I would like to believe that reactions take place within the cells.

Laragh: Apropos of that, though, didn't you show that there is both renin substrate and angiotensin in the CSF in significant concentrations?

Ganten: Yes, angiotensinogen is present in the CSF in very high concentrations.

Laragh: That being true, it isn't clear that the reaction is always intracellular, is it?

Ganten: No, not necessarily always. It is well possible that the reaction also occurs extracellularly, though renin is rarely detected in the CSF, and whenever it is detected, it is so low that I'm not quite sure whether this may be contamination from ependymal cells.

Laragh: Yes, but everything else is outside, right?

Ganten: No, everything else is inside the cells.

Laragh: No, no.

Ganten: Only, angiotensinogen has been demonstrated to exist outside the cells in the CSF. But angiotensinogen also occurs intracellularly, as Dr. Pruite has shown.

Laragh: Well, granted it's inside, but substrate is also outside the cell. And you find angiotensin II outside too. The circulating blood *in vivo* is full of renin, and in certain places it would get in contact with the areas that we know about, say the area of postrema. In other places, renin might get through the blood-brain barrier from the kidney, right?

Ganten: It is theoretically possible that, for example, in the area of postrema, which has no blood-brain barrier, circulating renin might come into contact with CSF angiotensinogen. But, the anatomical situation and the biochemical evidence is really against it, because there has never been a correlation between plasma renin or plasma angiotensin and CSF renin or CSF angiotensin or angiotensinogen. Rather, there is a reverse correlation. There is frequently a kind of negative feedback between the plasma and the brain renin angiotensin system.

Laragh: I think you've got a very convincing story, but still you've only got 24- to 48-hour postnephrectomized dogs, and renin can have a long half-life, especially perhaps in brain tissues, so that conceivably it is all exported there from the kidneys. I'd be happier if you had one group of experiments where they've been nephrectomized for three or four weeks. You know, anything might survive after nephrectomy for a day or so. It looks like the brain makes renin. You've got a very good story. But the ultimate proof may still be lacking.

Ganten: Well, we have had dogs in Montreal that survived nephrectomy for 10 to 14 days, and renin was still at control levels or even above in the brain. This was done, however, with a different methodology. So, I'm not sure whether we really measured the same renin as we measure now. In any case, I don't think that the nephrectomy experiments would really solve the problem and add much to what we already know. I'm convinced that renin and any protein, if it is well compartmentalized, can stay in the tissue for quite a long time, and I would not be more convinced after 14 days of nephrectomy than I am after three days. I don't think that really matters any more. The key issue, I believe, is the question as to whether the system is active *in vivo* or not, and this is independent of the question of whether the components are synthesized locally or not. In addition, of course, Dr. Murakami has recently reported definite proof that the amino acid sequence of brain renin is different from kidney renin. This shows that the enzyme is not simply taken up from the plasma but synthesized locally in the brain, and this also supports previous data on physicochemical differences between brain renin and plasma renin.

Laragh: Yes, I still think the other question is important - how it got there. One final question: When captopril lowers blood pressure in people or animals, to what extent is the central action relevant, or doesn't captopril get into the nervous system cells?

Ganten: Well, that's a difficult question. First of all, in order for captopril to have central effects, it doesn't have to get into the brain because circulating angiotensin has central effects. So, part of the captopril-lowering actions may be brought about by inhibition of plasma angiotensin effects on the brain. Secondly, we find changes in the activity of the brain renin angiotensin system following chronic oral captopril treatment and other converting enzyme inhibitors. This indicates that at least there are specific effects of the oral converting enzyme inhibitor treatment on the brain renin angiotensin system. All the observed changes point to a reduction of angiotensin II synthesis also in the brain.

Some data indicate that lipophilic compounds such as the Japanese SA446 do penetrate into the brain rather freely, and radioactivity has been picked up following oral treatment. In addition, central renin or angiotensin I reponses are withheld following oral converting enzyme inhibitor treatment. So I think the evidence is quite good that some of the compounds do penetrate into the brain. This does not answer the question, however, whether the blood-pressure-lowering effects of captopril, for example, are brought about by such central effects, such as in the low-renin hypertensives.

Corvol: It is usually assumed that converting enzyme is not a limiting step for the formation of angiotensin II in the plasma. What do you think about the renin angiotensin system in the brain? Do you think that the converting enzyme is or is not a rate-limiting step, especially when you see this very localized distribution of converting enzyme compared to the wide distribution of renin or angiotensin II?

Ganten: There's one piece of evidence that converting enzyme can be the rate-limiting step: If we take our *in vivo* enzyme activity paradigm and inject renin into the lateral brain ventricle, we get immediate angiotensin I generation. Angiotensin II generation lags behind, and this gap between angiotensin I and angiotensin II probably reflects the rate-limiting step of converting enzyme. But this is an artificial situation, of course. Renin is being injected into the cerebrospinal fluid in this experiment. We have no data so far, and it will be very difficult at the tissue level, the local level, to see whether angiotensin I is generated quickly and whether angiotensin II is lagging behind in the synthesis.

Inagami: In relation to your comment about the interaction of angiotensin II with GABA, you may have noticed that Haas in Zurich and we have also shown that the action of angiotensin II is to release inhibition of the neurons which is most likely due to the inhibitory action of GABA.

Ganten: Yes, our data fit very well with those reported by Haas and co-workers.

Denton: I noticed you used the term physiological at one stage in dealing with renin of the brain, or it may have been angiotensin in relation to its biological action. I think that about 50 actions have been reported for angiotensin, and quite a large number of them in the central nervous system. For example, recently there has been a proposal that renin or angiotensin injected into the cerebrospinal fluid in very large amounts can induce salt appetite. Against that background, I was wondering what sort of concept would you have of the biological observation that an animal may be depleted of water or salt and selectively in a cafeteria situation drink water or salt? Alternatively, it may be depleted of both water and salt, and then it will select one and then the other in whichever order it finds them. I was wondering, in this sort of a biological situation how you'd conceive a change - for example, in generation of angiotensin of the brain - contriving the sort of level of specificity of choice under these conditions.

Ganten: To answer that question, one really would have to be able to measure the activity of the renin angiotensin system in the tissue strictly quantitatively. At the present time, I do not think it's possible. We can measure specific renin, so-called 'true renin,' separately from other angiotensin-generating enzymes. We can measure converting enzyme, but not very specifically, and we can extract angiotensin from the brain. The clue to your question, however, would be quantitative measurements of brain angiotensin II in various pathophysiological states, as you mentioned. This hasn't been possible so far, so I can't really answer your question. I believe personally, to elaborate on that a little bit more philosophically, that it may be a mistake to look at brain angiotensin only in the context in which we are used to thinking of the kidney renin angiotensin system. Certainly, in certain pathophysiological situations as you mentioned, brain angiotensin seems to have similar effects as circulating angiotensin, e.g., stimulation of thirst and salt appetite. I certainly believe that brain angiotensin is also important for blood pressure control, because we don't know of any other peptide that leads to increase of blood pressure peripherally and centrally and is as potent as angiotensin II. If you take substance P for example, it is blood-pressure-decreasing peripherally and blood-pressure-increasing centrally. If you take kinins, they're equally blood-pressure-decreasing peripherally, but again blood-pressure-increasing centrally. If you take the opioid peptides, it's a very complex story which I can't go into detail now, but clearly they have both blood-pressure-decreasing and blood-pressure-increasing potential. Thus, angiotensin is the only peptide I can think of that acts synergistically, centrally, and peripherally with respect to volume homeostasis and blood pressure. This probably represents an important part of brain angiotensin effects, but I certainly believe it's not the only possible biological action of brain angiotensin. Studies have been done on angiotensin effects on memory, but I don't know how relevant they are pathophysiologically.

Denton: Can I put the question in another way? If renin or angiotensin will produce a specific physiological effect when they are infused into or injected into the lateral ventricle and one can block that effect with saralasin, would it be a reasonable assumption that saralasin is getting to the site where the angiotensin is acting to produce the behavioral effect? If so - if one then compares that situation with a physiological indication of the behavior such as salt appetite in sodium deficiency - would you then expect that saralasin introduced into the ventricle would similarly block the behavior?

Ganten: That's a question concerning exogenous angiotensin versus endogenous angiotensin effects, isn't it?

Denton: It's presumptive, yes. I'm asking the question, why saralasin introduced into the ventricle does not modify salt appetite evoked by sodium deficiency.

Ganten: I think there is a problem if you try to compare blockage of exogenously administered peptides with endogenously generated peptides. There appear to be different pathways involved. We have tried to block exogenously infused angiotensin peripherally with saralasin, and in parallel experiments we tried to block the circulating endogenous angiotensin. The results indicated that we need much higher doses, 10 to 50 times higher doses of the angiotensin receptor antagonist to block the endogenous system versus the exogenous system. In analogy, the receptor availability for the agonists and antagonists given exogenously may be even more complex at the brain level with the various sites of action and the various possibilities of interaction. So I know that there are these discrepancies to which you alluded. I can't explain why they occur at the present time, but I am not surprised.

Palkovits: You mentioned a high concentration of angiotensin in the hypothalamus, especially in the median eminence. What is the final destination of the angiotensin from here? We know only three ways – but three different ways. Could it be the neuroendocrine adenohypophysis, or the posterior pituitary, or the cerebrospinal fluid? What do you think?

Ganten: What about if it stays there, where it is?

Palkovits: The median eminence could not be the final destination. From the median eminence, it should get somewhere. Which of the three ways? What do you think?

Ganten: I don't know. I could imagine that it stays where it is locally.

Palkovits: The median eminence is only a pathway to the anterior pituitary or the posterior pituitary, or to the cerebrospinal fluid. There are only fibers and vessels there, so the median eminence could not be a target site. To where from here? – that's my question.

Ganten: I can't answer your question. Of course, angiotensin-positive material has been observed in the anterior and posterior pituitary, and angiotensin releases ACTH, antidiuretic hormone and, as Dr. Lang has recently shown, oxytocin. So the pituitary gland is a definite target organ for angiotensin in the median eminence.

IV. RENAL, ADRENAL, AND CENTRAL HORMONES IN HYPERTENSION

Jacques Genest and John H. Laragh

INTRODUCTION

The topics discussed in this section are not only most relevant to the pathophysiology of hypertension, but have also been especially productive for providing new insights into understanding mechanisms, thereby providing new strategies for treatment, as well.

As one can appreciate by scanning the titles of the topics discussed in this section, there are many hormonal mechanisms of great relevance involved in human hypertensive disorders. Indeed, in the past, whenever we have understood the cause or pathogenesis of a hypertensive condition, it has in fact turned out to be due to a hormonal abnormality. One need not cite compelling examples of this – Cushing's syndrome, primary aldosteronism or Conn's syndrome, and renovascular or Goldblatt hypertension.

In this section, exciting information is presented, which highlights to an increasing degree the important role of hormones in that still unsolved residue, that large group of people with so-called 'essential' hypertension. The participatory or pathogenic role of the renin-angiotensin-aldosterone system, of the brain hormones, vasopressin pro-opio-melanocortin and ACTH, of kidney tumors such as the renomedullary interstitial cell substance, and of as yet unidentified but potent adrenocortical mineralocorticoids are critically examined. Another topic that pervades the discussion is the often important role of sodium as a substrate for hypertensive mechanisms and of arteriolar vasoconstriction as a final determinant.

We are most pleased to present these provocative topics for your consideration. We can only hope that what is contained herein will lead to further fruitful studies to bring us ever closer to a final solution for at least another portion of the large problem of human hypertension.

A BIPOLAR ANALYSIS OF BLOOD PRESSURE PHENOMENA: THE VASOCONSTRICTION AND VOLUME FACTORS IN NORMOTENSION AND IN THE SPECTRUM OF HYPERTENSIVE DISORDERS AS REVEALED BY RENIN-SODIUM PROFILING OR PHARMACOLOGIC PROBES; PRORENIN AS A DETERMINANT OF RENIN SECRETION

JOHN H. LARAGH AND JEAN E. SEALEY

INTRODUCTION

Evidence from experiments in human hypertension and in animal models of the last 20 years has led us to formulate what we have called the vasoconstriction-volume hypothesis [1], an analytical approach that is useful clinically and conceptually. This hypothesis states that given normal cardiac function, the arterial blood pressure is ultimately determined by the reciprocal interplay of two factors: (1) the capacity and resistance of the contractile arterial chamber between the aortic valves and the capillaries, and (2) the volume of fluid in the chamber. The capacity can be defined as a function of the state of contractility, i.e., the degree of *vasoconstriction*. The total peripheral resistance also can be altered by changes in viscosity [2] or in arteriolar wall structure, but we assume that the dynamic changes observed are largely due to changes in the degree of vasoconstriction or dilation.

Long-term changes in *volume* are ordinarily determined on an osmotic basis by changes in the state of sodium balance. The critical volume is that in the arterial chamber, but this is only a small fraction of either the total blood volume or interstitial volume. However, for the most part, these volumes probably move together in the same directions.

To restate the situation, any given arterial pressure level is maintained by the contribution and interplay of these *vasoconstriction* and *volume* components, and any hypertensive state is maintained by excessive vasoconstriction or excessive volume or by an inappropriate excess of one relative to the other. It also follows that any induced change in blood pressure will be predicated on changes in one of these two factors. Although there are many external or afferent factors that can affect arterial hypertension, such as emotion, exercise, posture, catecholamines, peptide hormones, prostaglandins, cyclic AMP, venous return, or cardiac contraction, in the final analysis, if the blood pressure is to change, these various inputs must be translated into a quantitative change in either the vasoconstriction or the volume factor. Furthermore, if a stable pressure is to be restored, any change in either one of these two components of the basic blood pressure equation must sooner or later be countered by a reciprocal adjustment in the other. If this adjustment does not occur, an essential system of control has become inoperative, and a pathologic state exists.

The renin-angiotensin-aldosterone endocrine system imposes continuous surveillance over both the vasoconstriction and volume components of blood pressure, and by its secretions, adjusts one to suit the other in the service of homeostasis [3], reacting to all the physical and chemical inputs mentioned above. Because of its role as long-term governor of volume and vasoconstriction, this system participates in the pathologic states of hypertension, either primarily or as a secondary reactive response to defects elsewhere. Thus, to define the nature of the renin system participation in the hypertensive state is to probe the cause of the hypertension and thus to deduce specific therapeutic maneuvers.

This paper will address the pivotal role played by the renin-angiotensin-aldosterone system in a day-to-day regulation of blood pressure and in the pathogenesis of all forms of human hypertension. The elucidation of this endocrine control system in the last 20 years or so has enabled a clearer understanding of hypertensive phenomena, which collectively appear as a spectrum of disorders requiring differential diagnosis and different types of therapy. It is important to add that one of the most significant aspects of this new understanding is the recognition that the broad and indiscriminate entity termed 'essential hypertension' is not a single point on that spectrum but, rather, a considerable portion of it and is itself composed of physiologically different subunits.

THE RENIN SYSTEM DESCRIBED

The proteolytic enzyme renin is secreted into the plasma by the juxtaglomerular apparatus of the kidneys (Fig. 1). The signal for renin release appears to be a lowered renal perfusion [3-5]. When it is released in the bloodstream, renin encounters the substrate angiotensinogen, from which it splits off an inactive decapeptide, angiotensin I. During passage through the lungs, where a converting enzyme resides in unusually high concentration, the decapeptide is converted to the octapeptide angiotensin II, the first effector hormone of the system.

Angiotensin II has several effects that contribute to its pressor activity. First, it is a most potent circulating pressor agent, exerting a direct and powerful vasoconstrictive effect on the arteriolar bed. Second, it acts on the cortex of the adrenal gland to stimulate the production of the hormone aldosterone [6-9]. Aldosterone causes the kidney to retain sodium in exchange for potassium, thus raising extracellular and plasma fluid volume. Additional sodium retention and volume enhancement is achieved by a direct effect of angiotensin II, up to a certain dose level, on the kidneys to promote sodium reabsorption [10]. The sodium retained by all of these means amplifies the vascular sensitivity of the vasoconstrictive action of angiotensin II [9].

Renal perfusion pressure is restored by these hormonal events. This correction is detected by a renal arteriolar baroreceptor or a tubular chemoreceptor, and the

THE RENIN-ANGIOTENSIN-ALDOSTERONE SYSTEM

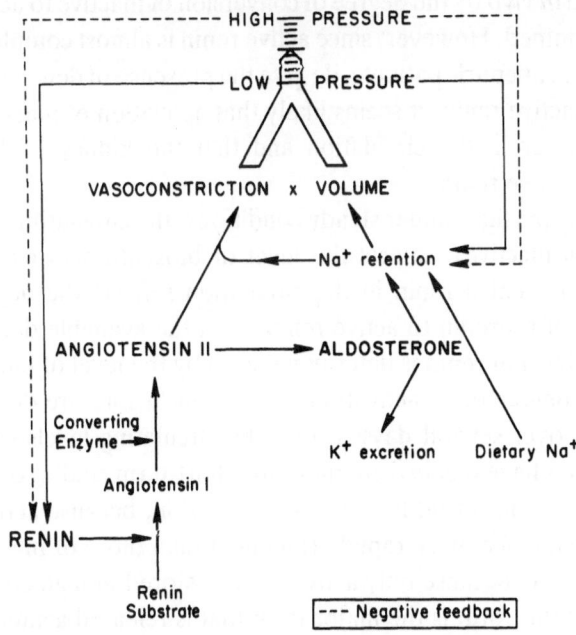

Figure 1. Renin-angiotensin-aldosterone system. Renin secreted in response to reduced arterial pressure on renal tubular sodium acts to release angiotensin II. Angiotensin II raises pressure and stimulates aldosterone secretion, leading to sodium and water retention and improved flow. These pressure and volume effects turn off more renin release. Dashed line indicates negative feedback. From Laragh, et al. [24].

signal for renin release is, in classic feedback fashion, turned off. Signals for turning renin release on or off also may be mediated in part by a renal beta-adrenergic receptor mechanism [11] connected to the autonomic and central nervous system and also in part by chemoreceptor sites sensitive to the renal tubular sodium supply in the region of the macula densa. Thus, the renin-angiotensin system responds to pressure and volume signals and negotiates its efferent control by acting on the two reciprocal supports of pressure – vaso-constriction and volume, a fine example of how hormonal changes can translate into mechanical events.

THE BIOCHEMICAL REGULATION OF RENIN PRODUCTION AND RELEASE: PRORENIN

Since the discovery that close to 90% of the circulating plasma renin is in an inactive form (i.e., prorenin), evidence has accumulated that renin is synthesized as a large-molecular-weight precursor and is converted to active renin prior to its secretion from the kidneys. While the biochemical evidence for this statement is far from complete, much of the data concerning inactive renin is consistent with such a view [12]. Whether regulation of the circulating level of active renin can be determined *in vivo* by the degree of conversion of inactive to active renin remains to be determined. However, since active renin is almost completely absent in the circulation of anephric patients, despite the presence of detectable but subnormal levels of inactive renin, it seems likely that activation of inactive renin does not normally occur in the circulation and that the kidney is the sole source of circulating active renin.

If one accepts that, under steady conditions, the circulating level of total renin (active plus inactive) reflects the level of biosynthesis of renin and that the proportion of active renin in the circulation reflects the degree of intrarenal conversion of prorenin to active renin, then the available data suggest that the circulating level of renin is determined both by the level of biosynthesis of renin and by the degree of its activation. These conclusions are derived from studies carried out over several days so that the circulating levels of both active and inactive renin have reached equilibrium. Short-term studies of circulating active and inactive renin reveal less useful information, because active renin levels in blood change much more rapidly (minutes) than those of inactive renin (days). This is probably because only active renin is stored in high concentration in the kidney, and this form is the major form that is released acutely.

Under most circumstances, when the circulating level of active renin changes, total renin changes in the same direction. For another example, long-term sodium depletion with diuretics causes an increase in both active and total renin, as does chronic treatment with the converting enzyme inhibitor, captopril [13]. Figure 2 illustrates the consistent relationship between plasma prorenin and active renin levels in a whole spectrum of human disorders and illustrates the marked increases in plasma prorenin levels that occurred in patients with renin-secreting tumors. Interestingly, as the levels of renin increase in the circulation, the proportion of active renin also increases, suggesting more efficient activation of prorenin. The opposite situation occurs in low-renin essential hypertension, in which the total renin level is low and the proportion of active renin is also subnormal [12]. The lowest levels of both active and total renin are found in patients with primary aldosteronism; these patients appear to have very low levels

→

Figure 2. Relationship between plasma active renin levels and the absolute level (A) or proportion (B) of plasma inactive renin. The solid circles labeled *A*, *B*, and *C* represent the three patients with renin-secreting malignancies. Solid dots represent normal subjects; open symbols, essential-hypertensive patients with low (□), normal (○), or high (△) renin-sodium profiles; solid squares, patients with aldosterone-producing adenomas; and solid triangles, patients with malignant or renovascular hypertensions. Lettered symbols refer to patients with other conditions associated with hyperreninemia; *a*, adrenocortical insufficiency; *b*, Bartter's syndrome; *c*, hepatic cirrhosis; *g*, ganglioneuroma; and *t*, trophoplastic disease. From Atlas SA, Hesson TE, Sealey JE, et al. Characterization of inactive renin ('prorenin') from renin-secreting tumors of non-renal origin: Similarity to inactive renin from kidney and normal plasma. (Submitted for publication).

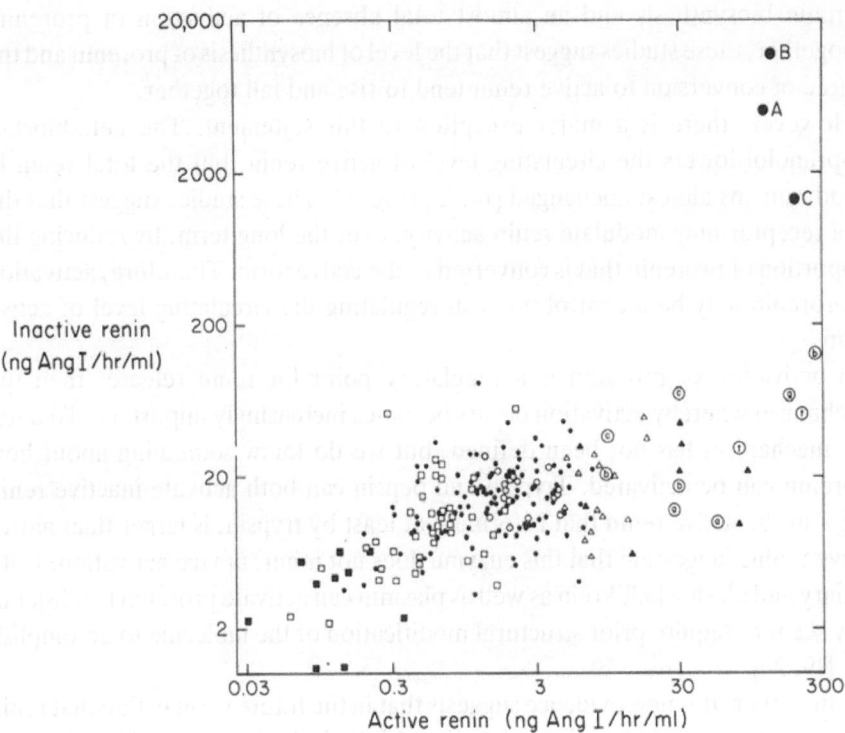

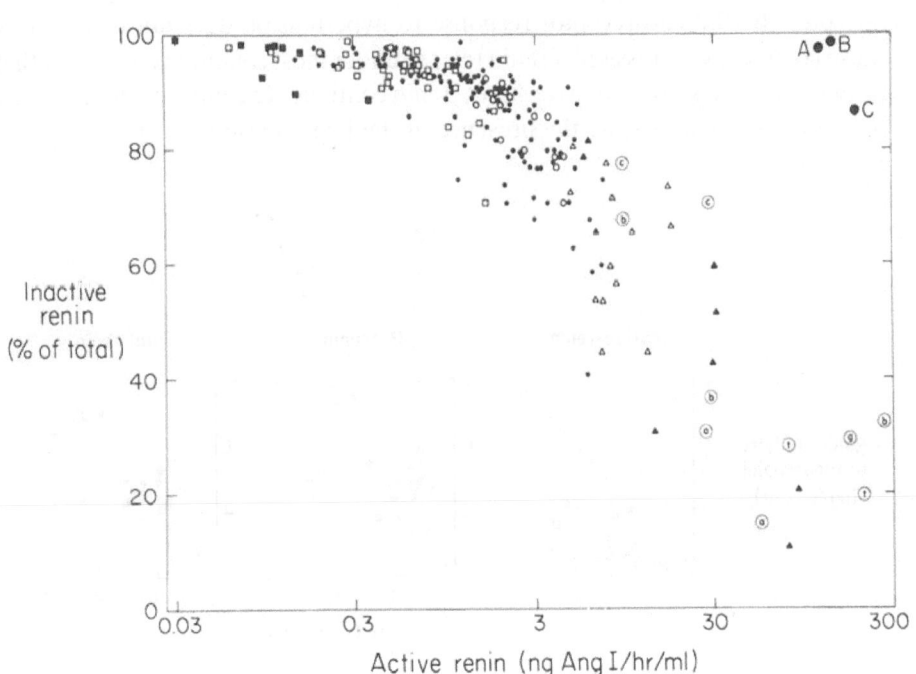

of renin biosynthesis and an almost total absence of activation of prorenin. Altogether, these studies suggest that the level of biosynthesis of prorenin and the degree of conversion to active renin tend to rise and fall together.

However, there is a major exception to this statement. The beta-blocker propranolol lowers the circulating level of active renin, but the total renin in blood remains almost unchanged [14, 15] (Fig. 3). These studies suggest that the beta receptor may modulate renin activity, over the long term, by reducing the proportion of prorenin that is converted to the active form. Therefore, activation of prorenin may be a control point in regulating the circulating level of active renin.

If activation of prorenin is a regulatory point for renin release, then the mechanism whereby activation occurs becomes increasingly important. To date, this mechanism has not been defined, but we do know something about how prorenin can be activated. Trypsin and pepsin can both activate inactive renin [16], but the active renin that is formed, at least by trypsin, is larger than native active renin, suggesting that this enzyme does not mimic *in vivo* activation. Both urinary and plasma kallikrein as well as plasmin can activate prorenin [17, 18], but they seem to require prior structural modification of the molecule to accomplish this [19, 20].

Altogether, this new evidence suggests that in the future we may find that renin release is modulated by an interplay of physiological, physical, and biochemical factors. By understanding how renin release is regulated, it may be possible to find out why the baroreceptor response to hypertension does not consistently cause complete suppression of renin release under most conditions, an effect that means that in most hypertensive states, renin continues to contribute to the blood pressure elevation, despite the presence of the hypertension.

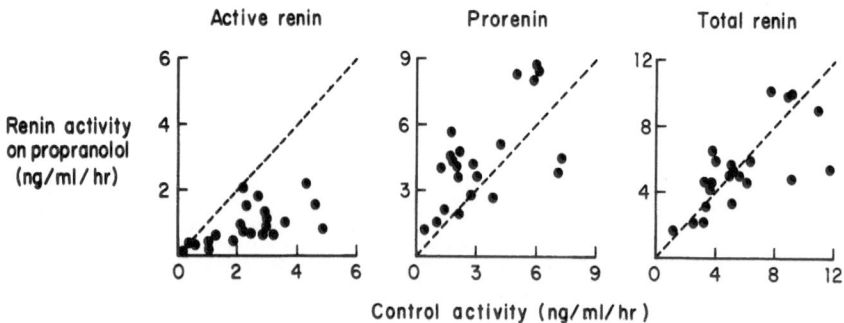

Figure 3. During propranolol therapy active renin always falls; prorenin usually rises; and total renin may rise, fall, or stay the same. Redrawn from Atlas, et al. [15].

REVEALING THE VASOCONSTRICTION AND VOLUME ELEMENTS IN HUMAN HYPERTENSIVE
STATES: MALIGNANT HYPERTENSION AND PRIMARY ALDOSTERONISM AS PROTOTYPES

The very first clue that an analysis of the varying degrees of vasoconstriction and volume factors in established forms of hypertension might prove to be meaningful arose from our research indicating that human malignant hypertension was associated with large excesses of renin activity and, as a consequence, large excesses of aldosterone [21, 22]. Most impressive was the fact that these patients often exhibited blood pressure levels no higher than those observed in primary aldosteronism, another hypertensive condition also accompanied by an over-secretion of aldosterone. Thus, these two disorders exhibit similar hypertension and similar aldosterone excess [22], but one (malignant hypertension) is associated with massive excess of renin-angiotensin vasoconstriction, whereas in the other (primary aldosteronism) renin production is virtually absent [23]. We were convinced that the presence as opposed to the absence of renin-vasoconstriction was the basis for the fundamental differences in pathophysiology between the two forms of hypertension and likely explained the gross differences in clinical course and prognosis of the two disorders [6, 21]. It also seemed reasonable to conclude that these two disorders might represent polar extremes of a spectrum of hypertensive pathophysiology [15] (Fig. 4).

Thus, in primary aldosteronism the hypertension is due to the aldosterone-induced excessive sodium-volume retention [23] and is therefore associated with overfilling of the circulation and a better flow to the capillaries and tissues. Conversely, in malignant hypertension there is intense generalized renin-mediated vasoconstriction with hemoconcentration, increased viscosity, poor flow to the microcirculation, acrocyanosis, and tissue ischemia. All of these are likely factors operating to cause the accelerated course of the disease with an early demise from irreversible vascular damage, especially in the heart, brain, and kidneys. Actually, the culpable role of renin excess in the vasoconstriction of malignant hypertension has been well verified by the dramatically corrective effects of either total nephrectomy or of the administration of several different types of antirenin system agents [4, 24]. In contrast, primary aldosteronism, though often exhibiting the same degree of blood pressure elevation, is usually a much more benign long-standing disease with little or no evidence of cardiovascular damage and a much better prognosis. Moreover, it can be totally corrected by sodium-volume depletion.

The study of these two forms of hypertension strongly suggested that, given equal degrees of hypertension, gross differences in *flow* and tissue perfusion can occur, and this could be a critical second dimension for analyzing and understanding any hypertensive condition. If vasoconstriction-mediated (in most cases from renin) and volume-mediated (sodium excess) forms of human hypertension do in fact exist, then it becomes apparent that any monodimensional analysis of a hypertensive person, based solely on manometric readings, may be overly sim-

THE VASOCONSTRICTION-VOLUME SPECTRUM IN HYPERTENSION

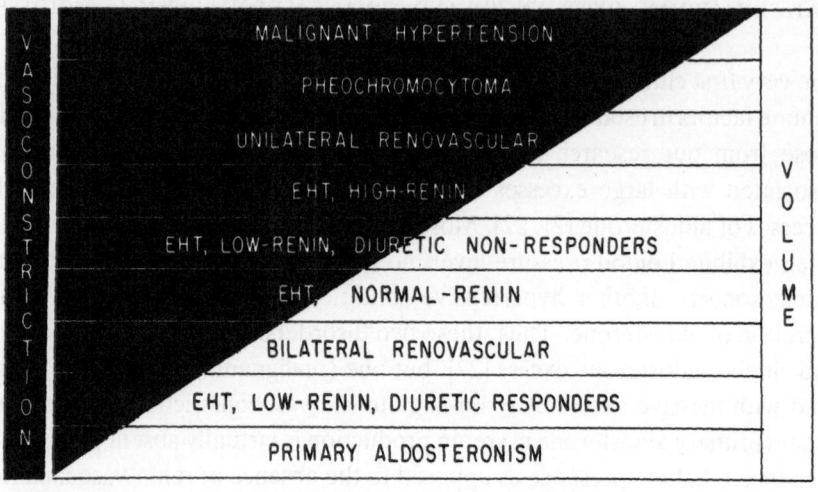

Figure 4. The vasoconstriction-volume spectrum of human hypertension. From Laragh, et al. [24].

plistic. These observations therefore raised the possibility that all hypertensive phenomena might compose a spectrum of abnormal vasoconstriction-volume participations [24] (Fig. 4). In this spectrum, malignant hypertension and primary aldosteronism would be the extremes, expressing a maximum excess of one of the two factors and a reciprocally minimal contribution of the other. If we accept this as true, then other hypertensive states, including essential hypertension and renovascular hypertensions, could also be profitably assayed pathophysiologically between these two polar extremes in terms of whether they might be mediated by vasoconstriction as opposed to volume factors or by an inappropriate mixture of the two. Were this to be the case, better understanding and more specific therapies could result.

TESTING THE VASOCONSTRICTION-VOLUME HYPOTHESIS

The approaches that we have used to test this vasoconstriction-volume hypothesis involve the identification and characterization of possible vasoconstriction factors; the demonstration of their participation or lack of participation in experimental models and in various forms of human hypertension; and the characterization of the interaction between vasoconstriction factors, occurring naturally or induced with naturally occurring or induced changes in sodium balance (i.e., with the volume factor).

The pursuit of these questions has been made possible not only by the development of precise methodology for measuring the hormone renin [25] as well as aldosterone [22, 26] but also by the discovery of a series of specific and potent pharmacologic probes capable of blocking the renal-adrenal pressor system at different biochemical steps (vide infra). These tools have made it possible to design experiments to quantify the vasoconstriction factor by blocking the renin system, while sodium balance is held constant and to quantify the volume factor in which sodium balance is manipulated, while blocking any dynamic response of the renin system.

ANGIOTENSIN AND NOREPINEPHRINE AS POSSIBLE VECTORS IN THE LONG-TERM VASOCONSTRICTION OF HUMAN HYPERTENSION: THEIR INTERACTION WITH THE SODIUM-VOLUME FACTOR

To seek the basis for a humoral vasoconstriction factor in common forms of chronic human hypertension means a search for those vectors physiologically capable of exerting their long-term effects. Further, since such arteriolar vaso-constriction is generalized, it is reasonable to presume that endocrine agents mediate this process via the central circulation. In this context, there are two well-known pressor substances, *noradrenaline* and *angiotensin II,* that can produce constrictive changes in the arterioles extremely similar to those occuring in established hypertension. However, measurements of circulating catecholamine in common forms of hypertension resulted in no consistent or convincing abnor-malities. As for angiotensin, a role for it had long been doubted, and it was even believed by some that a long-term infusion of it would produce tachyphylaxis with loss of activity.

However, after recognizing the existence of the renin-aldosterone system and its demonstrated role in the pathogenesis of malignant hypertension [6], we wondered if lesser, more subtle excesses of renin, leading to milder increases in angiotensin II levels, could be casually involved in mediating chronic, less fulmi-nant forms of human hypertension such as common essential hypertension.

For a fresh examination of this question, normal volunteers were recruited to a metabolic ward where they received constant diets of known sodium content [7]. We then compared the pressor effects of angiotensin II or norepinephrine infused continuously under identical 10-day protocols.

The results of an angiotensin infusion in a 35-year-old normal subject is representative of the group of subjects. Angiotensin raised the blood pressure to 130/65 from a control of 100/60 mm Hg. In the first four or five days, a markedly positive sodium balance was noted with about a 2-kg gain in weight. Aldosterone secretion rose from 200 to 800 μg/day. As the infusion proceeded, diminishing quantities of angiotensin were required to maintain the same level of blood pressure. After about five days, only a fifth of the starting dose was needed. Angiotensin's pressor potency actually increased with time, contradicting the oft-claimed tachyphylaxis. The diminishing amounts infused at the end of the 10 days

470

came close to producing blood levels similar to those occurring in normals. In addition, as the angiotensin infusion rate was reduced, aldosterone secretion sank back toward normal levels.

Most importantly, the increasing sensitivity to angiotensin was closely related to the state of sodium balance [7]; it developed after sodium retention had occured, caused by the angiotensin-induced aldosteronism. This and other studies show that the induced volume accumulation turns off the need for angiotensin vasoconstriction by amplifying the pressor response to it.

This see-saw sequence seems attractive teleologically, since it indicates that as the renin system defends blood pressure over the long-term, an initial vasoconstriction is increasingly replaced by improved volume or flow. Indeed, restoration of perfusion is probably a more rational final goal for the control system.

In sharp contrast, when we employed norepinephrine [7] in the identical protocol, it was difficult or impossible to sustain mild hypertension even with increasing dosages. Paroxysms of natriuresis were induced, and the blood pressure repeatedly tended to fall back to normal. With norepinephrine infusion, tachyphylaxis actually did occur – perhaps partly because of the lack of any auto-induced volume support limb; i.e., norepinephrine did not stimulate aldosterone secretion. Perhaps with a still longer time and with more attendant renal vasoconstriction or renal damage, circulating norepinephrine could be shown to be a long-term pressor agent. However, the tachyphylaxis that we found is in keeping with clinical experiences using this drug in intensive care units.

Thus, while this research provides no support for the idea that circulating norepinephrine could be a vector of chronic human hypertension, these findings do indeed nominate circulating angiotensin for such a role. Its involvement has a rather convincing physiologic coaptation. It interacts positively with sodium-volume status to support blood pressure; thus, an auto-induced volume expansion progressively turns down the initial corrective surge of angiotensin-vasoconstriction, with its attendant ischemia, and replaces it with a volume and flow support that is far more beneficial to the tissues over the long term.

This experiment, we believe, demonstrated how the renin system mediates blood pressure support in *normal* people via the reciprocating support of vasoconstriction and volume factors.

VASOCONSTRICTION AND VOLUME FACTORS IN EXPERIMENTAL RENOVASCULAR HYPERTENSIONS

Having demonstrated reciprocation of vasoconstriction and volume factors mediated by the renin system in normal people, we next looked for an animal model of hypertension to examine further relationships.

We chose experimental renovascular hypertension because there are two forms, both of which exhibit similar degrees of established hypertension (Fig. 4). One of these forms (the one-clipped kidney, opposite kidney intact) is known to be associated with a higher renin and relatively lower volumes, while the second form (one-clipped kidney, opposite kidney removed) is associated with higher volumes, due to reduced total GFR, and, consequently, with relatively lower plasma renin levels. The first form is the counterpart of classified surgically curable human renovascular disease; the second is a counterpart of the hypertension of renal insufficiency where renin is also usually suppressed.

It was easy enough to demonstrate that there were two pathophysiologic forms of experimental hypertension [27], i.e., vasoconstriction or volume-mediated. With the infusion of either highly specific antibodies to angiotensin II or saralasin (an angiotensin II antagonist), we could demonstrate that the hypertension of the two-kidney form was renin-dependent and that presumably there is little or no excess-volume factor in this model, because the opposite untouched kidney responded with a reactive pressure natriuresis. In the one-kidney model, renin secretion appeared to be playing no role whatsoever in the hypertension. We presumed that this one-kidney form, where renin was not participating, was instead sodium-volume dependent. However, after several weeks of stringent dietary sodium deprivation, the blood pressure remained high in these animals. But when we again challenged this model with angiotensin blockade, the blood pressure fell to normal [28], revealing the reciprocation of volume and vasoconstriction factors working to maintain renovascular hypertension. The fact that the one-kidney model is basically volume-dependent is intriguing. However, when the volume support was removed (sodium-deprivation), the hypertension remained, and renin secretion, which was suppressed by the volume excess, rose markedly to completely replace the volume support and keep the high blood pressure unchanged. This is proved by showing that the high blood pressure now becomes correctable by the administration of an angiotensin-blocking drug [28]. After dietary sodium repletion, the blocking drug again becomes totally ineffective. Thus, this animal model ordinarily uses volume to sustain the desired hypertension but readily recruits increased renin secretion for this purpose if sodium is withdrawn.

Accordingly, there are two forms of renovascular hypertension, either vasoconstriction or volume-mediated and these two components can reciprocally support the hypertension in the same model [29]. The goal of the system in this model always seems to be to achieve enough hypertension to maintain intrarenal normotension, by either of the two means, at some point distal to the partly occluded renal artery.

Accordingly, the one-kidney renovascular model appears to differ from patients with low-renin essential hypertension, because the renin-system response to volume depletion in the animal is strong enough to sustain the hypertension.

One might predict from these studies that if one could completely block both

472

the renin-vasoconstriction and the sodium-volume factors, the renovascular hypertension could be totally corrected or prevented. If this could be shown, then the equation

    B.P. = renin × aldo (Na), or more simply

    B.P. = (renin) × (volume)

might be applied to analyze the active components of renovascular hypertension.

These studies, suggesting that experimental renovascular hypertension can be totally corrected or prevented by completely blocking the renin-vasoconstriction and sodium-volume components, have recently been reaffirmed in studies of experimental renovascular hypertension in the dog [30].

The defense of arterial blood pressure by the renin-angiotensin-aldosterone system, as described by the clinical and experimental studies, is depicted by Figure 5. The renin system accomplishes this via long-term governance of arterial-bed vasoconstriction and by also determining the amount of fluid available to fill this chamber. Let us next consider whether the arithmetic of this analysis can be applied to study the spectrum of human hypertension.

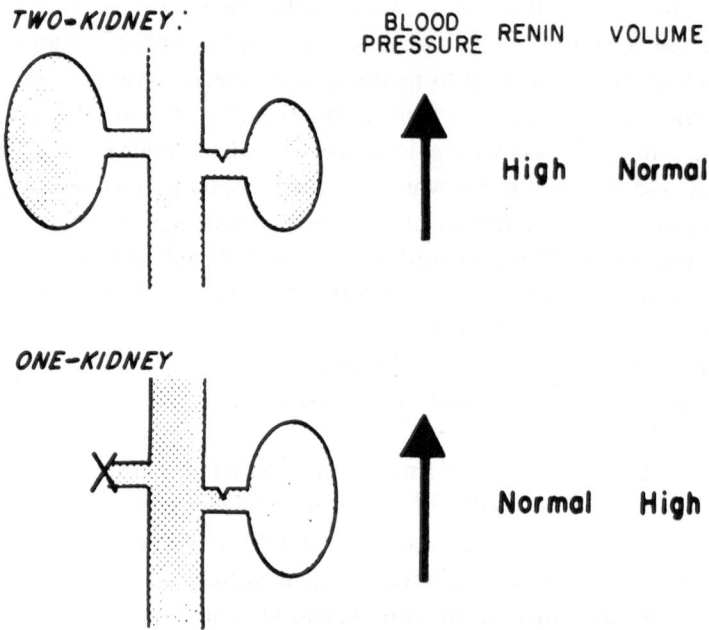

Figure 5. Animal models of renovascular (i.e., Goldblatt) hypertension. Although comparable blood pressure elevation occurs in the Goldblatt hypertension of either the one-kidney or the two-kidney type, different mechanisms are involved. Volume overexpansion from impaired renal excretory capacity is implicated in the one-kidney type, whereas renin-initiated vasoconstriction appears largely responsible for the two-kidney type. From Laragh, et al.: *Am J Med* 58:4, 1975.

VASOCONSTRICTION AND VOLUME FACTORS IN HUMAN HYPERTENSION

Malignant hypertension

It was quickly possible for us to verify and quantify the vasoconstriction and volume factors operating in malignant and in renovascular forms of human hypertension. In both of these forms under balance ward conditions, it was in fact possible to demonstrate reciprocation of the two factors resembling those observed in the animal models. In malignant hypertension, the blood pressure can be instantly corrected by infusion of an angiotensin antagonist [31] (Fig. 6). While this blockade is maintained, the infusion of sodium chloride over some 40 hours will restore the hypertension, this time on a volume basis.

Renovascular hypertension

In bilateral renovascular disease (Fig. 7), saralasin infusion will only partially correct the hypertension [31]. The additional component in this patient might be

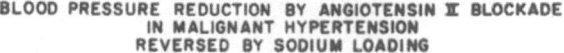
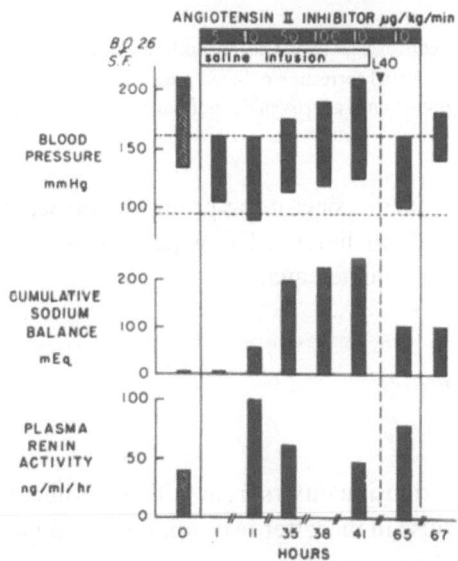

Figure 6. A patient with malignant hypertension studied under balance ward conditions, demonstrating first vasoconstriction and then volume support to the hypertension. Angiotensin blockade produced dramatic improvement in the blood pressure. However, as the blockade was maintained, when sodium chloride was infused over the next 40 hours, the blood pressure returned to the high control value, and volume replaced vasoconstriction in the support of the blood pressure (see text). From Brunner, et al. [31].

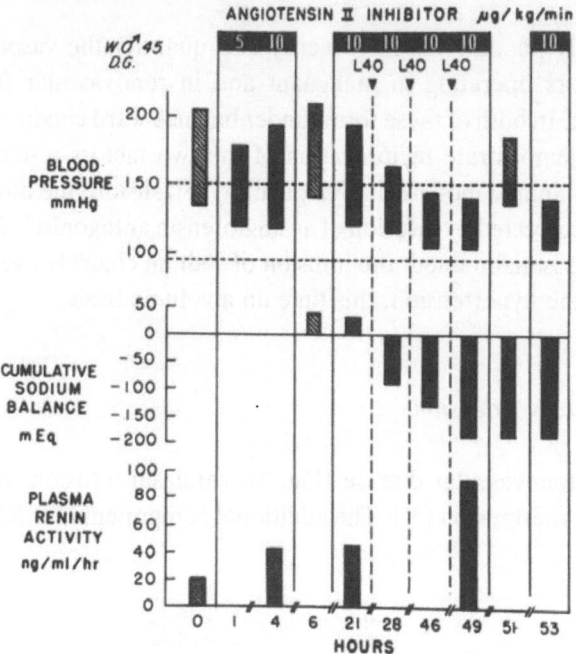

Figure 7. In a patient with renovascular hypertension, both vasoconstrictor and volume components are present. Saralasin produced partial correction of blood pressure, but complete correction could only be achieved following superimposition of a furosemide-induced diuresis (see text). From Brunner, et al. [31].

attributed to a volume factor, since it was promptly corrected by superimposing a furosemide-induced sodium diuresis. This hypertension can be analyzed in terms of the vasoconstriction-volume equation.

Essential hypertension

The volume factor
Human essential hypertension differs from both experimental and clinical reno-vascular disease, because in the latter two situations sodium depletion is ineffective in lowering blood pressure as described above. In essential hypertension, a low-sodium diet or diuretic therapy will lower blood pressure in about one third of patients with essential hypertension. Studies of many groups, including our own [32], have shown that it is the low-renin form in particular that responds to volume depletion. This by itself can be taken as evidence for a volume excess as the mediator of this form of essential hypertension. The low plasma renin levels are

also in keeping with how the renin control system would be expected to behave in reaction to a higher blood volume. Moreover, low-renin patients tend to exhibit higher blood volumes and other evidences of hemodilution [24]. It may very well be that patients with low-renin essential hypertension respond so well to diuretic therapy because their renin system reacts more sluggishly or incompletely to the sodium diuresis [32]. This is to be contrasted with the more complete renin-system response of experimental and clinical renovascular disease.

In contrast, in medium- or high-renin forms of essential hypertension, the blood pressure lowering response to diuretics is commensurately poorer, because in these forms the renin secretory reaction to the diuretic is much more brisk and successfully defends the pre-existing level of hypertension. The response in these patients resembles the renovascular situation. That the lack of response to a diuretic is due to a more lively renin-system defense can be shown in two ways. First, those failing to respond can be promptly normalized by adding a renin-system blocker, such as the angiotensin-converting enzyme inhibitor, teprotide [33]. Secondly, it has been shown that patients who fail to respond to diuretics exhibit much higher reactive plasma renin levels [34]. Thus, the vasoconstriction volume see-saw, as characterized in other clinical and animal studies, can also be shown to operate within the spectrum of so-called essential hypertension.

Altogether, this experience suggests that in essential hypertension, the volume factor is most predominant in low-renin forms and progressively less important in medium- and high-renin patients. Accordingly, the plasma renin level inversely reflects the volume status of the hypertensive individual. Conversely, the renin measurement directly reflects the degree of renin vasoconstriction.

The vasoconstriction factor as revealed through the use of pharmacologic probes
Propranolol suppresses renin secretion [11], saralasin inhibits the engagement of angiotensin II to its vascular receptor [31], and teprotide [33, 35] and captopril [36] block the formation of angiotensin II. The use of these four types of pharmacologic probes, dissecting the renin system at critical junctures, has built up a body of mutually reinforcing evidence, collectively indicating that renin-induced vasoconstriction is the factor sustaining all or part of hypertension in some 60 to 70 percent of patients with essential hypertension – those with high and most of those with medium (or 'normal') renin values. Equally persuasive, all four of these renin-system blocking agents are ineffective in lowering blood pressure in low-renin states, including patients with low-renin essential hyperten-sion, primary aldosteronism, and anephric patients [37]. It turns out that a properly measured plasma renin activity level is a good indicator of its active vasoconstriction, while the concurrent urinary sodium-excretion rate provides an index against which the appropriateness of the vasoconstriction to the patients' volume status can be rated [35].

THE VASOCONSTRICTION-VOLUME INTERPLAY IN NORMAL SUBJECTS

Does this same vasoconstriction-volume interplay operate in the same way in normal subjects? The answer is yes, as indicated by two representative studies. The first was performed by Morganti and colleagues on themselves [38]. They studied the blood pressure response to tilt, both before and after sodium depletion, in the control state and then after intravenous propranolol. In the sodium replete state, blood pressure was defended, accompanied by a mild rise in plasma renin, which, when blocked by propranolol, did not affect the pressure defense. However, after sodium-volume depletion, baseline renin levels were higher and then rose briskly in defense against the tilt. However, after propranolol was given in this situation, renin levels failed to rise with tilt, and the blood pressure fell precipitously. Thus, renin-vasoconstriction had become operative to defend or support arterial pressure when the volume support had been reduced.

In a second approach, Niarchos and his associates [39] used the nonapeptide-converting enzyme inhibitor, teprotide, to demonstrate active renin participation in normotension and at the same time to characterize their hemodynamic responses to acute angiotensin depletion. In normal volunteers on a normal salt intake, teprotide only reduced blood pressure in that subgroup with renin levels ranging towards the high side of the 'normal' range. However, after prior sodium-volume depletion with a reactive rise in baseline renin, all subjects responded to teprotide with a drop in blood pressure. Thus, these two studies indicate that the renin system supports normotension in a manner reciprocally related to the sodium-volume status, and this status is revealed by the control plasma renin level.

WHAT IS THE VOLUME COMPONENT THAT THE RENIN SYSTEM PERCEIVES AND REGULATES?

The above research raises some pervasive questions. First of all, what is the sodium-volume component that the renin system perceives and regulates? Secondly, is this the same volume that supports the arterial pressure? Thirdly, how does volume actually support or raise the blood pressure? Obviously, it does not lead to any significant or maintained changes in cardiac output, so it must exert its influence by raising the peripheral resistance. Presently, we only have some clues on these questions.

Dr. Marcia Bull and her associates have done a study in normal human volunteers to investigate the first question [40]. She wanted to find out whether it was the plasma volume or the whole blood volume, as opposed to the extracellular fluid volume or sodium space, that was being regulated by the renin system. To this end, normal volunteers, housed on the metabolic ward for two months, were fed constant low-sodium diets. Then blood and plasma were withdrawn in serial phlebotomies to reduce the plasma and blood volumes below normal. Salt was given orally and intravenously to produce a positive sodium balance, while the hypovolemia was maintained by continued phlebotomies. The positive sodium balance suppressed renin and aldosterone levels all the way back to normal. In other words, the renin system was turned off by a saline excess in the face of an impressive maintained reduction in plasma and in blood volumes.

This study suggests that the critical volume perceived is probably not the plasma or whole blood volume but is more likely a function of the interstitial volume somewhere in the body – perhaps a subcompartment within the kidney itself. How refilling this critical volume or space might support the arterial pressure remains unexplained. It is well-known that saline solutions can counteract shock and support pressure. This effect might occur by supporting arteriolar tone extrinsically or by increasing arteriolar cell volume or tonus.

SPACE MEASUREMENTS IN ESSENTIAL HYPERTENSION

While the critical volume that is monitored by the renin system may not yet be identified, what is already known about blood and extracellular volumes in essential hypertension can be instructive. For example, is clear that, in general, the higher the blood pressure, the lower the blood volume [41]. This raises some caveats not always heeded: Only patients with equivalent degrees of hypertension can be validly compared when looking for differences in blood volume. Also, sodium balance must be controlled while performing space measurements because this, too, affects total blood volume.

But even with these reservations and with all the inherent inaccuracies in space measurements, a tabulation of all such published studies [24] suggests again that the plasma renin level of individual hypertensive patients reflects their volume status. Thus, low-renin patients generally have the highest blood and extracellular fluid volumes among hypertensive patients, and they never exhibit reduced spaces. Moreover, at the other end of the spectrum, plasma volumes were significantly *reduced* in high-renin subjects in the only study reported to date. These findings are coherent with others showing that low-renin patients tend to exhibit lower hematocrit, plasma protein, and blood urea values, again reflecting their relative hemodilution [4, 42].

A PATHOPHYSIOLOGIC COMPARISON BETWEEN LOW- AND HIGH-RENIN ESSENTIAL HYPERTENSION

Altogether, the findings from this two-dimensional analysis of hypertensive patients allow a simulated comparison of two hypothetical hypertensive individuals who could present with equal degrees of hypertension, let us say 220/120. Let

478

Table 1. Pathophysiologic differences: high- and low-renin forms of hypertension

HIGH-RENIN (vasoconstricted)		LOW-RENIN (less vasoconstricted)
O	Arterioles	O
Higher	Peripheral resistance	High
High	Aldosterone	Low to high
Low	Plasma volume	High
Low	Cardiac output	High
High	Hematocrit	Low
High	Blood urea	Low
High	Blood viscosity	Low
Low	Tissue perfusion	High
Yes	Postural hypotension	No
	CLINICAL EXAMPLES	
High-renin essential		Low-renin essential
Renovascular and malignant		Primary aldosteronism
	VASCULAR SEQUELAE	
(+)	Stroke	(−)
(+)	Heart attack	(−)
(+)	Renal damage	(−)
(+)	Retinopathy-encephalopathy	(−)
	TREATMENTS	
No	Diuretics	Yes
Yes	Antirenin drugs	No
Yes	Direct vasodilators	±
Yes	Adrenergic blockers	±

us consider these two cases as the polar extremes of what we consider to be a spectrum (Table 1).

One patient has a very high and the other a very low renin level. That is to say, one has vasoconstriction hypertension and the other a volume-mediated hypertension. Clinically, the two forms may look alike. However, in flagrant forms, the high-renin patient might exhibit such intense vasoconstriction as to exhibit black hands and feet (e.g., malignant scleroderma). Such constriction can be dramatically reversed by antirenin therapy [43].

The known and expected differences between these two patients are depicted in Table 1. Most of the physiologic and biochemical differences listed have been demonstrated, but the proposed difference in tissue perfusion remain as a hypothesis to be proven because such measurements are not easy to make. As discussed already, the response to specific pharmacologic probes also differ markedly in the two forms, as does the propensity to vascular damage [27, 44, 45].

Thus, two different forms of hypertension with the same blood pressure do in fact occur, in which there are basic differences in biochemistry, pathophysiology, and pharmacologic responses, all of which are related to differences in volume and in flow. These abnormal patterns are revealed by the renin-sodium profile and verified by the responses to pharmacologic probes. In this construction, high-renin vasoconstriction disease might appropriately be termed 'dry' or low-flow ischemic hypertension, whereas low-renin volume hypertension (i.e., less vaso-constriction) is 'wet' or higher-flow essential hypertension.

This vasoconstriction-volume spectrum, within which all forms of human hy-pertensive disease are expressed, is depicted on the grid shown in Figure 4. This analytical framework is useful for revealing mechanisms in individual patients, because the vasoconstriction and volume components can be quantified simply by using renin-sodium profiling and/or the response to separately administered pharmacologic probes. The approach has practical value, because it separates out subgroups for simpler and more specific treatment for the long-term commitment involved and often enables treatment with only one agent. It also identifies at the beginning those patients who might be cured, by surgery or by angioplasty, of their renovascular or adrenocortical disease. The vasoconstriction-volume bipo-lar phenomena also reveals a pathophysiologic basis for the well-known differen-ces in risk and prognosis (i.e., of heart attack, stroke, and early demise) occurring among equally hypertensive people. Beyond this, the approach has added value because it separates out for further research those exceptions not explained by the model. For example, we have now identified a low-renin group not responsive to diuretics in whom we postulate another pressor mechanism at work to suppress renin secretion and maintain the hypertension.

SUMMARY

The data reviewed herein indicate that normotension and all hypertension is sustained by either excessive arteriolar vasoconstriction or excessive volume or by an inappropriate excess of one component relative to the other. All hyperten-sive phenomena can be profitably analyzed in terms of the relative contribution of vasoconstriction or volume factors. The identification and quantification of these components is now a simple matter using the renin-sodium profile and/or the separated response to specific antirenin or antivolume drugs. In this approach, the plasma renin value itself is a direct measure of renin-vasoconstriction and is often an inverse measure of the arterial volume factor. The urinary sodium value is an index of the appropriateness of the vasoconstriction to the volume status.

This bidimensional analysis of blood pressure phenomena identifies some key questions for future research, such as:

(1) How does a sodium-volume excess increase peripheral resistance and support or even raise blood pressure?

(2) What is the critical volume in question, and is it the same volume that is regulated by the renin system?

(3) How and why does overfilling of the circulation develop in volume-dependent forms of hypertension?

(4) Why is inappropriate renin-induced vasoconstriction so often the mediator of both the medium- and high-renin forms of essential hypertension (approximately 70% of the whole), and why does renin secretion fail to turn itself off in the face of the systemic hypertension?

(5) What are the discrete central and peripheral nervous system mechanisms for the coordination and defense of vasoconstriction and volume, and how are they coordinated with the known renin system governance of pressure and flow?

A body of evidence has been reviewed, indicating that all hypertensive phenomena ranging from mild disorders to fulminant malignant hypertension can be profitably analyzed by assessing the relative contribution of two final determinants of the arterial pressure - the vasoconstriction and volume components. Renin-sodium profiling and the separate application of specific pharmacologic probes provide the basic tools for quantifying the two components.

This bidimensional analysis has provided new understanding of pathophysiology of practical value for the evaluation, diagnosis, and treatment of individual patients in the whole spectrum of human hypertensive diseases. Beyond this, the new analytical scaffold identifies some key questions for future research.

REFERENCES

1. Laragh JH: Vasoconstriction-volume analysis for understanding and treating hypertension: The use of renin and aldosterone profiles. Am J Med 55:261-274, 1973.
2. Letcher RL, Chien S, Pickering TG, et al.: Direct relationship between blood pressure and blood viscosity in normal and hypertensive subjects. Role of fibrinogen concentration. Am J Med 70:1195-1202, 1981.
3. Laragh JH, Sealey JE: The renin-angiotensin-aldosterone hormonal system and regulation of sodium, potassium, and blood pressure homeostasis, in Orloff J, Berliner RW (editors): Handbook of Physiology - Renal (American Physiological Society). Baltimore, Waverly Press, 1973, pp 831-908.
4. Laragh JH, Baer L, Brunner HR, et al.: Renin, angiotensin and aldosterone system in pathogenesis and management of hypertensive vascular disease. Am J Med 52:633-652, 1972.
5. Laragh JH, Bühler FR, Seldin DW (editors): Frontiers in Hypertension Research. New York, Springer-Verlag, 1980.
6. Laragh JH, Angers M, Kelly WG, et al.: Hypotensive agents and pressor substances. The effect of epinephrine, norepinephrine, angiotensin II and others on the secretory rate of aldosterone in man. JAMA 174:234-240, 1960.
7. Laragh JH: The role of aldosterone in man: Evidence for regulation of electrolyte balance and arterial pressure by renal-adrenal system which may be involved in malignant hypertension. JAMA 174:293-295, 1960.
8. Genest J: Angiotensin, aldosterone and human arterial hypertension. Can Med Assoc J 84:403, 1961.
9. Ames RP, Borkowski AJ, Sicinski AM, et al.: Prolonged infusions of angiotensin II and

norepinephrine and blood pressure, electrolyte balance, aldosterone and cortisol secretion in normal man and in cirrhosis with ascites. J Clin Invest 44:1171-1186, 0000.

10. Laragh JH, Cannon PJ, Bentzel CJ, et al.: Angiotensin II, norepinephrine and renal transport of electrolytes and water in normal man and in cirrhosis with ascites. J Clin Invest 42:1179-1192, 1963.

11. Bühler FR, Laragh JH, Baer L, et al.: Propranolol inhibition of renin secretion. A specific approach to diagnosis and treatment of renin-dependent hypertensive disease. N Engl J Med 287:1209-1214, 1972.

12. Sealey JE, Atlas SA, Laragh JH: Prorenin and large molecular weight renins. Endocr Rev 1:365-391, 1980.

13. Sealey JE, Overlack A, Laragh JH, et al.: Effect of captopril and aprotinin on inactive renin. J Clin Endocrinol Metab 53:626-630, 1981.

14. Derkx FHM, van Gool JMG, Wenting GJ, et al.: Inactive renin in human plasma. Lancet 2:496, 1976.

15. Atlas SA, Sealey JE, Laragh JH, et al.: Plasma renin and 'prorenin' in essential hypertension during sodium depletion, beta-blockade and reduced arterial pressure. Lancet 2:785, 1977.

16. Atlas SA, Sealey JE, Dharmgrongartama B, et al.: Detection and isolation of inactive, large molecular weight renin in human kidney and plasma. Hypertension 3 (suppl 3):I30-40, 1981.

17. Sealey JE, Atlas SA, Laragh JH, et al.: Initiation of plasma prorenin activation by Hageman factor-dependent conversion of plasma prekallikrein to kallikrein. Proc Natl Acad Sci USA 76:5914, 1979.

18. Derkx FHM, Bouma BN, Schalekamp MPA, et al.: An intrinsic factor XII-prekallikrein-dependent pathway activates the human plasma renin-angiotensin system. Nature 280:315-316, 1979.

19. Hsuek WA, Carlson EJ, Israel-Hagman M: Mechanism of acid-activation of renin: Role of kallikrein in renin activation. Hypertension 3 (suppl I):I-22, 1980.

20. Leckie B, McGhee NK: Reversible activation-inactivation of renin in human plasma. Nature 288:702, 1980.

21. Laragh JH, Cannon PJ, Ames RP: Aldosterone secretion and various forms of hypertensive vascular disease. Ann Intern Med 59:117-120, 1963.

22. Laragh JH, Ulick S, Januszewicz W, et al.: Aldosterone secretion and primary and malignant hypertension. J Clin Invest 39:1091-1106, 1960.

23. Conn JW: Plasma renin activity in primary aldosteronism. Importance in differential diagnosis and in research of essential hypertension. JAMA 190:222, 1964.

24. Laragh JH, Letcher RL, Pickering TG: Renin profiling for modern diagnosis and treatment of hypertension. JAMA 241:151-156, 1973.

25. Sealey JE, Gerten-Banes J, Laragh JH: The renin system: Variations in man measured by radioimmunossay or bioassay. Kidney Int 1:240-253, 1972.

26. Sealey JE, Bühler FR, Laragh JH, et al.: Aldosterone excretion: Physiologic variations in man measured by radioimmunoassay or double isotope dilution. Circ Res 31:367-378, 1972.

27. Brunner HR, Kirshman JD, Sealey JE, et al.: Hypertension of renal origin: Evidence for two different mechanisms. Science 174:1344-1346, 1971.

28. Gavras H, Brunner HR, Vaughan ED Jr, et al.: Angiotensin-sodium interaction in blood pressure maintenance of renal hypertensive and normotensive rats. Science 180:1369-1372, 1973.

29. Gavras J, Brunner HR, Thurston H, et al.: Reciprocation of renin dependency with sodium-volume dependency in renal hypertension. Science 188:1316-1317, 1975.

30. Seymour AA, Davis JO, Freeman RH, et al.: Sodium and angiotensin in the pathogenesis of experimental renovascular hypertension. Am J Physiol 240:H788-792, 1981.

31. Brunner HR, Gavras H, Laragh JH, et al.: Hypertension in man. Exposure of the renin and sodium components using angiotensin II blockade. Circ Res 34/35 (suppl I):35-45, 1974.

32. Vaughan ED Jr, Laragh JH, Gavras I, et al.: Volume factor in low and normal renin essential

482

hypertension: Treatment with either spironolactone or chlorthalidone. Am J Cardiol 32:523-532, 1973.

33. Gavras H, Brunner HR, Laragh JH, et al.: An angiotensin converting enzyme inhibitor to identify and treat vasoconstrictor and volume factors in hypertensive patients. N Engl J Med 291:817-821, 1974.

34. Weber MA, Drayer JIM, Rev A, et al.: Disparate patterns of aldosterone response during diuretic treatment of hypertension. Ann Intern Med 87:558-563, 1977.

35. Case DB, Wallace JM, Keim HJ, et al.: Possible role of renin in hypertension as suggested by renin-sodium profiling and inhibition of converting enzyme. N Engl J Med 296:641-646, 1977.

36. Case DB, Atlas SA, Laragh JH, et al.: Clinical experience with blockade of the renin-angiotensin-aldosterone system by an oral converting enzyme inhibitor (SQ 14,225, captopril) in hypertensive patients. Prog Cardiovasc Dis 31:195-206, 1978.

37. Case DB, Wallace JM, Keim HJ, et al.: Estimating renin participation in hypertension. Superiority of converting enzyme inhibitor over saralasin. Am J Med 61:790-796, 1976.

38. Morganti A, Lopez-Ovejero JA, Pickering TG, et al.: Role of the sympathetic nervous system in mediating the renin response to head up tilt. Their possible synergism in defending blood pressure against postural changes during sodium deprivation. Am J Cardiol 43:600-604, 1979.

39. Niarchos AP, Pickering TG, Case DB, et al.: Role of the renin-angiotensin system in blood pressure regulation: The cardiovascular effects of converting enzyme inhibition in normal man. Circ Res 45:829-837, 1979.

40. Bull MB, Hillman RS, Cannon PJ, et al.: Renin and aldosterone secretion in man as influenced by changes in electrolyte balance and blood volume. Circ Res 27:953-960, 1970.

41. Tarazi RC: Hemodynamic role of the extracellular fluid in hypertension. Circ Res 38 (suppl 2):73-83, 1976.

42. Drayer JIM, Weber MA, Sealey JE, et al.: Low- and high-renin essential hypertension: A comparison of clinical and biochemical characteristics. Am J Med Sci 281:135-142, 1981.

43. Lopez-Ovejero JA, Saal SD, D'Angelo WA, et al.: Reversal of scleroderma vascular and renal crisis by oral angiotensin converting enzyme blockade. N Engl J Med 300:1417-1418, 1979.

44. Brunner HR, Sealey JE, Laragh JH: Renin as a risk factor in essential hypertension. Am J Med 55:295-302, 1973.

45. Laragh JH: Hypertension, vasoconstriction and the causation of cardiovascular injury: The renin-sodium profile as an indicator of risk, in Laragh JH, Bühler FR, Seldin DW (editors): Frontiers in Hypertension Research. New York, Springer-Verlag, 1981, pp 383-395.

DISCUSSION

Discussants: Sambhi, Laragh, MacGregor, Williams, Denton, Genest

Sambhi: It was my impression that much of your early work on prorenin was done with cryoactivation. Today you have consistently used the term 'trypsin-activated renin.' Was the data that you showed us on trypsin activation?

Laragh: Yes, it was.

Sambhi: Would you consider a reduction in cardiac output as one of the possible and important antihypertensive actions of beta blockers?

Laragh: I would certainly consider it, but it doesn't make any sense and let me tell you why. Beta blockers lower the cardiac output in everybody. They do it instantly; intravenously given beta blockers always take down the cardiac output in a minute or two, but the blood pressure usually does not drop. In fact, the many years of experience in treating angina pectoris with beta receptor blockers makes it pretty clear that it doesn't usually lower the pressure in normotensive people, but it lowers the cardiac output in everybody. Furthermore, if you take the whole spectrum of patients with high blood pressure, beta blockers lower the cardiac output to the same degree in low-renin patients but do not lower their pressure. Actually when Jim Black discovered the beta receptor blockers, he had no idea that they would lower blood pressure because theoretically beta blockers would be expected to *raise* the pressure by leaving everybody with unopposed alpha tone. That's why in anephric people the pressure goes up. Actually, malignant hypertension has been induced in anephric people receiving beta blockers and also in some patients receiving beta blockers for the treatment of schizophrenia. Beta blockers leave the recipient with unopposed alpha tone expressed by cold hands and feet, for example. It you didn't have the renin factor suppressed by the drug, your pressure would *rise* with a beta receptor blocker as it does in primary aldosteronism, in low-renin essential hypertension and in anephric man. The evidence becomes incontrovertible from the anephric human and animal model experiences because here you get a pressor response to beta blockers given intravenously. Thus, when there is no renin to suppress, blood pressure rises. Secondly, I don't see any a priori reason why lowering the cardiac output would lower pressure, and it doesn't.

Sambhi: I accept all that on acute basis - but in chronic terms there could be long-term hemodynamic adjustment.

Laragh: I don't know what the parameters that would do this could be. The cardiac output and the pulse rate are lowered by these drugs in everybody, but the blood pressure only goes down in those in whom renin is present and then is reduced by the beta blocker.

Sambhi: The next question was on your experiences with beta blockers in malignant hypertension.

Laragh: Beta blockers are tremendously effective in high-renin patients with malignant hypertension and about half of the patients in our original study were completely normalized with beta blockers alone. They are not powerful enough as anti-renin drugs to do the job all the time, although they usually produce significant benefits. They are not as powerful as drugs like captopril, and you have to add another agent about half of the time, but the evidence that the blood pressure drop is related to renin, I think, is quite impressive. However, I'm willing to listen if someone can tell me another way besides renin suppression that beta blockers might lower blood pressure.

MacGregor: We and others have shown that if you look at the percentage fall in blood pressure, propranolol and captopril lower blood pressure more in normotensive than in hypertensive subjects. Now, this to me implies that renin is actually participating less in essential hypertension in maintaining blood pressure than in normotensives, and I wondered if you'd like to comment on that.

Laragh: Your data and ours are extremely similar. I share your view that renin supports the blood pressure in normal people so I have no problem with that either. I think your interpretation that the renin participation in essential hypertension is fractionally *less* than in normals is a reasonable interpretation, but not one which we are attracted to. We believe that the system is still actively participating in many patients with hypertension when in fact it should turn itself off. I guess you believe that it's participating too, but it's trying not to because its fractional participation is somewhat less in hypertension than it is in normal people. I respect your point of view, but I still think the participation in the presence of hypertension is inappropriate.

Williams: You mentioned that maybe one of the main reasons for looking into this area is to piece out the heterogeneity of hypertension. Many of us are interested in doing that genetically. Have there been any good studies to help us see the relationship? For example, has anyone found that low-renin hypertension aggregates in some families and high renin hypertension in others?

Laragh: I believe the low-renin patient expresses a biologically different phenomenon than that observed in a high-renin patient. One or both of these phenomena could be genetic or acquired. I am sure that you realize that all of the massive epidemiologic data that we have has been based on a lumping phenomenon where everybody with hypertension has been lumped together simply because they have high blood pressure. A more thoughtful epidemiological analysis should fractionate hypertensive people into subgroups based on the other parameters such as the renin profile, because these people are not all alike, in my opinion, either biochemically, physiologically or pharmacologically. Therefore, the old aphorisms that essential hypertension is salt sensitive or is uniform in its prognosis are incorrect. We need to stratify this large group in order to make more meaningful analyses.

Denton: I noticed in your first patient that there was an increase in sensitivity of the pressor response with sodium retention, which is conventional. You didn't show us the measurements of blood angiotensin, but it was noteworthy that as the infusion rate decreased, the aldosterone concentration or secretion decreased. What impression have you had in terms of the idea of the induction of increased numbers of receptors in the adrenal with protracted exposure to angiotensin? I was also wondering if you might tell us something of your experience with the converting enzyme inhibitors, such as captopril, particularly in terms of the side effects on taste, and whether these occur in the seventh or the ninth nerve - whether you have any evidence on it.

Laragh: We did that study before receptor physiology was as sophisticated as it is today. I would predict from what we know that angiotensin induces increased receptor populations in the adrenal cortex, which in time might get to a point where you'd have an increased sensitivity. I think the important point about our study was that you could find a small dose of angiotensin which could still keep your pressure elevated when aldosterone has fallen back to normal.

Denton: It did fall to normal, then.

Laragh: Yes.

Denton: Though you had the infusion continued.

Laragh: Yes, it did. This phenomenon is retraced in nature because many patients in whom we can correct their hypertension by reducing their renin levels with a beta blocker, or saralasin, or with captopril, have medium or normal plasma renin values and entirely normal aldosterone levels in the control state and yet they get an antihypertensive effect when renin is suppressed or blocked.

Genest: You mentioned that when the blood pressure goes up there's a feedback to lower renin. Do you have any hard data that in any acute rise in blood pressure in the patient with high or low renin that there is an effect on plasma renin activity or angiotensin II.

Laragh: To answer your other question, Dr. Sambhi, the blood volume is increased in low renin essential hypertension as far as I can tell. Blood volume measurements really aren't worth too musch because they're too inaccurate and so are sodium space measurements. What Tom Pickering did is review every measured space ever made in low renin hypertension and the data show that whenever the measurements have been made, the cardiac output is higher and the blood volume and the extracellular sodium space are either above normal or on the high side of normal. Also, as a group they exhibit lower hematocrit, hemoglobin, and blood urea values. I think it's very difficult to claim they're not relatively hemodiluted, and overfilled when compared with medium or high-renin forms of hypertension. Perhaps this is why low-renin patients exhibit the best blood pressure responses to diuretic therapy.

REGULATION OF BLOOD PRESSURE BY VASOPRESSIN

C.I. JOHNSTON, Y. IMAI AND R.L. WOODS

INTRODUCTION

Vasopressin has two major biological actions important for blood pressure regulation: vasoconstriction (pressor) and antidiuresis (volume) (Fig. 1). Vasopressin shares these dual physiological effects with angiotensin, a potent vasoactive hormone, long known to be important in blood pressure homeostasis. However, vasopressin's role in blood pressure regulation has been neglected and its pressor activity regarded as a pharmacological effect rather than of any physiological relevance. Recent studies, summarized in reviews [1, 2], have suggested that vasopressin may be physiologically important in the control of blood pressure and may be part of an integrated hormonal system involving the renin angiotensin-aldosterone system (RAS), the sympathetic nervous system, and catecholamines. The sum of the vasoconstrictor activity of these vasoactive hormones may determine the level of blood pressure in states such as orthostasis, salt and volume depletion, hemorrhage, and some forms of hypertension.

Interestingly, it is also now apparent that there are at least two distinct types of vasopressin membrane receptors. The classical vasopressin receptor (V_1) is located in the kidney and is responsible for its antidiuretic action. This V_1 receptor uses adenylate cyclase and cyclic AMP as its second messenger [3]. The second vasopressin receptor (V_2), which is found in the vasculature and mediates the vasoconstrictor response, utilizes calcium to transduce the signal from membrane binding to physiological action (Fig. 1). The different vasopressin receptors have allowed the development of vasopressin analogues, which act as specific competitive inhibitors for either the vasculature or the antidiuretic receptors. Such compounds are now available to block either the pressor or antidiuretic response of vasopressin.

VASOCONSTRICTOR PROPERTIES OF VASOPRESSIN

Vasopressin is the most potent vasoconstrictor known *in vitro* [4] and more potent than angiotensin *in vivo*. It has a slightly longer duration of action than angiotensin so that if the area under the curve is used as a function of its vasoconstrictor

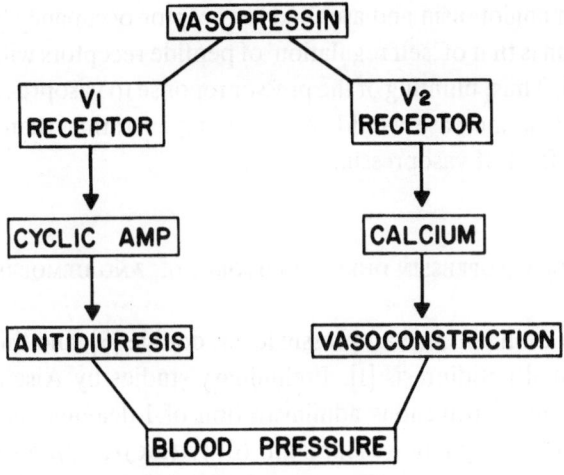

Figure 1. Physiological actions of vasopressin affecting blood pressure.

properties, it is some 10 to 50-fold more potent than angiotensin (Fig. 2).

The plasma levels reported for vasopressin in various physiological states [5] and even in hypertension are much lower than pressor levels achieved by exogenous vasopressin infusions [6]. Hence, for vasopressin to act as a direct vasoconstrictor agent in hypertension, some 'sensitization' needs to be postulated. This 'sensitization' may be made possible by removal of normal cardiovascular reflexes used to dampen the pressor activity of vasopressin or, alternatively, by changes in vascular reactivity to vasopressin. It has been clearly shown that under normal conditions the baroreceptor reflex arc and sympathetic nervous system considerably attenuate the pressor response to vasopressin [7, 8, 9]. Similarly, suppression of renin release and acute lowering of plasma renin by vasopressin has been well documented and again would dampen the apparent blood pressure response to vasopressin *in vivo* [8, 10].

Little is known about the vascular reactivity to vasopressin and its modulation. We have recently shown, using the rat bioassay blood pressure preparation, that both volume and salt status modulate the pressor response to vasopressin; but this was a nonspecific effect, as the pressor response to several other vasoconstrictor agents were also modified. The vascular response to vasopressin is also dependent on the ambient concentration of circulating vasopressin. The homozygous Brattleboro rat with genetic central diabetes insipidus (DI), which is totally devoid of vasopressin in its plasma, posterior pituitary, and hypothalamus, shows supersensitivity to injected exogenous vasopressin, whereas the normal rat infused with vasopressin to elevate plasma vasopressin levels has a blunted blood pressure rise to exogenous vasopressin (Fig. 3). This change in vascular reactivity was specific for vasopressin and did not occur in response to angiotensin. Such changes in vascular reactivity dependent on plasma levels have been previously described with angiotensin and ascribed to receptor occupancy [11]. An alternative explanation is that of 'self regulation' of peptide receptors with 'down and up' regulation [12]. Thus, blunting of the pressor reponse to vasopressin when plasma vasopressin levels increase would tend to dampen rather than accentuate the hypertensive effect of vasopressin.

PRESSOR ROLE OF VASOPRESSIN DURING DEHYDRATION AND HEMORRHAGE

During dehydration plasma vasopressin levels double [5], and this is sufficient to produce maximal antidiuresis [1]. Preliminary studies by Aisenbrey et al. [13] demonstrated that intravenous administration of 1-deamino penicillamine [2,-(o-methyl)tyrosine] arginine vasopressin, (dPtyr(me)AVP), a specific competitive vasopressin vascular receptor antagonist, acutely lowered the blood pressure in dehydrated rats. Andrews and Brenner [14] in further studies showed that a similar specific vasopressin vascular antagonist – 1-(β mercapto-β, β-cyclopenta methylene-propionic acid), 4 valine, 8-D-arginine vasopressin (cyclodVDAVP) – produced transient hypotension in dehydrated anesthetised rats but was without

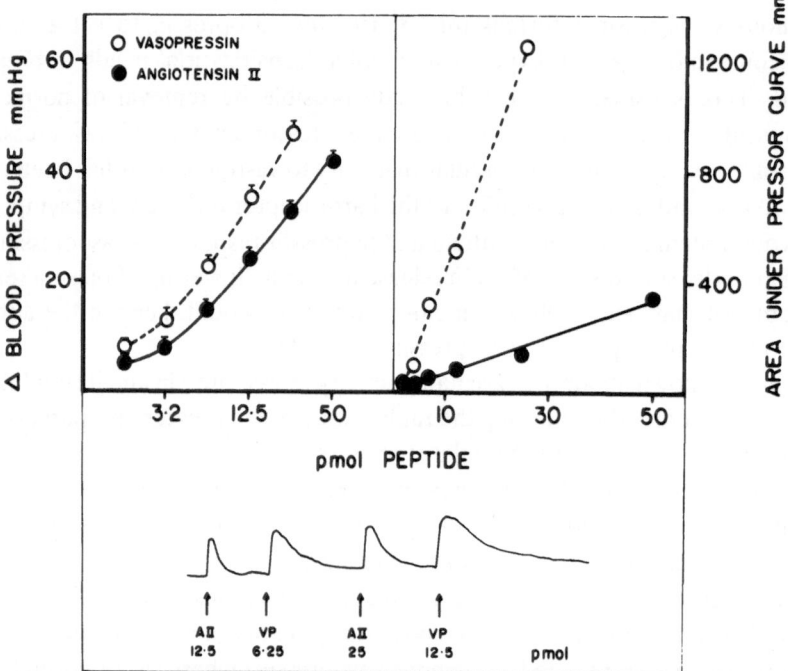

Figure 2. Dose-response blood pressure curves for vasopressin and angiotensin II in the anesthetised rat bioassay preparation. Curves on left represent rise in blood pressure (ΔBP); curves on right represent area under pressor response curve. Below, typical blood pressure responses to vasopressin (VP) and angiotensin (AII) in rat bioassay system.

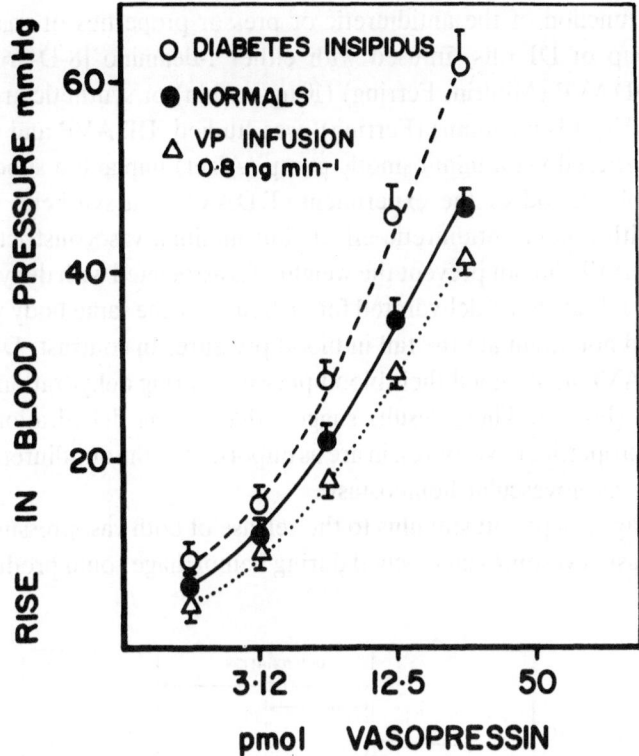

Figure 3. Change in dose-response blood pressure curves in rats of the Brattleboro strain with hereditary diabetes insipidus (DI), in normal Long-Evans control rats, and in rats infused intravenously with synthetic arginine[8]-vasopressin (VP) at 0.8 ng/min for 2 days.

effect in rats undergoing a water diuresis. These results suggest that despite the low circulating levels of vasopressin in dehydration, it is important in helping to maintain the blood pressure.

Studies in the Brattleboro rat with diabetes insipidus allow some quantitation of the role of vasopressin and have provided conclusive evidence for its involvment in the circulatory response to dehydration. Brattleboro rats and their unaffected litter mates of the Long-Evans strain were placed in metabolic cages and dehydrated. Brattlelboro rats were dehydrated for 24 hours to produce approximately 20% body weight loss (39 g), whereas to achieve a comparable body weight loss it was necessary to dehydrate Long-Evans rats for 48 hours. Following the period of dehydration, the rats were allowed to rehydrate. During the experiment, body weight, water balance, urine volume, osmolality, and blood pressure by tail plethysmography were measured. In normal rats body weight declined, urine flow decreased, and urine osmolality increased without change in arterial blood pressure (Fig. 4). In Brattleboro rats, despite equivalent body weight loss, decreases in urine flow and rise in urine osmolality, blood pressure fell significantly by 14 ± 3 mm Hg ($p<0.001$).

To establish whether the maintenance of the blood pressure during dehydration was a function of the antidiuretic or pressor properties of vasopressin, a further group of DI rats, infused with either 1-deamino [8-D-arginine] vasopressin, DDAVP (Minirin, Ferring) (10 ng/kg/min) or synthetic arginine[8]-vasopressin (AVP) (3 ng/kg/min) (Ferring), was studied. DDAVP and vasopressin were administered via a mini-osmotic pump (Alzet) implanted subcutaneously for the whole period of the experiment. DDAVP is a synthetic vasopressin analogue with potent antidiuretic effects but minimal vasoconstrictor activity. DDAVP or AVP did not prevent the weight loss associated with dehydration but enabled the DI rats to be dehydrated for 48 hours for the same body weight loss. DDAVP did not attenuate the fall in blood pressure. In contrast, DI rats given exogenous AVP maintained their blood pressure during dehydration, similar to normal rats (Fig. 5). These results suggest that during dehydration the vasoconstrictor properties of vasopressin are as important as the antidiuretic actions in maintaining cardiovascular homeostasis.

Hemorrhage is a potent stimulus to the release of both vasopressin and renin. Levels of plasma vasopressin reached during hemorrhage could produce marked

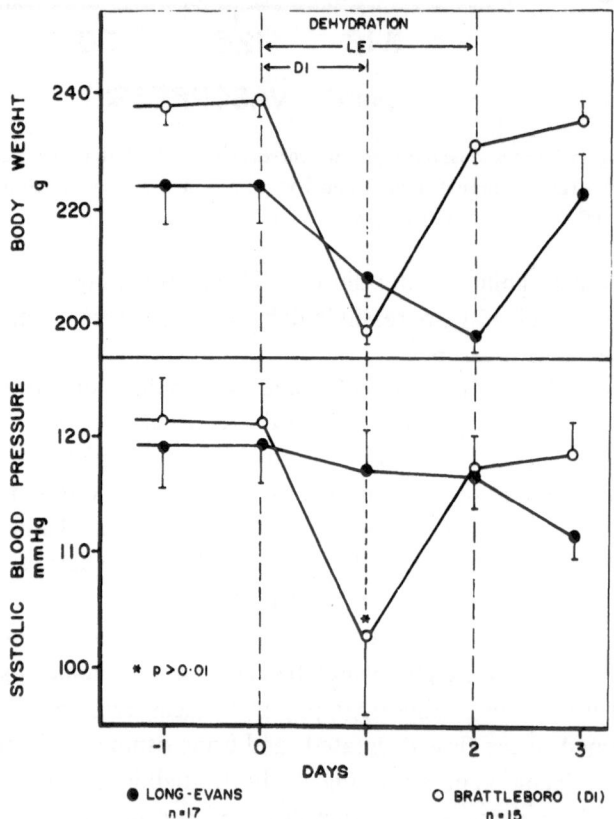

Figure 4. Body weight and systolic blood pressure in mm Hg in normal Long-Evans rats (●) dehydrated for 48 hours, compared with Brattleboro diabetes insipidus rats (○) dehydrated for 24 hours.

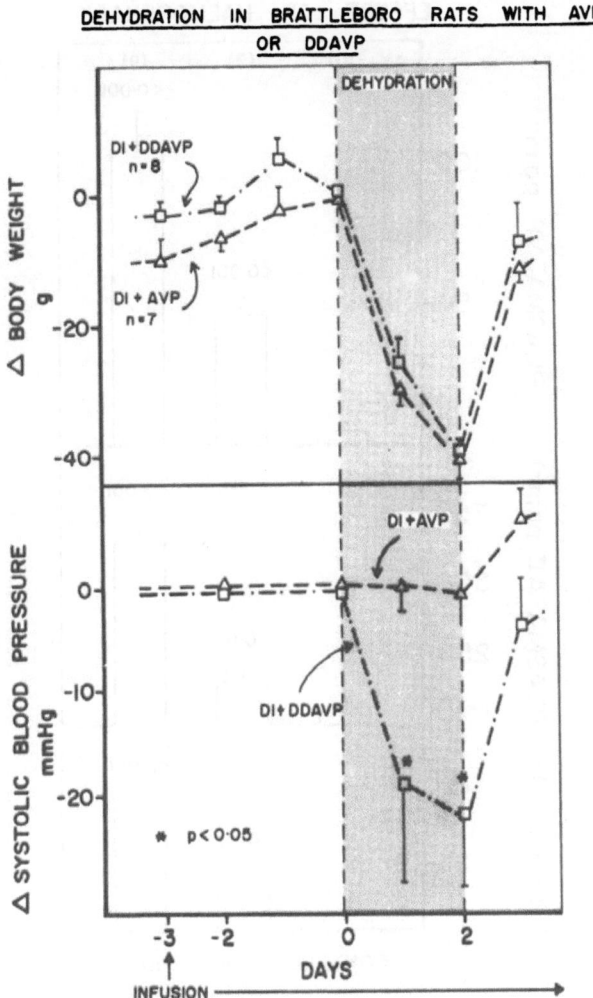

Figure 5. Change (△) in body weight and (△) systolic blood pressure (SBP) in mm Hg in groups of Brattleboro diabetes insipidus (△I) rats infused intravenously with either DDAVP (□) or synthetic arginine[8]-vasopressin (AVP) (△) during 48 hours dehydration. Only the rats receiving the vasopressin infusion were able to maintain their blood pressure during dehydration.

vasoconstriction. Figure 6 shows the hormonal responses of anesthetised rats to progressive hemorrhage of 15 and 30% of their blood volume. Both plasma vasopressin and angiotensin II reach very high levels and probably act to maintain blood pressure together [15]. This has recently been established using a compound to block the action of vasopressin and angiotensin both singularly and in combination [16]. The importance of vasopressin in the maintenance of blood pressure during hemorrhage has also been documented in studies using the Brattleboro rat [2, 17].

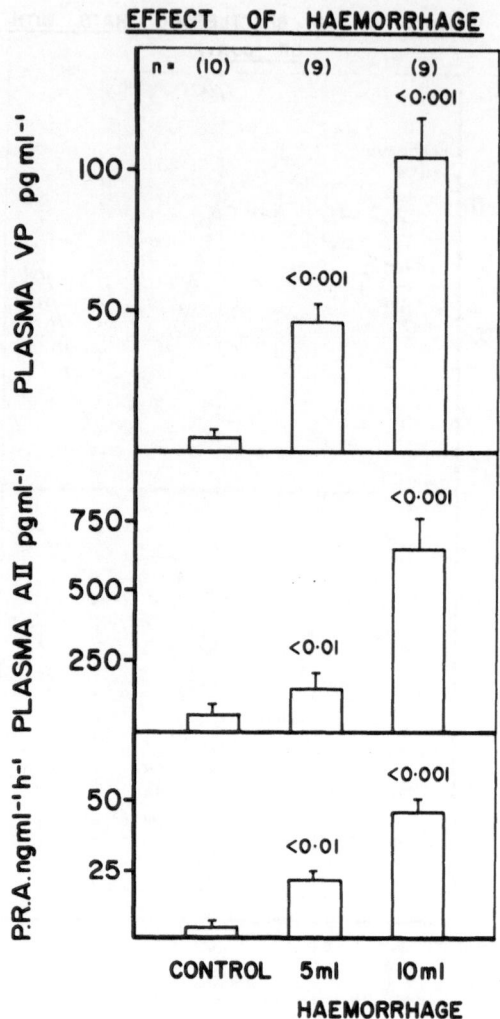

Figure 6. Effect of hemorrhage (5 ml, 15%, of blood volume and 10 ml, 30%, of blood volume) on plasma levels of vasopressin (VP), angiotensin II (AII), and plasma renin activity (PRA) in rats.

VASOPRESSIN IN THE PATHOGENESIS OF EXPERIMENTAL HYPERTENSION

Plasma vasopressin has been reported to be elevated in DOCA-salt hypertension [18]; the spontaneously hypertensive rat [19]; and 2-kidney, 1-clip (2K-1C) Goldblatt hypertension in rats [20, 21] and dogs [8]. It is also higher in malignant than benign forms [22]. However, in all these forms of hypertension, elevation of plasma vasopressin is small and could possibly be a consequence of the pathophysiological changes accompanying high blood pressure rather than a contributing cause.

We have confirmed the elevation of plasma vasopressin in both 2-kidney, 1-clip

(2K-1C) and 1-kidney, 1-clip (1K-1C) Goldblatt renal hypertension, as well as a form of malignant hypertension produced by complete aortic ligature between the two renal arteries (Fig. 7) [23].

We have also been able to produce experimental renal hypertension in the homozygous Brattleboro diabetes insipidus rat [24]. The onset, development, and severity of 2K-1C renal hypertension in the DI rat was identical to normal Long-Evans control rats (Fig. 8). In the 1K-1C renal hypertension model the onset and development of hypertension was similar, but the absolute level of blood pressure achieved was less (Fig. 9). Administration of DDAVP to correct the metabolic water balance of the DI rat resulted in an increase in the hypertensive blood pressure and cardiac hypertrophy to levels comparable with 1K-1C Long-Evans hypertensive rats [25]. This form of renal hypertension is known to be volume-dependent, and these results support this and suggest that vasopressin's antidiuretic activity by maintaining volume may be more important in the pathogenesis of this type of hypertension than its vasoconstrictor properties.

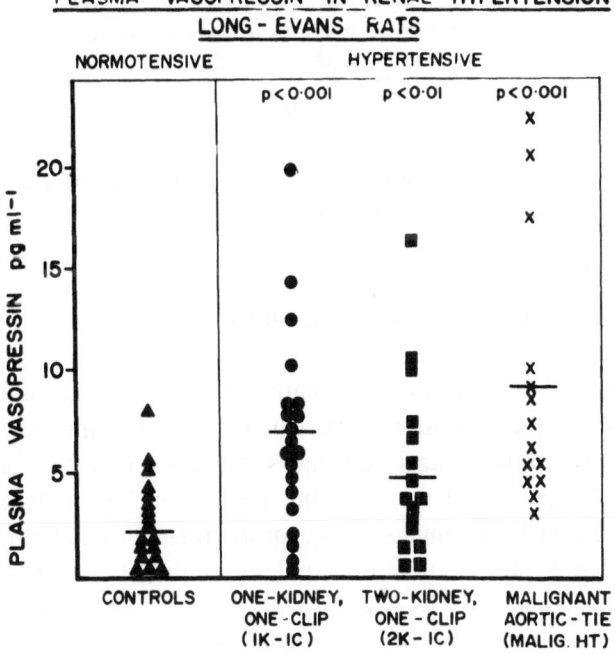

Figure 7. Plasma vasopressin levels in normal control rats, rats with 1K–1C and 2K–1C Goldblatt renal hypertension, and rats with malignant hypertension (HT) produced by complete ligation of the abdominal aorta between the renal arteries.

2K-IC HYPERTENSION

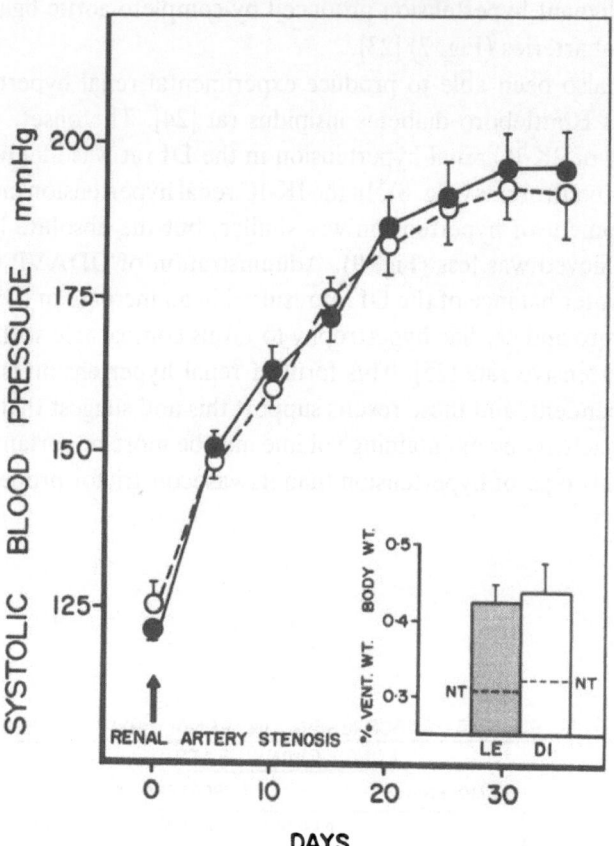

Figure 8. Blood pressure and cardiac hypertrophy in group of Long-Evans rats (●) and Brattleboro DI rats (○) after induction of 2-kidney, 1-clip Goldbattt renal hypertension.

VASCULAR EFFECTS OF VASOPRESSIN IN MALIGNANT HYPERTENSION

Plasma vasopressin levels are also greatly increased in malignant hypertension [22]. One of the characteristics of malignant hypertension is fibrinoid necrosis. Möhring [26] therefore suggested that vasopressin may be vasculotoxic and responsible for fibrinoid necrosis in some forms of malignant hypertension. The alternative theory to the humoral vasoconstrictor-induced etiology of fibrinoid necrosis is that it is the result of the rapid rate of rise of the blood pressure. The lesions are ischemic, and excessive vasoconstriction from any cause – humoral, nervous, or structural – probably precipitates the lesion.

Malignant hypertension can be reproducibly induced in the rat by complete ligation of the aorta between the two renal arteries. In a study with Brattleboro DI rats and Long-Evans rats, the incidence (50-60%) and severity of malignant

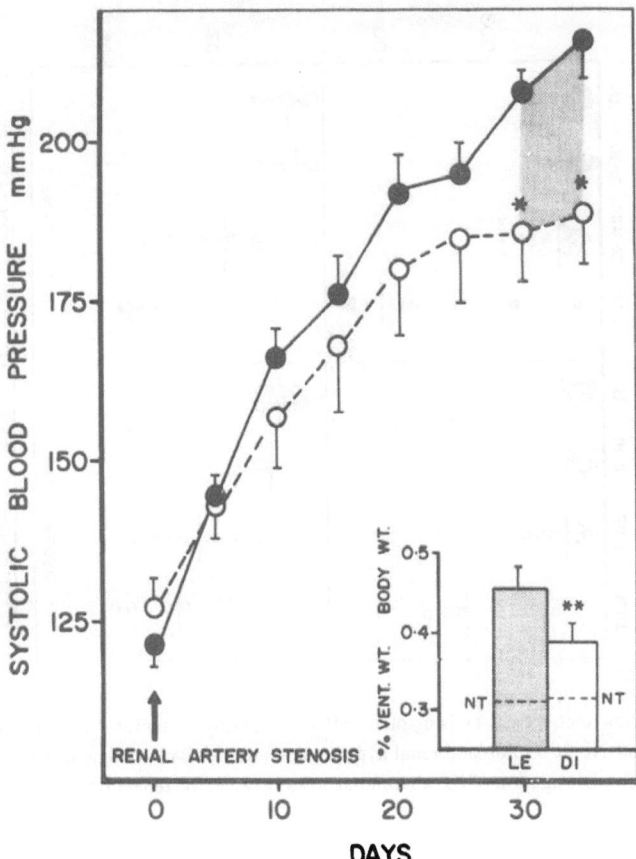

Figure 9. Blood pressure and cardiac hypertrophy in group of Long-Evans rats (●) and Brattleboro DI rats (○) after induction of 1-kidney, 1-clip Goldblatt renal hypertension. The hypertensive blood pressure and cardiac hypertrophy could be increased in the Brattleboro DI rats to levels comparable to Long-Evans hypertensive rats by the administration of DDAVP to correct their water balance.

hypertension in the two strains were the same [27]. Furthermore, fibrinoid necrosis was seen with equal frequency in Brattleboro rats with diabetes insipidus as in normal animals.

Lastly, it has been argued that in the DI rat the renin-angiotensin system often overcompensates for the lack of vasopressin. However, no evidence for excessive levels of renin or angiotensin could be found in several models of experimental hypertension (Fig. 10) [24].

496

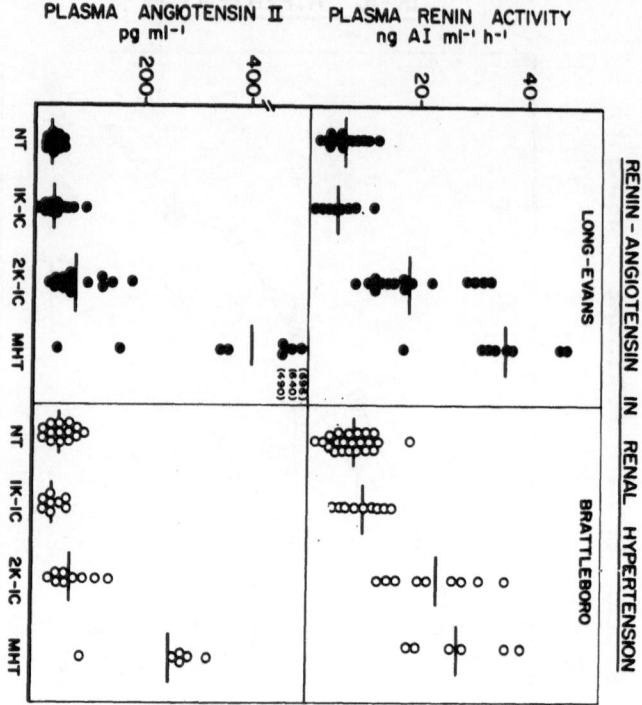

Figure 10. Plasma renin activity and angiotensin II levels in Long-Evans rats (●) or Brattleboro rats (○) with 1K–1C and 2K–1C Goldbladd renal hypertension and rats with malignant hypertension (MHT) produced by complete ligation of the abdominal aorta between the renal arteries.

CONCLUSIONS

There is increasing evidence that physiological concentrations of plasma vaso-pressin may exert significant cardiovascular effects. Under normal circumstances, the rise in blood pressure is buffered and prevented by compensatory mechanisms involving the baroreceptor reflex arc and suppression of plasma renin and angiotensin. In addition, vasopressin leads to bradycardia and a fall in cardiac output, probably mediated via a central nervous system action involving an increase in vagal tone. Therefore, rises in plasma vasopressin within the physiological range may increase the peripheral resistance without a change in arterial blood pressure.

In states of dehydration, orthostasis, hemorrhage, and hypotension, these modifying influences on vasopressin's vasoconstrictor responses appear attenuated. In these circumstances, vasopressin may help to maintain the blood pressure. Vas-opressin, together with angiotensin and catecholamines, thus act as an integrated vasoactive hormonal system to regulate blood pressure.

In experimental renal hypertension, vasopressin seems unlikely to act as a direct vasoconstrictor in the pathogenesis of hypertension. However, in more volume-dependent models of experimental hypertension (DOCA-salt hypertension and 1K-1C Goldblatt hypertension), the antidiuretic action of vasopressin is important in maintaining volume and thus may contribute to the absolute level of blood pressure.

ACKNOWLEDGMENTS

These studies were supported by a grant-in-aid from the National Health and Medical Research Council of Australia. R.L. Woods holds a Biomedical Graduate Research Scholarship from the N.H. & M.R.C. The technical assistance of D. Casley and J. Abrahams is gratefully acknowledged.

REFERENCES

1. Möhring J, Arbogast R, Dusing R, et al.: Vasopressor role of vasopressin in hypertension, in: (editors): Brain and Pituitary Peptides. Ferring Symposium, Munich 1979, Basel, Karger, 1980, pp 157-167.
2. Johnston CI, Newman M, Woods RL: Role of vasopressin in cardiovascular homeostasis and hypertension. Clin Sci 61:129s-139s, 1981.
3. Dousa TP: Cyclic nucleotides in the cellular action of neurohypophyseal hormones. Fed Proc 36:1867-1871, 1977.
4. Altura BM, Altura BT: Vascular smooth muscle and neurohypophyseal hormones. Fed Proc 36:1853-1860, 1977.
5. Robertson GL: The regulation of vasopressin function in health and disease. Recent Prog Horm Res 33:333-385, 1977.
6. Pullan PT, Johnston CI, Anderson WP, et al.: The role of vasopressin in blood pressure control and in experimental hypertension. Clin Sci Mol Med 55:251s-254s, 1978.
7. Cowley AW Jr, Monos E, Guyton AC: Interaction of vasopressin and the baroreceptor reflex system in the regulation of arterial blood pressure in the dog. Circ Res 34:505-514, 1974.
8. Pullan PT, Johnston CI, Anderson WP, et al.: Plasma vasopressin in blood pressure homeostasis and in experimental renal hypertension. Am J Physiol 239:H81-H87, 1980.
9. Montani J-P, Liard J-F, Schoun J, et al.: Hemodynamic effects of exogenous and endogenous vasopressin at low plasma concentrations in conscious dogs. Circ Res 47:346-355, 1981.
10. Vander AJ: Inhibition of renin release in the dog by vasopressin and vasotocin. Circ Res 23:605-609, 1968.
11. Thurston H, Laragh JH: Prior receptor occupancy as a determinant of the pressor activity of infused angiotensin in the rat. Circ Res 36:113-117, 1975.
12. Catt KJ, Harwood JP, Austera GI, et al.: Hormonal regulation of peptide receptors and target cell responses. Nature 280:109-116, 1979.
13. Aisenbrey G, Manning M, Schrier R: Specific inhibitor of the vascular effect of exogenous and endogenous arginine vasopressin (AVP). Kidney Int 19:229, 1981.
14. Andrews CE Jr, Brenner BM: Relative contributions of arginine vasopressin and angiotensin II to maintenance of systemic arterial pressure in the anaesthetised water-deprived rat. Circ Res 48:254-258, 1981.

15. McNeill JR, Wilcox WC, Pang CCY: Vasopressin and angiotensin: Reciprocal mechanisms controlling mesenteric conductance. Am J Physiol 232(3):262-266, 1976.

16. Cowley AW Jr, Switzer SJ, Guinn MM: Evidence and quantification of the vasopressin arterial pressure control system in the dog. Circ Res 46:58-66, 1980.

17. Laycock JF, Penn W, Shirley DG, et al.: The role of vasopressin in blood pressure regulation immediately following acute hemorrhage in the rat. J Physiol 292:267-275, 1979.

18. Möhring J, Möhring B, Petri M, et al.: Vasopressin and malignant deoxycorticosterone hypertension in rats. Clin Sci Mol Med 51:45s-48s, 1976.

19. Crofton JT, Share L, Shade RE, et al.: Vasopressin in the rat with spontaneous hypertension. Am J Physiol 135:H361-H365, 1978.

20. Möhring J, Möhring B, Petri M, et al.: Plasma vasopressin concentrations and effects of vasopressin antiserum on blood pressure in rats with malignant two-kidney Goldblatt hypertension. Circ Res 42:17-22, 1978.

21. Johnston CI, Pullan PT, Walter NMA: Vasoactive peptides in experimental renal hypertension. Klin Wochenschr 56 (suppl 1):81-85, 1978.

22. Möhring J, Möhring B, Petri M, et al.: Is vasopressin involved in the pathogenesis of malignant deoxycorticosterone hypertension in rats? Lancet 2:170-173, 1976.

23. Woods RL, Johnston CI: The role of vasopressin in hypertension: Studies using the Brattleboro rat. Am J Physiol 242(6):F727-F732, 1982.

24. Johnston CI, Abrahams JM, Woods RL: Renal hypertension in the Brattleboro diabetes insipidus rat. Ann NY Acad Sci, in press.

25. Woods RL, Johnston CI: Importance of antidiuretic properties of vasopressin in experimental renal hypertension. Clin Exp Pharmacol Physiol 8:519-523, 1981.

26. Möhring J: The case for humoral factors as well as pressure. Clin Sci Mol Med 52:111-117, 1977.

27. Woods RL, Abrahams JM, Kincaid-Smith P, et al.: Vascular lesions and angiotensin in malignant hypertension in the absence of vasopressin. Clin Exp Pharmacol Physiol 9:297-301, 1982.

DISCUSSION

Discussants: Muirhead, Johnston, Brody, Corvol, Laragh

Muirhead: Have you had a chance to unclip the renal artery of the hypertensive Brattleboro rat?

Johnston: No, we haven't done that as yet.

Brody: I'd like to amplify on your suggestion that nonvasoconstrictor effects of vasopressin might participate in the development of hypertension. Our laboratory has studied the Brattleboro rat and its relationship to DOCA/salt hypertension. We confirmed that DOCA/salt does not produce increased blood pressure in these animals.[1] However, if they were given vasopressin concurrently with DOCA/salt, in amounts that restored the normal fluid intake and excretion, DOCA/salt became hypertensive. This finding could not be explained by the direct vasoconstrictor action of vasopressin because when we took vasopressin away, blood pressure required several weeks to return to normal despite the very short half-life of the peptide.

We looked at several possibilities relating to the mechanism of these vasopressin interactions. We found that vasopressin induced an increase in renal vascular reactivity to a number of different vasoconstrictor agents, and that effect was a very early one, occurring before or at the onset of the increase in blood pressure produced by vasopressin in Brattleboro rats given DOCA/salt. Perhaps the most interesting finding was that the ability of vasopressin to raise arterial pressure in Brattleboro vasopressin-deficient animals was blocked by our anterior hypothalamic lesion in the AB3V area, suggesting the possibility of a central nervous system interaction.[2] We believe that these pieces of evidence suggest that vasopressin can play a permissive role in the production of DOCA/salt hypertension by mechanisms which may well be unrelated to its renal excretory or direct vasoconstrictor actions.

Johnston: Yes, I would agree with you. I don't know whether you are aware, but Saito in Japan was the first to show that the Brattleboro rat could be made hypertensive with DOCA salt, if one corrected its volume homeostasis by infusing DDAVP. I think that the changes in vascular sensitivity are relatively nonspecific. The infusions of very small amounts of vasopressin potentiate quite markedly the vasoconstriction from noradrenaline or sympathetic nerve stimulations, as well as offer vasoconstrictor substances such as angiotensin.

Corvol: Did you make a vasopressin dose-response curve in these Brattleboro rats, before and after volume expansion, to see whether or not you get a shift of the dose-response curve?

Johnston: We've done the first part, that is, we have performed dose-response curves in the Brattleboro rat without replacement. The Brattleboro rat is supersensitive to vasopressin, presumably on a mechanism of up regulation to receptors, but we have not as yet repeated it when they are volume-replete.

Laragh: You showed that vasopressin was a more potent constrictor than angiotensin. How did you set that up?

Johnston: I think it's been shown many times both *in vitro* and *in vivo*. We used the standard sympathetically blocked bioassay rat preparation.

Laragh: The point is, do you have to take the sympathetics away?

Johnston: Yes, for both.

Laragh: Then you always get about ten times more potent vasoconstriction from vasopressin if you take the sympathetics away.

Johnston: Right. With the sympathetics intact, angiotensin would, I think, cause a greater increase in blood pressure than vasopressin. But in the sympathetically blocked animal, vasopressin is a more potent pressor agent than angiotensin. This is because vasopressin interacts with the baroreceptors, leading to a marked bradycardia. Angiotensin, on the other hand, has a central vagal inhibitor action and this does not produce reflex bradycardia in response to the rise in blood pressure.

[1] Berecek KH, Murray RD, Gross F, et al.: Vasopressin and vascular reactivity in development of DOCA hypertension in rats with hereditary diabetes insipidus (DI). *Hypertension* 4: 3-12, 1981.

[2] Berecek KH, Barron KW, Webb R, et al: Vasopressin - central nervous system interactive in the development of DOCA hypertension. *Hypertension* 4 (Suppl II) 131-137, 1982.

THE RENOMEDULLARY INTERSTITIAL CELLS IN HYPERTENSION

JAMES A. PITCOCK AND E. ERIC MUIRHEAD

The renomedullary interstitial cells (RIC) are thought to be the source of the mediators of the antihypertensive action of the kidney [1, 2]. The numerous osmiophilic lipid droplets are the most distinctive morphologic feature of the RIC. If one accepts the concept that the RIC are endocrine cells, then it is tempting to feel that an enumeration of RIC granules might yield some information on the endocrine activity of the cells. Such an approach was quite sucessful during the early investigations of the juxtaglomerular cells when hypergranulation correlated quite well with increased secretion of renin. A number of studies of RIC have been published utilizing this concept, but their interpretation is still not clear.

One of the problems may be the methods used for quantitation. Data have been reported in a variety of ways, ranging from a simple subjective evaluation of increased or decreased granularity to counting granules on two-dimensional sections, reporting the results as granules per RIC cell or as granules per unit area. Similarly, the number of cells may be reported as numbers per unit area of a tissue section. In addition, some investigators have used light and others have used electron microscopy for their counting (Table 1).

Two-dimensional evaluation of what are basically three-dimensional structures has a variety of potential pitfalls. With experience, one can subjectively interpret a two-dimensional pattern in three-dimensional terms. However, such an interpretation can be erroneous. For example, one may think that one tissue has more granules than another when, in fact, the granules are merely bigger and therefore more likely to appear in the plane of section.

A number of procedures were developed in the last century by geologists for the evaluation of specimens by examining a two-dimensional cut surface. These principles have been extended, particularly by Weibel, for the evaluation of tissue sections [3]. The principle of DeLesse states that, on average, the area of a structure profile as a fraction of some baseline, such as total tissue, is equivalent to volume of that structure as a fraction of the baseline volume. This is the volume density, a measure of concentration. This is a relatively straightforward procedure, as areas can be measured in a variety of ways, such as planimetry, measuring intercepts of a grid, or more recently, electronically. The evaluation of the number of a structure in a given volume is considerably more complicated, so

Table 1. RIC in hypertension

References	Hypertensive model	Method	% Change granularity
Manda et al. [9] (1967)	Rat Uni-Nephrectomy + Doca-salt	EM – granules/cell	→ 74%
Muehrcke et al. [10] (1969)	Rat Uni-Nephrectomy + Doca-salt	LM + EM – granules/cell	→ 36%
Tobian et al. [11] (1969)	Rat 'Post-Salt'	LM – granules/area	→ 42%
Ishii and Tobian [12] (1969)	Rat 2-kidney, 1-clip	LM – granules/area	→ 26%
Tobian and Ishii [13] (1969)	Rat 'Post-Goldblatt'	LM – granules/area	→ 45%
Latta et al. [14] (1975)	Rat 2-kidney, 1-clip	LM – granules/cell	30%
Szokol et al. [15] (1979)	Rat 2-kidney, 1-clip + salt	LM – granules/cell	→ 40%
Perov and Postnov [5] (1976)	Rat 2-kidney, 1-clip	EM – mophometric	↑
Nekrosova et al. [16] (1973)	Rabbit 1-kidney, 1-clip	EM – granules/cell	→ 86%
Mandal et al. [17, 18] (1974–1975)	Rat – Spontaneous genetic	EM – granules/cell	→ 35%
Simpson [19] (1970)	Rat – Spontaneous genetic	LM – granules/cell	↑

that several approximations have been developed. We have used the formula of Weibel and Gomez, which requires assumptions about the shape and size distribution of the structures in question. These procedures have been applied to the RIC by only a few investigators, particularly, Bohman and Jansen [4], Perov and Postnov [5], and our group [6, 7].

Determination of an absolute figure, such as the number of RIC in a kidney, requires a knowledge of the volume in which RIC is found. We have tried to do this in the inner medulla of the rat. Such determinations are quite difficult, however, and one is likely to obtain data with a larger standard error.

All tissues, when fixed, tend to shrink or swell depending upon the fixative used and the specific tissue involved. Stereologic (morphometric) technics have been most thoroughly applied to bone where shrinkage (or swelling) is not much of a problem. The renal inner medulla, however, has a high but variable tissue osmolality. An iso-osmolar fixative tends to cause swelling in this tissue. A hyperosmolar fixative can correct for this, but one still has variations due to location within the inner medulla and variations due to experimental manipulation[8]. All of these problems may potentially confound the data. Small experimental changes may be missed, and small but statistically significant changes may be related to osmolality variations rather than to real structural changes.

Lipid granule enumeration has been used by workers to evaluate several physiologic and pathophysiologic states, particularly experimental hypertension. For example, water diuresis causes a decrease in the number of RIC granules. Most experimental hypertensive states have also been associated with a decrease in lipid granule count (Table 1). The degree of the apparent degranulation has not been great in some of the studies, making interpretation difficult. All of the studies involving severe or malignant hypertension, however, have also shown degranulation, often of severe degree, so that confounding problems of the enumeration method are probably not relevant. None of the studies in Table 1 evaluated the RIC cellularity of the inner medulla.

In our studies, we have evaluated not only RIC granulation but also cellularity and have tried to evaluate degenerative changes in the RIC by electron microscopic evaluation. We have particularly looked for loss of cytoplasmic processes and 'rounding up' of the cells, vacuolization of granules, loss of relationship between granules and cisterns, loss of other cytoplasmic organelles, granularity of cytoplasm, and rarely, overt necrosis.

Our studies (Table 2) have tended to confirm that degranulation is associated with hypertension, at least in rapidly developing and severe models. In addition, degeneration and decreased cellularity can be seen in these circumstances. The degeneration and decreased cellularity, in one model, correlated with decreased antihypertensive function of the renal medulla as evaluated by transplants into hypertensive recipients [20-22].

In a recent study of the Dahl rats genetically resistant and genetically sensitive to the hypertensive action of increased salt intake, we have also shown a marked

Table 2. State of RIC in hypertension

Model	No. RIC/grid	No. granules/RIC
Partial Nephrectomy-salt	5.2 ± 0.3	2.3 ± 0.14
	p < 0.005	P < 0.001
Partial Nephrectomy-H$_2$O	7.76 ± 0.4	5.0 ± 0.2
Malignant Hypertension Rabbit 1-Kidney 1-Clip	5.18 ± 0.41	1.29 ± 0.6
	p < 0.001	p < 0.001
Uninephrectomy Control	7.90 ± 0.81	6.72 ± 0.80
JGC Transplant Hypertension	5.48 ± 0.27	3.27 ± 0.18
	p < 0.005	p < 0.001
Uninephrectomy Control	7.06 ± 0.35	8.65 ± 1.04

decrease in cellularity and granulation of the sensitive rats, even when they are on a low-salt diet and are not overtly hypertensive (Fig. 1). The resistant rats degranulate on a high-salt intake, even without becoming overtly hypertensive [7]. These data and previous data cannot be interpreted as a simple, direct relationship to hypertension.

One interpretation would suggest that the number of healthy, well-granulated RIC would indicate the ability of the kidney to excrete a salt load in the absence of an increased hypertensive perfusion pressure. The granulation of the RIC would reflect the balance between lipid intake into the cell and utilization of lipid precursors to form mediators of the antihypertensive function. With intake into the cell held constant, degranulation of the RIC would indicate an attempt of the RIC to perform its antihypertensive function, possibly either by helping expedite salt and water excretion or by release of a peripheral antihypertensive hormone. The success of this attempt would depend on many other variables.

In models such as the unclipped kidney of a previously clipped Goldblatt rat and the Dahl resistant rat on a high salt intake, this attempt is successful and blood pressure remains or becomes normal [6-7]. In many of the models of experimental hypertension, the attempt is inadequate and the animal remains hypertensive. This could be because of genetically inadequate RIC, as in the Dahl S animal [7]; degeneration of the RIC, as in the partial nephrectomy-salt model [20]; or possibly, in other models, because of internal renal restraints.

REFERENCES

1. Muirhead EE: The role of the medulla in hypertension, in Stollerman GH (editor): Advances in Internal Medicine. Chicago, Year Book Medical Publishers, 1974, vol 19, pp 81-107.
2. Muirhead EE: Evidence for an involvement of renal papilla in hypertension, in Bohman S-O, Mandal AK (editors): Renal Papilla and Hypertension. New York, Plenum Press, 1980, pp 35-61.
3. Weibel ER: Stereological techniques for microscopic morphometry, in Hayat MA (editor):

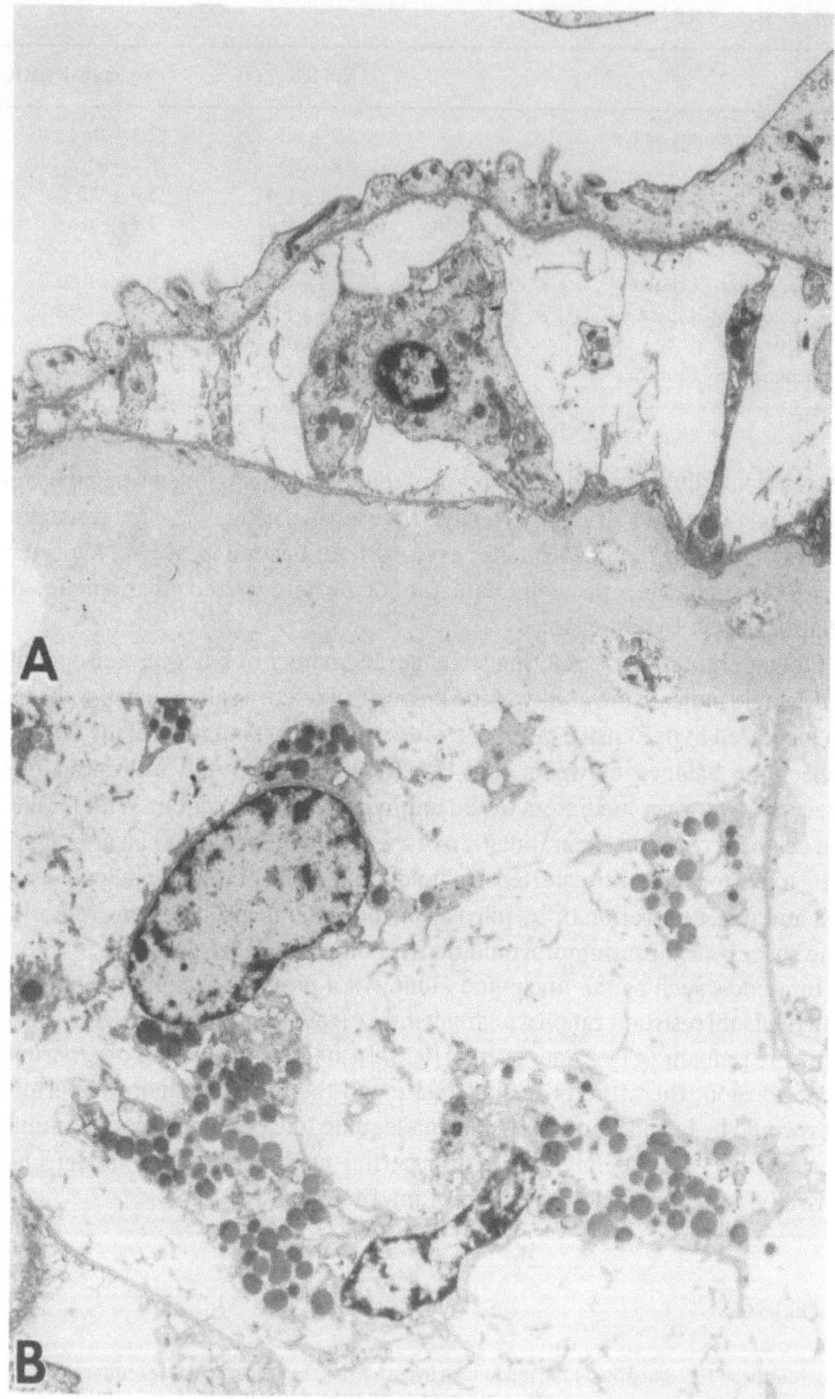

Figure 1A. The renomedullary interstitial cells of the sensitive Dahl rat are scanty in number, contain few osmiophilic granules, and appear somewhat smaller than those of the resistant Dahl rat, × 4900.
Figure 1B. The renomedullary interstitial cells of the resistant Dahl eat are numerous, well developed, and contain numerous osmiophilic granules, × 4900.

Principles and Techniques of Electron Microscopy: Biological Applications. New York, Van Nostrand Reinhold, 1970, vol 3, pp 237-296.

4. Bohman S-O, Jansen PKA: Morphometric studies on the lipid droplets of the interstitial cells of the renal medulla in different states of diuresis. J Ultrastruct Res 55:182-192, 1976.

5. Perov YL, Postnov YV: Lipid droplets of interstitial medullary cells of intact rat kidney with two-kidney Goldblatt hypertension. Virchows Arch (Cell Pathol) 22:163-172, 1976.

6. Pitcock JA, Brown PS, Byers LW, et al.: Degranulation of renomedullary interstitial cells during reversal of hypertension. Hypertension 3 (suppl 2):75-80, 1981.

7. Pitcock JA, Brown PS, Rapp JP, et al.: Morphometric studies on the renomedullary interstitial cells of Dahl hypertension-prone and hypertension-resistant rats, to be published.

8. Bohman S-O: The ultrastructure of the renal medulla and the interstitial cells, in Mandal AK, Bohman S-O (editors): The Renal Papilla and Hypertension. New York, Plenum, 1980, pp 7-29.

9. Mandal AK, Muehrcke RC, Epstein M: Relationship of the renomedullary interstitial cells to experimental hypertension. J Lab Clin Med 70:872-873, 1967.

10. Muehrcke RC, Mandal AK, Epstein M, et al.: Cytoplasmic granularity of the renal medullary interstitial cells in experimental hypertension. J Lab Clin Med 73:299-308, 1969.

11. Tobian L, Ishii M, Duke M: Relationship of cytoplasmic granules in renal papillary interstitial cells to 'post-salt' hypertension. J Lab Clin Med 73:309-319, 1969.

12. Ishii M, Tobian L: Interstitial cell granules in renal papilla and the solute composition of renal tissue in rats with Goldblatt hypertension. J Lab Clin Med 74:47-52, 1969.

13. Tobian L, Ishii M: Interstitial cell granules and solutes in renal papilla in post-Goldblatt hypertension. Am J Physiol 217:1699-1702, 1969.

14. Latta H, White FN, Osvaldo L, et al.: Unilateral renovascular hypertension in rats. Measurements of medullary granules, juxtaglomerular granularity and cellularity and area of adrenal zones. Lab Invest 33:379-390, 1975.

15. Szokol M, Schomig A, Thomazy V, et al.: On the lipid granularity of renomedullary interstitial cells in benign and malignant courses of renal hypertension. Exp Pathol 17:143-151, 1979.

16. Nekrosova AA, Sokolova RI, Lantsberg LA: Prostaglandin-like renal vasodepressor lipids and electrolyte exchange in the kidney, in Bergstrom S (editor): Advances in the Biosciences. International Conference on Prostaglandins. Elmsford, NY, Pergamon, 1973, vol 9, pp 307-312.

17. Mandal AK, Frohlich ED, Chrysant K, et al.: Ultrastructural analysis of renal papillary interstitial cells of spontaneously hypertensive rats. J Lab Clin Med 83:256-262, 1974.

18. Mandal AK, Frohlich ED, Chrysant K, et al.: A morphological study of the renal papillary granule: Analysis in the interstitial cell and the interstitium. J Lab Clin Med 85:120-131, 1975.

19. Simpson FO: Renal vasculature and hypertensive mechanisms. Circ Res 26 + 27 (suppl 2):235-244, 1970.

20. Pitcock JA, Brown PS, Brooks B, et al.: Renomedullary deficiency in partial nephrectomy-salt hypertension. Hypertension 2:281-290, 1980.

21. Muirhead EE, Pitcock JA, Brown PS, et al.: Possible link between converting enzyme inhibition and renomedullary interstitial cells. Fed Proc 40:2262-2267, 1981.

22. Muirhead EE, Rightsel WA, Pitcock JA, et al.: Juxtaglomerular cells grown as monolayer cell culture contain renin, angiotensin I converting enzyme, angiotensins I and II/III. Circ Res, in press.

DISCUSSION

Discussants: Haeusler, Muirhead, Tobian, Johnston, Sambhi, Abadesi

Haeusler: You have shown that for several types of renal hypertension both a decrease in the number of lipid granules of the interstitial cells and degenerative changes in these cells. Do you interpret this decrease in the number of granules as a consequence of increased release in order to counteract hypertension? If so, are the degenerative changes a sign of exhaustion of the cells?

Muirhead: The way we attempt to interpret this is that at a certain phase, degranulation is associated with increased function - the cells are intact. But there comes a time when the cells are markedly reduced and so damaged that they're nonfunctional.

Haeusler: Is the damage due to exhaustion or to a direct deleterious effect of either salt or high blood pressure?

Muirhead: In DOCA-salt hypertension, in partial nephrectomy, salt hypertension in one of the angiotensin-salt models, the amount of salt intake is fantastic - 15 milliequivalents a day in a 400-gram rat, and you can translate how much that would be for a man. Under those conditions, the interstitial cells are damaged whereas in controlled animals, without that salt intake, interstitial cells are intact. So there is a suggestion here that this very high salt intake may be damaging to the cells. Of course, we don't consider the whole picture.

Haeusler: Is there an increased precursor uptake or an increased turnover of lipid material in hypertension?

Muirhead: We have not done that. It's a good point.

Tobian: Just by way of confirmation, some years ago we published a paper where the interstitial cells were affected by diuresis, and we came to the same conclusion. In these fairly healthy cells, increased secretion was associated with degranulation. We saw the same kind of pattern as you did. The other point is that I certainly agree that the volume of the granules is the best way to count. We always counted granules per area, and I'm very leery of people who count granules per cell because they see only a small portion of a given cell. They miss all the cell's processes, and the only way they can tell it's a cell is that they happen to be in the area of the nucleus. It seems much more accurate to count granules per area rather than granules per apparent cell because that apparent cell will only be part of the cell.

Muirhead: Yes, what we do is to take serial sections through an area and then count. We do granule size - granule numbers per area - and that averages out to get a random distribution. This is what volume density is. Volume density is a percent of a given volume - like a hematocrit is a percent of red cells in the volume of blood. We consider it to be a little more accurate in terms of what's there.

Johnston: I wonder if I could just pursue the first point that Dr. Haeusler was making. I take it that you think that the cells secrete lipids in response to a rise in blood pressure and in an attempt to lower it. If you have a mechanism that's driving it so fast the cell gets exhausted, what then determines those models in which you get exhaustion and degeneration of the cell as against those models that are just as hypertensive but don't exhaust the cell?

Muirhead: Let me just allude to your first comment there. We struggled with what is the signal to the cells. I have a hard time accepting pressure as a signal. But it could be that flow associated with pressure is a signal in terms of something in the blood acting as a signal. What that is, we don't know. We suspect that more angiotensin is a bad signal because more angiotensin will tend to decrease flow, less angiotensin is a better signal, captopril blocks it. Now the second question about what determines degeneration, I'm not sure. All I'm saying is that we have some indication that very high salt intake in the rat is bad, and that very high angiotensin is bad. That's about as far as we can go right now.

Sambhi: One type of renal medullary lipid in your data was a direct renin inhibitor. Does it come from the granules also?

Muirhead: The granules are inert. The granules are made up of over 90% of inert triglycerides. All the granules appear to be doing is storing fatty acids.

Sambhi: So these lipids were then extracted from the kidney as a whole?

Muirhead: I think that the renin inhibitors are extracted from whole kidney, and therefore mostly from the cortex. I don't know whether anyone has extracted those particular inhibitors from the medulla alone.

Abadesi: This is a question related to cause and effect in the Dahl-S ratas. Do you see these changes if the Dahl-S rats are kept on a low-salt diet - in other words, are not hypertensive?

Muirhead: These changes were seen in Dahl salt rats that were not hypertensive and on a low-salt diet.

THE PITUITARY AND HYPERTENSION

J. Genest, J. Gutkowska, J. Julesz, E. Schiffrin, P. Hames, M. Chrétien, N.G. Seidah and M. Lis

INTRODUCTION

Many factors are involved in the mechanism of hypertension, and each of these can produce a specific type of hypertension. What needs to be elucidated is how these factors or a combination of some of them interact with one another to produce the condition known as primary or essential hypertension, which affects about 90% of the hypertensive population.

Three key factors control the blood pressure in the arterial system: a) the cardiac output, b) the blood and extracellular fluid volume, and c) the total peripheral resistance. There is a general consensus in view of the overwhelming evidence in favor of an increased peripheral resistance represented by an increased tonicity, responsiveness, and reactivity of the resistance vessels as the key and primary factor leading to essential hypertension [1, 2].

We know little about the factors controlling the basal resting tone of the contractile protein in the resistance vessels, but we know that an increase of free intracellular calcium is associated with increased tonicity and contractility of the arterioles, and that norepinephrine and angiotensin are the most potent physiological vasoconstrictor substances.

The evidence of an increased arteriolar reactivity to norepinephrine, especially from clinical and experimental studies, is overwhelming. Although some results are conflicting, studies dealing with the systemic circulation, the regional vascular beds, or isolated strips generally support an increased vascular reactivity in hypertensive states. This evidence is clearer from the study of precapillary territory, such as the bulbar conjunctiva [3] and in the nailfolds of patients with essential hypertension [4]. These studies show an increased vasomotor activity of the precapillary vessels and of the meta-arteriolar sphincters.

Additional and more important evidence comes from the use of the superior mesenteric artery preparation of McGregor in the rat [5]. If this preparation is perfused with an artificial medium, such as Tyrode or Krebs' solution, the pressor response to a standard ED_{50} dose of norepinephrine (i.e., the dose that will give half of the maximal response) will be an increase in blood pressure. This phenomenon is reproducible over a period of hours. The comparison of the reactivity of the mesenteric artery preparations from SH-rats and from rats with experimental, renal-saline, or DOCA-salt hypertension shows significantly greater responsiveness to the same ED_{50} dose of norepinephrine when compared to the response given by the same preparations from normal rats [5-7].

Furthermore, an increased pressor response to norepinephrine and other pressor agents can be demonstrated before the onset of hypertension in Goldblatt hypertensive dogs [8]. There is also a significantly increased reactivity of arterial strips and of the mesenteric artery preparation prior to the development of hypertension in the 2-K, 1-C Goldblatt dogs, in DOCA-salt hypertension in rats and pigs, in Grollman's hypertensive hamsters, and in hypertensive rabbits with aortic coarctation [9].

Michelakis et al. have demonstrated that plasma from hypertensive patients contains fractions that increase the vascular reactivity to pressor agents such as norepinephrine and angiotensin II when injected intravenously in nephrectomized rats. The increase in sensitivity is more marked with plasma from low-renin essential hypertensive patients and from subjects on a high-sodium intake [10].

The strongest evidence comes from the experiments of Nolla-Palades [11] and from those of Bohr and Berecek [12]. The former used rats made hypertensive by coarctation of the aorta and showed that strips from the femoral arteries protected by the aortic constriction from the increased arterial pressure had the same hyperresponsiveness to pressor agents, such as norepinephrine, as strips from the 'hypertensive' arteries [11]. The latter workers, Bohr and Berecek, obtained similar results in pigs rendered hypertensive by DOCA-saline administration and in which a hind leg was protected from the systemic hypertension by iliac or femoral occlusion [12].

Veins showed increased reactivity to pressor agents both in experimental, as well as in human hypertension. These changes cannot be secondary to an increase in blood pressure in the venous system and must therefore reflect a basic abnormality [13, 14].

This summary of clinical and experimental evidence demonstrates beyond doubt that there is vascular hyperreactivity in various hypertensive conditions, even in the prehypertensive stage. It is difficult to believe that it could be caused by factors other than circulating substances, and it constitutes a major argument against the view that the increased muscle mass in the media of the arteries is primarily responsible for their hyperreactivity and for the increased peripheral resistance [15]. Furthermore, similar degrees of vascular changes have been reported in normotensive patients [16].

Such hyperreactivity to norepinephrine is enhanced by a high salt intake and is decreased or prevented by acute and severe restriction or depletion of sodium [17, 18]. It is also enhanced by vasopressin by angiotensin II, and by aldosterone.

What then are the hormonal-metabolic factors responsible for the increased peripheral resistance as demonstrated by an increased arteriolar reactivity and responsiveness? Almost all the factors that can be involved – ACTH, progesterone, DOC, prostaglandins, kallikrein, and dopamine – are closely related in one way or another to aldosterone and sodium regulation. Others in this symposium will discuss in detail the clinical and experimental data relating the adrenal cortex, especially aldosterone to hypertension, and the disturbances of sodium regulation in hypertensive states.

Of greatest interest are the more recently described findings of a higher content of intracellular sodium in red cells, lymphocytes, and leukocytes and those related to abnormalities in sodium transport across cell membranes for which there are already four different transport systems described: (a) the Na^+/K^+-ATPase pump, (b) the Na^+/K^+ co-transport, (c) the Na^+/Li^+ counter-transport, and (d) the Na^+/Ca^{2+} countertransport. This area is a complex one with many conflicting results. Much work remains to be done to elucidate the nature of these disturbances and to clarify the various sodium transport mechanisms across cell membranes.

There is a great deal of excitement at present concerning deWardener's findings on the natriuretic hormone, which inhibits the Na^+/K^+-ATPase pump and which shows an inverse relationship to the G-6-PD activity [19, 20]. An increase in the circulating natriuretic hormone would explain, at the same time, the inability of the kidney to excrete sodium loads and the increase in intracellular sodium content. This has received wide attention on account of Blaustein's hypothesis that an increased intracellular sodium concentration would lead to an increase in free cytosolic calcium content, leading to increased tonicity and reactivity of the contractile protein [21]. But this remains to be demonstrated with hard data.

In my presentation, I would like to concentrate on the relationships between the pituitary and hypertension. Some of these relationships are described in Table 1. The evidence suggests that the ACTH may be involved in hypertension through its effects on aldosterone and sodium regulation. I would like to describe two recent studies from our Institute: [1] the effect of the N-terminal peptide fragment of pro-opiomelanocortin on aldosterone production from cultured cells from aldosteronomas, and [2] preliminary findings of plasma ACTH concentrations in patients with mild, stable essential hypertension.

Table 1. Reationship of pituitary to hypertension

1. Higher incidence of hypertension in acromegalic patients
2. Hypophysectomy:
    (A) Lowers blood pressure of spontaneously hypertensive, renal hypertensive, and of PHEO-NEDP rats to normal
    (B) Lowers blood pressure of normal and renal hypertensive dogs
    (C) Abolishes the increase in aldosterone secretion in rats in response to sodium depletion
3. No rise in aldosterone secretion after sodium depletion in patients with panhypopituitarism
4. Source of the aldosterone stimulating factor (A.S.F.)
5. ACTH-saline hypertension in sheep and in rats (prevented in the latter by DOC antibodies)

STUDIES OF THE EFFECT OF THE N-TERMINAL PEPTIDE FRAGMENT OF PRO-
OPIOMELANOCORTIN ON ALDOSTERONE PRODUCTION FROM CULTURED CELLS FROM
ALDOSTERONOMAS

This fragment, which is a glycopeptide of 76 amino acids in humans and 80 amino acids in pigs, has been isolated, and its amino acid sequence has been determined by Chrétien and Seidah at our Institute [22] (Fig. 1). The effect of this N-terminal peptide was studied for the production of aldosterone from cultured cells derived from adrenocortical adenomas from two patients with primary aldosteronism.

These two patients had typical clinical and biochemical features of primary aldosteronism. Adrenal adenomas were demonstrated by computer-assisted tomography scans and confirmed at surgery.

In the first patient reported by Lis et al. [23] and by Chrétien et al. [24], the adenoma weighed 14 g. The details for the culture of the cells from this adenoma have been previously described. Results show that both porcine and human N-terminal peptide of pro-opiomelanocortin were much more potent in stimulat-

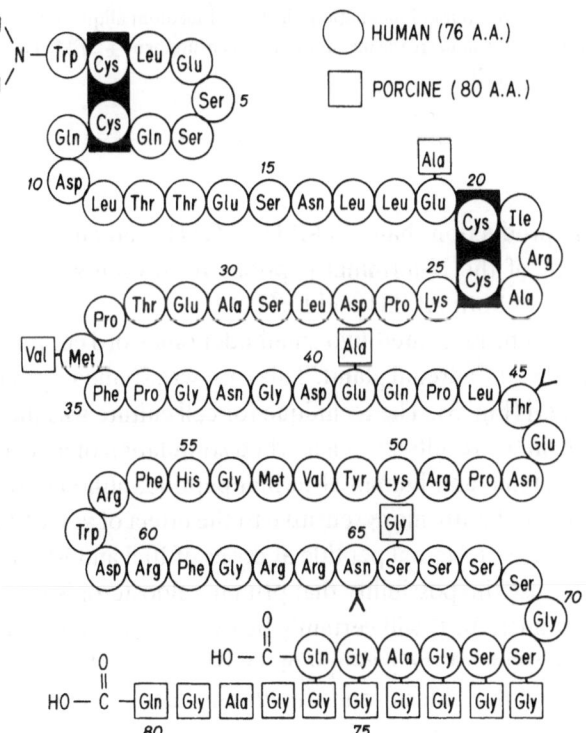

Figure 1. Amino acid sequence of the N-terminal peptide of human and porcine pro-opiomelanocortin, according to Seidah and Chrétien [22].

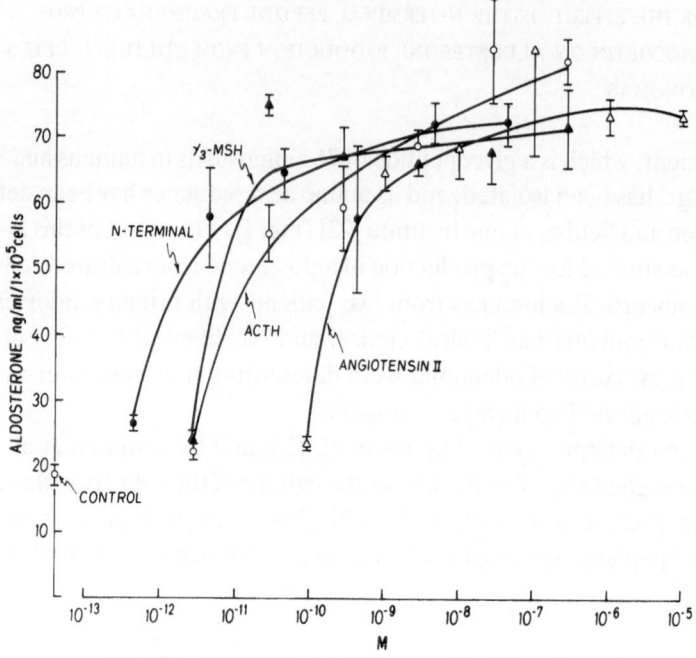

Figure 2. The isolated tumor cells were incubated as a monolayer in a 96-well cell culture plate in a total volume of 2.0 ml. After two hours of incubation, the 0.1-ml medium aliquots were collected for aldosterone determinations. All points are the means of three measurement ± SEM. The control value is the mean of 12 measurements [23].

ing aldosterone production than γ-3 MSH, ACTH, and angiotensin II (Fig. 2). The preparations of the N-terminal peptides from both species were demonstrated to be free of both ACTH and LPH.

The second patient presented two small adenomas of 1 cm in diameter and a small nodule in the left adrenal gland. This case was studied by Schiffrin et al. in our laboratory [25] (Fig. 3). The technique for cell culture was the same as in the first patient. Again the results show a marked stimulation of aldosterone production with both porcine and human N-terinal peptide, although in this case, the cells appeared to be slightly more sensitive to the effect of γ-3 MSH. But this was less potent than the N-terminal peptide at doses of 10⁻¹² and 10⁻¹¹ mol/L (Fig. 4).

These results raise the possibility that primary aldosteronism could be related to a pituitarydysfunction. It will certainly be of interest to compare the effect of this N-terminal peptide of the pro-opiomelanocortin on aldosterone production with the effects of the aldosterone-stimulating factor apparently of pituitary origin isolated by Sen et al. [26, 27].

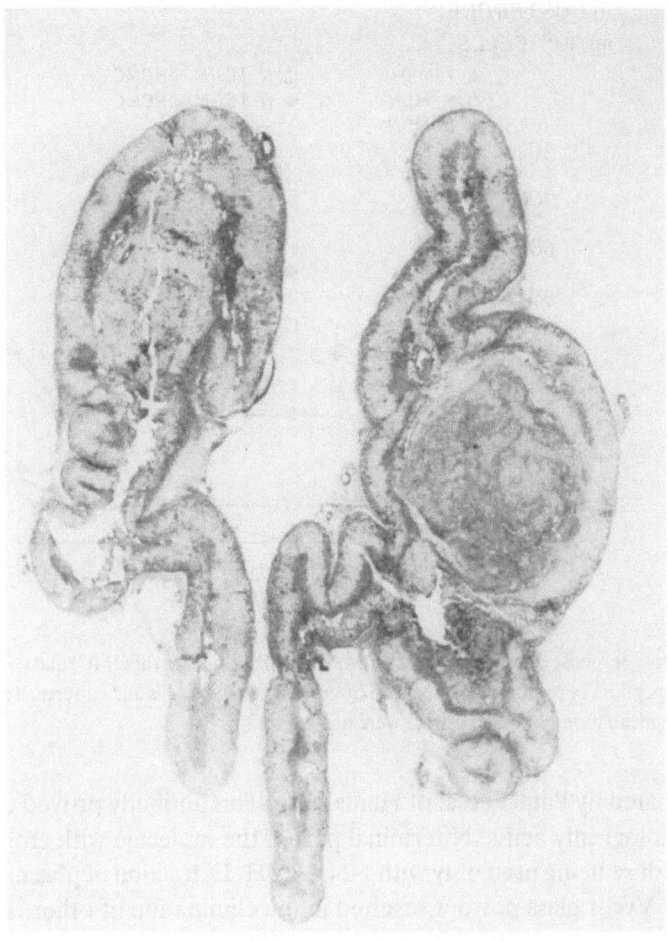

Figure 3. Photograph of the section of the left adrenal from a patient with primary aldosteronism. There were two distinct adenomas of 1 cm in diameter and at least one small nodule.

MEASUREMENT OF PLASMA ACTH CONCENTRATIONS IN PATIENTS WITH MILD, STABLE ESSENTIAL HYPERTENSION

Twenty-five healthy volunteers, aged 22-41 years, served as controls for 21 patients with mild, stable essential hypertension, aged 21 to 63 years. All hypertensive patients had blood pressures between 140-175/90-105 mm Hg, and they were thoroughly evaluated for possible secondary causes for their hypertension. Renal arteriography was done in all patients.

The method used for measurement of plasma ACTH was essentially that of Orth et al. with minor modifications. The ACTH antibody raised in rabbits against synthetic α-h, 39 ACTH coupled to bovine serum albumin, was gener-

514

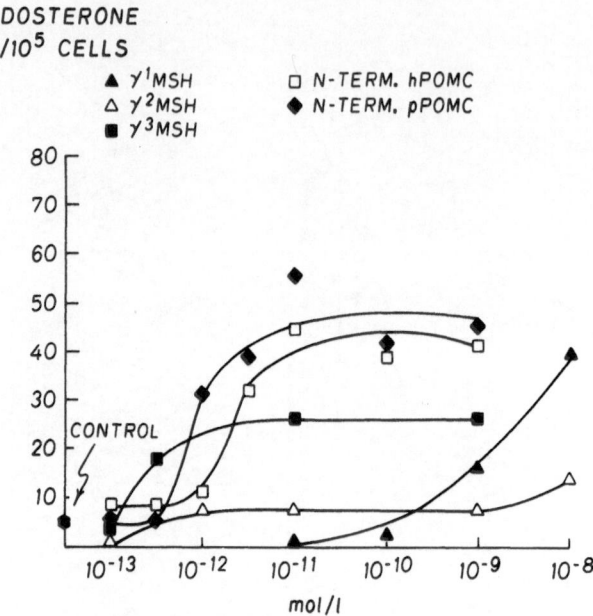

Figure 4. Dose-response curve of γ^1-MSH, γ^2-MSH, γ^3-MSH, human (hPOMC) and porcine (pPOMC) N-terminal peptides of pro-opiomelanocortin by adrenal adenoma cells and cultures. Results are means of duplicate incubation cell wells. Curves were had-drawn.

ously donated by Paul Vecsei of Heidelberg. This antibody proved to be specific for the biologically active N-terminal part of the molecule with cross-reactivity, the procedure being used only with 1-24 ACTH. Extraction of plasma at 4° C with 100-mesh Vycor glass powder resulted in the elimination of other cross-reactive fragments and most of the 1-18 and 1-17 ACTH.

Results of plasma ACTH in control subjects and patients with mild stable essential hypertension are illustrated in Figure 5. Mean plasma ACTH concentration in the control subjects ($N = 25$) was 10.8 pmol/L ± 4 S.D. with a range of 4.6-15.4 pmol/L (one pmol/L equals 4.9 pg/ml). The ACTH plasma concentration in the hypertensive patients was within normal range in three patients and below normal in 17 patients with a mean for the latter group of 4.8 mol/L ($P<0.005$) [28].

Administration of clonidine, a centrally active α-adrenergic agent, given at 200 mg orally in one dose resulted in a significant ($P<0.005$) decrease of plasma ACTH within 2 to 4 hours (Fig. 6). Alpha-methyldopa and propranolol were without effect.

The mechanisms responsible for the significantly lower plasma ACTH concentration in patients with mild and stable essential hypertension remain to be elucidated. It is possible that it may be part of homeostatic mechanism compensating for the hypersensitivity of the adrenal aldosterone production to angiotensin II in hypertensive patients, especially those with low renin [29, 30]. Our

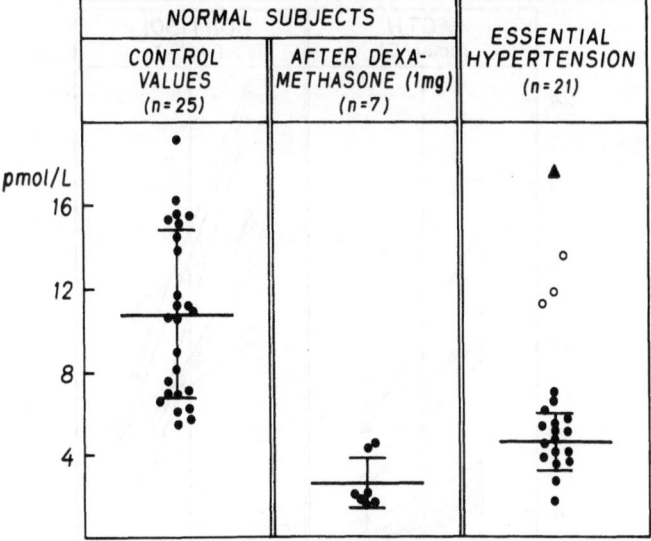

PLASMA ACTH CONCENTRATION IN
PATIENTS WITH MILD ESSENTIAL HYPERTENSION

Figure 5. Results of plasma ACTH concentration expressed as pmol/L in 25 control subjects, 7 of whom received dexamethasone (1 mg) and in 21 patients with mild and stable essential hypertension.

studies are being extended to other patients with essential hypertension of greater severity and to secondary hypertension.

SUMMARY

In summary, we have presented evidence demonstrating that the key and primary factor of hypertension is an increased peripheral resistance, first functional in nature and due to an increased tonicity, responsiveness, and reactivity of the resistance arterioles. This disturbance is, from all available evidence, related to disturbances in sodium regulation. In that relation, we have reported results of the stimulating effects of the N-terminal peptide of pro-opiomelanocortin on aldosterone production by cultured cells from aldosteronomas as well as some preliminary studies on the plasma ACTH concentration in patients with mild stable essential hypertension.

516

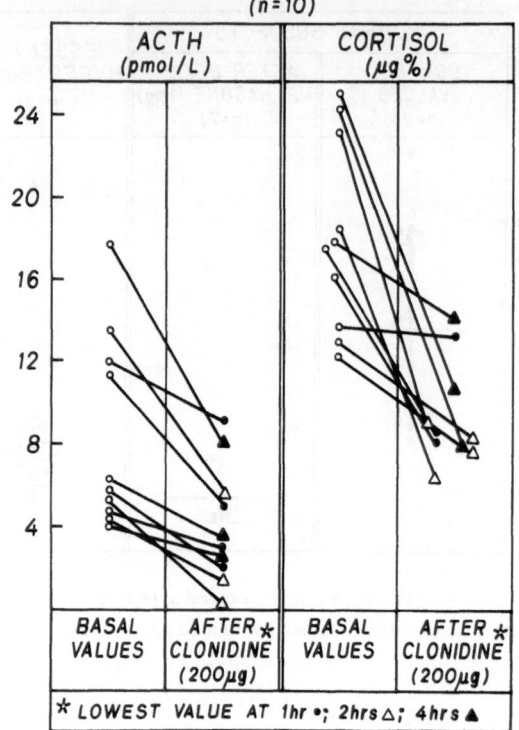

Figure 6. Effect of clonidine on plasma ACTH and cortisol concentration in 10 patients with mild, stable essential hypertension.

REFERENCES

1. Genest J, Nowaczynski W, Boucher R, et al.: Role of the adrenal cortex and sodium in the pathogenesis of human hypertension. Can Med Assoc J 118:538-549, 1978.
2. Genest J: Personal views on the mechanisms of hypertension, in Genest J, Kuchel O, Hamet M, et al. (editors): Hypertension: Physiopathology and Treatment, New York, McGraw-Hill, 1983.
3. Lee RE, Holze EH: Peripheral vascular hemodynamics in the bulbar conjunctiva of subjects with hypertensive cardiovascular disease. J Clin Invest 30:539-546, 1951.
4. Greisman SE: The reactivity of the capillary bed of the nailfold to circulating epinephrine and norepinephrine and norepinephrine in patients with normal blood pressure and with essential hypertension. J Clin Invest 31:782-788, 1952.
5. McGregor TD, Smirk FM: Vascular responses in mesenteric arteries from genetic and renal hypertensive rats. Am J Physiol 214:1429-1433, 1968.
6. Collis MG, Alps PJ: The renin-angiotensin system, dietary salt and increased sensitivity to noradrenaline in mesenteric vasculature preparations from renal/salt hypertensive rats. Cardiovasc Res 10:232-235, 1976. Cardiovasc Res 9:118-126, 1975. Arch Int Pharmacodyn Ther 211:107-114, 1974.

7. Beilin LJ, Wade DN, Honour AJ, et al.: Vascular hyperreactivity with sodium loading and with deoxycorticosterone induced hypertension in the rat. Clin Sci 39:793-810, 1970.

8. Ogden E, Brown LT, Page EW: The increased sensitivity of arterial muscle in the prehypertensive phase of experimental renal hypertension. Am J Physiol 129:560-564, 1940.

9. Greenberg S, McGowan C, Saida N: Vascular responses to vasoactive agents during the development of 2-K, 1-C Goldblatt hypertension in dogs. Circ Res 48:895-906, 1981. Clin Sci Mol Med 55:31s-36s, 1978.

10. Michelakis AM, Mizukoshi H, Huang C, et al.: Further studies on the existence of a sensitizing factor to pressor agents in hypertension. J Clin Endocrinol Metab 41:90-96, 1975.

11. Nolla-Palades J: Hypertension and increased hind limb vascular reactivity in experimental coarctation of the aorta. Circ Res 12:3-9, 1962.

12. Bohr DF, Berecek KH: Relevance of vascular structural and smooth muscle sensitivity changes in hypertension. Aust NZ J Med 6:26-34, 1976. Circ Res 42:764-771, 1978.

13. Overbeck HW: Hemodynamics of early experimental renal hypertension in dogs. Circ Res 31:653-661, 1972.

14. Greenberg S, Bohr DF: Venous smooth muscle in hypertension: Enhanced contractility of portal veins from spontaneously hypertensive rats. Circ Res 36 (suppl I):I208-I213, 1975.

15. Folkow B: Cardiovascular structural adaptation: Its role in the initiation and maintenance of primary hypertension. Clin Sci Mol Med 55:3-22, 1978.

16. Moritz R, Oldt MR: Arteriolar sclerosis in hypertensive and non-hypertensive individuals. Am J Pathol 13:679-728, 1937.

17. Friedman S: Hypertension: Physiopathology and treatment. Blood Vessels 16:2-16, 1979. Microvasc Res 3:416-425, 1971. Hypertension 1:572-582, 1979.

18. Reid WU, Laragh JH: Sodium and potassium intake, blood pressure and pressor response to angiotensin. Proc Soc Exp Biol Med 120:26-29, 1965.

19. De Wardener HE, MacGregor GA: Dahl's hypothesis that the saluretic substance may be responsible for a sustained rise in arterial pressure: Its possible role in essential hypertension. Kidney Int 18:1-9, 1980.

20. De Wardener HE, MacGregor GA: The natriuretic hormone, in Genest J, Kuchel O, Hamet P, et al. (editors): Hypertension: Physiopathology and Treatment, ed 2. New York, McGraw-Hill, 1983.

21. Blaustein MP: Sodium ions, calcium ions, blood pressure regulation and hypertension. Am J Physiol 232:C165-C173, 1977. Clin Exp Hypertens 3:173-178, 1901.

22. Seidah NG, Chrétien M: Complete amino acid sequence of a human pituitary glycopeptide in an important maturation product of pro-opiomelanocortin. Proc Natl Acad Sci USA 78:4236-4240, 1981. J Biol Chem 256:7977-7984, 1981.

23. Lis M, Hamet P, Gutkowska J, et al.: Effect of N-terninal portion of proopiomelanocortin on aldosterone release in human adrenal adenoma in vitro. J Clin Endocrinol Metab 52:1053-1056, 1981.

24. Chrétien M, Lis M, Larivière N, et al.: Primary aldosteronism: A pituitary adrenal dysfunction related to a new pituitary glycopeptide? (submitted for publication).

25. Schiffrin EL, Chrétien M, Seidah NG, et al.: Response of human aldosteronoma cells in culture to the N-terminal glycopeptide of pro-opiomelanocortin and γ^3-MSH, (submitted for publication).

26. Sen S, Bumpus FM: A hypertensive micromolecule from human urine. Acta Physiol Lat Am 24:496, 1975.

27. Sen S, Valenzuela R, Smeby R, et al.: Localization, purification and biological activity of a new aldosterone-stimulating factor. Hypertension 3 (suppl 1):81-86, 1981. Hypertension 3:4-10, 1981.

28. Julesz J, Gutkowska J, Genest J: Plasma ACTH in essential hypertension, (submitted for publication).

29. Brown RD, Wisgerhof M, Carpenter PC, et al.: Adrenal sensitivity to angiotensin II and

518

undiscovered aldosterone stimulating factors in hypertension. J Steroid Biochem 11:1043-1050, 1979.

30. Rayfield EJ, Rose LI, Dluhy RG, et al.: Aldosterone secretory and glucocorticoid excretory responses to α 1-24 ACTH (Cortrosyn) in sodium-depleted normal man. J Clin Endocrinol Metab 36:30-35, 1973.

DISCUSSION

Discussants: Melby, Genest, Tobian, Denton, Bohr, Laragh

Melby: In our experieence, using γ³-MSH, we're able to markedly increase aldosterone biosynthesis by dispersed model layer culture tumor cells from patients with aldosterone adenomas and also from glomerulosa cells from rats. But we also get ACTH stimulation in man and rat of cortisol biosynthesis. I'm wondering, have you specifically looked at the stimulation of the glucocorticoids with your fragments and have you also measured γ³-MSH?

Genest: Obviously, this has to be done. Already a group has demonstrated that γ³-MSH potentiated the effect of ACTH on cortisone release. We are on the lookout for patients with primary aldosteronism for further such studies on adrenal cell cultures and we plan to investigate the effects of various fragments of the pro-opiomelanocortin on cell cultures of rat adrenals.

Tobian: I thought, when you showed your picture of the molecule that γ³-MSH was almost part of ACTH. Is it part of a long chain and then it gets clipped down?

Genest: There are three forms of MSH, α, β, γ. The main reason why they are called MSH is because they have the same hexapeptide sequence in the three of them. The α-MSH is the 1-13 ACTH. The β-MSH is the 41-58 peptide in the β-lipoprotein, and the γ¹- and γ²-MSH are the 51-62 peptide in the N-terminal, the γ²-being acetylated a AA-51. The γ³-MSH is the peptide 51-76 of the N-terminal.

Denton: You kindly referred to our work on ACTH hypertension but you called it ACTH saline hypertension. I wasn't quite clear why you used the term saline.

Genest: Because lately some people reviewing your work referred repeatedly to the fact that these sheep were on a high saline intake. I didn't have time to check the original papers and that was surprising. But in these reviews I can give you the references. They referred to ACTH-saline hypertension.

Denton: I see, they got it wrong, actually it's not sodium dependent. The sodium-depleted animal still becomes hypertensive with ACTH.

Genest: I'm sorry.

Bohr: I agree with your bias about vascular sensitivity being increased in these various types of hypertension, but I missed the connection between that and your pituitary story or was there one?

Genest: The pituitary is part of the search for factors involved in the increased peripheral resistance. The lower ACTH values may be a secondary facet related to factors involved in the peripheral resistance.

Laragh: Would you be willing to speculate about how the findings with your fragment fit with your other observation, that the ACTH is often low in hypertension?

Genest: One possible explanation is that the adrenal glomerulosa cells secreting aldosterone were more sensitive to angiotensin than in normotensive animals or in humans. Maybe it is part of the compensatory homeostatic mechanism that the ACTH is lower because of this hyperresponsiveness of the adrenal cells to angiotensin II, or because angiotensin infusions to normal subjects decrease plasma ACTH concentration.

Laragh: I was wondering whether some other fragment could be replacing ACTH that you don't pick up by your longer fragment, and that would give you a lower ACTH because something else was higher. Do you think that's possible?

Genest: That is possible. This is a new door open that may answer the questions about the unknown pituitary factor involved in the aldosterone response.

STRESS, ACTH, AND HYPERTENSION

D.A. Denton, J.P. Coghlan, M. McKinley, J. Nelson, B.A. Scoggins,
R. Weisinger and J.A. Whitworth

INTRODUCTION

It is well recognized that blood pressure is responsive to emotional influences, and that psychosocial events can aggravate or ameliorate existing hypertension in man and can cause hypertension in animals. Henry and Cassell [1] have reviewed experimental and clinical data, which they believe are consistent with the hypothesis that repeated arousal of the defense-alarm response may be one important mechanism involved in the etiology of essential hypertension. It is proposed that in man arousal follows when previously socially-sanctioned patterns of behavior, especially those to which the organism has become adapted during critical early learning periods, can no longer be used to express normal behavioral urges. Adaptation difficulties, as in the example of status ambiguity, may result in years of repeated arousals of vascular autonomic and hormonal function due to the perception of classes of events as being threatening. Progressive and eventually irreversible vascular disturbances result. The psychologically significant defense alarm response has been proposed by Charvat et al. [2] as having a significant role in essential hypertension. Mechanisms have been identified whereby hypothalamic impulses may modify hindbrain response to carotid sinus inflow, preventing the fall in blood pressure that characteristically follows baroreceptor stimulation [3].

Evidence from human studies, consonant with the hypothesis of psychosocial influence on blood pressure, include the observations of Graham [4] on high blood pressure (180 mm Hg or more) in over 30% of a victorious battalion resting in the Libyan desert. Their blood pressure returned to normal after a few weeks. An epidemic of high blood pressure was also recorded in the siege and bombardment of Leningrad [5]. The comprehensive studies of Scotch and Geiger [6] showed a considerable difference between blood pressure in urban and rural Zulu populations in South Africa. Mean blood pressure and frequency of hypertension were greater in urban than in rural populations. Scotch [7] puts much emphasis on the fact that in rural Zulu, women having a large number of children is associated with normal blood pressure. This was also recorded by Miall and Oldham [8] in Wales, and Boe et al. [9] in Norway.

The reverse was seen in urban Zulu women. In rural Zulu areas, status is related to ability to produce children. But in urban conditions, where women are often the wage earners and alcoholism, divorce, job competition, and humiliation are frequent, children often compounded these problems. Social stress is proposed as being the cause for the difference in the incidence of hypertension. In a study of individuals in the US exposed to high-stress situations, Cobb and Rose [10] examined the prevalence of hypertension and peptic ulcer in 4,325 male air-traffic controllers working in control towers and centers as compared with 8,435 second-class airmen. Although differences in age and licencing procedures may have influenced the analysis, the prevalence of hypertension was four times higher in air-traffic controllers. Furthermore, there was some evidence of higher prevalence of hypertension in towers where traffic density was high. This was also true of peptic ulcer prevalence.

In animal studies, sustained high blood pressure has been produced by Pavlovian conditioning techniques in dogs, by interference with basic sex responses in monkeys and baboons [5], during aversive operant conditioning in chimpanzees [11] and in mice under conditions of crowding and social interaction in the absence of appropriate experience in early life of reactions to con-specifics due to rearing in isolation [1]. Folkow and Rubinstein [12] have shown that mild intermittent stimulus via an electrode planted in the defense area of the lateral hypothalamus, if continued for weeks intermittently, may eventually lead to mild persistent hypertension, although no evident disturbance apart from alertness was seen during stimulation.

It is clear that if stress is a contributory cause of essential hypertension concomitant with other factors, there are diverse physiological pathways whereby any chronic effect could occur. Whereas the neurogenic and sympathetico-adrenal pathways rightly claim high profile in some scenarios of causation, there are other physiological mechanisms worthy of intense scrutiny in this context.

In the overall reaction to stress situations, a major element of physiological response is in the hypothalamic-pituitary-adrenal axis with the release of ACTH. Major effects might result from the long-term episodic but frequent excess release of this peptide in circumstances similar to those mentioned above. I wish to raise two questions that involve fruitful areas for future research in man.

There is a substantial body of evidence, epidemiological, physiological, biochemical, and clinical, pointing to a major causative role of excess salt intake in the etiology of hypertension. By excess we mean grossly in excess of physiological requirement for replacement of obligatory loss and reproduction as exemplified by level of intake and normal health in unacculturated societies. Physiological evidence indicates that the 'set point' of sodium status involves turnover in the range of 3-10 mmol/day - probably reflecting the dietetic history of primates and hominoids over the course of evolution from the Oligocene onwards. By contrast, in contemporary technological society, intake may range from 50-500 mmol/day. A second tenet is that only a minor proportion of society (perhaps 15-20%) has a genetically determined susceptibility to develop hypertension in the face of excess

522

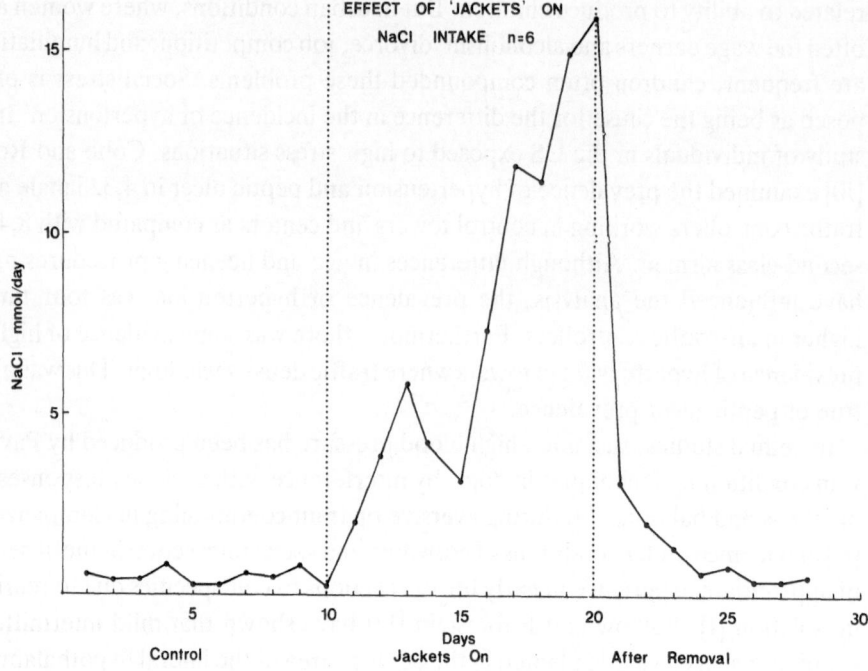

Figure 1. The effect of strapping jackets on the backs of caged wild rabbits on voluntary intake of 500 mM NaCl solution. Over the first 5 days, the rabbits succeeded in dislodging the jackets after a period of some hours, but thereafter, they remained attached over 24 hours.

salt intake. The evidence of this view of the etiology of hypertension is presented in detail elsewhere [13].

If it were true, then it is a matter of some importance that stress and ACTH can directly cause large salt appetite and also that ACTH, in itself, is a hypertensinogenic agent. There is clear-cut data on these effects in experimental animals.

MATERIALS AND METHODS

In wild rabbits, we found that fixing jackets on their backs was an extremely stressful maneuver, and this caused a very large rise in voluntary salt intake. However, it reversed when the jackets were removed. The amount (mean, 15 mmol/day) represents turnover of about 30% of ECF sodium per day. The effect is placed in perspective by consideration of the rabbit's salt-drinking behavior when adrenalectomized and deprived of salt for 1-3 days. The animals take 9-12 hours to correct deficit, which is done in precise fashion - no overdrinking occurring. With 3 days of adrenal insufficiency, this usually involves approximately 15 mmol, so that the response to stress by the sodium-replete animals was similar.

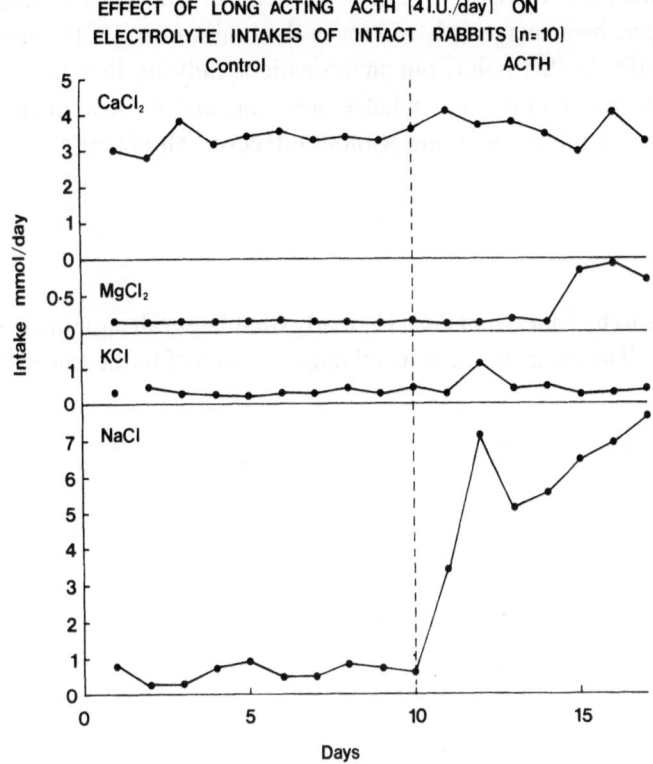

EFFECT OF LONG ACTING ACTH [4 I.U./day] ON
ELECTROLYTE INTAKES OF INTACT RABBITS [n= 10]

Figure 2. The effect of long-acting ACTH (Organon 4 IU/day) on appetite for electrolyte solutions (500 mEq/L) by adrenal-intact wild rabbits. Intake reverts to basal by 2–3 days.

The administration of large doses of ACTH to the animals also causes a large salt appetite, but mean intake (about 6-7 mmol/day) is only about half of that caused by very severe stress. If the hormones cortisol and corticosterone are given to contrive blood levels similar to that with ACTH, the response is only about half that seen with ACTH. From this starting point, a remarkably interesting fact emerged.

If ACTH were given to an adrenalectomized rabbit, a large increase in salt appetite occurred, although not as great as in the adrenal-intact animal. This suggested that the peptide may have a direct action on the brain - analogous to the de Wied experiments on conditioned avoidance behavior. Furthermore, and of singular importance, if in an adrenalectomized animal basal maintenance DOCA were continued and thus no change of sodium balance occurred, but the cortisol support was halved causing rise in endogenous ACTH production, there was a clear-cut increase in salt appetite. This result with endogenous ACTH - physiologically produced rather than exogenously administered - raises the following questions. Does the endogenous ACTH enter the circulation and then cross the blood-brain barrier to have the effect? Does it travel up the vessels of the pituitary stalk, as has been suggested, and reach the brain, or is ACTH generated in the brain itself? At this point, our investigations indicate that the 4-10 fragment, which acts in conditioned avoidance behavior, and the 4-10 analogue, which is superactive in this context, are without effect on salt appetite.

RESULTS

It remains to be added that ACTH greatly stimulates salt appetite in the rat and in the sheep. Turnover of salt induced ranges from half to the total of extracellular

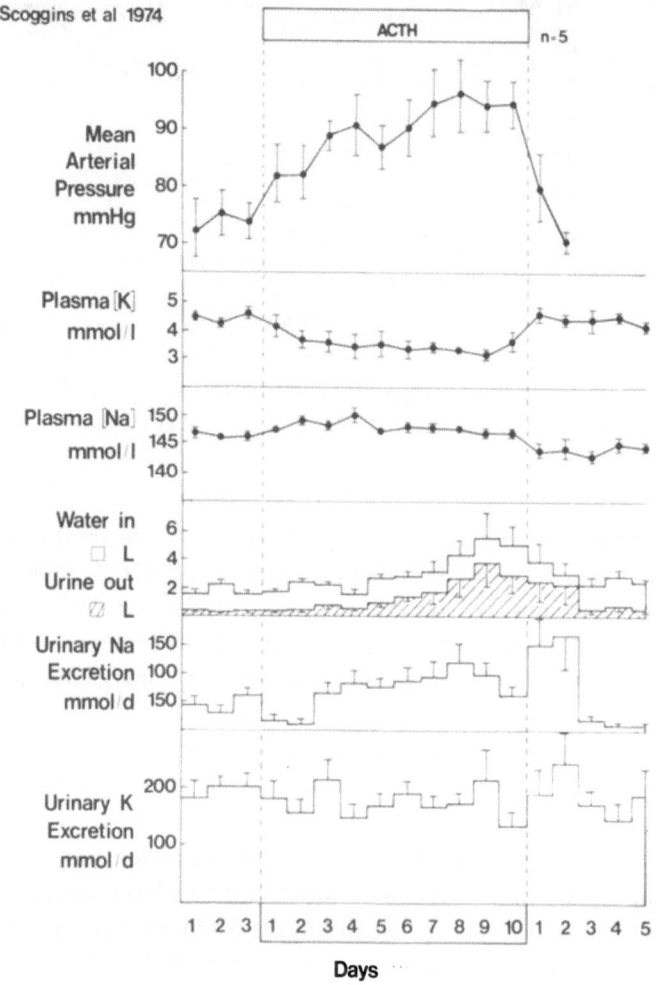

Figure 3. The effect of 10 days administration of ACTH (20 μg/kg/day of Synacthen) on mean arterial pressure, plasma [K] and [Na], urinary electrolyte excretion, water intake, and urine volume in 5 sheep (figure redrawn from Scoggins et al. 1974).

sodium content in sheep to total body sodium content each day in rats. However, in neither species does ACTH stimulate salt appetite in the adrenalectomized animal.

There is a body of data that reflects the other side of the coin in our proposal in relation to ACTH and to the effect on sodium homeostasis. That is, as well as generating salt appetite, a balanced appraisal requires recognition that ACTH may cause increased sodium loss. There are data that show unequivocally that after 4-5 days of a high level of ACTH administration, major degenerative changes occur in the glomerulosa of the adrenal, concurrent with fasciculate hypertrophy.

This deleterious effect on glomerulosa is validated functionally by the demonstration that aldosterone hypersecretion in response to sodium deficiency and angiotensin is much blunted. On the other hand, to preempt an obvious question, it is quite clear from appropriate time sequence balance studies in our laboratories that the salt appetite-inducing effect of ACTH precedes any increase in urinary sodium excretion.

DISCUSSION

In the face of this data on several species, it would be most interesting to know the influence of ACTH on salt appetite in man, but no systematic study has been done. Differences in salt preference, which may reflect corresponding differences in intake, do exist. For example, Desor and colleagues found that black children and adolescents in the U.S. showed a much greater preference for salt than age-matched white children and both black and white adults. The cause for this and any relation to greater prevalence of hypertension in the black population is unknown. If there is a genetically based ethnic difference, it would seem to be of great importance.

It has been known from early days of treatment of rheumatoid arthritis with ACTH that hypertension may occur. A systematic study in sheep has shown that ACTH administration can cause a consistently reproducible sustained mild to moderate hypertension. If a 'cocktail' of the principal and commonly measured hormones in the adrenal effluent is given (viz., cortisol, corticosterone, deoxycorticosterone, deoxycortisol, and aldosterone), there is only a small rise in blood pressure, though other characteristic metabolic effects of ACTH occur [14].

However, adding two other components, we identified a high concentration in adrenal venous effluent – 17α20αdihydroxyprogesterone and 17αhydroxyprogesterone, which is converted in blood to 17α20αdihydroxyprogesterone – causing a rise in blood pressure comparable to that with ACTH. Curiously, these steroids have no hypertensinogenic action in their own right. Further studies have shown that they do not have *in vivo* mineralocorticoid or glucocorticoid activity, and this is confirmed in *in vitro* binding systems. Accordingly, we have termed

526

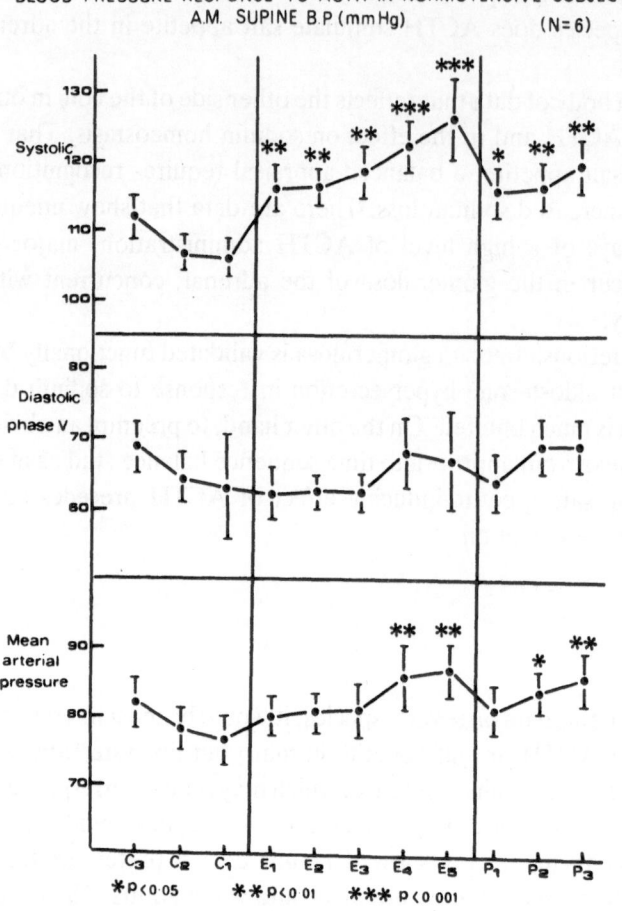

Figure 4. The effect of ACTH (2 μg/kg/day, Synacthen) on blood pressure in 6 normotensive subjects (A.M., supine).

them 'hypertensinogenic' steroids. At present, we have no idea whether they exert their effect on blood pressure through a classical genomic action or through nongenomic effects [14].

Significant among many physiological changes that occur with the development of hypertension with ACTH are increases in cardiac output, heart rate and stroke volume, plasma volume, water turnover, and CSF sodium and osmotic pressure, but there is no increase in total peripheral resistance over 5 days. However, if a beta blocker is administered prior to ACTH, blood pressure still increases, with the change now being an initial increase of peripheral resistance rather than an increase of cardiac output.

Recently, our group [15] showed that ACTH administration to normal subjects and patients with mild essential hypertension caused a modest increase of 20 mm

Hg in systolic blood pressure over 5 days, accompanied by similar metabolic changes as in the sheep. This includes the large rise in 17α20αdihydroxy-progesterone as well as the other steroids. The corresponding 'cocktail' infusion experiments with and without inclusion of 17α20αdihydroxyprogesterone have yet to be done in man. We do not know whether the hypertensinogenic mechanism is analogous to that of the sheep.

Overall, the question emerging from this analysis is whether psychosocial stress, at least in some personality patterns, may result in chronic, though, very probably episodic, activation of the hypothalamic-pituitary-adrenal axis; in integral, over a period of time, this has quantitative effects on salt intake and on hemodynamic mechanisms. The increased salt intake could cause hypertensinogenic effects in those genetically susceptible and aggravate any direct hypertensinogenic effects that ACTH-stimulated steroids might have. Furthermore, such effects could also synergize with those due to any increased catecholaminergic activity.

REFERENCES

1. Henry JP, Cassell JC: Psychosocial factors in essential hypertension. Recent epidemiological and animal experimental evidence. Am J Epidemiol 90:171, 1969.
2. Charvat J, Dell P, Folkow G: Mental factors and cardiovascular diseases. Cardiologica 44:124-141, 1964.
3. Smith OA, Nathan MA, Clarke NP: Central nervous system pathways mediating blood pressure changes, in Wood JE (editor): Hypertension. Neural Control of Arterial Pressure. Proceedings of the Council on High Blood Pressure Research. New York, American Heart Association, 1968, vol 16.
4. Grahàm JDP: High blood pressure after battle. Lancet 1:239-240, 1945.
5. Miashnikov AL: Significance of disturbances of higher nervous activity in the pathogenesis of hypertensive disease, in Cort JH, Fencl V, Hejl Z, et al. (editors): Symposium on the Pathogenesis of Essential Hypertension. New York, p 153.
6. Scotch NA, Geiger HG: The epidemiology of essential hypertension: A review with special attention to psychologic and sociocultural factors. II. Psychologic and sociocultural factors in aetiology. J Chronic Dis 16:1183-1213, 1963.
7. Scoth NA: Sociocultural factors in the epidemiology of Zulu hypertension. Am J Public Health 53:1205-1213, 1963.
8. Miall WE, Oldham PD: Factors influencing arterial blood pressure in the general population. Clin Sci 17:409, 1958.
9. Boe J, Humerfelt S, Wedervarg F: The blood pressure in population; blood pressure readings and height and weight determination in adult population of the city of Bergen. Acta Med Scand (Suppl 321):157, 1957.
10. Cobb S, Rose RM: Hypertension, peptic ulcer and diabetes in air traffic controllers. JAMA 224:489, 1973.
11. Meehan JP, Fineg J, Mosely JD: The effect of restraint and training on the arterial pressure of the immature chimpanzee. Fed Proc 23:515, 1964.
12. Folkow B, Rubinstein EH: Cardiovascular effects of acute and chronic stimulations of the hypothalamic defense area in the rat. Acta Physiol Scand 68:48-57, 1966.

528

13. Denton DA: The Hunger for Salt. New York, Springer-Verlag, 1982.
14. Coghlan JP, Butkus A, Denton DA, et al.: Steroid receptors and hypertension. Circ Res 46(6):188-193, 1980.
15. Whitworth JA, Saines D, Thatcher R, et al.: Blood pressure, renal and metabolic effects of ACTH in normotensive man. Clin Sci 61:2695-2725, 1981.

DISCUSSION

Discussants: Laragh, Denton, Melby, Sambhi, Bohr, Palkovits

Laragh: If you were looking for this phenomenon in humans, how would you go about looking for it? Should you measure 17-alpha, 20-alpha-hydroxyprogesterone in the blood as a index of ACTH hypertension? Would that work out?

Denton: Well, I think that is certainly one initial step, and we are doing that. I don't think we've got adequate data at this stage to make a statement on it. I would add that at this point we haven't seen any spectacular rises in hypertension.

Laragh: In humans, and in animal models too, you can produce hypertension with cortisol and in fact it was done years ago in the rat, dog, and the rabbit. How does cortisol hypertension differ from ACTH hypertension? Obviously it does.

Denton: If you give an amount of cortisol-equivalent and contrive the same blood level as with ACTH, in the sheep you get only a minor change in blood pressure. There is, therefore, something occurring additionally with ACTH. If we add those other steroids in, including DOCA, we get a small additional rise, but it's only when we add in the 17-alpha, 20-alpha that we get the full picture as with ACTH. Any speculation about the role in man must await determination of whether we can reproduce in man the phenomenon we see in sheep, because it does point to some very curious action of 17-alpha, 20-alpha which does not appear on the basis of binding studies to be either a minero- or glucocorticoid.

Laragh: Can you show that 17-alpha, 20-alpha is a vasoconstrictor in an assay?

Denton: No.

Laragh: What happens in ACTH hypertension to plasma renin?

Denton: It goes down, but plasma volume definitely goes up.

Laragh: Even though you can get it with zero salt intake?

Denton: Yes, it appears to be a redistribution.

Laragh: How does ACTH stimulate salt appetite?

Denton: I suppose the direct answer is that I don't know. But of course there's another body of data. For example, the remarkable salt appetite rabbits get in pregnancy and lactation. This will involve turnover in the sodium-replete animal of the total sodium content of extracellular fluid per day. We find that in order to reproduce this phenomenon, we require to have the action of five steroid and peptide hormones. In effect, the animal is initially primed with estrogen and progesterone in physiological amounts or, alternatively, pseudopregnancy is induced, and we then add ACTH, prolactin and oxytocin again in physiological amounts. This reproduces the biological phenomenon. What this is pointing to, I think, is that it is actually a transcription translation process which is induced by a change in sodium in cells, as has been proposed by a lot of the workers on mitogenesis. The fact that the steroid hormones will induce appetite points to a fairly complex neurochemical mechanism underlying it, in contrast to the mechanism of thirst. Now, you're really asking the question of how ACTH acts on cells and, of course, there are many debates on that and also specifically how it acts on neurons, and I don't know the answer at this point.

Laragh: But it would be interesting to speculate that when any of us are under stress and make our ACTH go up as with athletic events or stressful examinations, etc., that we eat salt and don't know it. Do you think that's possible?

Denton: I think it's going to be very interesting to investigate it though the obvious difficulties in validating it in the human are evident.

Laragh: Does the 17-alpha, 20-alpha-hydroxyprogesterone come from the adrenal gland?

Denton: Yes, definitely.

Melby: It does not come from the human adrenal gland. You probably know that we did look at the human adrenal venous effluent. 17-alpha-hydroxyprogesterone does, but it's rate-limited by the next enzyme, 21-hydroxylase, and you can only go up so much. But in man, you couldn't achieve the levels that you've achieved in the sheep.

Laragh: Where does the 21 hydroxylation occur?

Melby: In the adrenal cortex.

Laragh: But not in man, though.

Melby: Yes – of course it does. He's talking about 20-alpha hydroxylation peripherally in the sheep and also in the adrenal. This doesn't occur to any extent in man.

Denton: There's a rise with ACTH in man in the 17-alpha, 20-alpha with ACTH. We measured it.

Melby: I don't doubt that. But I jut say that in the adrenal venous effluent you can't show it. You have to make it from 17-alpha-hydroxyprogesterone in the periphery.

Denton: But, of course, the virture of the sheep model may be that it points to the feasibility of a comparable process in man. We'll get an idea when we do the cocktail infusion experiment in the human.

Sambhi: Would you consider this whole process to be rather independent of the kidney? Do you believe that the kidney may not necessarily get involved at this initial stage? And my second question is, have you tried to get rid of one of the kidneys in some of your models? I assume it will accelerate the ACTH hypertension.

Denton: Yes, the renin and angiotensin go down with hypertension, as Dr. Laragh mentioned. It is also true that if you reduce sodium intake or you deplete them, you can still get the hypertension - albeit somewhat less. So it's not a classical sodium retention DOCA type. The third thing is that if you reduce renal mass and you increase salt intake, you can aggravate the hypertension. So it can be modified by those kinds of physiological events.

Bohr: Was my interpretation correct that these are cardiac output hypertensions – at least the three-day run that you showed us was cardiac output – and if that's correct, does it continue to be cardiac output on the long run, and what happens with beta blockers?

Denton: The answer to the first question is yes, over five. I think it's been measured up to ten days. It is increased cardiac output. If you give a beta blocker, you still get the hypertension without the rise in cardiac output, and peripheral resistance goes up.

Laragh: Yes, that also occurs in primary aldosteronism where administration of a beta blocker drops the cardiac output. However, the peripheral resistance goes up, and so the pressure goes even higher, just as it does in other low-renin states. After beta blockade you can vary the nature of a hypertension shifting the cardiac output to resistance ratio to the right. But blood pressure stays up, or goes higher. This is exactly what happens when you give a beta blocker in primary aldosteronism where there's no renin to suppress. The blood pressure rises. You have to suppress renin to suppress the blood pressure with these drugs. The reasoning checks out.

Denton: My hypothesis as to why it goes up is that there is a center that has been reset and it's going to use some response or another, cardiac output or total peripheral resistance, to get the pressure up to the called-for reset value.

Laragh: I understand your proposition, but my answer to it is that in high-renin hypertension your postulated center is nonexistent because then the blood pressure goes down when you give a beta blocker. It's only in low-renin forms that this 'center' hypothesis holds. If I were to give the beta blocker to a high-renin form of hypertension, the blood pessure would drop, but in the low-renin from it doesn't drop, so whatever the resetting center is, renin has to be changed to change the blood pressure.

Palkovitz: You mentioned the possible role of brain-borne ACTH in hypertension. Could you comment on it a little bit? I'm asking because anatomically it's very nice to see the ACTH-synthesizing cells in the basal hypothalamus projecting directly to the baroreceptor center.

Denton: I think this is one of the most fascinating questions in neurobiology at the moment. The real issue is whether those peptides - e.g., the ACTH – are there as a warehousing operation, having been brought from somewhere else and stored there, or whether it's a factory. And I think the solution to these problems is going to depend on hybridization histochemistry, which is going to be much more precise than immunohistochemistry. It uses radiolabeled cDNA probes to determine whether or not transcription is actually occurring and there is a message there. That, I think, is going to be the crucial way towards into the resolution of this type of problem. We'll know a vast amount more about the role of these peptides when we use the recombinant methods to determine what's actually going on in the brain.

Laragh: I would like to add that this is the first model of hypertension that I know of where stress has been biochemically linked to the process via the secretion of ACTH, which we know is a stress-responding hormone, so maybe at last the psychosomatists will have something tangible to relate to.

MINERALOCORTICOIDS IN HYPERTENSION: 19-NOR-CORTICO-STEROIDS IN EXPERIMENTAL AND HUMAN HYPERTENSION

JAMES C. MELBY, SIDNEY L. DALE, MONIKA HOLBROOK AND GEORGE T. GRIFFING

INTRODUCTION

The isolation of 19-nor-DOC by Gomez-Sanchez [1] from the urine of rats developing adrenal regeneration hypertension and, more recently, the isolation of 19-nor-DOC from human urine by Dale et al. [2] have markedly renewed interest in this group of steroids, which has been known for many years. 19-nor-DOC is a potent mineralocorticold with a high affinity for mineralocorticoid receptors in rat adrenal cytosol [3] and has a sodium-retaining activity up to five times that of DOC. This steroid has been shown to be markedly hypertensinogenic in the rat by Hall et al. [4]. Dale et al. [2] have demonstrated that 19-nor-DOC production in humans can be markedly stimulated by corticotropin. From this same laboratory, Griffing et al. [5] have shown that corticotropin enhances the production of 19-nor-DOC and dexamethasone suppression of corticotropin markedly suppresses it, whereas alterations in sodium balance had a much lesser effect. Griffing et al. [5] also reported an increased excretion of 19-nor-DOC in some patients with hypertension and primary aldosteronism. 19-nor-DOC was synthesized over 25 years ago, but its biological significance has never been understood until the studies of Gomez-Sanchez [1]. Kagawa and Van Arman [6] found the sodium-retaining activity or 19-nor-DOC to be between two and five times that of deoxycorticosterone itself. Since 19-nor-DOC is produced by both humans and rats. It would be of considerable interest to know the tissue of origin of this steroid.

Recent observations from this laboratory by Dale et al. [3] identified 19-hydroxy-11-deoxycorticosterone (19-OH-DOC) in the incubation medium of enucleated rat adrenal glands during the early sodium-retaining phase, at a time when 19-nor-DOC had been isolated from urine. 19-Nor-DOC could not be isolated from the enucleated rat adrenal glands media. 19-Oxo-DOC was not isolated from the media in these experiments. Labelled pregnenolone was used as the substrate for conversion to 19-OH-DOC in these experiments. Conversion of labelled pregnenolone to 19-nor-DOC was not demonstrated. Because of the failure to demonstrate conversion to 19-nor-DOC but facilitated conversion to 19-OH-DOC, the possibility that 19-OH-DOC is a precursor of 19-nor-DOC became a real one.

In 1955, Mattox [7] isolated 19-OH-DOC from bovine adrenal extracts. Using labelled DOC as a substrate, three independent laboratories found *in vitro* conversion to 19-OH-DOC by bovine and hog adrenals [7-9]. Levy and Kushinsky [10] perfused progesterone as well as DOC in a bovine adrenal system and found conversion of progesterone to both 19-OH-DOC and 19-OH-cortisol. The percent conversion of substrate averaged 1.5. Griffiths [8] obtained a 30% conversion of DOC to 19-OH-DOC in the golden hamster adrenal. Neher and Wettstein isolated 19-OH-11-deoxycortisol as well as 19-OH-corticosterone from beef and pork adrenal glands [9]. 19-OH-DOC has not been isolated from human adrenals thus far except that 19-hydroxylase activity has been demonstrated in the fetal adrenal [8]. Neither 19-oxo-DOC nor 19-carboxy-DOC have been isolated from the adrenal cortex of any mammalian species thus far. 19-OH-DOC has little sodium-retaining activity. In a study by Perrone et al. [11], it has been shown that by using short-circuit current as a measure of sodium transport in the toad bladder, 19-OH-DOC had no significant effect on sodium transport, whereas 19-nor-DOC increased sodium transport to a degree not different from that of aldosterone.

It is our present working hypothesis that 19-OH-DOC or any oxygenated intermediate are precursors of 19-nor-DOC, which is formed peripherally. This reaction is not unknown biologically. This is essentially what occurs to 19-hydroxy-androstenedione secreted by the adrenal and 19-hydroxy-steroids when incubated with peripheral tissues. It has already been demonstrated that estrogens may be synthesized through the formation of 19-nor-testosterone as follows:

Testosterone → 19-hydroxytestosterone → 19-oxo-testosterone → 19-carboxy-testosterone → 19-nor-testosterone → estradiol 17β

Should the synthesis of the 19-nor-corticosteroids, including 19-nor-DOC, occur through a similar biosynthetic sequence, it would appear as follows: DOC → 19-OH-DOC within the adrenal cortex → 19-oxo-DOC → 19-carboxy-DOC → 19-nor-DOC. As shown in Figure 1, this pathway for the formation of 19-nor-

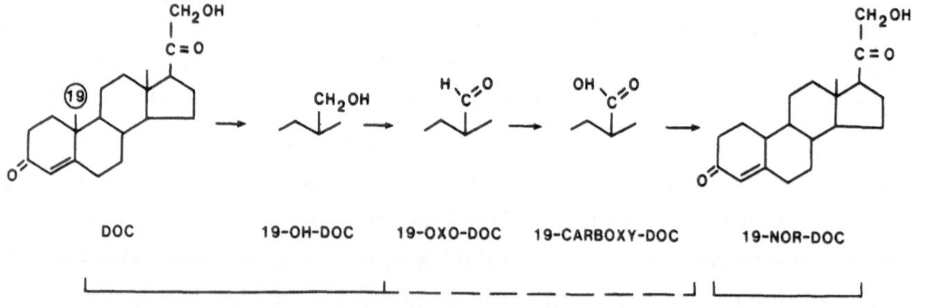

Figure 1. Postulated pathway for the biosynthesis of 19-nor-DOC from DOC. It is probable that 19-oxo and 19-carboxy (OIC) are obligatory intermediates and may be synthesized by the adrenal cortex or peripherally.

Table 1. Peripheral conversion of radiolabelled (H³) 19-OH-DOC to 19-nor-DOC (H³) in vitro

Rat tissue	Percent conversion
Aorta	34.9
Muscle	20.1
Gut	25.4
Fat	39.9
Kidney	12.7
Heart	20.5

DOC peripherally could have considerable biological significance. It indicates that tissues distal to the adrenal cortex and not affected by the same secretogogues could determine the rate of formation of a potent mineralocorticoid in the instance of 19-nor-DOC.

Preliminary studies in this laboratory indicate clearly that 19-nor-corticosteroids are not of adrenal origin and are formed peripherally via the decarboxylation of the corresponding 19-acidic compound. In Table 1, percent conversion of radiolabelled substrate, H³-19-OH-DOC, by six rat tissues to H³-19-nor-DOC, was demonstrated. Fat and aortic tissues exhibited the highest conversion rates.

METHODS

The measurement of urinary 19-nor-DOC excretion is extremely complex and laborious at present, because the technology for the development of a radioimmunoassay of 19-nor-DOC involves the chemical synthesis of a radioligand of high specific activity. Production of a radioligand is currently underway in collaboration with Dr. Marcel Gut of the Worcester Foundation for Experimental Biology and Medicine. A brief description of the isolation and measurement of 19-nor-DOC follows:

19-Nor-DOC, in the neutral fraction of human urine, was isolated and quantitated as the acetate derivative using ultraviolet absorption of the peak emerging from a high-pressure liquid chromatographic column. Identification of 19-nor-DOC in a pooled collection of urine after ACTH administration included identical chromatographic mobilities as the parent compound and acetate derivative compared to authentic 19-nor-DOC and mass spectral analysis of the acetate derivative. Values obtained for control and post-ACTH urines were 528 ± 100 (SE) ng/24 h and 8851 ± 824 ng/24 h, respectively. One patient with primary aldosteronism excreted 1894 ng/24 h.

All solvents were distilled prior to use over anhydrous potassium carbonate with the exception of HPLC-grade methanol and water used in high-pressure liquid chromatography (HPLC). Authentic 19-nor-DOC was a generous gift from

Dr. Marcel Gut of the Worcester Foundation for Experimental Biology and Medicine, Shrewsbury, Massachusetts. 1,2-³H-Deoxycorticosterone (SA = 46 cI/ mmol) was obtained from New England Nuclear Corporation. Mass spectral analysis was performed using a Finnegan 3200 mass spectrograph by direct insertion probe with the ion source temperature at 90° C and electron ionization energy at 70 eV through the courtesy of Dr. Kenneth I.H. Williams of the Worcester Foundation. HPLC was carried out using a Dupont 850 liquid chromatograph equipped with a Zorbax ODC (octadecylsilane) C-18 column, 4.6 mm ID × 25 cm, and an ultraviolet spectrophotometer.

Urine, equivalent to one half or more of the entire 24 h collection, was extracted twice with equal volumes of ethyl acetate after the addition of 100,000 dpm of 1,2-³H-DOC. The ethyl acetate extracted was washed successively with 1/10 volume of 0.1 N sodium hydroxide in 1/10 volume water. The organic layer was reduced to dryness *in vacuo* and the residue chromatographed on a 375-micron silica gel gF 254 (Brinkman Instruments) thin-layer plate, using as the mobile phase chloroform=ethanol (97/3 v/v). DOC standard was applied at each edge of the plate. After development, the standard was located by ultraviolet light, and an area of the sample 0.5 cm above and 1.5 cm below the standard was eluted by suspending the silica gel in 5 ml water and extracting with 50 ml of methylene chloride. 19-Nor-DOC migrates slightly slower than DOC in this system ($R_{DOC} = 0.95$). After evaporation of the methylene chloride, the residue was chromatographed as above, only the mobile phase was chloroform/acetone (95/5). DOC and 19-nor-DOC have the same mobilities in this system. The area corresponding to 19-nor-DOC was eluted as above and subjected to HPLC using 62% methanol/water as the eluting solvent. The fraction from 20 to 34 min was collected and reduced to dryness *in vacuo*. Retention time of 19-nor-DOC is 26.3 minutes and of DOC is 29 minutes.

DERIVATIVE FORMATION

The residue from HLPC was acetylated overnight in acetic anhydride/pyridine (2/1 v/v). After the addition of 1 ml of 95% ethanol, the sample was evaporated to dryness with nitrogen and the residue rechromatographed on silica gel in the chloroform/acetone (95/5) system using DOC-acetate standard. DOC-Ac and 19-nor-DOC-Ac have identical running rates in this system. The area in the unknown sample corresponding to the standard was eluted as previously described and the residue subjected to HPLC using 70% methanol/water as the mobile phase. The 19-nor-DOC-Ac peak (20.5 min) was collected (10-20 min fraction) and pooled for mass spectral analysis. The DOC-Ac peak (25.8 min) was collected (24-27 min fraction) and the tritium counted in a liquid scintillation counter to correct for procedural losses, since labelled 19-nor-DOC is not commercially available. Quantitation of 19-nor-DOC-Ac was accomplished by measuring and comparing peak heights at 254 nm absorption of standard 19-nor-DOC-Ac from 0.2 to 1 μg with that of the sample.

The remaining 19-nor-DOC-Ac from the urinary pool was deacetylated by dissolving in 1 ml of a solution containing 700 mg potassium bicarbonate, 15 ml methanol, and 10 ml water, and allowing the sample to hydrolyze overnight. The 19-nor-DOC was extracted with methylene chloride after addition of 5 ml water. The methylene chloride was reduced to dryness and the residue chromatographed on a celite thinlayer plate, which was impregnated by development in 15% formamide in acetone. The area corresponding to 19-nor-DOC was eluted and subjected to HPLC using 65% methanol/water as the mobile phase. Identical retention times of 19.0 minutes were observed for the deacetylated pool and standard 19-nor-DOC.

CHEMICAL STUDIES

19-nor-deoxycorticosterone excretion in healthy and hypertensive subjects

(These results are seen in Fig. 2 and 3)
In this study, 19-nor-DOC production could be markedly stimulated by ACTH, but changes in sodium intake or dexamethasone administration did not alter the urinary excretion of the free 19-nor-DOC in the neutral extract of human urine. In addition, some hypertensive subjects had elevated levels of 19-nor-DOC excretion comparable to levels produced by ACTH administration. 19-nor-DOC excretion increased during low-sodium periods and decreased during the high-sodium periods in four out of six subjects, although the mean levels of 19-nor-DOC excretion were not significant from the baseline. This, of course, could be due to the small sample size (n = 6). 19-nor-DOC excretion decreased during ACTH suppression with dexamethasone, and this was accompanied by natriuresis, potassium retention, and a fall in mean body weight. The fall of 19-nor-DOC exretion below baseline levels after dexamethasone administration may be indicative of the ACTH dependence of the product of this steroid. 19-nor-DOC's mineralocorticoid activity is thought to be comparable to that of aldosterone in normal subjects and hypertensive subjects in this study. Urinary free aldosterone was found to be 350 ± 125 ng/24 h in normal subjects and 950 ± 590 ng/24 h in patients with primary aldosteronism, whereas the urinary free 19-nor-DOC was found to be 459 ± 120 ng/24 h in the normal subjects in this study, reaching levels of 10,000 ng = 24 h or higher in hypertensives.

Conclusions from the data on studies in hypertensives and normal subjects in this first major study on 19-nor-DOC production in humans were that ACTH is the major activator of 19-nor-DOC production, and lesser effects are produced by changes in dietary sodium balance and ACTH suppression with dexamethasone. The fact that the urinary 19-nor-DOC excretion did not decrease to lower values

536

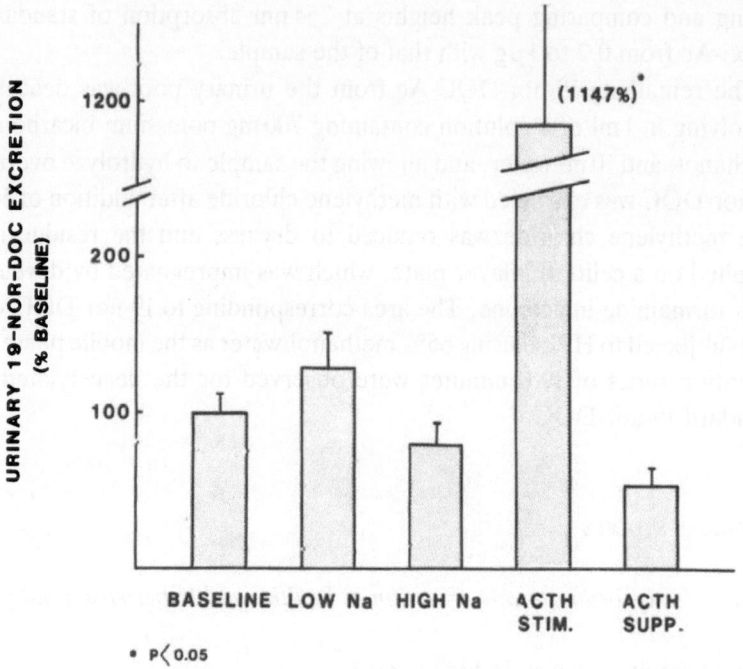

Figure 2. Urinary excretion of free 19-nor-DOC in six healthy subjects before and during sodium deprivation (10 mEq/day on day 4); sodium loading (250 mEq/day on day 4); ACTH stimulation (day 2) and dexamethasone suppression (day 2).

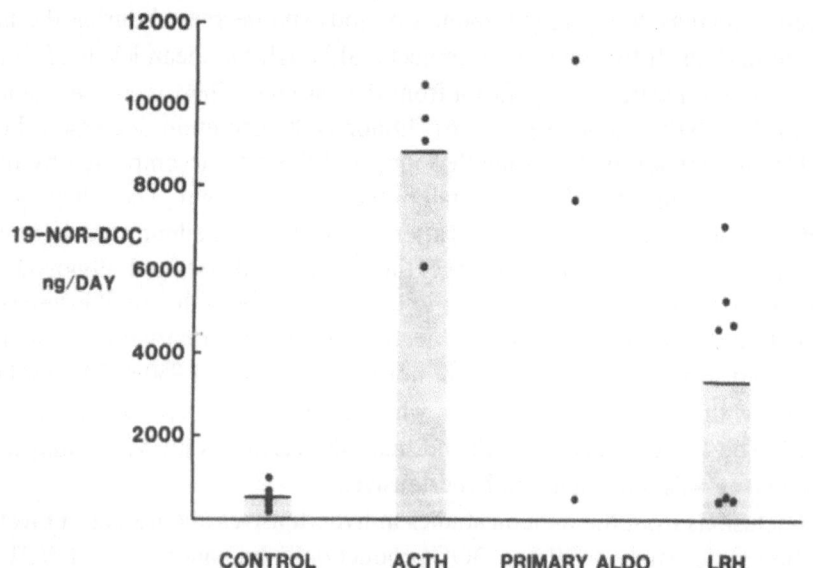

Figure 3. Urinary free 19-nor-DOC excretion (ng/24h) in healthy subjects, patients with primary aldosteronism, and patients with essential hypertension and suppressed plasma renin activity.

during the high-sodium period has important implications for hypertensive patients. Residual levels of relatively nonsuppressible potent mineralocorticoids could contribute to hypertensive disease in the sodium-surfeit state. It is possible, then, that 19-nor-DOC may be important in the regulation of systemic arterial pressure and deserves intensive further study in normal subjects and in human hypertension.

19-nor-DOC excretion in spontaneously hypertensive rats [12]

The spontaneously hypertensive strain of rat (SHR), developed by Okamoto and Aoki [13], has since been studied extensively and has been suggested as a model for the investigation of essential hypertension in man. One factor thought by many investigators to be contributive to the pathogenesis of the hypertension in SHR is an abnormally functioning hypothalamic-pituitary-adrenal, gonadal, and thyroid axis [14]. Hypophysectomy, adrenalectomy, or castration have been shown to prevent or retard the development of hypertension in SHR [15, 16].

Adrenal corticosteroid levels have been reported to be the same, lower, or elevated at various stages during and after establishment of hypertension in SHR and to be hypersensitive to stress compared with normotensive controls [17-19]. There is growing evidence that some genetically programmed alteration of adrenal steroidogenesis occurs in SHR. Whether this alteration is adrenal in origin or at the adrenal-pituitary axis has not definitely been shown. Incubation of SHR adrenals has not demonstrated any abnormality of production in the major corticosteroids produced by the rat [20, 21]; however, not all of the labelled precursors added could be accounted for in the products measured.

We measured 19-nor-DOC in the urinary neutral fraction of SHR and compared it to the excretion in the normotensive WKY counterpart in both male and female animals during development of hypertension. 19-Nor-DOC excretion was significantly elevated in the 4- and 5-week-old SHR compared with the same age WKY. The values obtained in the 3- to 4-week-old animals exhibited quite a large range, especially in the WKY rats. SHR 19-nor-DOC levels returned to WKY rat levels in the 5- to 6-week-old animals and remained at this level in the 6- to 7-week-old rats (date not shown).

In contrast to the male SHR, as seen in Figure 4, the female SHR excretes more 19-nor-DOC and for a longer period of time, remaining elevated in the 5- to 6-week-old animal compared with the WKY rat controls. Female SHR levels return to the WKY rat levels at 6 to 7 weeks of age, just before the onset of hypertension at 8 weeks of age.

Blood pressures measured in 10-week-old male SHR and WKY, and female SHR and WKY, were 171 ± 4.8 SE versus 140 ± 6.8 SE and 172 ± 5.6 SE versus 132 ± 4.5 SE mm Hg, respectively.

19-Nor-DOC excretion is elevated in the SHR compared with the normotensive WKY strain of rat. Furthermore, it is elevated at an early age, when hypertension is clearly not present. Studies have indicated the pituitary-adrenal-gonadal axis to be implicated in the development of hypertension in SHR. Selye [22] has reviewed the work of many investigators in producing metacorticoid hypertension after removal of mineralocorticoid in a rat sensitized by uninephrectomy, salt, and the mineralocorticoid (usually DOC-Ac). Usually, production of metacorticoid hypertension [23] requires a prolonged period (up to 3 months) of administration of the mineralocorticoid. However, Selye [22] has shown in rats sensitized by uninephrectomy, excess salt, DOC, and growth hormone or LAP (lyophilized anterior pituitary powder) that metacorticoid hypertension can be established in as little as 12 days.

It could not be ascertained whether 19-nor-DOC is elevated in SHR rats prior to the age of 21 days or whether the pregnant SHR rat (and/or fetus) produces excess 19-nor-DOC, since 3 weeks of age is the earliest the rat can be weaned from its mother. It is well known that estrogen production increases during pregnancy and that 19 hydroxylation of androgen is a prerequisite for estrogen formation. It remains to be established if the same factor(s) that increases estrogen production during pregnancy also stimulates the 19-hydroxy pathway of the adrenal, which could lead to increased 19-nor-DOC production. If 19-nor-DOC production is elevated prior to weaning (or in the fetal stage), a sufficient period of time of exposure to this mineralocorticoid could result in metacorticoid hypertension in the SHR, even though the excretion of this steroid declines to normal levels prior to the developments of hypertension.

The WKY strain of rat, the genetically similar stock column used by Okamoto and Aoki [13] to develop the SHR, has been primarily used as a control for studies involving SHR. The validity of using the WKY as a control has been discussed [24]. The usual blood pressure used by many investigators for the determination of hypertension is 150 mm Hg. Hartle et al. [25] reported the mean blood pressure in the WKY rats used in their study as 151 mm Hg, which was significantly different than their SHR of 202 mm Hg. It is possible that the high values of blood pressure and 19-nor-DOC found in two of our male WKY animals may have been due to the genetic tendency toward SHR, since at 3 weeks of age blood pressure measurements via the tall cuff method are very difficult to obtain. This difference did disappear, however, at 4 to 5 weeks of age.

The reason for the return of 19-nor-DOC levels to those of the WKY strain of rat prior to the development of clear-cut hypertension at 8 weeks of age is not known. Since no definite abnormality in the known secretory products of the adrenal has been demonstrated [20, 21], it may be that, with advancing age, further hydroxylation of the steroid nucleus occurs (at C-11 or C-18), resulting in different metabolic end-products. To our knowledge, the 19-nor-derivative of 18-hydroxydeoxycorticosterone (18-OH-DOC) has never been synthesized. Since 18-OH-DOC can produce hypertension in the rat [26, 27] and has been implicated in some forms of human hypertension [28], and since removal of the

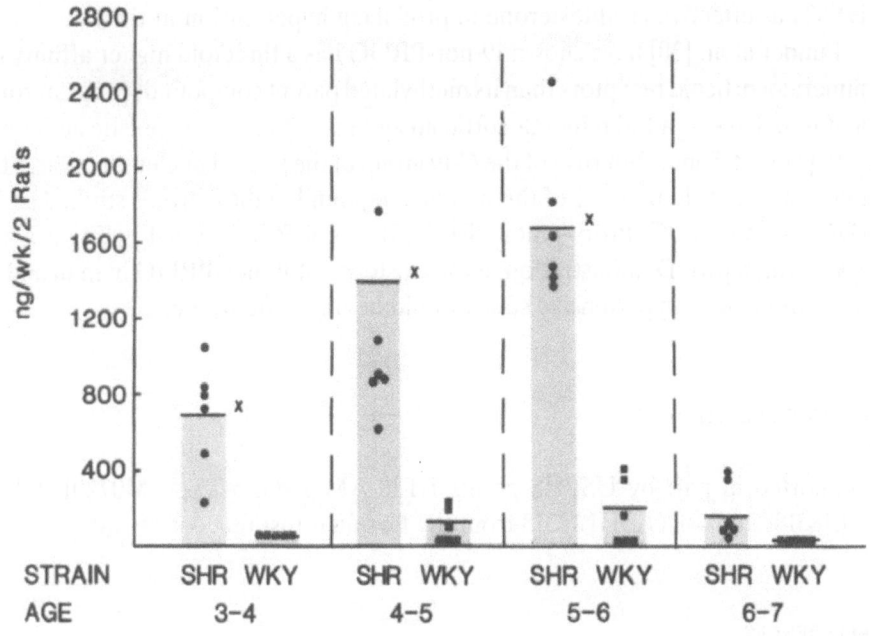

Figure 4. Urinary 19-nor-DOC excretion (ng/wk/two rats) in female weanling SHR and WKY control rats prior to onset of hypertension.

19-methyl group enhances mineralocorticoid activity of DOC, it should be of considerable interest to investigate the biological properties of this compound.

It is well-known that the major route of elimination of steroid metabolites in the rat is via the feces. The amount of 19-nor-DOC excretion measured in the present study may represent only a small fraction of that produced by the rat. If the difference in excretion of 19-nor-DOC in SHR versus WKY rats is representative of total production, it is conceivable that exposure to this mineralocorticoid for a sufficient length of time could produce metacorticoid-like hypertension.

It is concluded that 19-nor-DOC secretion/excretion and peripheral blood levels should be examined in a large sample of patients with primary systemic arterial hypertension.

19-nor-progesterone (19-nor-PROG)

Although the existence of 19-nor-PROG as a naturally occurring biological substance remains to be determined, the probability for its existence and its precursor(s) is high. 19-OH-PROG and 19-nor-PROG have been chemically synthesized, and studies have been published demonstrating the hypertensive mineralocorticoid receptor and sodium-retaining effects of 19-nor-PROG. Komanicky et al. [29] from our laboratory first demonstrated that 19-nor-PROG

540

is 55% as effective as aldosterone in producing hypertension in the rat.

Funder et al. [30] have shown 19-nor-PROG has a threefold higher affinity for mineralocorticoid receptors than its methylated parent compound, progesterone, and to behave as a full mineralocorticoid agonist with no antagonistic activity as with progesterone. Removal of the C-19 group of the steroid nucleus increases the mineralocorticold potency of the parent compound in the steroids studied so far (DOC → nor-DOC, Prog → nor-PROG, B → nor-B, F → nor-F) (Kagawa and Van Arman [6]). Demonstration of the existence of 19-nor-PROG in man and its measurement in hypertensive states would be highly desirable.

ACKNOWLEDGMENTS

Supported in part by USPHS grants 1-T30-AM21683, 5-T32-AM07201, 5-PO-HL18318, and 5-ROL-HL18318 from the National Institutes of Health.

REFERENCES

1. Gomez-Sanchez CE, Holland OB, Murray BA, et al.: 19-Nor-deoxycorticosterone: A potent mineralocorticoid isolated from the urine of rats with regenerating adrenals. Endocrinology 105:708, 1979.
2. Dale SL, Holbrook MM, Melby JC: 19-Nor-deoxycorticosterone in the neutral fraction of human urine. Steroids 37:103-110, 1981.
3. Dale SL, Holbrook MM, Melby JC: Identification of 19-hydroxy-deoxy-corticosterone in regenerating rat adrenal incubations. Steroids 36:601-610, 1980.
4. Hall CE, Gomez-Sanchez CE, Holland OB, et al.: Influence of 19-Nor-deoxycorticosterone on blood pressure, saline consumption, and serum electrolytes, corticosterone, and renin activity. Endocrinology 105:600, 1979.
5. Griffing GT, Dale SL, Holbrook MM, et al.: 19-Nor-deoxycorticosterone excretion in health and hypertensive subjects. Trans Assoc Am Physicians 94:301-309, 1981.
6. Kagawa CM, Van Arman CG: Sodium retaining activity of 19-nor-steroids in adrenalectomized rats. Proc Soc Exp Biol Med 94:444, 1957.
7. Mattox VR: Isolation of 19-hydroxy-11-deoxycorticosterone from beef adrenal extracts. Mayo Clin Proc 30:180, 1955.
8. Griffiths K: Hydroxylation of II-deoxycorticosterone by adrenals of various species. J Endorinol 26:437, 1963.
9. Neher R, Wettstein A: Isolierung und Konstitutionermittlung Weiterer Pregnanverbindungen aus Nebennieren. Helv Chir Acta 39:2062, 1956.
10. Levy H, Kushinsky S: Conversion of radiolabelled progesterone to 19-hydroxy-11-deoxy-corticosterone and 19-hydroxy-cortisol by perfusion of bovine adrenals. Arch Biochem Biophys 59:290, 1955.
11. Perrone R, Schwartz JH, Bengele HH, et al.: The mineralocorticoid activity of 19-nor-deoxycorticosterone and 19-OH-deoxycorticosterone in the toad bladder. Am J Physiol 241(5):E406-409, 1981.
12. Dale SL, Holbrook MM, Komanicky P, et al.: Urinary 19-nor-deoxycorticosterone (19-nor-DOC) excretion in the spontaneously hypertensive rat (SHR). Endocrinology, in press.

13. Okamoto J, Aoki K: Development of a strain of spontaneously hypertensive rats. Jpn Circ J 27:282, 1963.
14. Wexler BC: Arterial lesions and hypertension induced by saline, unilateral nephrectomy, and deoxycorticosterone in spontaneously hypertensive (SHR) rats. Paroi Arterielle 5:99, 1979.
15. Aoki K, Tankawa H, Fiyinami T, et al.: Pathological studies on the endocrine organs of the spontaneously hypertensive rat. Jpn Heart J 4:426, 1963.
16. Jams SG, Wexler BC: Retardation in the development of spontaneous hypertension in SH rats by gonadectomy. J Lab Clin Med 90:997, 1977.
17. Sowers J, Tuck M, Asp ND, et al.: Plasma aldosterone and corticosterone responses to adrenocorticotropin, angiotensin, potassium and stress in spontaneously hypertensive rats. Endocrinology 108:1216, 1981.
18. Moll D, Dale SL, Melby JC: Adrenal steroidogenesis in the spontaneously hypertensive rat (SHR). Endocrinology 96:416, 1975.
19. Freeman RH, Davis JO, Aharon NV, et al.: Control of aldosterone secretion in the spontaneously hypertensive (SHR) rat. Paroi Arterielle 5:99, 1979.
20. De Nicola AF, Oliver JT, Birmingham MK: In vitro metabolism of progesterone by the adrenals of spontaneously hypertensive rats. Experientia 25:880, 1969.
21. Rapp JP, Dahl LK: Adrenal steroidogenesis in rats bred for susceptibility and resistance to the hypertensive effects of salt. Endocrinology 88:52, 1971.
22. Selye H (editor): Experimental Cardiovascular Disease. New York, Springer-Verlag, 1970, vol 1, p 21.
23. Freedman SM, Freedman CL: Self-sustained hypertension in the albino rat: A hypothesis to explain it. Can Med Assoc J 61:596, 1949.
24. McMurthy JP, Wexler BC: Hypersensitivity of spontaneously hypertensive rats (SHR) to heat, ether and immobilization. Endocrinology 108:1730, 1981.
25. Hartle DK, Kapski GF, Baron J: Alterations in the contents of cytochrome P-450 and adrenal ferredoxin in adrenals of spontaneously hypertensive rats. Biochem Biophys Res Commun 77:955, 1977.
26. Oliver JT, Birmingham MK, Bartova A, et al.: Hypertensive action of 18-hydroxydeoxycorticosterone. Science 182:1249, 1973.
27. Rapp JP, Knudsen KD, Iwai J, et al.: Genetic control of blood pressure and corticosteroid production in rats. Circ Res 32:139, 1973.
28. Melby JC, Dale SL, Grekin RJ, et al.: 18-Hydroxy-11-deoxycorticosterone (18-OH-DOC) secretion in experimental and human hypertension. Recent Prog Horm Res 28:287, 1972.
29. Komanicky P, Melby JC: Experimental hypertension induced by 19-nor-progesterone treatment in the rat. Endocrinology 109:1164-1167, 1981.
30. Funder JW, Mercer J, Ingram B, et al.: 19-Nor deoxycorticosterone (19-nor-DOC): Mineralocorticoid receptor affinity higher than aldosterone, electrolyte activity lower. Endocrinology 103(4):1514-1517, 1978.

DISCUSSION

Discussants: Laragh, Melby, Abernathy, Sambhi, Inagami

Laragh: I want to start by asking you whether those SHR animals have hypokalemia prehypertension.

Melby: No, they don't. We see less of a tendency to lower potassium than we do to retain sodium, and we see equal tendencies to produce hypertension. You can't equate the effect on potassium metabolism with hypertensinogenicity or the effect on sodium transport. Now, according to some investigators that would be entirely wrong because it's totally dependent upon a change in electrical gradient. Nevertheless, these agents show very little effect on potassium. With 19-nor-progesterone we do as well as with DOCA or aldosterone in producing hypertension, and only with aldosterone in this group of four steroids did we see hypokalemia. However, 19-nor-progesterone is less potent than aldosterone itself.

Laragh: So aldosterone is the only kaliuretic steroid of those four, even DOCA isn't kaliuretic.

Melby: They have some tendency, but only nearly as potent as aldosterone.

Albernathy: This concerns obesity in hypertension. Have you studied this problem since the increased peripheral conversion by adipose sites?

Melby: We are collecting urines to do the free fraction in obese children and fat adults, before and during dietary deprivation. Of course, it would be tempting to believe that this steroid abnormality is worse in the obese, but we do not have that information.

Laragh: Dr. Melby you've astonished us with a very powerful steroid that looks like it has a great deal of relevance and we look forward to your progress.

Sambhi: You said that you have only preliminary data on two things. Since you have the labeled compound now, have you looked at the comparative receptor-binding to aldosterone yet?

Melby: If you don't use its carrier protein the receptor-binding is around 70 to 80% of aldosterones, if you use the carrier proteins it falls to about 60% of aldosterone. Now Gomez-Sanchez thought it was much higher than that and that's because he didn't have any protein in the system, but you have to have some protein.

Sambhi: That is impressive. And the binding-protein is bound to protein very avidly. Would you make a guess if it's a specific protein or just bond to albumin?

Melby: No, I would guess it's bound to corticosteroid-binding globulin the same way DOCA is because it has many of the features of DOCA-just like progesterone. They're both bound to the same.

Inagami: Is it not stimulated by angiotensin II?

Melby: It is not, as far as we can tell.

RENAL AND CNS FACTORS IN NACL-INDUCED HYPERTENSION

Louis Tobian

The mechanism of NaCl-induced hypertension depends upon the presence of two factors. The first is the presence of excess sodium in the body. The second factor is that accumulation of excess sodium in the body causes increased blood pressure. Only when both of these links are present, will salt-induced hypertension occur. Sodium accumulation in the body, is a function of the amount of sodium in the diet and the ability of the kidney to excrete that sodium.

Let us consider evidence for the second link – that increase in body sodium leads to hypertension. There is good clinical evidence for this link. In renal parenchymal disease, for instance, sodium balance is achieved with high levels of body sodium. Patients with the disease have a high prevalence of hypertension. In primary hyperaldosteronism, sodium balance is achieved during the 'escape' phase with a high level of body sodium, and this frequently causes hypertension. Dialysis patients provide another example for the second link. As they proceed from dialysis to dialysis, the body sodium level swings up and down, and blood pressure swings up and down in the same pattern.

Onesti and Kim conducted experiments to investigate the excess sodium-hypertension link [1]. They obtained blood pressure and cardiac output measurements on subjects so that peripheral vascular resistance could be calculated. A number of their subjects had end-stage renal disease. During a series of dialyses, their body sodium increased for a number of weeks. Most of these subjects had a corresponding rise in blood pressure; the authors state that the primary cause of this rise was an increase in peripheral vascular resistance. In these subjects, the increase in body sodium resulted mainly in vasoconstriction.

In about 20% of subjects, blood pressure however, rose after salt-loading, solely because of an increase in cardiac output. The peripheral resistance in these subjects remained at the baseline level. It is possible, however, that their level of resistance was actually elevated in relation to the increased cardiac output. Generally, the blood pressure rose because of an increase in peripheral vascular resistance. Recent evidence suggests that this is due to passive structural narrowing as well as to active smooth muscle shortening.

About 20% of the patients with end-stage renal disease, did not show the pattern described above; an increase in body sodium did not lead to a rise in pressure. This finding indicates that the 'second factor' must be in salt-induced hypertension. Thus, salt-induced hypertension depends on both factors operating in the chain of causation.

What are the mechanisms by which the increase in body sodium leads to a rise in blood pressure and to vasoconstriction? The answers to these question are still uncertain, but there is much recent information available. In key experiments conducted by Takeshita and Mark [2], Dahl S rats were fed a high-sodium diet; then developed increased peripheral vascular resistance in the hindquarters. The sympathetic nerves to their hindquarters were cut, thereby decreasing salt-induced vascular resistance by 50%. This result was a strong indication that the sympathetic nerves play an important role in salt-induced hypertension.

In another experiment, the same investigators gave 6-OH dopamine peripherally to baby Dahl S rats in order to destroy most of the peripheral sympathetic nerves [2]. These rats were then fed a high-salt diet, which did not induce any hypertension, again suggesting the importance of sympathetic nerves in salt-induced hypertension.

Since cutting the sympathetic nerves eliminated only half the increase in peripheral vascular resistance we were prompted to explore other causes of increased vascular resistance.

For feeding Dahl S and R rats a high-salt diet for a month, we perfused the blood of these rats at a constant flow, through the hindquarters of another R-rat that was used as a bioassay organ [3]. After one month of high-salt feeding, the S rats were hypertensive, and the R rats were normotensive. We then detected vasoconstrictor or vasodilator humoral agents in the following way: when the hindquarters were perfused with R blood at a constant flow, we detected a certain level of vascular resistance; if they were perfused with S blood, we detected a 17% higher vascular resistance, suggesting that there is a vasoconstrictor humoral agent in the blood of the S rats that promotes salt-induced hypertension. This agent is not likely to be angiotensin II since the S rats had a 39% lower level of plasma renin than the R rats. Subsequent experiments suggest that the rat must have a high-salt diet producing hypertension in order for the vasoconstrictor agent to appear. If the S rat is on a low-salt diet and has a normal blood pressure, the vasoconstrictor agent is absent. If the kidney of salt-fed S rats is removed, about an hour before the perfusion, humoral vasoconstrictor activity is greatly reduced.

Searching further for factors that influence salt-induced hypertension, we investigated the effect of lesions on the central nervous system [4]. A group of Dahl S rats was fed a high-salt diet and became hypertensive over the course of many weeks. A group of Dahl R rats was also fed salt over the same time period but did not become hypertensive. A second group of Dahl S rats was injected with 6-hydroxydopamine in the lateral brain ventricle and developed only half of the expected hypertension when fed a high-salt diet. The 6-hydroxydopamine destroys only catecholamine-containing neurons in the brain. This experiment indicated that S rats will not get the full expression of salt-induced hypertension unless catecholamine-containing neurons in the brain are intact.

The paraventricular nucleus located, on either side of the third brain ventricle, was also investigated [4]. This nucleus secretes vasopressin; it has neural connections with the vasomotor center and receives neural signals from the kidney. The nucleus, therefore, seemed likely to be involved in salt-induced hypertension. In Dahl S rats with sham lesions of these nuclei, a high-salt diet gradually produced hypertension. Dahl R rats with sham lesions had no change in blood pressure. On the other hand, when S rats had both paraventricular nuclei completely destroyed by anodal lesions, they had only about half the level of hypertension on salt feeding that was seen in the rats with sham lesions. The results indicate that one must have two intact paraventricular nuclei in the brain in order to get the full expression of salt-induced hypertension.

Similarly, we produced an electrolytic lesion in Dahl S rats in the anterior inferior end of the third brain ventricle, the so-called 'AV3V' area. We then fed the rats an 8% salt diet. The S rats with the lesion had a greatly attenuated rise in blood pressure, less than half the rise seen in S rats with sham lesions. This study indicates that the nuclei and nerve tracts in the periventricular region around the anterior inferior and of the third brain ventricle must be intact in order to achieve the full expression of salt-induced hypertension. This area includes the OVLT region, which has receptors for angiotensin II.

Other lesions in specific areas of the brain can also exacerbate hypertension. Goto et al. induced bilateral lesions of the suprachiasmatic nuclei, which lie on either side of the third brain ventricle in the ventral part of the anterior hypothalamus [4]. The suprachiasmatic nuclei secrete vasopressin, but the vasopressin does not reach the pituitary. These nuclei have many neural connections with several hypothalamic nuclei. The S rats with sham lesions had the usual rise in blood pressure when fed a high-salt diet. However, in the rats with bilateral suprachiasmatic nuclei lesions, the blood pressure rose even higher during the high-salt diet (p<.001), and several lesioned rats died prematurely with severe hypertension. These nuclei, then, tend to keep the blood pressure down. When they are destroyed, a particularly severe salt-induced hypertension appears, accelerating mortality rates in these rats and increasing the heart weight: body weight ratio by 15% (p<.001).

In still another study of the CNS in relation to salt-induced hypertension, we studied genetic susceptibility. If 500 ng of angiotensin II are injected into the lateral brain ventricle, a transient increase in blood pressure is seen regularly. Ikeda et al. injected S rats and R rats on a low-salt diet with angiotensin II [5]. Both groups were normotensive prior to injection. They found that a small amount of angiotensin II in the lateral brain ventricle caused a rise in blood pressure which was twice as great in S rats as in R rats. They also produced a transient rise in pressure by injecting a small amount of hypertonic saline into the lateral brain ventricle in both groups of rats. Again, the rise in blood pressure was twice as great in the normotensive S rats as it was in the normotensive R rats.

These two studies suggest that pressor response in S rats are poised to react in a particularly strong fashion whenever the pressor stimuli are introduced. Similarly, Gotoh et al. studied hypertensive patients whose blood pressure rose when they were fed salt [6]. In these patients, the investigators found a 5 mEq/L increase in the sodium concentration of the cerebrospinal fluid when these patients switched from low- to high-salt diets.

In another study, one group of S rats was fed a high-salt diet, and they became hypertensive; another group of S rats was fed the same high-salt diet, with the addition of equimolar KCl, and they had much smaller increases in pressure [7]. We wondered whether the central nervous system pressor responses could be influenced by adding potassium to the diet. Goto et al. placed Dahl S and R rats on a low-salt diet, which resulted in a normal blood pressure through young adulthood [8]. They then injected a small amount of angiotensin II into the lateral brain ventricle as a pressor stimulus. As before, the S rats had a greater increase in pressure than the R rats. Next, the investigators added either potassium chloride or potassium citrate to the diet of selected groups of S and R rats. They found that potassium feeding had a profound effect on the hyperactive pressor response to angiotensin II in S rats, bringing it down nearly to the low level seen in the R rats. Using small amounts of hypertonic NaCl in the lateral brain ventricle as a stimulus, Goto et al. examined the pressor responses in the S rats, which again were much greater than in R rats [8]. However, when the S rats had been given either potassium chloride or potassium citrate in the diet, the hyperactive pressor response of the S rats was brought down almost to the low level seen in the R rats. Thus, Goto et al. found that either of these potassium salts, when added to the diet, will almost normalize the hyperactive pressor responses in S rats. This may explain, in part, the prevention of NaCl-induced hypertension by the feeding of potassium salts.

As discussed above, the first link in the chain of causation in salt-induced hypertension is a transient increase in body sodium. This extra body sodium is the result of both increased salt intake and the inability of the kidney to excrete salt. One factor in genetic susceptibility to salt-induced hypertension, then, could be that such individuals who are genetically susceptible to hypertension have more trouble excreting salt rapidly, even though their kidneys may not have obvious pathologic lesions. In the Indiana study, the relatives of hypertensive individuals excreted salt more slowly after a salt challenge, supporting this hypothesis [9]. The hypothesis can be investigated in the Dahl rats, since they can be studied at a time when both S rats and R rats have a blood pressure within the normal range. In our study, both S and R rats were fed a low-sodium diet, and both groups were normotensive. We then obtained an isolated kidney from each S and R rat, put it into a chamber without ischemia, and perfused it with blood from two neutral Sprague-Dawley rats.

In 1951, Selkurt observed that as pressure in the renal artery rises, the kidney excretes increasing amounts of sodium [10]. Our findings confirm this [11]. The

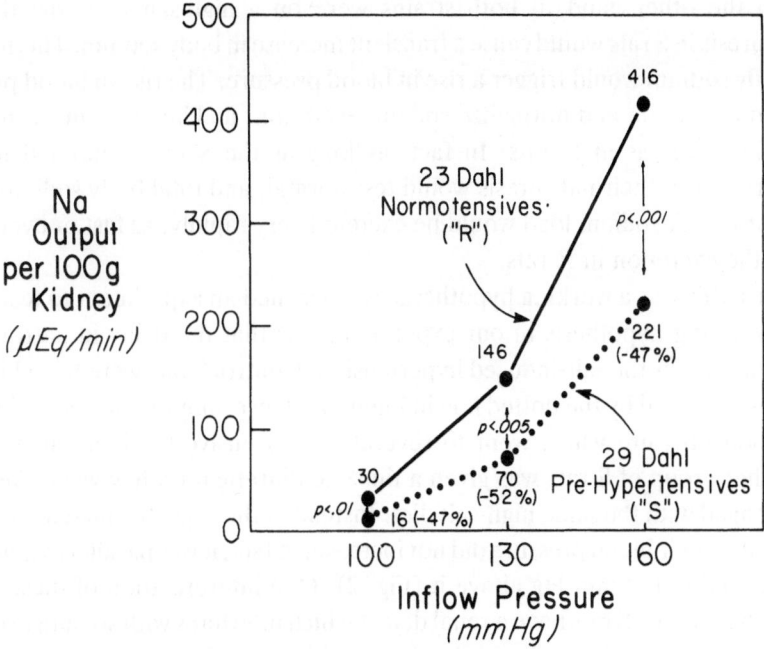

Figure 1. Sodium excretion of isolated kidneys from S and R rats at varying inflow pressures. The distance between the large black dot (the mean value) and the tip of the arrowhead represents the standard error of the mean.

top-line of Figure 1 represents isolated kidneys from R rats. As inflow pressure rose, R rats progressively excreted increasing amounts of sodium. The bottom line of Figure 1 represents kidneys from prehypertensive S rats. Again, as renal artery pressure increased, progressively more salt was excreted. Note that there was a distinct shift in the pressure natriuresis curve for the S kidneys. It took more pressure to excrete a given amount of sodium in the S kidneys than it did in the R kidneys. In this type of a study, one can also compare the sodium excretion at equal levels of inflow pressure. At 100, 130, and 160 mm Hg, the S kidneys put out about half as much sodium per minute as did the R kidneys (Fig. 1). It is also possible to overcome this defect of natriuresis in S kidneys by applying a greater renal arterial pressure. Thus, if one perfused the S kidney at 160 mm Hg, that kidney would excrete 50% more sodium than an R kidney perfused at a normal pressure of 130 mm Hg. This study allowed us to extend Dahl's working hypothesis, according to which the shift in the pressure natriuresis curve in S rats partially accounts for their great susceptibility to salt-induced hypertension. However, as long as both S and R rats are on the low-salt diet, this shift in the pressure natriuresis curve would be of little consequence. There is so little salt taken in on this low-salt diet that even with the handicap in sodium excretion, there would be almost no increase in body sodium and thus insufficient stimulus to cause a rise in blood pressure in the S rats.

On the other hand, if both strains were on a high-salt diet, the delay in natriuresis in S rats would cause a transient increase in body sodium. This increase in body sodium would trigger a rise in blood pressure. The rise in blood pressure would accelerate and normalize sodium excretion, making it occur at the same rate in S rats as in R rats. In fact, as long as the S rats continued to have hypertension, their natriuresis would test normal, and total body sodium would be normal. A sodium load would be excreted very rapidly, as fast or even faster than the excretion in R rats.

Since this was a working hypothesis, we designed an experiment to test it [12]. The working hypothesis in our experiment was that the delay in natriuresis is responsible for the salt-induced hypertension. Control S rats were fed a high-salt diet as indicated by the dotted line in Figure 2; they promptly showed an increase in blood pressure which went to severely hypertensive levels in eight weeks. Another group of S rats was given a thiazide diuretic for a few weeks and then challenged with the same high-salt diet. Instead of the expected increase in blood pressure, their blood pressure did not increase; in fact, it was parallel to that of the R rats and only 5 mm Hg above it (Fig. 2). One interpretation of these results could be that the S rats have a renal defect which interferes with sodium excretion even though they do not have obvious renal lesions. Thus, when they receive a sodium challenge, they have a transient increase in body sodium; this produces a higher blood pressure. On the other hand, the S rats receiving thiazide had their sodium excretion facilitated and accelerated by the drug. Hence, when they received the sodium challenge, they were able to excrete the sodium in a normally rapid manner. There was no accumulation of body sodium and hence no stimulus for a rise in pressure. As long as they had the facilitation of the thiazide, their kidneys excreted sodium fast enough to prevent any accumulation of body sodium [9].

We then sought to determine why the S kidney had a reduced rate of sodium excretion [12]. We had either an S rat or an R rat perfusing a normal Sprague-Dawley kidney at a constant pressure. We found that when the normal kidney was perfused with R blood, it excreted about 130 μEq of sodium per 100 g per minute. When the kidney was perfused with S blood, it excreted about half as much sodium per minute. There appeared to be a humoral effect in S blood which retarded the rate of natriuresis in the neutral 'normal' kidney by about 50%.

Still searching for reasons why the S kidney is slow to excrete, we developed a technique for quick freezing rat kidneys [13]. We plunged them into liquid nitrogen to achieve almost instantaneous freezing. When the kidneys were thawed to -5μC, we dissected out the renal papilla and determined the prostaglandin E_2 concentration in the renal papilla of both R rats and S rats. When both strains of rats were on a .3% low-salt diet, the S rats had a 60% reduction in prostaglandin E_2 concentration in the papilla compared with the R rats. When both strains were fed a 4% high-salt diet for 4 weeks or for 11 weeks, prostaglandin E_2 concentration in the papilla doubled in the R rats and doubled in the S rats,

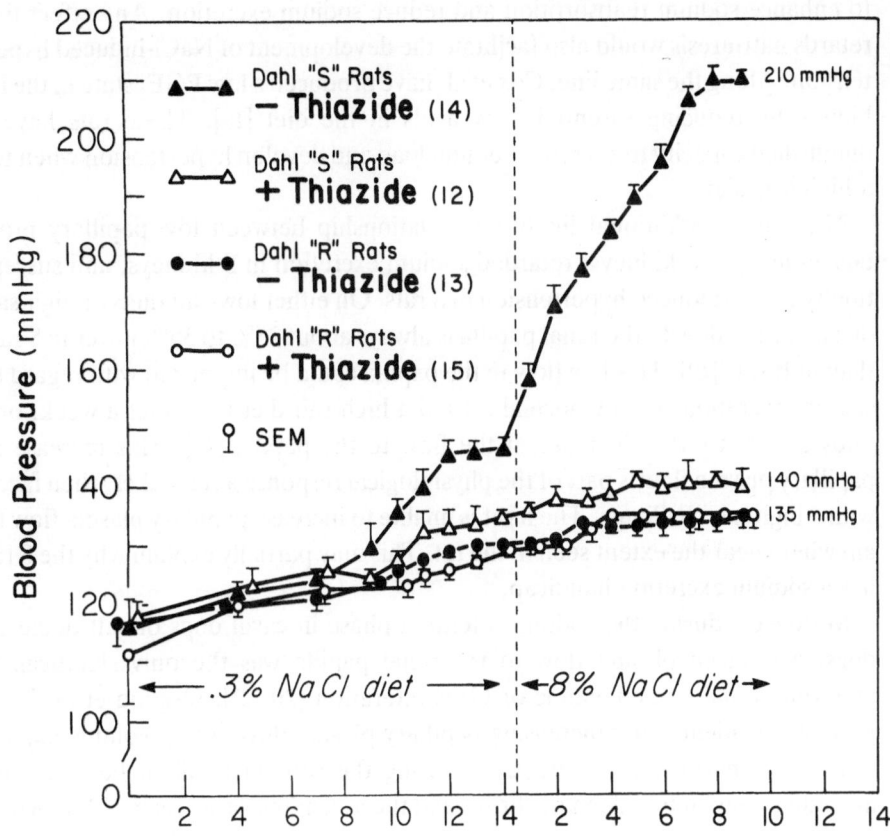

Figure 2. Blood pressure of Dahl S and R rats as influenced by high and low levels of sodium in the diet, and by treatment with a thiazide diuretic agent.

but the concentration was always about 50% lower in the S rats compared with the R rats. For some reason, there seemed to be an intrinsically low concentration of prostaglandin E_2 in the renal papilla of S rats.

It is known that the prostaglandin in the renal medulla has an influence on sodium reabsorption, at least in the ascending limb of the loop of Henle and in the collecting tubule and collecting duct. One piece of evidence for this influence is that intravenous indomethacin will double the sodium concentration in the rat papilla 20 minutes after injection [14]. The reason for this would appear to be that the indomethacin had severely reduced the level of prostaglandin, and this reduction in prostaglandins had increased transport of sodium by the ascending limb and collecting tubule and duct, thereby exaggerating the countercurrent mechanism. Utilizing isolated tubules, Stokes has shown that increasing prostaglandin E_2 retards sodium transport in the ascending limb of Henle and in the collecting tubules [15, 16]. Wilson et al. have shown a similar effect the in collecting duct [17]. Thus, the reduced prostaglandin E_2 is S rat papilla would tend to enhance sodium reabsorption and reduce sodium excretion. Any effect that retards natriuresis would also facilitate the development of NaCl-induced hypertension. Along the same line, Cox et al. have produced a low PGE_2 state in the rat kidney by reducing essential fatty acids in the diet [18]. These rats have a diminished capacity to excrete a sodium load and develop hypertension when fed a high-salt diet.

There is an additional likely interrelationship between low papillary prostaglandin E_2 in S kidneys, retarded sodium excretion in S kidneys, and susceptibility to salt-induced hypertension in S rats. On either low-salt diets or high-salt diets, plasma flow to the renal papilla is always about 25% to 35% lower in S rats than in R rats [19]. This low flow in the papilla could be important with regard to sodium excretion. In any normal rat fed a high-salt diet for about a week, one finds a 32% to 45% increase in the flow to the papilla [19]. This increase in papillary plasma flow is part of the physiological response a rat makes when faced with a high salt challenge. The S rat is unable to increase papillary plasma flow to anywhere near the extent seen in the rat. This may partially explain why the S rat has a sodium excretion handicap.

Moreover, during the sodium retention phase in caval dogs or salt-depleted dogs, a reduced plasma flow to the renal papilla was the only significantly abnormal renal hemodynamic or GFR alteration [20, 21]. Osgood et al. have produced evidence that increasing papillary plasma flow during volume expansion favors natriuresis by greatly reducing the sodium gradient between the ascending thin limb of deep nephrons and the ascending vasae rectae [22]. When this gradient was abolished, passive sodium reabsorption from the thin ascending limb was also largely abolished, thereby favoring increased natriuresis by the deep nephrons [22]. In the sodium-retaining caval dogs or sodium-depleted dogs, the low plasma flow to the papilla presumably was largely responsible for the increased papillary osmolality, which removed more water from the descending limb [20, 21].

In the volume-expanded rats, the high plasma flow to the papilla was presumably largely responsible for the reduced papillary osmolality, which removed less water from the descending limb [22]. The physiologic pattern appears to be low papillary plasma flow, high papillary osmolality, enhanced sodium retention; or high papillary plasma flow, low papillary osmolality, enhanced sodium excretion. In this connection, it is noteworthy that the Dahl S rats always have greatly reduced papillary plasma flows compared with Dahl R rats, regardless of whether the diet contains low or high amounts of NaCl [19]. This should favor an enhanced passive reabsorption of sodium out of the thin ascending limb of the deep nephrons, which would significantly diminish natriuresis. Furthermore, the papillary prostaglandins also have a place in this scenario. We have recently found strong evidence that prostaglandins act as vasodilator substances upon the vessels supplying the rat renal papilla [23]. Thus, the low level of PGE_2 in the papillae of S rats would encourage relative vasoconstriction and reduced papillary flow. As mentioned above, this would increase the tendency to sodium retention which, in turn, would increase susceptibility to salt-induced hypertension.

We attempted to determine if we could correct the low papillary prostaglandin E_2 level in S rats by feeding rats large amounts of its precursor, linoleic acid. We expected this might influence the course of salt-induced hypertension [13]. To test this hypothesis, we placed two groups of S rats on 20% high-fat diets containing 5% NaCl. One group had 1.5% linoleic acid in their diet, more than enough to prevent essential fatty-acid deficiency. The other group had 16% linoleic acid in their diet. This study compared a 'normal' linoleic intake with a 'high' linoleic intake. The S rats with the normal linoleic intake promptly developed hypertension when they were fed a high-salt diet. The S rats on the high linoleic intake had a much different course. Their increase in blood pressure was delayed for about six weeks; when their blood pressure did increase, it only went up to about half the extent of the normal linoleic group. In fact, it rose to just about the level found in the S rats on a low-sodium diet at this relatively advanced age (Fig. 3). Moreover, the 16% linoleic diet tripled the prostaglandin E_2 content in the S

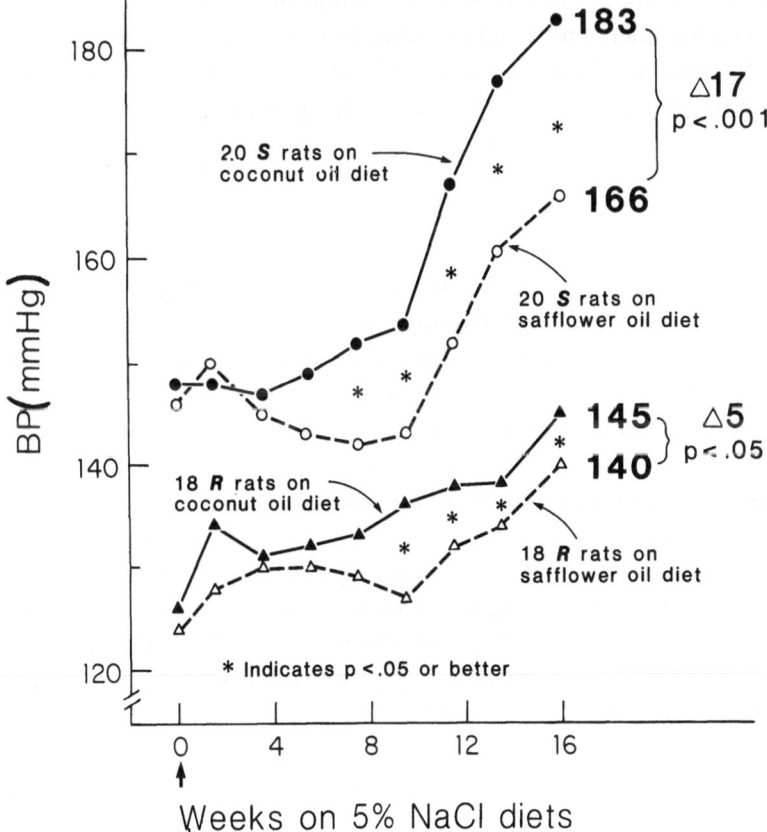

Figure 3. Blood pressures of Dahl S and R rats as influenced by 5% NaCl diets containing coconut oil (1.5% linoleic acid diet) or safflower oil (16% linoleic acid diet).

papilla, bringing it to approximately normal levels. Seemingly, the increased amount of linoleate in the diet increased the prostaglandin concentration in renal papilla and greatly retarded the extent of salt-induced hypertension.

It is useful to bring together the pieces of evidence pointing to abnormal humoral factors in salt-induced hypertension. In the Dahl S rat, there is evidence for circulating humoral agents that retard natriuresis in an isolated 'neutral' kidney [12]. There is also evidence for a circulating vasoconstrictor agent in the blood of hypertensive, salt-fed Dahl S rats [3]. Additional evidence shows that S rats have a reduced level of two types of humoral agents: ouabain-sensitive agents, which retard sodium efflux in lymphocytes, and furosemide-sensitive humoral agents, which retard sodium efflux in lymphocytes. This work was presented at the American Society of Nephrology meeting in December 1982 [24].

Furthermore the most recent evidence suggests that plasma factors in hypertensive salt-fed S rats can confer mild hypertension and a 40% increased pressor sensitivity to i.v. norepinephrine and angiotensin II onto normotensive recipient Dahl S rats [25]. Daily i.v. injections of these plasma factors into the recipient S rat will bring about these statistically significant changes.

Taken together, these findings constitute solid evidence that circulating humoral factors do exist in the plasma of S rats and that these factors may play a key role in the mechanisms of NaCl-induced hypertension.

SUMMARY

In genetically susceptible human beings and in genetically susceptible Dahl S rats, moderate amounts of NaCl will bring on increased arteriolar narrowing (active and passive) and hypertension. The first link in the hypertension chain is the tendency to sodium accumulation in the body, largely caused by generous amounts of salt in the diet and by the reduced ability of the kidneys to excrete salt rapidly. The arteriolar narrowing gradually takes place as the generous salt intake continues. The regulatory systems are reset to achieve a higher average level of arterial pressure. Increased arteriolar narrowing is the primary change, but cardiac output also tends to be slightly high early in the hypertension, and the veins show decreased compliance. This resetting of the blood pressure level is an integrated response and is only partially understood. However, it is highly likely that control centers in the brain, in the sympathetic nervous system, in the kidney, and in the renal juxtaglomerular cells are reset in an integrated fashion to achieve this higher level of arterial pressure. Signal-receiving receptors which control total body sodium are also part of the integrated response resulting in hypertension, and the circulating humoral agents mentioned above are an additional factor in the response. It is likely that renin, as well as the sympathetics, the other circulating humoral agents, and the sodium regulators all play integrated roles simultaneously. The future unraveling of the complex system which leads to hypertension will undoubtedly permit better prevention and better therapy for this life-shortening condition.

REFERENCES

1. Onesti G, Kim KE, Greco JA, et al.: Blood pressure regulation in end-stage renal disease and anephric man. Circ Res 36,37(Suppl 1):1, 1975.
2. Takeshita A, Mark AL: Neurogenic contribution to hindquarters vasoconstriction during high sodium intake in Dahl strain of genetically hypertensive rats. Circ Res 43(Suppl 1):1, 1978.
3. Tobian L, Pumper M, Johnson S, et al.: A circulating humoral pressor agent in Dahl 'S' rats with salt hypertension. Clin Sci 57:345s, 1979.
4. Goto A, Ikeda T, Tobian L, et al.: Brain lesion in the paraventricular nuclei and cate-cholaminergic neurons minimize NaCl hypertension in Dahl salt-sensitive rats. Clin Sci 61(Suppl 7):53-55, 1981.
5. Ikeda T, Tobian L, Iwai J, et al.: Central nervous system pressor responses in rats susceptible and resistant to NaCl hypertension. Clin Sci Mol Med 55:225, 1978.
6. Gotoh E, Ohnishi T, Fujishima S, et al.: Relation of sodium concentrations in cerebrospinal fluid to systemic blood pressure levels in salt-sensitive and nonsalt-sensitive, essential hypertensive patients. Proceedings of the Eighth Scientific Meeting of the International Society of Hypertension, abstract 158. Milan, Italy, 1981.
7. Dahl LK, Lietl G, Heine M: Influence of dietary potassium and sodium/potassium molar ratios on the development of salt hypertension. J Exp Med 136:318, 1972.
8. Goto A, Tobian L, Iwai J: Potassium feeding reduces hyperactive central nervous system pressor responses in Dahl salt-sensitive rats. Hypertension 3(Suppl 1):3, 1981.
9. Grim CE, Luft FC, Miller JZ, et al.: Effects of sodium loading and depletion on normotensive first-degree relatives of essential hypertensives. J Lab Clin Med 94:764, 1979.
10. Selkurt EE: Effects of pulse pressure and mean arterial pressure modifications on renal hemodynamics and electrolyte and water excretion. Circulation 4:541, 1951.
11. Tobian L, Lange J, Azar S, et al.: Reduction of natriuretic capacity and renin release in isolated blood-perfused kidneys of Dahl hypertension-prone rats. Circ Res 43(Suppl 1):92, 1978.
12. Tobian L, Lange J, Iwai J, et al.: Prevention with thiazide of NaCl-induced hypertension in Dahl 'S' rats: Evidence for a Na-retaining humoral agent in 'S' rats. Hypertension 1:316, 1979.
13. Tobian L, Ganguli M, Johnson MA, et al.: Influence of renal prostaglandins and dietary linoleate on hypertension in Dahl S rats. Hypertension 4(Suppl II):149-153, 1982.
14. Ganguli M, Tobian L, Azar S, et al.: Evidence that prostaglandin synthesis inhibitors increase the concentration of sodium and chloride in rat renal medulla. Circ Res 40(Suppl 1):135-139, 1977.
15. Stokes JB, Tisher CC, Kokko JP: Structural-functional heterogeneity along the rabbit collecting tubule. Kidney Int 14:585-593, 1978.
16. Stokes JB: Effect of prostaglandin E_2 on chloride transport across the rabbit thick ascending limb of Henle. Selective inhibitions of the medullary portion. J Clin Invest 64:495-502, 1979.
17. Wilson DR, Honrath U, Sonnenberg H: The role of prostaglandins in the response of medullary collecting duct (MCD) reabsorption to isotonic volume expansion (VE), abstract. Eight International Congress of Nephrology, Athens, 1981, p 175.
18. Cox JW, Rutecki GW, Francisco LL, et al.: Studies of the effects of essential fatty acid deficiency in the rat. Circ Res 51:694-702, 1982.
19. Ganguli M, Tobian L, Dahl L: Low renal papillary plasma flow in both Dahl and Kyoto rats with spontaneous hypertension. Circ Res 39:337, 1976.
20. Faubert PF, Chou SY, Porush JG, et al.: Papillary plasma flow and tissue osmolality in chronic

caval dogs. Am J Physiol 242(4):F370-378, 1982.

21. Spitalewitz S, Chou SY, Faubert PF, et al.: Effects of chronic salt depletion on intracortical blood flow distribution and papillary plasma flow in the dog, abstract. Clin Res 28:462A, 1980.

22. Osgood RW, Reineck HJ, Stein JH: Further studies on segmental sodium transport in the rat kidney during expansion of the extracellular fluid volume. J Clin Invest 62:311, 1978.

23. Ganguli M, Tobian L, Ferris T, et al.: Prostaglandin inhibition decreases plasma flow to the renal papilla in rats. Fed Proc 41:1590, 1982.

24. Tobian L, Norman B, Johnson MA, et al.: Plasma factors in Dahl S and rats which affect Na efflux. Kidney Int 23:177, 1983.

25. Hirata Y, Tobian L, Simon G, et al.: Humoral factors in Dahl salt-sensitive rats: Effects of chronic injection of erythrocytes and serum. Fed Proc 42: March, 1983.

DISCUSSION

Discussants: Sambhi, Tobian, Yamori, Abernathy, Mark, Blaustein, MacGregor, Johnston, May

Sambhi: Was there a difference to start with in the weight of the kidneys of the S and R rats, particularly if you compare it to the total body weight? I think Dr. Yamori and Dr. Simpson did a study recently looking at the kidney weight comparing the Japanese population with the New Zealand population, and among other factors it showed that the Japanese population had smaller kidneys so they had smaller total capacity to get rid of the salt load. Was there any difference between the S and R kidney weight?

Tobian: Well, in terms of the total kidney: total body weight ratio, there's not much difference, but there are some specific differences. The papillae are a little bit lighter in the S rat, even though the whole kidney is not lighter. The S rats have some fewer glomeruli which are longer, so the total glomerular filtering surface seems to be about the same, but there is that slight difference. Those are the two main differences just in terms of the morphology, but the total kidney weight is about the same, as is total filtering surface.

Yamori: We have been very much interested in the relationship between salt and hypertension and we confirmed that in Japan the salt intake is closely related to the blood pressure level. Dr. Simpson tried the same study in New Zealand but he failed to prove the relationship between salt intake and high blood pressure. We thought that in Japan the salt intake might affect the people more, because the Japanese are smaller and have smaller kidneys. Therefore, the effect of the salt would be greater. However, the result was just the opposite to our speculation. So the Japanese people, in spits of the smaller body size, have larger kidneys than the New Zealand people. We did some experiments in rats and found that the salt intake accelerated the enlargment of the kidney in uninephrectomized rats. Even 8 strains of rats with genetic hypertension available now in the world seem to be of two different types – the strain with smaller kidneys and the strain with larger kidneys.

Tobian: Dr. Eric Hall, in many studies over the years, has shown that high salt intake in the rat will increase kidney size – mostly in Sprague-Dawley type rats.

Abernathy: Going back to the pressure natriuresis effect in rats, you tried the pressure natriuresis effect in SHR and did not find the same thing as with the Dahl-S rats. Is that true?

Tobian: That's right and I think the SHR rat is really a different kind of hypertensive rat. By giving them thiazide from the time of weaning, we have reduced body sodium about 5 or 6 percent and we didn't reduce the blood pressure 1 mm Hg compared to SHRs, not on thiazide. I know that you can raise the blood pressure of an SHR rat with a high salt diet, but, at least with the way we did it, you can't lower it 1 mm Hg using thiazide to reduce body sodium by about 6 percent. We found no natriuretic defect; we found no ability to cure the blood pressure with a thiazide. So I think it fits in with what you're saying.

Abernathy: Other workers have not duplicated your results in the Dahl-S rats by using an artificial perfusion medium containing ox red cells.

Tobian: Yes. We perfuse with blood and they perfuse with something else, either a Kreb's perfusion or some other type. This is the way it came out for us. The kidney does normally get perfused with blood. That is its normal means of operation.

Mark: I was fascinated by the observation that suprachiasmatic lesions actually aggravated the hypertension. What effect does that lesion have in the R rats and what are your thoughts about the mechanism of that aggravation of the hypertension by those lesions?

Tobian: I don't think we did that in our 8 rats. The suprachiasmatic nucleus has a number of connections with areas that are active in vasomotion and I can't really dissect it further than that. In any of these lesions, you always have to wonder whether it's the nucleus itself, or whether it's nerves passing through the area. We can't even be sure of that, so I would have to say that I really don't know the answer right now.

Mark: Based on your studies on the pressure natriuresis curves and the impairment in the vasodilator responses in the medulla, one would predict that the increase in blood volume, salt and water content with high salt feeding, at least initially, would be greater in the S rats than in the R rats. Now, I know that's a difficult thing to measure, but my understanding is that there is no evidence yet for a greater salt and water expansion in the S rats even in the pre-hypertensive phase of high salt diet. Is that true?

Tobian: I think that's right. If there's a salt load, there's some initial way of keeping homeostasis that will work for a short time, but not necessarily for a longer period. We're actually trying to look into some of the aspects of this. For instance, there's a delay in the onset of salt-induced hypertension. A rat can come into Na balance in just a few days, but that rat will not necessarily have hypertension then. It takes a number of weeks sometimes for the hypertension to appear. It could be that some initial means for reducing body sodium ceases to work, and then you have to get hypertensive in order to keep your body sodium at the right level.

Sambhi: You were the originator of the hypothesis that the animal's vascular wall might get water-logged and salt loaded in hypertension, particularly if you salt load these animals. Have you tried to analyze the vascular wall sodium in these S and R rats?

Tobian: Well, I really haven't, but I still believe that a lot of hypertensives do have this increased sodium and water in the wall. I know that I was very interested in Dr. Mulvaney's study of the very tiny vessels in the SHR rat. They also seem to have some increased intracellular sodium.

Blaustein: When you used blood from an S rat perfusing into a kidney, you got less sodium output than when you used blood from an R rat; yet we know that you get an exaggerated natriuresis with plasma from S rats that are hypertensive. I assume this was the pre-hypertensive stage that you were looking at. That may just be the difference in the condition (pre-hypertensive versus hypertensive stage).

Tobian: What was the evidence for plasma causing an exaggerated natriuresis?

Blaustein: The evidence is an exaggerated natriuresis, for example, with an extract of urine from hypertensive patients. In the study by Viskoper et al.[1] in which an extract of urine was taken from normotensive and hypertensive patients, it was found that the material from hypertensive individuals caused an exaggerated natriuresis to a salt load.

Also, I would like to come back to the problem of whether the kidneys or some plasma or blood factor appears to play a role in the control of sodium metabolism. I think that the evidence shows that you can take an abnormal kidney in the S rat and transplant it into a normal rat or an R rat and be able to produce hypertension on a high salt diet. Conversely, you can take the kidney from an R rat and transplant it into an S rat and not be able to produce hypertension. This suggests that it's not the plasma factor that contributes primarily to the salt defect, but it's the kidney itself.

Tobian: Yes, unless the kidney somehow induces the plasma factor. I admit that's a problem for me and the best way that one can put it together would be that something about that kidney ultimately induces the plasma factor. One can't downplay kidneys in hypertension.

Blaustein: I don't mean to. I think the kidney is the primary factor and I think that you've been one of the principal people to demonstrate it.

Sambhi: If you infuse plasma from a hypertensive individual into a normotensive individual, do you indeed get exaggerated natriuresis?

MacGregor: The question I would like to ask is whether the intact Dahl rats do have an exaggerated natriuresis as do patients with essential hypertension.

Tobian: There have been claims to that effect, but it's not a clearcut action like you often see in man. It's not an actual exaggerated natriuresis such as some people have claimed in the SHR rat and, in fact, it depends on how you do it. You can have it go one way or the other way, just depending on how you do the loading.

Blaustein: Certainly a salt load in a hypertensive individual produces an exaggerated natriuresis.

Overbeck: You demonstrated two humoral effects – one on the perfused hindquarters bed which was a vasoconstriction, and the other on the perfused kidney which was an attenuation of natriuresis, I believe. Do you have any data that would indicate whether that might be the same factor in both cases or whether it's a different factor?

Tobian: It's pretty hard to do both studies in the same rat, but I'm very definitely thinking along those lines. The only thing that makes me think they might not be the same is that one of them showed up on a low-salt diet and the other one didn't – so they might be slightly different. But again, it's hard for me to really believe that they're totally unrelated so it may be that there really is a relationship.

Johnston: Maybe I could just add to the confusion about what Dr. Blaustein was saying. I took it that your data showed that the Dahl-sensitive rat uses pressure natriuresis to get rid of its sodium load whereas the resistant rat uses not only pressure but has some other plasma factor. Because in the cross-perfusion experiments you showed that the plasma of that rat could get rid of more sodium. So I presume that it uses two mechanisms whereas the Dahl-sensitive rat has predominantly only the pressure.

Tobian: It wouldn't necessarily mean that one used one and one the other; the mix could be different.

[1] Viskoper JR, et al.: *Nephron* 8:540-548, 1971.

The R rat doesn't need to use pressure natriuresis as much because he's got something else – the S rat might need pressure more because he has less of the other. In other words they might both have both mechanisms, but maybe in a different mix.

Johnston: And that explains I think the difference between the cross-perfusion and the renal output experiments. I also wanted to ask you about CNS lesions and the amelioration, or the attenuation, or even the acceleration of the hypertension. I was wondering whether there were any other differences as far as appetite, sodium intake or body weight increases, when you produce the lesions in the rats?

Tobian: The 6-hydroxy-dopamine rat really eats less and so we had to pair-feed them – but the other rats were in pretty good shape and they were growing just about the same amount. Now the AV3V rat has a lot of aspects about it that are different. For instance, it's hypernatremic and one can give a little vasopressin and can get Na concentration close to normal. It is distinctly different in that it doesn't have diabetes insipidus, but has more than blood pressure differences. It has altered thirst mechanisms and some alteration in AVP secretion.

May: Your statement that potassium mitigates sodium hypertension intrigued me. Could you elaborate on that and perhaps discuss it a little bit?

Tobian: There's all sorts of evidence that feeding potassium to hypertensives will drop their blood pressure. Meneely found that when he gave a high salt diet and added potassium, he didn't drop the blood pressure so much, but he increased longevity quite a lot. We've done a little experiment suggesting that potassium citrate feeding reduces the vascular lesions in the kidney in hypertension. And then Dahl and a number of others have added potassium to high salt diets in rats and it mitigated hypertension in some. It's one of these fields that is not totally developed yet.

For three million years, up until 10,000 years ago, probably every man on earth who didn't live on the seacoast was on a low-salt diet. So that's the normal diet of man. This recent diet that we've been eating for four or five hundred years is distinctly peculiar. Man was intended to have mechanisms to cope with the salt-poor world he lived in.

The one in five who might be susceptible to hypertension now was in great shape two million years ago. He could conserve sodium better than his friends; he didn't need as much salt. So what was a big biological advantage a couple of million years ago is a handicap now when he's able to get a lot of salt that he couldn't possibly get two million years ago, even if he wanted it.

Unidentified discussant: Just to confirm what you said. I think some research dentists point out that the conformation of our teeth is mostly made for chewing herbivorous types of diet, and it's only recently that we have started eating meat which contains a lot of salt.

Tobian: I think the evidence on prehistoric man is that he was mostly eating vegetables and fruits and nuts and he just got a little bit of meat every now and then.

MacGregor: What about lions? I mean, if you're carnivorous, and you eat a wild beast, that must be several thousand millimoles of sodium. There must be mechanisms to get rid of sodium as well as retain it in carnivorous mammals.

Tobian: I'm talking about human beings and virtually a no-salt culture of up to five milliequivalents a day. We see from studies in remote areas at the present time that if one eats less than about 50-60 milliequivalents a day, you don't get very much hypertension even if you're susceptible. You can take somebody who's practically eating his fill of wild beast and still eating fruit and vegetables, and he will probably only be getting about 30 milliequivalents a day – not five but 30 – which is still way below what he needs to get hypertension.